EXTRAHEPATIC DRUG METABOLISM AND CHEMICAL CARCINOGENESIS

EXTRAHEPATIC DRUG METABOLISM AND CHEMICAL CARCINOGENESIS

Proceedings of the International Meeting on Extrahepatic Drug Metabolism and Chemical Carcinogenesis held in Stockholm, Sweden, on 17-20 May, 1983

Editors

Jan Rydström
Johan Montelius
and
Margot Bengtsson

1983

ELSEVIER SCIENCE PUBLISHERS
AMSTERDAM · NEW YORK · OXFORD

ISBN 0-444-80538-9

Published by:
Elsevier Science Publishers B.V.
P.O. Box 211
1000 AE   Amsterdam, The Netherlands

Sole distributors for the USA and Canada:
Elsevier Science Publishing Company Inc.
52 Vanderbilt Avenue
New York, N.Y. 10017

Printed in The Netherlands

FOREWORD

The tremendous progress which has characterized toxicological research during the last two decades has involved mainly research on hepatic systems. In depth characterization of isolated proteins, e.g., cytochrome P-450, has provided powerful tools for the elucidation of the mechanisms of action of drug-metabolizing systems and has allowed conclusions to be drawn which may also apply to extrahepatic systems. Based on this knowledge, hypotheses for metabolic activation and chemical carcinogenesis in general have been advocated which have been questioned only rarely. Epidemiological evidence indicates that more than 95% of all human cancers in the Western world are extrahepatic and that up to 80% of these are related to diet, environmental factors, and, indirectly, endogenous factors. Obviously, there is a need for more extensive research on the relationship between cancer in a specific extrahepatic organ and the generation of potential carcinogens and other relevant processes in that organ. The logical approach is thus to use our extensive knowledge of the hepatic system as a platform.

The International Meeting on Extrahepatic Drug Metabolism and Chemical Carcinogenesis held in Stockholm, 17-20 May 1983, from which the present proceedings are derived, was the first meeting which has specifically addressed the problems and approaches peculiar to extra-hepatic carcinogenesis. Topics included characterization and regulation of cytochrome P-450 and other detoxication enzymes, DNA-adduct forma-tion and repair, and model systems of extrahepatic carcinogenesis. The success of the meeting and the exceptionally good response from lecturers and other participants indicates the importance of stressing the often unique problems in extrahepatic carcinogenesis. A second meeting on similar topics is therefore planned to take place in USA in 1986.

Jan Rydström

Scientific Advisory Committee

P.L. Grover
J.-Å. Gustafsson
C.F. Jefcoate
D.W. Nebert
S. Orrenius
J. Rydström

CONTENTS

Preface

COMPARATIVE ASPECTS OF EXTRAHEPATIC AND HEPATIC DRUG METABOLISM AND
CHEMICAL CARCINOGENESIS

Selectivity of lesions produced by 7,12-dimethylbenz[a]anthracene
    in rat
    Charles Huggins   3

Initiation of carcinogenesis with chemicals - a biological per-
    spective
    Emmanuel Farber   11

Differences between kidney and liver in the regulation of micro-
    somal testosterone hydroxylase activities in inbred mice
    Roy Hawke, Lynn Raynor, Gurmit Singh and Allen Neims   23

The role of rabbit cytochrome P-450, form 5, in the pulmonary and
    hepatic metabolism of aromatic amines to mutagenic products
    Iain G.C. Robertson, Tore Aune, Cosette J. Serabjit-Singh,
    Jane E. Croft, John R. Bend and Richard M. Philpot   25

Comparison of coumarin 7-hydroxylase activities in kidney and
    liver of DBA/2J and C57BL/6J mice
    Pekka Kaipainen, Daniel W. Nebert and Matti Lang   27

Effect of various solvents on the xenobiotic biotransformation
    in the liver and the kidneys of the rat: a comparative study
    Tuula Heinonen, Eivor Elovaara, Säde Laurén, Harri Vainio
    and Jorma Järvisalo   29

Profile of drug metabolizing enzymes in the nuclei and microsomes
    of hepatic and extrahepatic tissues from monkeys
    Gian Maria Pacifici and Anders Rane   33

Comparative kinetic aspects of aromatics metabolism by rabbit
    lung and rat liver microsomes
    Dmitriy I. Metelitza, Sergey A. Usanov, Alexander N. Eriomin
    and Irina V. Tishchenko   39

MULTIPLICITY, REGIOSPECIFICITY AND LEVELS OF P-450, EPOXIDE HYDRO-
LASE AND CONJUGATING ENZYMES IN DIFFERENT TISSUES

Modulation of the levels of cytochrome P-450 isozymes in rabbit
    lung
    Barbara A. Domin, Richard M. Philpot, Betty L. Warren and
    Cosette J. Serabjit-Singh   43

Characterization of purified cytochrome P-450 in the rat lung
Minro Watanabe, Ikuko Sagami and Tetsuo Ohmachi   51

Evidence for the presence and reactivity of multiple forms of cyto-
chrome P-450 in colonic microsomes from rats and humans
Henry W. Strobel, S.N. Newaz, Wan-Fen Fang, Paul P. Lau,
R.J. Oshinsky, Daniel J. Stralka and Fred F. Salley   57

Characterization of cytochrome P-450 in the rat ventral prostate
Tapio Haaparanta, James Halpert, Lena Haglund, Hans Glaumann
and Jan-Åke Gustafsson   67

Localization of carcinogen-metabolizing enzymes in human and animal
tissues
Jeffrey Baron, Thomas T. Kawabata, Jan A. Redick, Shirley A.
Knapp, Donald G. Wick, Robert B. Wallace, William B. Jakoby
and F. Peter Guengerich   73

Immunohistochemical evidence for a heterogeneous distribution of
NADPH-cytochrome P-450 reductase in the rat and monkey brain
Lena Haglund, Christer Köhler, Tapio Haaparanta, Menek Gold-
stein and Jan-Åke Gustafsson   89

Microsomal and cytosolic epoxide hydrolases: total activities, subcellular distribution and induction in the liver and extrahepatic tissues
Joseph W. DePierre, Johan Meijer, Winnie Birberg, Åke Pilotti,
Lennart Balk and Janeric Seidegård   95

Metabolism of chemical carcinogens by prostaglandin H synthase
T.E. Eling, G.A. Reed, J.A. Boyd, R.S. Krauss and K. Sivarajah   105

Prostaglandin synthase catalyzed metabolism of p-phenetidine to
reactive products
Peter Moldéus, Roger Larsson, David Ross, Bo Andersson, Magnus
Nordenskjöld, Anver Rahimtula and Björn Lindeke   113

Peroxidase-dependent covalent binding of 7,12-dimethylbenz(a)-
anthracene metabolites to rat adrenal microsomes
Johan Montelius and Jan Rydström   123

Activation of the organospecific carcinogen, methylazoxymethanol,
via dehydrogenase enzymes: prevention of colon tumorigenesis
in rats and human studies
Morris S. Zedeck, Martin Lipkin and Queng Hui Tan   131

The role of extrahepatic and hepatic sulfation and glucuronidation
in chemical carcinogenesis: an overview
Gerard J. Mulder and John H.N. Meerman   143

Species and tissue differences in the occurrence of multiple forms
of rat and human glutathione transferases
Bengt Mannervik, Claes Guthenberg, Helgi Jensson, Margareta
Warholm and Per Ålin   153

Identification of novel glutathione S-transferases in kidney and
lung and the inducibility of various isozymes in liver and
other organs
F. Oesch, U. Milbert, T. Friedberg and C.R. Wolf   163

Isozymes of glutathione transferase in rat testis
Claes Guthenberg, Per Ålin, Ing-Mari Åstrand, Süha Yalçin and
Bengt Mannervik   171

Peroxisome proliferation, fatty acid β-oxidation and cancer initiation by phenoxyacetic acid herbicides
H. Vainio, E. Hietanen, K. Linnainmaa and E. Mäntylä   177

Induction of extrahepatic glutathione S-transferases and NAD(P)H:
quinone reductase by anticarcinogenic hindered phenols, lactones and Sudan III
Mary J. de Long, Hans J. Prochaska and Paul Talalay   181

Glutathione and GSH-dependent enzymes in the human gastric mucosa
Claus-Peter Siegers, Renate Hoppenkamps, Ernst Thies and
Maged Younes   183

Extrahepatic distribution of microsomal glutathione transferase
in the rat
Ralf Morgenstern and Joseph W. DePierre   185

Inhibitors for identification of glutathione transferase subunits
in the rat
Süha Yalçin, Helgi Jensson and Bengt Mannervik   187

A comparison of the glutathione transferases (GST) of three extrahepatic organs with different functions - the adrenal, the
lactating mammary gland and the male reproductive system
D.J. Meyer, L.G. Cristodoulides, O. Nyan, R. Schuster Bruce
and B. Ketterer   189

Glutathione transferase in human brain
Maria Olsson, Claes Guthenberg and Bengt Mannervik   191

Non-microsomal activation of styrene to styrene oxide
Giorgio Belvedere, Francesco Tursi and Harri Vainio   193

Biotransformation of ethylloflazepate (Victan) in plasma and
rat tissues
Horace Davi, Eric Marti, Andree Bondon and Werner Cautreels   201

Metabolism of promutagens to ultimate mutagens by the rat ventral
prostate and covalent binding of benzo(a)pyrene to prostatic
microsomal proteins
Peter Söderkvist, Leif Busk, Rune Toftgård and Jan-Åke Gustafsson   205

The metabolic activation of AFB_1 in rat and man
Simon Plummer, Alan R. Boobis, Clare Kahn and Donald S. Davies   207

X

Drug metabolizing enzymes in resting human lymphocytes
Janeric Seidegård and Joseph W. DePierre   209

Covalent binding of benzo(a)pyrene to cytochrome P-448 and other
proteins in reconstituted mixed function oxidase systems
Cecilia Schelin, Bengt Jergil and James Halpert   211

The dose dependent metabolism of anethole, estragole and p-propylanisole in relation to their safety evaluation
Susan A. Sangster, John Caldwell, Andrew Anthony, Andrew J. Hutt
and Robert L. Smith   213

DT-diaphorase in mouse epidermis, induction of the enzyme by methylcholanthrene
Olve Rømyhr, Vemund Digernes and Olav Hilmar Iversen   215

Inhibition of xenobiotic and steroid metabolism by aminoglutethimide in human placentas from smoking and non-smoking mothers
Markku Pasanen and Olavi Pelkonen   217

Metabolic conversion of styrene to styrene glycol in the mouse.
Occurence of the intermediate styrene-7,8-oxide
Marianne Nordqvist, Elisabeth Ljungquist and Agneta Löf   219

Subcellular distribution of epoxide hydrolase activity in the liver,
lung, kidney and testis of the C57 Bl male mouse
Johan Meijer, Winnie Birberg, Åke Pilotti and Joseph W. DePierre   221

Effect of polychlorinated naphthalenes and biphenyls on polysubstrate monooxygenase and UDP-glucuronosyltransferase activities
in rat lung
Eero Mäntylä, Antero Aitio and Markku Ahotupa   223

Comparison of the patterns of benzo(a)pyrene conjugates formed
in vivo in the liver and kidney of the Northern pike (*Esox lucius*)
Lennart Balk, Susanne Månér and Joseph W. DePierre   225

Does human placental PAH metabolism protect the conceptus?
David K. Manchester, Natalie B. Parker, Karen Gottlieb and
C. Michael Bowman   227

Separation of multiple forms of cytochrome P-450 from rabbit
kidney cortex microsomes
Masamichi Kusunose, Kiyokazu Ogita, Emi Kusunose, Satoru
Yamamoto and Kosuke Ichihara   229

Cytochrome P-450 from intestinal microsomes of rabbits treated with
3-methylcholanthrene
Kosuke Ichihara, Kiyomi Ishihara, Emi Kusunose, Masatoshi Kaku
and Kiyokazu Ogita   231

Aryl hydrocarbon hydroxylase (AHH) activity in human placenta and
its relation with air pollution
Filiz Hincal   233

Mechanisms of extrahepatic bioactivation of aromatic amines: the
role of hemoglobin in the N-oxidation of 4-chloroaniline
Ines Golly and Peter Hlavica   235

Bio-alkylation of benzo(a)pyrene in rat lung and liver
James W. Flesher, Kevin H. Stansbury, Abdelrazak M. Kardy and
Steven R. Myers   237

Urinary metabolite patterns as indicators of activation and inactivation reactions in the biotransformation of m-xylene and
ethylbenzene
Eivor Elovaara, Kerstin Engström and Harri Vainio   239

Dimethylsulfoxide induced activation of renal microsomal ethoxycoumarin O-deethylation
Aniti Zitting, Sinikka Vainiotalo and Eivor Elovaara   241

Drug-metabolizing enzymes in *Drosophila melanogaster* in relation
to genotoxicity testing
Aalbert J. Baars, Marijke Jansen and Douwe D. Breimer   243

Enhancement of extrahepatic drug metabolism by phenoxyacid herbicides and clofibrate
Markku Ahotupa, Eino Hietanen, Eero Mäntylä and Harri Vainio   245

Characterization of epoxide hydrolase from the human adrenal
gland
Dimitrios Papadopoulos, Janeric Seidegård, Antonis Georgellis
and Jan Rydström   247

Genetic variation and regulation of the cytochrome P-450 system
in the fruit fly, *Drosophila melanogaster*
Inger Hällström and Agneta Blanck   249

Inhibition of rat lung cytochrome P-450 by chloramphenicol
Birgitta Näslund, Ingvar Betner and James Halpert   251

Immunochemical and biochemical evidence of the presence of cytochrome P-450 monooxygenase components in rabbit heart and
aorta
Cosette J. Serabjit-Singh, Barbara A. Domin, John R. Bend and
Richard M. Philpot   253

INTESTINAL METABOLISM AND ENTEROHEPATIC CIRCULATION OF CARCINOGENS

Enterohepatic circulation and catabolism of mercapturic acid path-
way metabolites of naphthalene
Jerome Bakke, Craig Struble, Jan-Åke Gustafsson and Bengt
Gustafsson   257

Disposition and metabolism of mutagens-carcinogens *in vivo* -
involvement of the intestinal microflora
J. Rafter, L. Möller, L. Nilsson, L. Ball, I. Brandt, G. Lar-
sen, M. Blomstedt, B. Gustafsson and J.-A. Gustafsson   267

Enterohepatic circulation of the aromatic hydrocarbons benzo(a)-
pyrene and naphthalene
P.C. Hirom, J.K. Chipman, P. Millburn and M.A. Pue   275

Xenobiotics, the intestinal flora, and carcinogenesis
Rory P. Remmel and Peter Goldman   283

Studies with amaranth and ouabain in germfree rats
David Hewick and Sylvia Wilson   293

Metabolism of 1-nitropyrene in germ-free and conventional rats:
role of the gut flora in generation of mutagenic metabolites
L.M. Ball, J.J. Rafter, J.-Å. Gustafsson, B.E. Gustafsson
and J. Lewtas   295

Kinetic aspects of 2-acetylaminofluorene uptake, metabolism,
excretion and enterohepatic circulation
Lennart C. Eriksson, Joann Spiewak, Waheed Roomi and
Emmanuel Farber   297

The metabolism of benzo(a)pyrene in the intestine and the effect
of dietary fats
Jon D. Gower and E.D. Wills   299

Effect of diethyl maleate pretreatment on glutathione levels in
stomach, liver and blood of rats treated with gastric damage
inducing agents
Paolo Di Simplicio, Antonella Naldini and Maria Teresa Bianco   303

Effect of cholesterol on phenobarbital inducibility of biotransformation enzymes in the small intestinal mucosa and liver of
the rat
Eino Hietanen and Markku Ahotupa   305

Xenobiotic metabolism in the small intestinal mucosa of children
Eino Hietanen, Tuula Heinonen, Marja-Liisa Ståhlberg and
Markku Mäki   307

Inhibition of the mutagenic activity of 2-amino-3-methylimidazo-
(4,5-f)quinoline (IQ) by rat intestinal mucosa
Giovanna Caderni, Maura Lodovici and Piero Dolara   309

The effect of high fat diet on the disposition of benzo(a)pyrene
in the gut
Susan Bowes and Andrew G. Renwick   311

The cytostatic hexamethylmelamine, administered orally to rats,
is metabolized in the liver and the gut wall
Pierre Klippert, Paul Borm, Abram Hulshoff, Marie-José Mingels,
Gerard Hofman and Jan Noordhoek   315

Biotransformation of hexamethylmelamine in rat isolated intestinal
epithelial cells and hepatocytes. Role of mitochondrial cytochrome P-450
Paul Borm, Pierre Klippert, Marie-José Mingels, Abram Hulshoff
Ank Frankhuijzen-Sierevogel and Jan Noordhoek   319

PITUITARY CONTROL AND ROLE OF CYTOCHROME P-450 IN ENDOCRINE ORGANS

Metabolism of polycyclic hydrocarbons in the mammary gland and the
hormone mimetic action of the carcinogens
Thomas L. Dao, Charles E. Morreal and Dilip K. Sinha   325

Benzo(a)pyrene reproductive toxicity and ovarian metabolism
Donald R. Mattison, Maria S. Nightingale, Ken Takizawa,
Ellen K. Silbergeld, Haruhiko Yagi and Donald M. Jerina   337

Hormonal regulation of cytochrome P-450 dependent monooxygenase
activity and benzopyrene metabolism in rat testes
I.P. Lee, K. Suzuki, J. Nagayama, H. Mukhtar and J.R. Bend   351

Regulation of the metabolism of 7,12-dimethylbenz(a)anthracene in
the rat ovary by gonadotropins
Margot Bengtsson, Donald R. Mattison and Jan Rydström   363

Effects of ACTH on metabolism and toxicity of 7,12-dimethylbenz(a)-
anthracene in cultured rat adrenal cells
Einar Hallberg and Jan Rydström   371

Are pituitary factors acting as modifiers of liver carcinogenesis
in the rat?
Agneta Blanck, Tiiu Hansson, Lennart Eriksson and Jan-Åke
Gustafsson   373

Feminization of hepatic xenobiotic metabolism by ectopic pituitary
grafts or by continuous infusion of human growth hormone in
male rats
Agneta Blanck, Anders Åström, Tiiu Hansson, Joseph W. DePierre
and Jan-Åke Gustafsson   375

RECEPTORS AND INDUCTION OF DRUG-METABOLIZING ENZYMES

Several P-450 genes regulated by the *Ah* receptor
Daniel W. Nebert, Robert H. Tukey, Peter I. Mackenzie,
Masahiko Negishi and Howard J. Eisen   379

The *Ah* receptor: species and tissue variation in binding of
2,3,7,8-tetrachlorodibenzo-p-dioxin and carcinogenic aromatic
hydrocarbons
Allan B. Okey, Michelle E. Mason and Lynn M. Vella   389

Soluble receptor proteins in control of gene expression
Jan-Åke Gustafsson, Örjan Wrange, Lorenz Poellinger, Johan
Lund, Farhang Payvar and Keith Yamamoto   401

Is the primary function of the *Ah* locus to regulate cytochrome P-450?
Joyce C. Knutson and Alan Poland   409

Molecular biology of cytochrome P-450
   Ronald N. Hines, Edward Bresnick, Curtis Omiecinski and
   Joan Levy   419

Bone marrow toxicity induced by oral benzo[a]pyrene: protection
   resides at the level of the intestine and liver
   Catherine Legraverend, David E. Harrison, Francis W. Ruscetti
   and Daniel W. Nebert   423

Assignment of the *Ah* locus to mouse chromosome 17
   Sirpa O. Kärenlampi, Catherine Legraverend, Peter A. Lalley,
   Christine A. Kozak and Daniel W. Nebert   425

DRUG METABOLISM, DNA-ADDUCT FORMATION AND DNA REPAIR

Metabolism and activation of polycyclic hydrocarbons in mammary
   and other tissue
   P.L. Grover, D.H. Phillips, C.S. Cooper, W.H. Swallow,
   A. Weston, P. Vigny, M. O'Hare, A.M. Neville and P. Sims   429

7,12-dimethylbenz[a]anthracene-DNA interactions in mouse embryo
   cell cultures and mouse skin
   Anthony Dipple, Josef T. Sawicki, Robert C. Moschel and C. Anita
   H. Bigger   439

A kinetic approach to polycyclic hydrocarbon activation
   Colin R. Jefcoate, Maro Christou, Gabriela M. Keller, Christopher R. Turner and Neil M. Wilson   449

In vivo metabolism of benzo(a)pyrene: formation and disappearance
   of BP-metabolite-DNA adducts in extrahepatic tissues versus
   liver
   Marshall W. Anderson and John R. Bend   459

Spectroscopic studies of benzo(a)pyrene-7,8-dihydrodiol-9,10-
   epoxides covalently bound to DNA
   Bengt Jernström, Per-Olof Lycksell, Astrid Gräslund, Anders
   Ehrenberg and Bengt Nordén   469

Kinetics of DNA adduct formation and removal in liver and kidney
   of rats fed 2-acetylaminofluorene
   Miriam C. Poirier, John M. Hunt, B'Ann True and Brian A. Laishes   479

Metabolism of azo and hydrazine derivative to reactive intermediates
   R.A. Prough, M.I. Brown, C.A. Amrhein and L.J. Marnett   489

A role for active oxygen-induced DNA damage in tumor promotion
   Peter Cerutti, Joseph Friedman and Robert Zimmerman   499

Aromatic amine induced DNA damage in mouse hepatocytes
   Mona Møller, Irene B. Glowinski and Snorri S. Thorgeirsson   507

Possible significance of a direct interaction between NAD(P)H
and N-acetoxy-2-aminofluorene on the binding to human lymphocyte DNA
Janeric Seidegård and Ronald W. Pero   509

Guanosine and deoxyguanosine adducts of nitrogen mustards and
ethyleneimines - formation and destruction
Kirsti Savela, Seija Kallama and Kari Hemminki   511

A sensitive reversed-phase H.P.L.C. method for the determination
of RNA contamination in the analysis of DNA-carcinogen interactions
Keith R. Huckle   513

DNA repair as a determining factor in the transplacental organo-
tropic effect of N-methyl-N-nitrosourea
Alexei J.Likhachev, Valerii A. Alexandrov, Vladimir N. Anisimov,
Vladimir G. Bespalov, Mikhail V. Korsakov, Anton I. Ovsyannikov,
Irina G. Popovic, Nikolai P. Napalkov and Lorenzo Tomatis   515

Singel-strand breaks in DNA of various organs of mice induced by
administration of styrene
S.A.S. Walles and I. Orsén   517

Investigation of absorption, metabolism and DNA binding of
particle adsorbed PAH in the isolated perfused and ventilated
rat lung
Sam Törnquist, Lars Wiklund and Rune Toftgård   519

Genetic control of N-acetoxy-2-acetylaminofluorene (NA-AAF) induced unscheduled DNA synthesis and NA-AAF binding to DNA
determined in mononuclear leukocytes of twins
Ronald W. Pero, Carl Bryngelsson, Tomas Bryngelsson and
Åke Nordén   521

Age and diet dependent binding of ^{14}C-dimethylnitrosamine metabolites to mouse liver chromatin
Maria Klaude and Alexandra von der Decken   523

IN VIVO AND IN VITRO MODEL SYSTEMS OF CHEMICAL CARCINOGENESIS

Metabolism of N-nitrosamines and effects of formaldehyde on
DNA repair in cultured human tissues and cells
Roland C. Grafström and Curtis C. Harris   527

Early changes in gene expression during hepatocarcinogenesis
Snorri S. Thorgeirsson, Peter J. Wirth and Ritva P. Evarts   541

Mechanisms of initiation and promotion of carcinogenesis in mouse
epidermis
Stuart H. Yuspa   547

Metabolic activation of aromatic amines and the induction of
liver, mammary gland and urinary bladder tumors in the rat
Charles M. King, Ching Y. Wang, Mei-Sie Lee, Jimmie B. Vaught,
Masao Hirose and Kenneth C. Morton   557

Comparisons of benzo(a)pyrene metabolism and DNA-binding between
species and individuals: observations in rodent trachea and
human endometrium
David G. Kaufman, Marc J. Mass, Bonnie B. Furlong and B. Hugh
Dorman   567

Mechanisms involved in multistage chemical carcinogenesis in
mouse skin
T.J. Slaga   577

NMRI NU/NU mouse skin fibroblasts: regain of arylhydrocarbon
hydroxylase inducibility of transformed cell lines after a
tumor phase
Mariitta Laaksonen, Rauno Mäntyjärvi, Osmo Hänninen and
Asta Rautiainen   587

Modulating effects of 2,3,7,8-tetrachlorodibenzo-p-dioxin on skin
carcinogenesis initiated by 7,12-dimethylbenz(a)anthracene in
CF-1 swiss mice
Pierre Lesca   589

Role of diethylstilbestrol (DES) quinone formation in hamster
kidney tumor induction
Joachim G. Liehr, Beverly B. DaGue and Annie M. Ballatore   591

In vitro cultivation of embryonic rat tongue cells and induction
of GGT positive clones by benzo(a)pyrene: a good model system
for oral carcinogenesis studies
K.V. Kesava Rao, A.V. D'Souza and S.V. Bhide   593

Rabbit alveolar macrophage - mediated mutagenesis of polycyclic
aromatic hydrocarbons in V79 chinese hamster cells
Lennart Romert and Dag Jenssen   597

Inhibitory effects of some thiol compounds on the metabolic
activation of dimethylnitrosamine (DMN) and dimethylhydrazine
(DMH) in guinea-pig hepatocytes and enterocytes
Stanislav Yanev, Gabrielle Hauber, Michael Schwenk and
Herbert Remmer   599

Accumulation of carcinogens and drugs in cells as determined by
fluorescence microscopy
Erich Zeeck and Herbert Kowitz   601

Prediction of carcinogenic and mutagenic potencies using the
PLS method
Ulf Edlund, Sven Hellberg, Dan Johnels, Bo Nordén and Svante
Wold   603

Benzo(a)pyrene metabolism in human hair follicle cells: possible
   indicators for individual differences in susceptibility to
   chemical carcinogens
   Math W.A.C. Hukkelhoven, Lisette W.M. Vromans and Alphons J.M.
   Vermorken   605

Elucidation of the antineoplastic potency of vitamin C on
   benzo(a)pyrene induced tumors in rats
   George Kallistratos, Erhard Fasske, Andreas Donos, Vassiliki
   Kalfakakou-Vadalouka and Angelos Evangelou   609

Bronchiolar epithelial cell necrosis and selective impairment of
   pulmonary microsomal monooxygenases in mice by naphthalene and
   1,1-dichloroethylene
   Theodore E. Gram, Klaas R. Krijgsheld, Samuel S. Tong, Edward
   G. Mimnaugh, Michael A. Trush and Michael C. Lowe   613

Effect of inducers of AHH on proliferation of mitogen-stimulated
   human lymphocytes. Benzanthracene-induced increase in proliferation of cells showing low response to mitogen and its
   toxicity in cells showing high response to mitogen
   Andrzej L. Pawlak, Krzysztof Wiktorowicz and Renata Mikstacka   615

Benzo(a)pyrene metabolizing enzymes and lymophocyte stimulation
   in patients with bronchial carcinoma
   Christel Bluhm and Edgar E. Ohnhaus   617

Studies on a nasal cavity carcinogen: metabolism and binding of
   phenacetin in the mucosa of the upper respiratory tract
   Eva Brittebo and Maria Åhlman   619

Metabolism and binding of chlorobenzene in the mucosa of the
   upper respiratory tract
   Ingvar Brandt and Eva Brittebo   621

The renal metabolism of a glutathione conjugate of the carcinogen
   hexachloro-1,3-butadiene: evidence for the formation of a
   mutagenic metabolite in the rat kidney
   Trevor Green, John A. Nash, Jenny Odum and Edwin F. Howard   623

Dose- and sex-related variation in the disposition and hepatic
   effects of cinnamyl anthranilate in the mouse
   John Caldwell, Andrew Anthony, Ian A. Cotgreave, Susan A.
   Sangster and J. David Sutton   625

Author index   627

COMPARATIVE ASPECTS OF EXTRAHEPATIC AND HEPATIC DRUG METABOLISM AND CHEMICAL CARCINOGENESIS

© 1983 Elsevier Science Publishers B.V.
Extrahepatic Drug Metabolism and Chemical Carcinogenesis,
J. Rydström, J. Montelius and M. Bengtsson eds.

SELECTIVITY OF LESIONS PRODUCED BY 7,12-DIMETHYLBENZ[a]-ANTHRACENE IN RAT

CHARLES HUGGINS

The Ben May Laboratory for Cancer Research, The University of Chicago, Chicago, Illinois 60637 (U.S.A.)

7,12-Dimethylbenz[a]anthracene (DMBA) is of special and fascinating interest for many reasons: i, a single feeding or intravenous injection of DMBA rapidly elicits mammary adenocarcinoma in 100 percent of rats at risk under stipulated conditions (1) which are easily satisfied; ii, a single large but tolerable dose of DMBA results in massive destruction in the middle of the adrenal cortex comprising zona fasciculata and zona reticularis, whereas zona glomerulosa and adrenal medulla are uninjured and adrenal insufficiency does not result from this pharmacologic dissection; iii, DMBA and other foreign aromatics induce menadione reductase (EC 1.6.5.2) in mammary glands, mammary cancer, lipocytes and liver; iv, DMBA significantly inhibits the incorporation of [3H]TdR into DNA in adrenal, ileum and testis; v, in testis DMBA destroys diploid cells whereas haploid cells are uninjured; DMBA is radiomimetic.

7,12-Dimethylbenz[a]anthracene

The year 1938 was the year of synthesis and bioassay of DMBA. In one of the most elegant, hence useful, contributions to science, Bachmann and Chemerda (2) announced the synthesis of three new derivatives of BA: 7,12-dimethyl-; 7,12-diethyl-; 7,8,12-trimethylbenz[a]anthracene. It was found that DMBA and TMBA are powerful carcinogens in rat and mouse whereas DEBA does not produce cancer. A new era was introduced in cancer research by the discovery of DMBA.

In the tests for carcinogenic activity carried out by Kennaway (3), the usual procedure was to apply one drop of 0.3 percent solution of the compound in benzene twice weekly to the interscapular region of stock mice. In concurrent experiments, 3-methylcholanthrene (3-MC) was tested in parallel and it gave tumors of which the majority began to appear after 75 days. It was found (4) that DMBA applied by the usual procedure produced tumors about twice as rapidly as 3-MC did; the direct application of carcinogen directly to the cells of the skin of living mouse had caused cutaneous cancer in situ in 35 days. Moreover, the application of 7, 12-DMBA showed unusual results: i, multiplicity of tumors to an extent greater than that produced by other carcinogens; ii, epilation over an especially large area.

Mammary Adenocarcinoma

The mammary glands of young adult female Sprague-Dawley (S-D) rats, age 50-60 days, are foremost among the cells of living creatures in the induction of cancer by irradiation (5, 6) or chemical carcinogens (1). The most potent of the mammary carcinogens (7) is DMBA.

Many aromatic compounds with divergent molecular structures (8) possess in common the ability to induce mammary cancer selectively in rats. The carcinogenic effect is related to the participation of a polynuclear aromatic hydrocarbon possessing a prerequisite geometric configuration with DNA in a molecular complex. There is a remarkable similarity in three-dimensional geometric pattern between carcinogenic polynuclear aromatic hydrocarbons and the base pairs of DNA. The aromatic carcinogens have an identical thickness (3.6Å) with the base pairs.

DMBA is the quintessential mammary carcinogen. The optimal dose of DMBA (dissolved in sesame oil, 1 ml) to induce mammary cancer by intragastric intubation is 20 mg. Members of a series (7) of 40 S-D females, age 50 days, were given DMBA, 20 mg, by a single gastric intubation: i, every rat survived; ii, every rat developed mammary adenocarcinoma; iii, all of the mammary cancers were detected in 28-60 days.

DMBA in homogenized form is useful in cancer research. Under stated conditions (1) every female rat given one intravenous injection of DMBA, 30-35 mg/kg, at age 50 days will develop mammary adenocarcinoma or leukemia.

Selective Adrenal Destruction by DMBA

Huggins and Yang (8) observed that a single feeding of any of 8 carcinogens causes mammary cancer in S-D rats. Among the mammary carcinogens was DMBA. It was soon found out that DMBA and its congeners possess unique properties that set them apart from the generality of other powerful mammary carcinogens including 3-MC. Among the distinctive attributes of the DMBA group (9) is the capacity to destroy specifically and selectively the middle layer of the adrenal glands of adult rat. The vulnerable layer comprises zona fasciculata and zona reticularis; nonvulnerable regions of the adrenal are zona glomerulosa and the adrenal medulla. The rat with adrenal apoplexy does not appear ill and needs no supportive therapy with corticosteroids or saline drink because the aldosterone-secreting cells of zona glomerulosa are not injured and as a consequence the rat does not develop adrenal insufficiency.

Huggins and Morii (10) discovered the adrenocorticolytic property of the DMBA group in adult rats in studies on experimental cancer of the breast at the lab bench. At routine examination of rats bearing mammary cancer, which had been elicited by a single feeding of DMBA given a few weeks earlier to adult animals, it was observed that most of the adrenals contained calcified masses resembling grains of sand; the adrenal stones had the crystal structure of hydroxyapatite. The adrenals of adult rats with mammary cancer which had been evoked by carcinogens, other than members of the DMBA group, were not calcified. Retrospective studies were initiated immediately. Soon it was apparent that hemorrhage of gross proportions occurred in all adult rats in the adrenal within 72 hr after the animals had been given a large dose of DMBA (10). The destruction was not immediate but usually occurred 24-30 hr after administering the carcinogen. It was remarkable that DMBA did not injure the adrenal glands of juvenile rats or of mice of any age.

By definition, adrenal apoplexy is hemorrhage visible in the gross in the adrenal glands. In early stages, adrenal apoplexy is manifest as one or several small patches of extravasated blood, visible to the unaided eye, on the surface of the adrenal gland; later these patches coalesce to form a large turgid brilliant red structure reminiscent of a red light in the fog.

The adrenal cortex of rat must be in a susceptible state to permit damage by DMBA. Recent stimulation by corticotrophin (ACTH) is mandatory for DMBA-induced corticolysis to occur. Spared from injury are the adrenals of weanling rats and those of adults some three or more weeks after hypophysectomy.

At 0 hr a single feeding of DMBA, 30 mg, was provided to members of
two groups of rats, respectively, age 25 or age 50 days. There were 10
rats in each group and the adrenals were harvested at + 72 hr. Adrenal
necrosis and hemorrhage were found in 10 rats in the "age 50 day" group and
in no rat in the "age 25 day" group.

ACTH renders the adrenal cortex of infant rats susceptible to destruction
by DMBA, whereas bovine somatotrophin (BGH) was ineffective in this regard.
In an earlier experiment (11) rats were injected with ACTH, 8 IU daily, from
age 20 to 26 days and then 30 mg of DMBA was fed; at +72 hr the adrenals
were examined. All of the rats which received ACTH followed by DMBA
developed bilateral adrenal necrosis; the adrenals of none of the rats which
received DMBA or ACTH singly were damaged.

Menadione Reductase

The enzymes that detoxify compounds foreign to the organism are of three
sorts: i, enzymes engaged in biosynthesis of ascorbic acid; ii, insoluble
enzymes, absent from the cytosol, which are bound to microsomes or the
membranes of the smooth endoplasmic reticulum; iii, soluble enzymes
including menadione reductase.

Williams-Ashman and Huggins (12) discovered in rats that within 3 days
after a single oral dose of DMBA the oxidation of reduced pyridine nucleotides by vitamin K_3 is accelerated two-fold in the perirenal fat and in the
mammary gland.

The remarkable increase in the levels of menadione reductase in the
mammary glands after feeding carcinogenic polynuclear hydrocarbons
prompted a study of some properties of this enzyme. The diaphorase remained in solution after centrifugation of the extracts at 100,000 x $\underline{g}$ for
1 hr at 2°. The enzymatic oxidation of NADH and NADPH by vitamin K_3
was inhibited by dicumarol. The experiments showed that the mammary
gland diaphorase (EC 1.6.5.2) has many properties in common with the
soluble DT diaphorase described by Ernster et al. (13) and the vitamin K
reductase isolated by Märki and Martius (14).

DMBA Depresses the Incorporation of [3H]-Thymidine into DNA

[3H] TdR and DMBA were injected i.v. sequentially (15) in male S-D rats age 25 days or 50 days, respectively. The injection of DMBA prior to [3H]TdR considerably depressed but did not eliminate the incorporation of tritium into DNA of rat testis, intestine and adrenal. In the younger group the uptake of tritiated thymidine by the growing testis was considerably greater than that seen in older animals; even so, the concentration of radio-activity in terminal ileum was five times that in testis. Fractionation of the testis demonstrated that the decrease of tritium incorporation was associated exclusively with the perchloric acid-insoluble fraction. In the foregoing experiments it was found that DMBA injected 4 hr before [3H]TdR caused a profound inhibition of radioactivity during a 21-24 hr period thereafter, whereas DMBA injected 4 hr after [3H]TdR showed only a slight effect.

In Testis DMBA Destroys Diploid Cells Whereas Haploid Cells are Uninjured

After a single dose, i.g. or i.v., of 40 mg of DMBA the testis of rat was severely and selectively damaged whereas the ovary of sisters was spared from injury. After many weeks complete recovery of the testis ensued. The destructive effect of DMBA on testis was not shared by other powerful carcinogenic hydrocarbons including 3-MC.

The primary sites of destruction inflicted by DMBA on testis were spermatogonia and primary spermatocytes (16), the only germinal cells in testis which synthesize DNA. No other cells in the germinal epithelium were damaged by DMBA. The severe atrophy of testis which ensued (Fig. 1) after some weeks was secondary to destruction of DNA-synthesizing cells in the seminiferous cell line. Moreover, interstitial cells of testis were not injured by the hydrocarbon.

The selective destructive effects of cells in testis induced by DMBA are reminiscent of those inflicted by x-rays. In a classic description of the effect of ionizing radiation on the testis of rats, Regaud and Blanc (17) found that there was destruction of spermatogonia whereas spermatozoa were undamaged; this fact explains the "period of incubation" after which lesions in the germinal epithelium were observed by these workers.

8

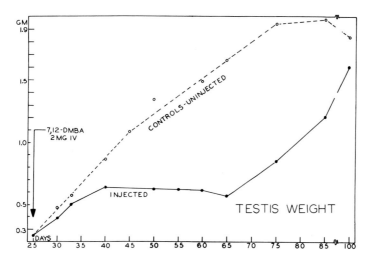

Fig. 1. Growth of testis in rats given an i.v. injection of 2 mg of DMBA (40 mg/kg) at age 25 days related to that of uninjected controls.

ABBREVIATIONS

i.g., intragastric; i.v., intravenous; ACTH, corticotrophin; BA, benz[a]anthracene; BGH, bovine somatotrophin; DEBA, 7,12-diethyl-benz[a]anthracene; DMBA, 7,12-dimethylbenz[a]anthracene; 3-MC, 3-methylcholanthrene; MR, menadione reductase; NADH, reduced nicotinamide adenine dinucleotide; NADPH, reduced nicotinamide adenine dinucleotide phosphate; S-D, Sprague-Dawley; [^{3}H]TdR, tritiated thymidine; TMBA, 7,8,12-trimethylbenz[a]anthracene.

REFERENCES

1. Huggins, C. B. (1979) Experimental Leukemia and Mammary Cancer, University of Chicago Press, Chicago.

2. Bachmann, W. E. and Chemerda, J. M. (1938) J. Am. Chem. Soc. 60, 1023.

3. Kennaway, E. L. (1930) Biochem. J. 24, 497.

4. Bachmann, W. E., Kennaway, E. L. and Kennaway, N. M. (1938) Yale J. Biol. Med. 11, 97.

5. Hamilton, J. G., Durbin, P. W. and Parrott, M. (1954) J. Clin. Endocrinol. Metab. 14, 1161.

6. Shellabarger, C. J., Cronkite, E. P., Bond, V. P. and Lippincott, S. W. (1957) Radiation Res. 6, 501.

7. Huggins, C. B., Grand, L. C. and Brillantes, F. P. (1961) Nature 189, 204.

8. Huggins, C. B. and Yang, N. C. (1962) Science 137, 257.

9. Huggins, C., Morii, S. and Pataki, J. (1969) Proc. Natl. Acad. Sci. USA 62, 704.

10. Huggins, C. B. and Morii, S. (1961) J. Exp. Med. 114, 741.

11. Morii, S. and Huggins, C. B. (1962) Endocrinol. 71, 972.

12. Williams-Ashman, H. G. and Huggins, C. B. (1961) Med. Exp. 4, 223.

13. Ernster, L., Ljunggren, M. and Danielson, L. (1960) Biochem. Biophys. Research Comm. 2, 88.

14. Mårki, F. and Martius, C. (1960) Biochem. Z. 333, 111.

15. Jensen, E. V., Ford, E. and Huggins, C. (1963) Proc. Natl. Acad. Sci. USA 50, 454.

16. Ford, E. and Huggins, C. (1963) J. Exp. Med. 118, 27.

17. Regaud, C. and Blanc, J. (1906) Compt. rend. Soc. biol. 61, 163.

© 1983 Elsevier Science Publishers B.V.
Extrahepatic Drug Metabolism and Chemical Carcinogenesis,
J. Rydström, J. Montelius and M. Bengtsson eds.

INITIATION OF CARCINOGENESIS WITH CHEMICALS - A BIOLOGICAL PERSPECTIVE

EMMANUEL FARBER, M.D., PH.D.
Departments of Pathology and Biochemistry, University of Toronto,
Toronto, Ontario, (Canada) M5G 1L5

INTRODUCTION

Chemical carcinogenesis, the development of cancer with chemicals, is a biological process which is both initiated and promoted by chemicals. Since altered functioanl behaviour of cells is central to the wole carcinogenic process, since the functional behaviour of cells is the resultant of the interactions between their genome and their environment, and since the environment of cells is established and mediated through the structure and function of the organ or tissue in which the cells reside, it is probable that what cells do metabolically and physiologically during cancer development is as much a reflection of the alterations in the whole organ as in the individual carcinogen-induced inititated cells.

It continues to be evident that the cell remains "the smallest integrating unit in biology: a pseudo-intelligent computer that receives, screens, changes, reacts to and adapts to a host of environmental signals, all of this activity apparently designed, through evolution, for cell survival and host survival" (1). Any meaningful discussion of "Drug metabolism and chemical carcinogenesis" must somehow integrate the chemistry and biochemistry with the biological change in the targets, the cell and its suroundings.

In this presentation, I would like to emphasize two fundamental aspects: (a) the role of cell proliferation in initiation, and (b) the nature of initiated cells in their role as precursors for the cellular evolution to cancer. Since this Conference is on drug metabolism, it seems appropriate to concentrate on the first few steps in the carcinogenic process. However, it must be emphasized that the later steps, not covered except peripherally in this presentation, are much closer and perhaps more relevant to the development of cancer.

INITIATION

Chemical carcinogenesis continues to be characterized as a "two stage process". While historically interesting, the only justification for a 2-stage designation is that cancer or better, the early precancerous changes, can be induced in many systems, including the skin, liver, urinary bladder and colon, by two discrete operations - the application of a chemical carcinogen, often as a single dose and the creation of a "promoting environment", often by repeated or prolonged exposure to a chemical, including carcinogens..

The uptake, metabolism, including "activation" and "detoxification", interactions with DNA and other cellular constituents, the repair of DNA lesions by excision or by other mechanisms and the modulation of these various activities by genetic variations, diet, drugs and other chemicals and by other concomittant pathologic processes will be discussed in great detail by the majority of participants and need not be discussed in detail further in relation to "drug metabolism".

Cell Proliferation in Initiation. There is general agreement that activated forms of carcinogens and their interactions with DNA (and perhaps other macromolecules) are important in initiation. However, there is increasing data to show that these events may have no biological meaning in relation to carcinogenesis without cell proliferation. Although cell proliferation has been discussed periodically over many years in regard to initiation and carcinogenesis (2-5), no precise delineation for its role in initiation was evident until stepwise liver systems began to be developed about 10 years ago. In tissues and organs that normally show continual cell proliferation (skin, intestine, bone marrow and lymph nodes), no unequivocal demonstration of a role for cell proliferation in initiation could be made (2). The main problem related to obtaining a base line with no proliferation and then being able to turn on cell proliferation at will. Since this is easily done in the liver, it was in this organ that its importance was first clearly established. Using foci of enzyme altered hepatocytes as a short term indicator for initiation, Scherer and Emmelot (6,7), Pitot and coworkers (8) and Schulte-Hermann and colleagues (9) clearly showed the importance of cell proliferation early in carcinogenesis. Using a different indicator for initiation, a resistant hepatocyte (10) Cayama et al (11), Columbano et al (12), Tsuda et al (13) and Ying et al (14,15) demonstrated clearly the dependence of initiation with over 30 chemical carcinogens upon a round of cell proliferation. Also, some of these studies showed a time dependence. With several carcinogens, cell proliferation, as induced either by partial hepatectomy (PH) or by the induction of cell death, was required within 48 to 72 hours in order to permit initiation. Delays of 48 hours or longer were associated with a drastic decrease in the level of initiation and in the incidence of hepatocellular carcinoma. There is some evidence that carcinogenesis in the pancreas (16) and urinary bladder (17), two quiescent tissues, is also dependent on an early round of cell proliferation.

It is therefore highly probable that chemical carcinogenesis in organs quiescent at some phase or phases in their normal developmental span will be quite dependent upon cell proliferation for initiation. Experimentally, this may be induced by a mitogen or by cell injury. Clinically, the latter is a much more likely method. Thus, pancreatic damage in chronic alcoholism, urinary bladder damage in bilharziasis (schistosomiasis) or perhaps some other forms of cystitis and liver damage with hepatic viruses or with hepatotoxins are three examples of how cell damage, cell proliferation and chemical carcinogenesis may be interrelated.

There are two other aspects that should be mentioned. Chemicals carcinogenic for a quiescent organ almost always induce cell damage and thus provide a round of cell proliferation for initiation. This is evident in liver, pancreas and bladder. Again, carcinogens generally are inhibitors of cell proliferation. Therefore, a carcinogen may either inhibit or induce cell proliferation depending upon its nature. These opposing possibilities must be considered in any analysis of chemical carcinogenesis.

What is the role of cell proliferation in initiation? One of the simplest hypotheses relates to DNA replication. If a permanent change in base composition of DNA is related to initition, then the role of cell proliferation in providing DNA replication is easily understood. Although this hypothesis is conceptually simple and attractive, its testing poses major difficulties at this time (15). Any suppression of DNA replication has many other biochemical metabolic consequences as a result of arresting the cell cycle. One or more of these might be important in the contribution of cell proliferation to initiation.

We all know that the passage of cells through the different phases of the
cell cycle is associated with many enzymatic and biochemical changes
including changes in cytochromes P450 and the associated drug
metabolizing enzymes in the microsones, as part of the phase I system, in
some phase II enzymes, in enzymes of nucleotide, RNA and DNA metabolism
and synthesis, in polymerization and depolymerization of filaments, to
name but a few. How any one or more of these may influence the
initiation process with chemicals has yet to be explored. For example,
one report indicates that the repair of certain lesions induced in DNA by
N-methyl-N-nitro-N-nitrosoguanidine (MNNG) may be delayed during cell
replication (18). This relates especially to O-6-methylguanine, on
altered base that has received major attention as a likely mutation-prone
lesion. Such a change could conceivably have a major impact on
initiation through a mechanism additional to DNA replication. Also, it
is quite possible that changes in DNA, other than a mutation, may be
important in initiation. Translocations and transpositions gene
rearrangements or gene amplifications are some possibilities. Clearly,
given the great importance of cell proliferation in the transfer or
translation of carcinogen-metabolic effects to the first major biological
effect, initiation, it would appear that this aspect of chemical
carcinogenesis would be a fruitful area for exploration in depth.

Nature of Initiated Cells in their Role as Precursors for the Cellular
Evolution to Cancer. According to current concepts of chemical
carcinogenesis, the first major biological consequence of initiation is
the genesis of altered cells that now become, as a group, the precursors
from which the malignant neoplastic process evolves. Logically, the
nature of the initiated cells would seem to be a problem highly relevant
to "Drug Metabolism" as it relates to "Chemical Carcinogenesis".
Regardless of the molecular or biochemical mechanism or mechanisms of how
an activated chemical induces a rare altered cell, what kind or kinds of
altered cells can act as the progenitors of cancer? Is the basic change
some alteration in the control of cell proliferation such as to allow the
rare initiated cell to proliferate or is it some other type of
biochemical alteration?

With respect to cell proliferation, there seems to be a common
feeling that here lies a primary defect in initiated cells. Since the

major phenotypic expression of cancer is some altered control of cell proliferation, since chemical carcinogens can participate in a process leading to cancer, since chemical carcinogens need only exert an effect for a brief period early in the carcinogenic process and since initiation is followed by expansion by cell proliferation of initiated cells, it seems almost axiomatic that chemical carcinogens might induce some fundamental change in growth control during their first biological effect, initiation.

Despite the strength of this feeling, there is no evidence for its support. In virtually every known system studied in which chemicals are the initiating agents, no significant proliferation of cells in an initiated tissue is seen without some identifiable or probable promoting influence. If this is valid, then an initiating carcinogen induces an "enabling phenomenon" for cell proliferation, not cell proliferation itself. Consistent with this tentative conclusion are the results of an ongoing study by Rotstein in our laboratory. He has found that initiated cells show if anything a prolongation of the cell cycle time due to lengthening of the S phase with no change in the duration of the G_1, G_2 or M phases of the cell cycle. A common perception, derived from increasing attention on mechanisms of action of promoting agents, is that the promoting environments act as selective mitogens to stimulate directly the proliferation of the altered initiated cells. One formulation visualizes some change in receptors for endogenous or exogenous mitogens that allows the selective growth of the initiated cells to form papillomas, polyps, nodules, etc. The evidence for this hypothesis is lacking so far.

Several alternative hypotheses seem equally attractive. One, for which there is increasing evidence, is based on the well known inhibition of cell proliferation by many carcinogens (19). By inducing a rare cell resistant to this effect of carcinogens, one can readily account for the initiating effect of most carcinogens (13). In this formulation, the resistant initiated cell can respond to a normal mitogen such as one generated by partial hepatectomy in the liver in the presence of a carcinogen that is inhibitory to the proliferation of all the uninitiated cells. This concept is the basis for the resistant hepatocyte model for liver carcinogenesis.

In addition to this hypothesis, that of "differential inhibition", at least two more formulations are possible - differential stimulation and differential recovery (20).

With this approach, we have been able to develop a model for the rapid generation of hepatocyte nodules so as to study their organization, structure, and biochemistry as well as their biological history. As with previous studies, the nodules demonstrate at least two options - remodeling to normal appearing liver and persistence with further evolution to cancer. The vast majority of nodules exercise the first option, remodeling (21).

A major question concerns the basis for the two options - is this simply a stochastic phenomenon or is a small subset of the rare initiated cells different at the time of induction? In its presumed "shotgun" effect at initiation, do the active carcinogens induce a very rare change such that the nodules derived from these cells behave differently than do the majority?

With maximum initiating doses of carcinogens in the liver, about 1 hepatocyte per 10^5 or 10^6 hepatocytes is initiated. Of this number, about 5-10 per 10^3 persist - i.e. 5 to 10 hepatocytes per 10^8 - 10^9 original cells are so altered by the initiating carcinogen to make them highly relevant to the ultimate development of cancer. Although the quantitation is not highly accurate, it does provide an order of magnitude.

A Common Biochemical Phenotype of Hepatocyte Nodules. Ideally, one would like to isolate and analyze the few initiated cells in the liver and elsewhere before they begin to expand into nodules etc. This may be possible now with improved cell sorters. However, a note of caution. If the few persistent nodules (or papillomas) are a reflection of some special effect of the carcinogen, pooling all of the initiated cells will obscure their special features.

Alternatively, the approach we have taken is to induce an expansion of each initiated cell to form nodules and to study their biochemistry and biology. In this way, the few persistent nodules can be readily obtained by allowing the animal to remodel the vast majority of the nodules. Since this small subset is much more related to the evolution to cancer than are the majority of nodules, it now becomes feasible to begin to follow the later steps in the carcinogenic process.

Work by Cameron, Eriksson, Roomi, Lee, Ho and Tatematsu in our laboraotry and collaborative work with Sharma and Murray have disclosed the presence of a common biochemical programming of the hepatocyte nodules that is most easily related to their acquisition of resistance to cytotoxic effects of many xenobiotics including carcinogens (22).

The nodules show a <u>pattern</u> of enzymatic and biochemical changes so far unique. Phase I enzymes including cytochromes P450 are very much reduced while many other components, especially phase II, are elevated (Table 1). These include glutathione, at least one glutathione-S-transferase (B) and at least one UDP-glucuronyl transferase (23) as well as DT-diaphorase, epoxide hydrolase and gamma-glutamyl transferase.

This pattern has now been found in hepatocyte nodules not only induced in the resistant hepatocyte model with several different carcinogens, but also when generated by phenobarbital, choline deficient diet or orotic acid. Also, this pattern is stable, since persistent nodules when transfered to the spleen, show the same phenomenon. These nodules have never been exposed to a carcinogen or a promoting environment for many months (24).

TABLE 1

PROPERTIES OF HEPATOCYTE NODULES

A - MICROSOMES
- Low cytochrome P450 and mixed function oxygenases
- Low NADPH-cytochrome C reductase
- High epoxide hydrolase
- High UDP-glucuronyl transferase

B - CYTOSOL
- High glutathione
- High glutathione-S-transferase (B, etc.)
- High DT-diaphorase
- Marked increase in 21Kd protein

C - MEMBRANES
- High γ-glutamyl transferase

In addition, recent evidence shows that the nodules have a very special protein pattern in their cytosol. Four proteins, including a 21 Kd fraction, show large elevations and others are decreased. Again, this is seen in nodules regardless of the nature of the initiating carcinogen or the promoting environment.

Thus, the expanded initiated cells show a remarkably uniform pattern of enzymes and proteins and peptides, many of which have an apparent role in the resistance of this population to carcinogen activation and/or cytotoxicity.

Studies in whole animals have shown that the biochemical pattern is reflected in the pharmacodynamics of a carcinogen, 2-acetylamino-fluorene. Decreased activation, more efficient conjugation and more efficient excretion in the urine are among the obvious differences between control animals and animals with nodules in their livers.

The constancy of the patterns and the nature of the changes have suggested to us that the steps in carcinogenesis we have discussed in this presentation are physiological, not abnormal or "pathological" and that they might represent a form of adaptation to xenobiotics that may have survival value (25). The possible relevance of this to the ultimate development of cancer remains a fascinating challenge.

SOME GENERAL CONSIDERATIONS

There is now abundant evidence that cancers of any cell type in humans and in experimental animals show a bewildering diversity. Cytological, biochemical, biophysical, ultrastructural, genetic, chromosomal and physiological "markers" are present in an inconstant form in cancers of many different kinds. Is this diversity present throughout the carcinogenic process or is it mainly a property of "late stage" cancer with advanced progression? This is not a trivial question by any means, since our understanding of how a carcinogenic process develops is very much dependent upon the nature of the answer.

The liver has become the "flagship" of the biochemical approach to chemical carcinogenesis by virtue of the availability of models. The studies of synchronized systems, such as in the resistant hepatocyte model, clearly show that early and later altered hepatocyte populations (hepatocyte nodules) seen with many initiating chemicals are remarkably uniform in respect to many phenotypic properties. This similarity is also seen in nodules in other models that do not use dietary 2-AAF plus partial hepatectomy for promotion. In models in which promotion is achieved by dietary phenobarbital, or by choline deficient - low methionine diet or by dietary orotic acid, the biochemical pattern is remarkably the same. Based upon this unusual commonality and upon its stability, as judged by the studies on persistant nodules transplanted to the spleen (24), we are impressed by the similarities in lesions during the carcinogenic process.

We consider that this commonality may be a reflection of similarities in the selection of an appropriately altered initiated hepatocyte. Since the early initiated cells show no autonomy and since

even later precancerous hepatocyte populations show very little, we think that even the later lesions are dependent upon the selection or promoting environment. It is thus attractive to consider that the commonality in the biochemical patterns is a reflection of a commonality in the selection of the new cells for further evolution to cancer. As new cell populations evolve progressively toward increasing autonomy and growth, diversity in phenotypic expression of older properties unrelated to these new ones would appear more and more until extreme diversity would be expected ultimately. The current liver models, especially the resistant hepatocyte model, may allow for a more definitive analysis of the biochemistry of the new cell populations as they approach the malignant phenotypic.

The characterization of the new cell populations in the liver models, especially in relation to the ultimate development of cancer offers a model with which carcinogenesis in other organs or tissues can be compared. The available information on the development of cancer in different organs suggests that many similarities exist in principle between the liver and other organs (25).

ACKNOWLEDGEMENTS

This research was supported by grants from the National Cancer Institute of Canada, the Medical Research Council of Canada (MT-5594) and the National Cancer Institute, NIH (CA-21157).

REFERENCES

1.   Farber, E. (1973) Cancer Res. 33, 2537.

2.   Grisham, J.W., Kaufmann, W.K. and Kaufman, D.G. (1983) Surv.
        Synth. Path. Res. 1, 49.

3.   Rajewsky, M.F. (1972) Z. Krebsforsch. 78, 12.

4.   Warwick, G.P. (1971) Fed. Proc. 36, 1760.

5.   Craddock, V.M. (1976) in:Cameron, H.M., Linsell, D.S. and
        Warwick G.P. (eds.) Liver Cell Cancer, Elsevier/North Holland
        Biochemical Press, Amsterdam, pp. 153-201.

6.   Scherer, E. and Emmelot, P. (1976) Cancer Res., 36, 2544.

7.   Scherer, E. and Emmelot, P. (1977) Mutat. Res., 46:155.

8.   Pitot, H.C., Barsness, L., Kitagawa, T. (1978) in:Slaga, T.J.,
        Sivak, A. and Boutwell, A.K. (eds.) Carcinogenesis: Mechanisms
        of Tumor Promotion and Carcinogenesis, Vol 2. Raven Press, New
        York, pp. 433-442.

9.   Schulte-Hermann, R., Ohde, G., Schuppler, J. and
        Timmermann-Trosiener, I. (1981) Cancer Res., 41, 2556.

10.   Solt, D. and Farber, E. (1976) Nature, 263, 701.

11.   Cayama, E., Tsuda, H., Sarma, D.S.R. and Farber, E. (1978)
        Nature, 275, 60.

12.   Columbano, A., Rajalakshmi, S. and Sarma, D.S.R. (1981)
        Cancer Res., 41, 1079.

13.   Tsuda, H., Lee, G. and Farber, E. (1980) Cancer Res., 40, 1157.

14.   Ying, T.S., Sarma, D.S.R. and Farber, E. (1981) Cancer Res.,
        41, 2096.

15.   Ying, T.S., Enomoto, K., Sarma, D.S.R. and Farber, E. (1982)
        Cancer Res., 42, 876.

16.   Scarpelli, D.G. and Rao, M.S. (1981) Cancer, 15, 1552.

17.   Cohen, S.M., Murosaki, G., Fukushima, S. and Greenfield, R.E.
        (1982) Cancer Res., 42, 65.

18.   Smith, G.J., Grisham, J.W. and Kaufman, D.G. (1981) Cancer Res.,
        41, 1373.

19.   Farber, E. (1976) in:Cameron, H.M., Linsell, D.A. and Warwick,
        G.P. (eds.) Liver Cell Cancer. Elsevier/North Holland
        Biomedical Press, Amsterdam, pp. 243-277.

20.   Farber, E. (1982) in:Becker, F.F. (ed.) Cancer: A Comprehensive
        Treatise. 2nd edition. Vol. 1, Plenum Publishing Corporation,
        New York, pp. 485-506.

21.   Enomoto, K. and Farber, E. (1982) Cancer Res. 42, 2330.

22.   Eriksson, L., Ahluwalia, M., Spiewak, J., Lee, G., Sarma,
       D.S.R., Roomi, M.J. and Farber, E. (1983) Environ. Hlth
       Perspectives 49, 171.

23.   Bock, K.W., Lilienbaum, W., Pfell, H. and Eriksson, L.C. (1982)
       Cancer Res., 42, 3747.

24.   Finkelstien, S.D., Lee, G., Medline, A., Tatematsu, M., Makowka,
       L. and Farber, E. (1983) Am. J. Pathol. 110, 119.

25.   Farber, E. and Cameron, R. (1980) Adv. Cancer Res., 31, 125.

© 1983 Elsevier Science Publishers B.V.
Extrahepatic Drug Metabolism and Chemical Carcinogenesis,
J. Rydström, J. Montelius and M. Bengtsson eds.

DIFFERENCES BETWEEN KIDNEY AND LIVER IN THE REGULATION OF MICROSOMAL TESTOSTERONE HYDROXYLASE ACTIVITIES IN INBRED MICE

ROY HAWKE, LYNN RAYNOR, GURMIT SINGH AND ALLEN NEIMS
Department of Pharmacology and Therapeutics, University of Florida, College of Medicine, Gainesville, Florida 32610 (U.S.A)

INTRODUCTION

We have compared liver and kidney microsomes with regard to catalytic specificity and the relative importance of gender and genetics in the regulation of constitutive cytochromes P-450 involved in the site-specific hydroxylation of testosterone.

MATERIALS AND METHODS

All animals were studied at age 77 days; where indicated, mice were castrated or sham-operated at age 56 days. Treatment with testosterone propionate or oil-vehicle involved daily sc injections of 100 µg of the hormone for 7 days beginning at age 70 days. Cytochrome P-450 was measured spectrophotometrically. Testosterone hydroxylation was routinely assayed in 100 mM potassium phosphate buffer, pH 7.4, at a testosterone concentration of 131 mM (0.5 µCi). After extraction of metabolites into methylene chloride, products were resolved by TLC, located by autoradiography, and quantitated by liquid scintillation.

RESULTS AND DICUSSION

Liver microsomes catalyzed the formation of several hydroxylated derivatives, four of which are listed in Table 1. These four comprise more than 55% of total metabolites. Although 6β-hydroxytestosterone is the major product, 15α- and 16α-hydroxytestosterone were most interesting. The rate of formation of 16α-hydroxytestosterone was higher in males and was reversibly induced by testosterone. The rate of formation of 15α-hydroxytestosterone was higher in microsomes from females, but only in certain strains (e.g., AKR/J, not BALB/cJ). This strain difference between females was controlled by one or at most a few genes. 15α-Hydroxylase activity in liver was induced by pharmacological doses of estradiol in BALB/cJ males and females and AKR/J males, and suppressed by treatment with testosterone in AKR/J females.

The situation in kidney microsomes was quite different. Cytochrome P-450 content exhibited a 5-7 fold male predominance in kidney. Many hydroxylations which were prominent in liver were virtually absent in kidney preparations. Microsomes from females were virtually inactive toward testosterone. The major activity in kidneys from males of both strains was 15α-hydroxylase, the level of which was nearly as high or higher than that in liver. These results are in sharp contrast to the strain-specific female predominance of 15α-hydroxylase in liver. Castration decreased renal 15α-hydroxylase activity in males to < 1% of control values, but cytochrome P-450 and 16α-hydroxylase only decreased to about one-half. Treatment of castrated males with testosterone reversed these effects. Treatment of females with testosterone increased P-450 to about one-half of the male value, but had less effect on 16α-hydroxylase and only a minimal effect on 15α-hydroxylase activity. Athough several experiments remain to be done, the results suggest neonatal androgen imprinting of 15α-hydroxylase activity with continuing adult androgen requirement for expression of activity.

The role of 15α-hydroxylation of steroids is unknown, but stringent regulation seems to exist. Gustafsson and Ingelman-Sundberg have described female-specific 15-hydroxylation of sulfated steroids in rat liver (1), while Solomon and colleagues have reported that the fetoplacental unit serves as a source of 15α-hydroxysteroids in late human pregnancy (2).

TABLE 1

HYDROXYLATION OF TESTOSTERONE BY HEPATIC AND RENAL MICROSOMES FROM AKR/J AND BALB/cJ MALE AND FEMALE MICE

Strain	Sex	Source	P-450 (nmol/mg protein)	Rate of Production of Hydroxytestosterone[a]			
				15α	16α	6β	15α
				(nmol/10 min/mg protein)			
AK	♂	Liver	0.71	1.37	3.87	27.6	1.19
AK	♀	Liver	0.63	4.64	1.15	32.3	1.94
BL	♂	Liver	0.82	1.68	4.80	18.6	1.09
BL	♀	Liver	0.76	1.96	2.34	18.7	1.00
AK	♂	Kidney	0.37	2.70	0.35	u.d	u.d
AK	♀	Kidney	0.05	u.d	u.d	u.d	u.d
BL	♂	Kidney	0.23	3.47	0.19	u.d	u.d
BL	♀	Kidney	0.05	u.d	u.d	u.d	u.d

[a]All values are means from 3 to 10 animals; standard deviations were 10-25% of means. u.d, undetectable.

REFERENCES

1. Gustafsson, J.-A. and Ingelman-Sundberg, M., J. Biol. Chem. 250:3451-3458 (1975).
2. Giannopoulos, G., Bowman, J. and Solomon, S., J. Clin. Endocrinol. Metab. 35:345-351 (1972).

© 1983 Elsevier Science Publishers B.V.
Extrahepatic Drug Metabolism and Chemical Carcinogenesis,
J. Rydström, J. Montelius and M. Bengtsson eds.

THE ROLE OF RABBIT CYTOCHROME P-450, FORM 5, IN THE PULMONARY AND HEPATIC METABOLISM OF AROMATIC AMINES TO MUTAGENIC PRODUCTS

IAIN G.C. ROBERTSON, TORE AUNE, COSETTE J. SERABJIT-SINGH, JANE E. CROFT, JOHN R. BEND AND RICHARD M. PHILPOT

Laboratory of Pharmacology, National Institute of Environmental Health Sciences, National Institutes of Health, P. O. Box 12233, Research Triangle Park, North Carolina 27709 (U.S.A.)

INTRODUCTION

A major isozyme of cytochrome P-450 in rabbit lung, form 5, is highly active in the metabolism of aromatic amines to mutagenic products (1). The effects of inducers on the hepatic content of form 5 have been investigated and the role of this isozyme in the metabolism of 2-acetylaminofluorene (AAF) to mutagenic products established.

MATERIALS AND METHODS

Assay for mutagenic activity. Mutagenic activity was detected with a modified *Salmonella* assay (1). Immunochemical assays were done as reported or cited (2).

High pressure liquid chromatography (HPLC). Separation of metabolites of AAF was done by HPLC using a μBondapak C_{18} column; details to be reported elsewhere.

RESULTS

Treatment of rabbits with phenobarbital (PB) increases the hepatic metabolism of 2-aminofluorene (AF) to mutagenic products. Form 5-catalyzed metabolism (determined by antibody inhibition) and the content of form 5 (measured by single radial immunodiffusion, "Western blotting", and amounts of antibody needed for 50% maximum inhibition) increase to the same extent, 10- to 12-fold (Table 1). In contrast, treatment of rabbits with β-naphthoflavone decreases the hepatic content of form 5 (data not shown).

TABLE 1

CORRELATION OF THE HEPATIC CONTENT AND ACTIVITY OF CYTOCHROME P-450, FORM 5

Treatment	Activity Inhibited[a]	I-50[b]	SRID[c]	Western Blotting[d]
None	5 (70%)	0.04	25	3
Phenobarbital	60 (89%)	0.47	269	38

[a] Amount of activity inhibited by antibody to form 5 (revertants/μg, % total).
[b] Amount of antibody (mg IgG/mg protein) needed for 50% maximum inhibition.
[c] Single radial immunodiffusion (pmol form 5/mg protein).
[d] Immunostaining intensity (peak area/μg protein).

The formation of mutagenic products from AF in pulmonary and hepatic, and from AAF in hepatic, microsomal preparations follows typical saturation kinetics, whereas the pulmonary metabolism of AAF increases linearly with increasing substrate concentration. Inhibition of mutagenic activity by paraoxon indicates that deacetylation is involved in the metabolism of AAF with either preparation (Table 2). As measured by HPLC, AF is the major product formed from AAF in pulmonary and hepatic preparations and N-hydroxy-AAF is a minor product formed only in the hepatic preparation (Table 3). (No N-hydroxy-AAF is formed by the pulmonary preparations even when paraoxon is present).

TABLE 2			TABLE 3		
INHIBITION OF AAF MUTAGENICITY			FORMATION OF METABOLITES FROM AAF		
Tissue	Paraoxon[a] $(10^{-5}M)$	Antibodies to form 5[a]	Tissue	AF[a]	N-Hydroxy-AAF[a]
Lung	9.3	8.9	Lung	480	not detected
Liver	3.8	36.0	Liver	1300	82

[a]Percent of control activity.   [a]Rate (pmol/min/mg protein).

DISCUSSION

Form 4, the major isozyme of cytochrome P-450 that is induced in rabbit liver by polycyclic aromatic hydrocarbons, catalyzes the metabolism of 2-aminoanthracene to mutagenic products (3) and the N-hydroxylation of AAF (4). With antibody inhibition studies, we have demonstrated that 90% of the pulmonary and 50-70% of the hepatic metabolism of AF and AAF to mutagenic products is catalyzed by form 5 (1). We have now shown that the hepatic content of form 5 is increased to the extent that it catalyzes 90% of the metabolism of AF to mutagenic products following treatment of rabbits with PB. Further, the metabolism of AAF in pulmonary microsomal preparations does not involve the formation of N-hydroxy-AAF, a pathway that contributes to the metabolism of AAF in hepatic microsomal preparations. The major pathway in both preparations is deacetylation followed by monooxygenation.

REFERENCES

1. Robertson, I.G.C., Philpot, R.M., Zeiger, E. and Wolf, C.R. (1981) Molec. Pharmacol., 20, 662-668.

2. Robertson, I.G.C., Serabjit-Singh, C., Croft, J.E. and Philpot, R.M. (1983) Molec. Pharmacol., (in press).

3. Norman, R.L., Muller-Eberhard, U. and Johnson, E.F. (1979) Biochem. Biophys. Res. Comm., 89, 195-201.

4. Johnson, E.F., Levitt, D.S., Muller-Eberhard, U. and Thorgeirsson, S.S. (1980) Cancer Res., 40, 4456-4459.

© 1983 Elsevier Science Publishers B.V.
Extrahepatic Drug Metabolism and Chemical Carcinogenesis,
J. Rydström, J. Montelius and M. Bengtsson eds.

COMPARISON OF COUMARIN 7-HYDROXYLASE ACTIVITIES IN KIDNEY AND LIVER OF DBA/2J AND C57BL/6J MICE

PEKKA KAIPAINEN[1], DANIEL W. NEBERT[2] AND MATTI LANG[3]

[1]Department of Pharmocology and Toxicology, college of Veterinary Medicine, 00550 Helsinki 55, (Finland) [2]NICHHD, NIH, Dev. Pharmacol Branch. Bethesda MD, 20205 (USA) and [3]Eflab Res. laboratories, Pulttitie 9, 00810 Helsinki 81 (Finland).

INTRODUCTION

A genetic difference exists in coumarin 7-hydroxylase activity among certain inbred strains of mice (1).

We have shown that in the case of liver this difference is due to a particular cytochrome P-450 isoenzyme, highly specific towards coumarin 7-hydroxylation (2).

The aim of our present investigation was to find out whether a cytochrome P-450 specific for coumarin 7-hydroxylation exists not only in liver but also in kidney, and whether similar genetic differences in the enzyme activity exist for both organs.

For this purpose the cytochrome was purified from the livers of both mouse strains and antibodies were raised in rabbits against these pure fractions. The immunological and catalytic properties of coumarin-7-hydroxylases in kidney and liver of DBA/2J (D_2) and C57BL/6J (B_6) mice were compared.

MATERIALS AND METHODS

In all experiments phenobarbital pretreated animals were used. Purification of the cytochrome P-450 specific for coumarin hydroxylation, development of the antibodies and determination of microsomal coumarin 7-hydroxylase activity in the presence and absence of antibody were carried out as previously described by Lang et al (3).

Ouchterlony double diffusion analysis was performed in a 1 % agarose gel containing 0,2 % Emulgen 911 (4).

Tissue localization of the cytochrome P-450 isoenzyme was carried out by fluorescene microscopy using a goat anti-rabbit IgG fraction, labelled with fluorescein.

RESULTS

The purified cytochrome P-450 fractions from the livers of both mouse strains showed an apparent homogeneity on SDS-polyacrylamide gel electrophoresis with a specific content of 14 nmol cytochrome P-450 per mg protein.

Microsomal cytochrome P-450 contents and coumarin 7-hydroxylase activities in kidney and liver of D_2 and B_6 mice:

	cyt. P-450 nmol/mg prot.	enzyme activity (pmol/min) $(nmol\ P\text{-}450)^{-1}$	$(mg\ prot)^{-1}$
Liver D$_2$	1.4	380	600
microsomes B$_6$	1.2	120	150
Kidney D$_2$	0.1	500	51
microsomes B$_6$	0.22	62	14

Antibody mediated inhibition of coumarin 7-hydroxylase:

Kidney: D$_2$, a strong inhibition by both antibodies

B$_6$, no inhibition

Liver: D$_2$, a strong inhibition by both antibodies

B$_6$, only the antibody against B$_6$ cytochrome caused inhibition.

Ouchterlony double diffusion analysis:

- 100 % crossreactivity between D$_2$ and B$_6$ liver microsomes with both antibodies
- 100 % crossreactivity between liver and kidney microsomes of D$_2$ mouse, when the antibody against D$_2$ cytochrome was used
- 50 % cross reactivity between liver and kidney microsomes of B$_6$ mouse when the antibody against B$_6$ cytochrome was used.

Immunofluorescence staining: centrilobular location of the antigen in liver. Tubular location in kidney.

CONCLUSIONS

According to our results, the genetic difference in coumarin 7-hydroxylation previously observed in mouse liver exists also in mouse kidney. We have demonstrated interorgan and inter strain differences in the immunological and catalytical properties of cytochromes P-450.

ACKNOWLEDGEMENTS

This study was supported by the Finnish Academy of Natural Sciences (Suomen Akatemian Luonnontieteellinen toimikunta) Grant No: 7312/22/81

REFERENCES

1. Wood, A.W and Conney, A.H. (1974) Science, Vol. 185, pp. 612-613.
2. Lang, M., et al (1982) in: Hietanen, E., Laitinen, M. and Hänninen, O. (Eds.), Cytochrome P-450, Biochem., Biophys and Env. Implications, Elsevier / North Holland Biomedical Press, Amsterdam, pp 391-394.
3. Lang et al. Manuscript submitted for publication.
4. Thomas, P.E., Lu, A.Y.H., Ryan, D., West, S.B., Kawalwek, J., and Levin, W, (1976) J. Biol. Chem. 251, 1385-1391.

© 1983 Elsevier Science Publishers B.V.
Extrahepatic Drug Metabolism and Chemical Carcinogenesis,
J. Rydström, J. Montelius and M. Bengtsson eds.

EFFECT OF VARIOUS SOLVENTS ON THE XENOBIOTIC BIOTRANSFORMATION IN THE LIVER AND THE KIDNEYS OF THE RAT: A COMPARATIVE STUDY

Tuula Heinonen, Eivor Elovaara, Säde Laurén, Harri Vainio and Jorma Järvisalo

Department of Industrial Hygiene and Toxicology, Institute of Occupational Health, Haartmaninkatu 1, SF-00290 Helsinki 29, Finland

The kidneys are generally regarded as the main excretory site for xenobiotics, whereas the liver is considered the main site of biotransformation. However, the kidneys seem to have drug metabolizing enzymes similar to those of the liver, but the activities per mg of protein are lower and both the induction and the inhibition of the enzymes in the kidneys differ from those in the liver (1,2,3,4,5,6).

The aims of this study were to compare the drug metabolism of the liver to that of the kidneys and to study the effect of the molecular structure of xenobiotics on the biotransformation of drugs in these organs. To fulfill these aims we exposed male Wistar rats to common industrial solvents, with different molecular structures by inhalation for 2 weeks, 5 days/week, 6 hours/day. The solvents were: cyclohexane (C_6H_{12}; 300, 1,000 or 2,000 ppm); n-heptane (C_7H_{16}; 100, 500 or 1,500 ppm); xylene (($CH_3)_2C_6H_4$; 50, 400 or 750 ppm); ethylbenzene ($C_6H_5CH_2CH_3$; 50, 300 or 600 ppm); vinyl toluene ($CH_3C_6H_5CH=CH_2$; 50, 100 or 300), furfuryl alcohol ($2-(C_4H_3O)CH_2OH$; 25, 50 or 100 ppm); and methyl cellosolve ($CH_3OCH_2CH_2OH$; 50, 100 or 400 ppm). Each group contained 5 animals. The following determinations were performed from the liver and the kidneys: the content of cytochrome P-450; the content of glutathione; the activity of 7-ethoxycoumarin O-deethylase; and the activity of UDPglucuronosyltransferase.

In the two tissues tested, all the solvents caused only moderate changes in the contents of free glutathione or cytochrome P-450, and the activity of 7-ethoxycoumarin O-deethylase was only slightly affected in the liver (Fig. 1). In kidneys, however, the activity of this enzyme was enhanced

30

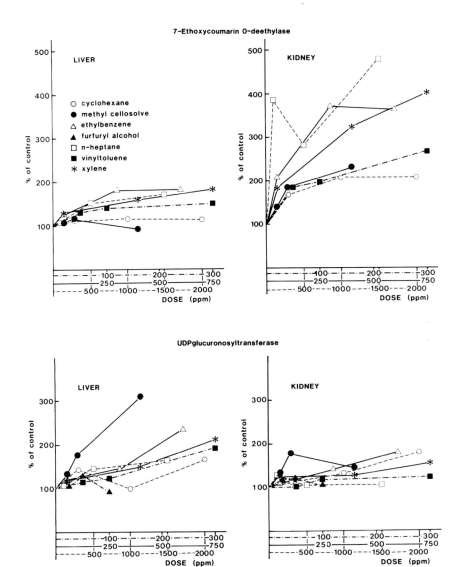

Fig. 1. The activity of 7-ethoxycoumarin O-deethylase and
UDPglucuronosyltransferase in the liver and kidneys of the rat
after exposure to different industrial solvents.

over 300 % by exposure to n-heptane (with max. dose of 1,500 ppm), and over 200 % by exposure to ethylbenzene or xylene (with max. doses of 600 ppm and 750 ppm, respectively), and to a lesser extent by the other solvents tested (Fig. 1). The most usual effect of these solvents on the parameters tested in the liver was the enhancement of the activity of UDPglucuronosyl-transferase, especially with methyl cellosolve (over 200 % with max. dose of 400 ppm), ethylbenzene (over 100 % with max. dose of 600 ppm), xylene (about 100 % with max. dose of 750 ppm), or vinyltoluene (about 100 % with max. dose of 300 ppm). This increase was not merely due to perturbation of the cellular membranes, because the increased activity was also seen after the liver microsomes were treated with detergent (at least in the case of vinyltoluene, cyclohexane, or methyl cellosolve).

In general, the effects of the solvents studied on the xenobiotic biotransformation in the liver resembled that in the kidneys. However, the activity of UDPglucuronosyltransferase typically increased most in the liver, and the activity of 7-ethoxycoumarin O-deethylase increased most in the kidneys. Ethylbenzene, xylene, and n-heptane caused the most prominent effects (increases) in the kidneys, whereas in the liver the solvents which most affected were vinyltoluene, xylene, ethylbenzene, and methyl cellosolve.

REFERENCES

1. Armbrecht, H.J., Birnbaum, L.S., Zenser, T.V., Mattammal, M.B. and Davis, B.B. (1979) Arch. Biochem. Biophys. 197, 277.

2. Kluwe, W.M. and Hook, J.B. (1980) Fed. Proc. 39, 3129.

3. Vainio, H. and Hietanen, E. (1980) in: Jenner, P. and Testa, B. (Eds.), Concepts in Drug Metabolism, Marcel Dekker, Inc, New York, part A, pp. 251-284.

4. Yasukochi, Y., Okita, R.T. and Masters, B.S.S. (1980) in: Coon, M.J., Conney, A.H., Estabrook, R.W., Gelboin, H.V., Gillette, J.R. and O'Brien, P.J. (Eds.), Microsomes, Drug Oxidations, and Chemical Carcinogenesis. Academic Press, New York, vol. 2 pp. 764-768.

5. Lock, E.A. and Ishimael, J. (1981) Toxicol. Appl. Pharmacol. 57, 79.

6. Kluwe, W.M., Herrmann-Kluwe, C.L. and Hook, J.B. (1982) J. Appl. Toxicol. 2, 226.

ᶜ 1983 Elsevier Science Publishers B.V.
Extrahepatic Drug Metabolism and Chemical Carcinogenesis,
J. Rydström, J. Montelius and M. Bengtsson eds.

PROFILE OF DRUG METABOLIZING ENZYMES IN THE NUCLEI AND MICROSOMES OF HEPATIC
AND EXTRAHEPATIC TISSUES FROM MONKEYS

GIAN MARIA PACIFICI[1] AND ANDERS RANE[2]

[1]Department of General Pathology, Medical School, University of Pisa, 56100
Pisa (Italy) and [2]Department of Clinical Pharmacology at the Karolinska Institute, Huddinge Hospital, 141 86 Huddinge (Sweden)

INTRODUCTION

Recent work has demonstrated that nuclear membranes of the rat liver are metabolically active and contain cytochrome P-450 (1,2,3), N-demethylase, aryl
hydrocarbon hydroxylase (AHH) (1) and O-deethylase activity (4). The kinetics
of AHH and the effect of phenobarbital, 3-methylcholanthrene and β-naphtoflavone on this enzyme has been described (5). Subsequent studies also demonstrated
that nuclear envelopes contain epoxide hydrolase (3,6,7,8) and UDP-glucuronyltransferase (9,10). These data were derived from the rat. We have recently
demonstrated epoxide hydrolase (EH) in the hepatic nuclear fraction in man (11)
and Rhesus monkeys (12) which seems to be the only information so far in primates.

Even less is known about nuclear drug metabolizing enzymes in extrahepatic
tissues (5,7,10). The present investigation was aimed to study the nuclear and
microsomal drug metabolizing enzymes in kidneys and lungs and, for comparative
purposes, the liver. Baboons and Rhesus monkeys were chosen as experimental
animals because they are in many respects appropriate models for man, particularly from a drug metabolic point of view.

MATERIALS AND METHODS

Chemicals. ^{3}H-styrene oxide (purity > 99.5 %), ^{3}H-benzo(a)pyrene (purity
> 99 %) and 1-^{14}C-naphtol (purity > 98 %) were purchased from the Radiochemical
Center (Amersham, England). Styrene oxide and styrene glycol were obtained
from Aldrich (Beerse, Belgium). Unlabeled benzo(a)pyrene, 1-naphtol, 7-ethoxy-
coumarin, 7-OH-coumarin and various cofactors were purchased from Sigma (St
Louis, USA). Unlabelled and tritium labelled benzo(a)pyrene-4,5-oxide were received from the NCI Chemical Carcinogen Ref Stand Repository, a function of the
Div of Cancer Cause and Prevention, NCI, NIH (Bethesda, Md).

Animals. Tissue specimens from three adult healthy male baboons and two
healthy Rhesus monkeys were used. The tissues were immediately frozen on dry
ice and stored at -80° C until assay.

Fractionation techniques: Tissue specimens were homogenized in 3 vol of 0.25 M sucrose-3 mM $MgCl_2$, adjusted to pH 7.4 with Tris. The nuclear and microsomal fractions were isolated by differential centrifugation (11) and the final pellets resuspended in 0.1 M Tris-HCl (pH 7.4) containing 30 % glycerol and stored at -20° C for 1 to 2 weeks. The purity of nuclear pellets was checked by phase contrast microscopy.

Enzyme assays: Previously described asssys for EH activity towards styrene oxide and benzo(a)pyrene-4,5-oxide (13) AHH (14), 1-naphthol glucuronidation (15) and 7-ethoxycoumarin O-deethylase (16) were employed. All assays were carried out under conditions linear with time and protein.

RESULTS

Table 1 reports the activities of EH, AHH, O-deethylase and 1-naphthol glucuronidation in the nuclei and microsomes of the liver, lungs and kidneys from three baboons. For all enzymes the hepatic microsomal activities exceeded by far the activities in the kidneys and lungs. The difference was particularly great for the oxidation reactions. The nuclear to microsomal ratio for the various enzyme activities are shown in table 2. This ratio was consistently lower in the liver than in the other organs for all enzymes except UDP-glucuronyltransferase. The kinetic constants of EH in the three tissues from baboons are summarized in table 3 and Eadie-Hofstee plots of the data are shown in Fig 1. Table 4 shows the enzyme activities in the nuclear and microsomal fractions of the liver from two Rhesus monkeys.

Table 1

ENZYMATIC ACTIVITIES ($\bar{x} \pm$ SEM) IN THE NUCLEI AND MICROSOMES OF THE LIVER, KIDNEYS AND LUNGS FROM THREE BABOONS

	LIVER		KIDNEYS		LUNGS	
	N^a	Mc^b	N^a	Mc^b	N^a	Mc^b
Epoxide hydrolase[c] (SO)[e]	1.0 ± 0.4	25.9 ± 2.5	0.6 ± 0.1	1.8 ± 0.05	0.2 ± 0.02	0.8 ± 0.1
Epoxide hydrolase[c] (BPO)[f]	1.4 ± 0.2	37.0 ± 2.2	0.7 ± 0.1	5.2 ± 0.04	0.7 ± 0.1	5.2 ± 1.2
AHH[d]	80.7 ± 9.6	1437 ± 493	45.1 ± 7.7	88.6 ± 21.6	20.2 ± 0.9	69.8 ± 6.5
O–Deethylase[d]	48.9 ± 9.1	1267 ± 95	19.1 ± 7.0	42.2 ± 4.7	9.6 ± 2.6	18.4 ± 1.3
Naphtol glucuronidation[c]	7.9 ± 0.3	24.5 ± 0.7	3.7 ± 0.8	10.2 ± 0.6	0.12 ± 0.03	0.15 ± 0.02

[a]Nuclei. [b]Microsomes. [c]nmol/min/mg protein. [d]pmol/min/mg protein. [e]Styrene oxide. [f]Benzo (a) pyrene–4,5–oxide.

Table 2

NUCLEAR/MICROSOMAL RATIOS (x ± SEM) OF THE ACTIVITY OF VARIOUS ENZYMES IN THE LIVER, KIDNEYS AND LUNGS FROM THREE BABONS

	LIVER	KIDNEYS	LUNGS
Epoxide hydrolase (SO)	0.04 ± 0.02	0.36 ± 0.07	0.27 ± 0.08
Epoxide hydrolase (BPO)	0.04 ± 0.01	0.13 ± 0.01	0.15 ± 0.02
AHH	0.07 ± 0.03	0.58 ± 0.05	0.29 ± 0.03
O-Deethylase	0.04 ± 0.004	0.41 ± 0.14	0.51 ± 0.10
Naphtol glucuronidation	0.32 ± 0.01	0.36 ± 0.07	0.71 ± 0.10

Table 3
KINETIC PARAMETERS ($\bar{x} \pm$ SEM) OF EPOXIDE HYDROLASE IN THE NUCLEI AND MICROSOMES OF THE LIVER, KIDNEYS AND LUNGS FROM THREE BABOONS.

Substrate		LIVER		KIDNEYS		LUNGS	
		Nuclei	Microsomes	Nuclei	Microsomes	Nuclei	Microsomes
Styrene oxide	Km^a	0.15 ± 0.02	0.08 ± 0.01	0.90 ± 0.46	0.05 ± 0.01	0.18 ± 0.01	0.11 ± 0.01
	$Vmax^b$	1.23 ± 0.04	25.4 ± 0.5	1.47 ± 0.71	1.97 ± 0.15	0.33 ± 0.02	0.82 ± 0.18
Benzo (a) pyrene—4,5— oxide	Km	0.03 ± 0.01	0.05 ± 0.01	0.05 ± 0.01	0.13 ± 0.03	0.05 ± 0.01	0.16 ± 0.04
	$Vmax$	1.62 ± 0.28	52.4 ± 3.0	0.62 ± 0.05	7.77 ± 1.35	0.81 ± 0.09	7.69 ± 1.30

[a]mM. [b]nmole/min/mg protein.

Table 4
ENZYMATIC ACTIVITIES IN THE NUCLEI AND MICROSOMES OF THE LIVER FROM TWO RHESUS MONKEYS

	Rhesus Monkey 1		Rhesus Monkey 2	
	N^a	Mc^b	N^a	Mc^b
Epoxide hydrolase[c] (SO)[e]	3.0	16.5	2.4	14.3
Epoxide hydrolase[c] (BPO)[f]	—	20.9	0.7	19.0
AHH[d]	93.0	908	47.9	1296
O—Deethylase[d]	90.1	1040	52.5	2019

[a]Nuclei. [b]Microsomes. [c]nmol/min/mg protein. [d]pmol/min/mg protein.
[e]Styrene oxide. [f]Benzo (a) pyrene—4,5—oxide.

Fig 1 Epoxide hydrolase with styrene oxide (left) and benzo(a)pyrene 4,5-oxide (right) as substrate in tissues from 3 baboons. Data presented as Eadie-Hofstee plots.

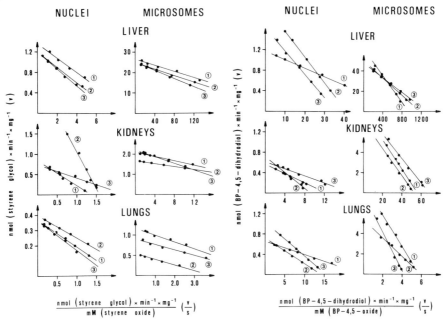

DISCUSSION

The nuclei from all investigated tissues catalyzed the enzymatic reactions tested. The rate of these reactions was consistently lower in the nuclear fraction than in microsomes of each tissues. The liver contained higher nuclear and microsomal activities than the corresponding organelles from kidneys and lungs. Interestingly, the nuclear/microsomal ratios of the tested enzyme activities were higher in the extrahepatic tissues than in the liver except for the UDP-glucuronyltransferase ratio which appeared comparable in liver and kidneys.

The kinetic analysis of EH revealed that the nuclei had higher K_m values than the microsomes when styrene oxide was used as substrate. The reverse was found for benzo(a)pyrene-4,5-oxide which may indicate the presence of different enzyme forms in each organelle or in the two subcellular particelles.

Microscopic analysis of the nuclear preparations revealed that these fractions were free from cytoplasmic contaminants. Therefore, the relatively high nuclear rates of the various enzyme reactions in the extrahepatic tissues can not be accounted for by the presence of microsomal contaminants.

The total protein content of the nuclear fraction is higher than in the microsomes. Therefore, the relative importance of the nuclear activities when expressed on the basis of g tissue equivalent is greater than indicated by the nuclear/microsomal ratios. The biological meaning of the nuclear drug metabolism enzyme systems is still unclear. Anyway, it seems obvious that the nuclei can contribute to the overall cellular metabolic clearance of the xenobiotics. This contribution is seemingly tissue dependent but it may also depend upon the subcellular distribution of the drug in the intact tissue.

ACKNOWLEDGEMENTS

This work was supported by CILAG Foundation.

REFERENCES

1. Kasper, C.B. (1971) Biochemical distinctions between the nuclear and microsomal membranes from rat liver hepatocytes, J.Biol.Chem. 246,577

2. Rogan, E. and Cavalieri, E. (1978) Differences between nuclear and microsomal P-450 in induced rat liver, Mol. Pharmacol. 14,215

3. Mukhtar, H., Elmamlouk, T.H., Philpot, R.M. and Bend, J.R. (1979) Rat hepatic nuclear P-450 and epoxide hydrolase membranes prepared by two methods: Similarities with the microsomal enzyme, Mol.Pharmacol.15, 192

4. Romano, M., Clos, V., Assael, B.M. and Salmona, M. (1982) Perinatal development of cytochrome P-450, NADPH-Cytochrome C-reductase and ethoxycoumarin deethylase in rat liver nuclear membranes, Chem. Biol.Interact.42,225.

5. Bresnick, E. Vaught, J.B., Chuang, A.H.L., Stoming, T.A., Bockman, D. and Mukhtar,H. (1977) Nuclear aryl hydrocarbon hydroxylase and interaction of polycyclic hydrocarbons with nuclear components, Arch.Biochem.Biophys.181, 257

6. Bornstein,W.A., Chuang, H., Bresnick,E., Mukhtar,A. and Bend, J.R.(1979) Epoxide hydrase activity in liver nuclei: Hydration of benzo(a)pyrene-4,5-oxide and styrene oxide, Chem.Biol.Interact. 21,343

7. Mukhtar,H.,Elmamlouk,T.H. and Bend,J.R. (1979) Epoxide hydrolase and mixed-function oxidase activities of rat liver nuclear membranes, Arch.Biochem. Biophys., 192,10

8. Gazzotti, G.,Garattini, E. and Salmona,M.(1981) Nuclear Metabolism. II: Further studies on epoxide hydrolase activity, Chem.Biol.Interact.35,311

9. Bansal,S.K., Zaleski,J. and Gessner,T, (1981) Glucuronidation of oxygenated benzo(a)pyrene derivatives by UDP-glucuronyltransferase of nuclear envelope, Biochem.Biophys.Res.Commun, 98,131

10. Elmamlouk,T.H., Mukhtar,H. and Bend, J.R. (1981) The nuclear envelope as a site of glucuronyltransferase in rat liver: properties and effect of inducers on enzyme activity, J.Pharmacol.Exp.Ther. 219,27

11. Pacifici,G.M., Colizzi, C., Giuliani, L. and Rane,A. (1982) Nuclear epoxide hydrolase in the human fetal and adult liver. Pharmacology, submitted

12. Pacifici, G.M., Lindberg,B., Glaumann, H. and Rane,A. (1982) Styrene oxide metabolism in Rhesus monkey liver: enzyme activities in subcellular fractions and in isolated hepatocytes. J.Pharmacol.Exp.Ther.submitted

13. Jerina,D.M., Dansette, P.M., Lu,A.Y.H. and Levin,W. (1977) Hepatic microsomal epoxide hydrolase: a sensitive radiometric assay for hydration of arene oxides of carcinogenic aromatic hydrocarbons, Mol.Pharmacol.,13,342

14. Van Cantfort,J. De Graeve, J. and Gielen, J.E. (1977) Radioactive assay for aryl hydrocarbon hydroxylase. Improved method and biological importance, Biochem.Biophys.Res.Comm. 79,505

15. Bock, K.W., Brunner,G., Hoensch,H., Huber, E. and Josting,D. (1978) Determination of UDP-glucuronyltransferase in needle-biopsy specimens of human liver. Eur.J.Clin.Pharmcol.14,367

16. Greenlee, W.F. and Poland,A. (1978) An improved assay of 7-ethoxycoumarin O-deethylase activity: Induction of hepatic enzyme activity in C57BL/6 J and DBA/2 J mice by phenobarbital, 3-methylcholantrene and 2,3,7,8-Tetrachlorodibenzo-p-dioxin,J.Pharmacol.Exp.Ther. 205,596

© 1983 Elsevier Science Publishers B.V.
Extrahepatic Drug Metabolism and Chemical Carcinogenesis,
J. Rydström, J. Montelius and M. Bengtsson eds.

COMPARATIVE KINETIC ASPECTS OF AROMATICS METABOLISM BY RABBIT LUNG AND RAT LIVER MICROSOMES

Dmitriy I.Metelitza, Sergey A.Usanov, Alexander N.Eriomin,
Irina V.Tishchenko
Institute of Bioorganic Chemistry, Minsk 220600, USSR

INTRODUCTION

Aromatic compounds can be metabolized not only in hepatic, but in some extrahepatic tissues also. A very important factor in carcinogenesis caused by polycyclic hydrocarbons is the relative rates of synthesis of the reactive intermediates. The steady state level of the arene oxides would be expected to be different in various tissues because of differences in the relative activities of the enzymes involved in the polycyclic hydrocarbons metabolism.

The aim of the present study is the systematic comparative investigation of the kinetic aspects of naphthalene metabolism by rabbit lung and rat liver microsomes in the wide temperature range. We also studied the effect of enzyme induction by phenobarbital (PB) and 3-methylcholanthrene on the ability of rabbit lung and rat liver to hydroxylate naphthalene.

MATERIALS AND METHODS

Rabbit lung and rat liver microsomes were prepared as previously described (1,2). Cytochrome P-450 LM_2 have been purified from liver microsomes PB-treated rabbits (3). Naphthalene hydroxylation was followed as described in (4) and that of aniline based on the rate of p-aminophenol formation (5).

RESULTS

Table 1 shows the kinetics parameters of naphthalene oxidation by rabbit lung and rat liver microsomes. It is evident that the lung cytochrome(s) P-450 are more efficient in naphthalene monooxygenation than hepatic ones. Indeed, when calculated per nmol of cytochrome P-450, the initial rates of naphthalene oxidation by intact and induced enzymes are much higher for the lung.

TABLE 1

KINETIC PARAMETERS OF NAPHTHALENE MONOOXYGENATION

Microsomes	Rabbit lung			Rat liver		
	K_m,mM	$[P-450]$ [a]	V_{max} [b]	K_m,mM	$[P-450]$ [a]	V_{max} [b]
Intact	0.125	0.12	393	0.145	0.68	54.3
PB-induced	0.068	0.26	228	0.166	1.36	49.0
MC-induced	0.044	0.18	265	0.142	0.92	43.5

[a] nmol per mg of protein

[b] nmol of 1-naphthol $/ s^{-1}$ per nmol of cytochrome P-450

The temperature dependence of naphthalene hydroxylation are characterized by the break in the Arrhenius plots for hepatic and lung microsomes from untreated and PB-treated animals. The break are observed at 17-20°C. However, the break is not observed at the Arrhenius plots for naphthalene hydroxylation by lung microsomes from MC-treated rabbits. The temperature dependence of aniline oxidation in NADPH- and cumene hydroperoxide-dependent systems are also characterized by the constant energy of activation. In addition, copper ion complexes with amino acids having a superoxide dismutase activity inhibit the aromatic compounds oxidation in lung and liver microsomes. Moreover, the nature of inhibition is practically the same for enzymes from both tissues.

Thus, the data obtained leave no doubts as to similarity in the organization and functioning of the monooxygenase systems of lung and liver microsomes.

REFERENCES

1. Matsubara, T., Prough, R.A., Burke, M.D., Estabrook, R.W. (1974), Cancer Res., 34, 2196

2. Tishchenko, I.V., Usanov, S.A., Metelitza, D.I. (1979), Izv. Acad. Nauk BSSR, 1, 93

3. Eriomin, A.N., Usanov, S.A., Metelitza, D.I., Akhrem, A.A. (1980), Bioorg. Khim., 6, 757

4. Akhrem, A.A., Usanov, S.A., Metelitza, D.I. (1975) Doklady Acad. Nauk SSSR, 223, 1014

5. Fujita, T., Mannering, G., (1973) J.Biol.Chem., 239, 2370

MULTIPLICITY, REGIOSPECIFICITY AND LEVELS OF P-450, EPOXIDE HYDROLASE AND CONJUGATING ENZYMES IN DIFFERENT TISSUES

© 1983 Elsevier Science Publishers B.V.
Extrahepatic Drug Metabolism and Chemical Carcinogenesis,
J. Rydström, J. Montelius and M. Bengtsson eds.

MODULATION OF THE LEVELS OF CYTOCHROME P-450 ISOZYMES IN RABBIT LUNG

BARBARA A. DOMIN, RICHARD M. PHILPOT, BETTY L. WARREN AND COSETTE J. SERABJIT-SINGH

Laboratory of Pharmacology, National Institute of Environmental Health Sciences, National Institutes of Health, P.O. Box 12233, Research Triangle Park, North Carolina 27709 U.S.A.

INTRODUCTION

The cytochrome P-450-dependent metabolism in a tissue is a composite of the activities of the individual isozymes, the concentrations of which can be significantly altered by response to exogenous agents. Thus, the ability to quantitate the individual isozymes and to measure all the changes in content after exposure to known inducers would significantly increase our understanding of the metabolism of carcinogenic and other toxic agents. We have modified recent immunochemical detection methods to examine the modulation of cytochrome P-450 isozymes in rabbit lung in response to exposure to polycyclic aromatic hydrocarbons and we are able to monitor at least 80% of the total rabbit pulmonary cytochrome P-450 which consists of isozyme forms 2, 5, and 6. In addition, we have developed a new technique for assaying isozyme content by direct application of microsomal protein to nitrocellulose paper.

MATERIALS AND METHODS

Microsomal preparations were electrophoresed on 7.5% sodium dodecyl sulfate polyacrylamide gels, and the proteins were transferred to nitrocellulose paper by the method of Towbin et al. (1) (Western blot). Immunochemical detection of isozymes was performed according to the above procedure with modifications as described in the text. For direct application of microsomal proteins to nitrocellulose paper, samples were diluted in 10 mM Tris-HCl, pH 7.4, 0.9% NaCl and pipetted into the wells of a "Hybridot" apparatus purchased from Bethesda Research Laboratories. Immunostained nitrocellulose papers were scanned with a soft laser Zeineh densitometer.

RESULTS

Immunochemical detection. Modifications of the horseradish peroxidase immunostaining procedure (1) that significantly decreased the background stain without decreasing the sensitivity were as follows: 1) blocking of non-specific sites on the nitrocellulose paper was maximal with the use of 3% bovine serum albumin (BSA) for 15 min at 40°C. The presence of BSA was not required at any step subsequent to this initial blocking step. 2) Exposure to the primary antibody for 1 hr at 25°C was maximum. 3) Rabbit anti-goat IgG (1:100

dilution) was used as the second antibody in place of conjugated peroxidase an-
ti-peroxidase (PAP). 4) The addition of PAP in the subsequent step was at a
1:2000 dilution. 5) 3,3'-Diaminobenzidine (0.3 mg/ml, 0.002% H_2O_2) for 30 min,
was used for staining. These modifications, in particular the use of a 10-fold
more dilute PAP preparation, significantly reduced the background staining such
that the sensitivity of the assay after soft laser scanning permitted detection
of 50 fmoles of purified form 2 with linearity to 1.0 picomole.

Effects of benzo(α)pyrene (BP). Changes in the contents of form 6 (pulmonary)
and forms 4 and 6 (hepatic) with time after administration of 10 mg/kg BP (a
dose causing maximum induction) are shown in Figures 1 and 2, respectively.
Rates of O-deethylation of 7-ethoxyresorufin (7-ERF), attributable to these isozymes, are also shown. Form 6 is detectable in untreated rabbit lung, and increases in this isozyme can be seen as little as 8 hr after BP administration,
with the maximum increase of 20-fold occurring at 48 hr. We could not detect
the presence of form 4 in rabbit lung even when form 6 was maximally induced
by BP. 7-ERF activity increased in parallel with the increase in form 6 except
that 7-ERF activity increased only 10-fold. There was no detectable change in
total P-450 content. In rabbit liver, treatment with BP increased forms 4 and
6 and 7-ERF activity (Figure 2) with similar time courses, the maximum occurring at 48 hr. However, Figure 3 shows a delay in the increase of total P-450
such that at 16-24 hr after treatment, 7-ERF activity was 70% of maximum increase before there was any change in total P-450 content. As noted for the
lung, the extent of the increase in 7-ERF activity did not correlate with that
of the increases in forms 4 and 6. As the lag in total P-450 increase suggested the possibility of a concurrent decrease in other P-450 isozymes, the effect of 10 mg/kg BP treatment on forms 2 and 5 in hepatic microsomes was determined (Figure 4). At 12 hr, both forms were significantly decreased and by
48 hr were less than 50% of control values. The dose response curve for BP was
similar for lung and liver such that the percent maxima of the increases in
forms 4 and 6 in liver, form 6 in lung, and 7-ERF activities in liver and lung
were the same at given doses of BP. In contrast, the dose response curve for
TCDD induction of 7-ERF activity showed that a 10-fold higher dose was required
for lung than for liver to obtain the same percent of maximum induction.

Effects of phenobarbital and polychlorinated biphenyls. Polychlorinated biphenyls (PCB), like TCDD, also caused up to 20-fold induction of form 6 in
rabbit lung while phenobarbital (PB) did not increase any of the P-450 isozymes. It did, however, have repressive effects. Figure 5 shows the effects
of PB and Aroclor 1260 (ARC) on the form 6-mediated metabolism of 7-ERF

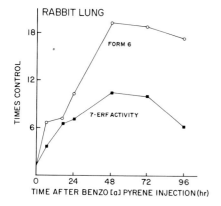

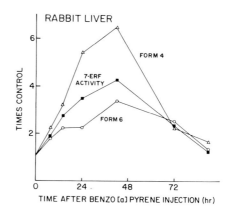

Figure 1. Time course in rabbit lung after benzo(α)pyrene (10 mg/kg) i.p. injection. Microsomal preparations were electrophoresed, blotted onto nitrocellulose paper, and immunostained with anti-body to form 6 as described in the text. Form 6 (O), 7-ERF activity (■). These are single animal determinations and are expressed as times control value.

Figure 2. Time course in rabbit liver after benzo(α)pyrene (10 mg/kg) i.p. injection. Form 6 (O), form 4 (△), 7-ERF activity (■). These are single animal determinations and are expressed as times control values.

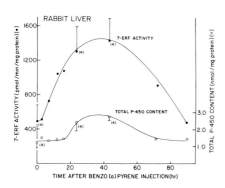

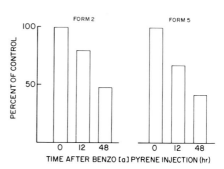

Figure 3. Time course in rabbit liver after benzo(α)pyrene (10 mg/kg) i.p. injection. 7-ERF activity (●), total P-450 content (O). Number of animals is two unless otherwise indicated in parentheses with bars representing standard deviations.

Figure 4. Effects with time of 10 mg/kg benzo(α)pyrene i.p. injection on forms 2 and 5 in rabbit lung. Results are the mean of 3 single animal determinations and are expressed as percent of control.

46

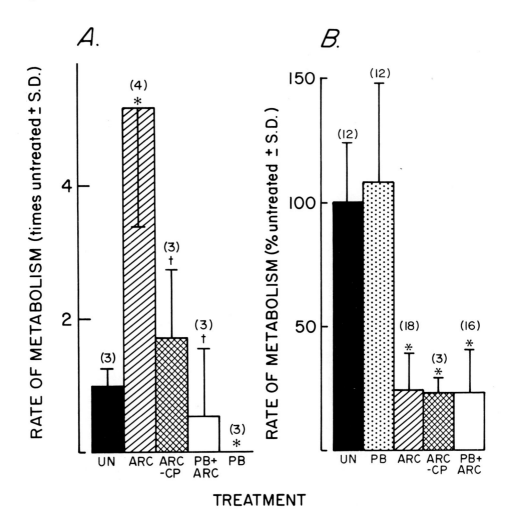

Figure 5A. Pulmonary microsomal 7-ERF activity after simultaneous administration of phenobarbital and Aroclor 1260. No treatment (UN), Aroclor 1260 (ARC), Aroclor 1260 minus coplanar isomers (ARC-CP), phenobarbital (PB), Aroclor 1260 plus phenobarbital (ARC + PB). Doses were 200 mg/kg ARC or ARC-CP and 160 mg/kg PB. (*) $p < 0.01$ versus untreated value and (+) $p < 0.05$ versus Aroclor value by Student's unpaired two-tailed t-test.

Figure 5B. Pulmonary microsomal benzphetamine-N-demethylation activity after simultaneous administration of phenobarbital and Aroclor 1260. Symbols and doses are the same as described for Figure 5A.

(A) and on form 2-mediated *N*-demethylation of benzphetamine (B). Not only did PB at 160 mg/kg decrease the pulmonary content of form 6, it also blocked the inductive effects of the ARC coplanar isomers. ARC and ARC from which the co-planar isomers (hydrocarbon-like inducers) were removed decreased form 2 in rabbit lung (5B) and this was unchanged with co-administration of PB.

Direct application assay of cytochrome P-450 isozymes. Figure 6A shows the immunostained Western blot (0.028 (lane 1) to 0.56 (lane 6) pmoles) of purified form 2. This technique has a limit of detection of 0.05 pmoles and a linearity range up to 1.0 pmole. Figure 6B shows the immunostained spots obtained from direct application of 10 (spot 1) to 100 (spot 8) fmoles purified form 2 onto nitrocellulose paper. Spot 7 is a buffer blank. As little as 2 fmoles can be detected with direct spotting with linearity to 100 fmoles. This is 10-fold more sensitive than Western blotting. Individual isozyme content in microsomal samples can be readily obtained with a monospecific antibody using this technique. Estimates for form 2 content obtained through direct spotting, single radial immunodiffusion, or Western blotting of hepatic microsomes from untreated and phenobarbital-treated rabbits showed excellent agreement for all of these methods.

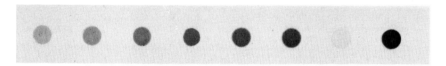

Figure 6A. Western blot of purified cytochrome P-450, form 2. Femtamoles of P-450 on gels are 28 (lane 1), 56 (lane 2), 140 (lane 3), 280 (lane 4), 420 (lane 5), and 560 (lane 6).

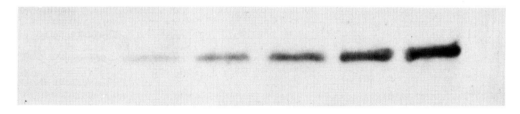

Figure 6B. Direct application of purified cytochrome P-450, form 2, to nitrocellulose paper. Femtamoles of P-450 on spots are 10, 20, 30, 40, 50, 60, 0 and 100.

DISCUSSION

Recent developments in immunochemical detection of proteins transferred from gels to nitrocellulose paper enable us to directly measure the isozyme content in microsomal samples, even the content of minor forms. Form 6 has been previously detected in rabbit lung following treatment with TCDD (2, 3) and PCBs (4). We are able to detect form 6 in untreated rabbit lung as a small proportion of the total cytochrome P-450 (1-3%). Form 6 is induced after BP treatment in a dose- and time-dependent manner with maximum induction occurring at a dose of 10 mg/kg at 48 hr. It is interesting that form 6 is increased 20-fold by treatment with BP while the form 6-associated 7-ERF activity is increased only 10-fold. Forms 4 and 6 increase (3- to 6-fold) in a time- and dose-dependent manner in the liver following treatment with BP. These responses are similar to those of form 6 in the lung. Form 4 was not detected in the lung even after BP, TCDD, or PCB treatments which maximally induced form 6. The liver 7-ERF activity is increased 4-fold, much less than would be expected from the increases in forms 4 and 6. This discrepancy between the maximum increases in activity and the increases in isozyme content is also seen with other inducers such as TCDD and PCB coplanar isomers where up to 20-fold increases in form 6 in the lung are accompanied by 5-fold to 10-fold increases in 7-ERF activity. The responses of isozyme-mediated activity and isozyme content to dose and time are concommitant but the extent of the response is different. The most reasonable explanation for this is that some other component of the cytochrome P-450 system, such as the reductase, is rate limiting for activity. Indeed, the spectral determination of P-450 content of isomers separated by DEAE cellulose chromatography of pulmonary microsomes from TCDD-treated rabbits show form 6 to be 26% of the total cytochrome. This is in agreement with the isozyme content estimate by immunoquantitation.

The significant time delay in the increase of total P-450 content in liver following BP treatment is partially accounted for by the decreases in forms 2 and 5. Although these contribute a small percentage of the total P-450, the fact that they do decrease during this time lag suggests the possibility that other isozymes, such as form 3, could also be decreasing. Thus, a lack of change in total P-450 content could be masking significant opposing effects on isozyme content.

In contrast to the changes following BP treatment, where a single dose results in the same percent maxima for form 6 in lung and liver and form 4 in liver, treatment with TCDD requires a 10-fold higher dose for lung than for liver to obtain the same percent of maximal induction. This dose differential between these two inducers could reflect a difference in tissue distribution.

Unlike the polycyclic aromatic hydrocarbons, PB has an inductive effect in liver (forms 2 and 5) but not in lung. It does, however, decrease the content of form 6 in lungs by greater than 50%. More important, PB blocks the induction of pulmonary form 6 by the coplanar isomers of PCBs. The PCB mixture from which the coplanar isomers have been removed significantly decreases the content of pulmonary form 2; administration of PB does not alter this effect. Indeed, the lack of inductive effect of PB on pulmonary isozymes permits a clear demonstration of the repression of form 2 by the non-coplanar isomers of PCBs.

It is clear that multiple changes in isozyme content can occur after treatment with inducers and these changes can be inductive or repressive or both. These fine perturbations in isozyme profile could be extremely important in the determination of the final direction of drug metabolism in tissues. Delineation of the constitutive profile of isozymes and of the changes in these profiles with exposure to exogenous agents holds the promise of being able to predict the metabolism and possibly the carcinogenic effects of drugs. Since greater than 80% of the rabbit lung cytochrome P-450 system can be accounted for by forms 2, 5, and 6, the pulmonary P-450 profiles are the most clearly understood at this time and will provide valuable information for the examination of P-450 profiles in more complex systems such as the liver.

The immunoquantitation technique of microsomal samples directly applied to nitrocellulose paper has the same sensitivity as radial immunodiffusion and has several advantages such as lack of interference by extraneous protein, decreased time of assay, and increased sample capabilities. Thus, it should prove to be a valuable tool in the assay of specific isozymes in crude samples.

REFERENCES

1. Towbin, H., Staehelin, T. and Gordon, J. (1979) Proc. Natl. Acad. Sci. U.S.A., 76, 4350-4354.

2. Leim, H., Mueller-Eberhard, U. and Johnson, E.F. (1980) Mol. Pharmacol., 18, 565-570.

3. Dees, J.H., Masters, B.S.S., Muller-Eberhard, U. and Johnson, E.F. (1982) Cancer Res., 42, 1423-1432.

4. Serabjit-Singh, C.J., Albro, P.W. and Philpot, R.M. (1982) Fed. Proc., 41, 1497.

© 1983 Elsevier Science Publishers B.V.
Extrahepatic Drug Metabolism and Chemical Carcinogenesis,
J. Rydström, J. Montelius and M. Bengtsson eds.

CHARACTERIZATION OF PURIFIED CYTOCHROME P-450 IN THE RAT LUNG

MINRO WATANABE, IKUKO SAGAMI AND TETSUO OHMACHI
Research Institute for Tuberculosis and Cancer, Tohoku University, 4-1, Seiryo-machi, Sendai 980 (Japan)

INTRODUCTION

Contrasted to liver, lung seems to be one of the target organs to carcinogenic polycyclic hydrocarbons, such as benzo[a]pyrene (BP), in rodents and human species. BP requires metabolic activation by the mixed-function oxidases (MFO) system to form chemically reactive metabolites that are mutagenic and carcinogenic (1,2). Cytochrome P-450 is the terminal oxidase of MFO system which metabolizes BP in the presence of NADPH-cytochrome P-450 (cytochrome c) reductase (fp$_T$). In rat liver there are multiple forms of cytochrome P-450 and each form may have different substrate specificities. This paper aims to describe the characteristics of the highly purified form of lung cytochrome P-450MC from 3-methylcholanthrene (MC)-treated rats, compared with purified hepatic cytochrome P-450MC (P-450c (3)).

MATERIALS AND METHODS

Purification. Pulmonary P-450MC from MC-treated Buffalo male rats was purified by the previously published methods (4,5). Hepatic P-450MC from MC-treated rats and fp$_T$ from phenobarbital-treated rats were purified by the published procedures, respectively (6,7). Rat liver epoxide hydrolase (EH) was purified by the modified method of published procedures (8).

Analytical procedures. Assays of spectrophotometrical and immunochemical properties and of peptide compositions on sodium dodesyl sulfate-polyacrylamide gel electrophoresis (SDS-PAGE), of amino acid compositions of the hemoprotein, and of catalytic activity in the reconstituted system were performed with the published method (5,9).

Analysis of ^{14}C-BP metabolites. Incubation was performed in air for 10 min. After the termination of the reaction 3000 nmol vitamin E was added to each reaction mixture. High-pressure liquid chromatography (HPLC) was used to analyze organic solvent soluble metabolites and synthetic derivatives of BP using a Japan Spectroscopic Liquid Chromatograph Trirotar, and a Dupont Zorbax octadecyltrimethoxysilane column (4,5 nm internal diameter × 0.25 m). Unlabeled synthetic BP metabolites solution was added to the pooled organic extract and the mixture was dried under nitrogen. The precipitate was dissolved in 50 μl of a mixture of 10% tetrahydrofuran in methanol and injected into the

TABLE 1

COMPARISSON IN PROPERTIES OF PURIFIED CYTOCHROME P-450MC

	Lung	Liver
Specific content of purified forms (nmol/mg protein)	12.5	17.0
Minimum molecular weight on SDS-PAGE ($M_r. \times 10^{-3}$)	54	56
Peptide composition after partial proteolysis with		
Staph. aureus V8 protease	different	
Papain	different	
α-Chymotrypsin	similar	
Amino acid composition (mol %)		
Glycine	8.85	7.96
Leucine	11.13	12.05
Other amino acids	similar	
Maximum of reduced CO-complex (nm)	447.5	447.5
Spin state of heme iron	low	low
Catalytic activity in reconstituted system (mol/min/mol P-450)		
Benzo[a]pyrene 3-hydroxylation	11.9	17.1
7-Ethoxycoumarin O-deethylation	23.5	40.0
Benzphetamine N-demethylation	6.3	8.8
Ouchtalony double diffusion with antibody against hepatic P-450MC	single fused line	
Inhibitory patterns by antibody against hepatic P-450MC		
Benzo[a]pyrene 3-hydroxylation	similar	
7-Ethoxycoumarin O-deethylation	similar	

column. A linear gradient from 60% to 85% methanol containing 0.1% phosphoric acid was used. The flow rate was 1.0 ml/min. The monitoring wavelength was 254 nm. Fractions were collected every 30 sec, 5 ml Aquasol was added, and the fractions were counted in a Beckman LS-100 liquid scintillation counter.

RESULTS AND DISCUSSION

It was observed that the content of P-450 in the lung was very low, compared with that in the liver from the corresponding species. Only one paper has been published on the purification of P-450 from the rat lung (10). As summarized in Table 1, a major form of pulmonary P-450MC was purified approximately 313 fold from lung microsomes of MC-treated rats. The purified pulmonary P-450MC, in which no activity of epoxide hydrolase was detected, contained 12.5 nmoles of P-450 per mg protein and the minimum molecular weight was estimated by SDS-PAGE to be 54,000 which was clearly different from hepatic P-450MC. The peptide patterns on SDS-PAGE and the amino acid composition of pulmonary P-450MC were also different from those of hepatic P-450MC, indicating the presence of an unique P-450MC in the rat lung. On the other hand, there was no clear difference in the immunological properties between pulmonary and hepatic P-450MC. In the reconstituted systems containing purified pulmonary P-450MC and NADPH-cytochrome P-450 reductase, high activity of BP hydroxylation was detected.

For the separation of BP metabolites formed in the reconstituted-MFO systems containing different forms of P-450 from rat liver, HPLC was used (11,12). The profile of BP metabolites formed by pulmonary P-450MC in the presence of purified epoxide hydrolase was shown in Fig. 1. The portions of the radioactivity eluted with authentic BP diols (9,10-, 4,5- and 7,8- diol), diones (1,6-, 3,6- and 6,12- dione), and phenols (9- and 3- phenol). An unidentified fraction was also detected between the portions of 9,10-diol and those of 4,5-diol. Table 2 shows the amount and percentage of each metabolite formed by pulmonary and hepatic P-450MC in the presence or absence of purified epoxide

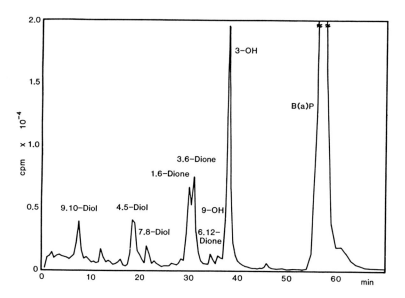

Fig. 1. HPLC pattern of BP metabolites formed by pulmonary P-450MC in the presence of epoxide hydrolase

TABLE 2

BP METABOLITES FORMED BY HEPATIC P-450MC OR PULMONARY P-450MC

BP metabolites	Hepatic P-450MC (pmol/min/nmol P-450)		Pulmonary P-450MC	
	-EH[a]	+EH	-EH	+EH
9,10-Diol	301(6.4)[b]	486(8.6)	228(3.5)	514(9.7)
4,5-Diol	276(5.9)	758(13.3)	369(5.6)	727(13.7)
7,8-Diol	115(2.4)	194(3.4)	182(2.8)	226(4.3)
Σ Diols	692(14.7)	1438(25.3)	779(11.9)	1467(27.7)
1,6-Dione 3,6-Dione	1388(29.0)	1616(28.4)	1706(25.9)	1554(29.2)
6,12-Dione	212(4.4)	156(2.7)	164(2.4)	144(2.7)
Σ Diones	1600(33.4)	1772(31.1)	1870(28.3)	1698(31.9)
9-Phenol	606(12.7)	140(2.5)	804(12.2)	177(3.3)
3-Phenol	1894(39.5)	2335(41.1)	3145(47.7)	1981(37.2)
Σ Phenols	2500(52.2)	2475(43.6)	3949(59.9)	2158(40.5)
Total	4677(100)	5685(100)	6598(100)	5323(100)

[a] The reactions were performed in the presence or absence of epoxide hydrolase.
[b] The numbers of parenthesis are the percent of total BP metabolites.

hydrolase. By the addition of epoxide hydrolase to the reconstituted enzyme system the amount of BP-9-phenol decreased apparently, with increasing the amount of BP-4,5-diol. In summary no clear difference in the amount of BP metabolites formed was observed between pulmonary and hepatic P-450MC. The amount of BP-7,8-diol, which was considered as a proximate carcinogen in BP carcinogenesis, was relatively low, compared to the levels reported previously (12).

ACKNOWLEDGEMENTS

This research was supported, in part, by a Grant-in Aid for Cancer Research from the Ministry of Education, Science and Culture, Japan, and by a grant from the Japan Tobacco and Salt Public Corporation. BP metabolites were received from the NCI Chemical Carcinogen Reference Standard Repository, a function of the Division of Cancer Cause and Prevention, NCI, NIH, Bethesda, U.S.A.

REFERENCES

1. Jerina, D.M., Yagi, H., Lehr, R.E., Thakker, D.R., Schaefer-Ridder, M., Karle, J.M., Levin, W., Wood, A.W., Chang, R.L. and Conney, A.H. (1978) in: Gelboin, H.V. and Ts'o, P.O.P. (Ed.), Polycyclic Hydrocarbons and Cancer: Environment, Chemistry, and Metabolism, Academic Press, New York, p. 173.

2. Gelboin, H.V. (1980) Physiol. Rev., 60, 1107.

3. Ryan, D.E., Thomas, P.E., Korzeniowski, D. and Levin, W. (1979) J. Biol. Chem., 254, 1365.

4. Tamura, Y., Abe, T. and Watanabe, M. (1981) J. Toxicol. Sci., 6, 71.

5. Sagami, I. and Watanabe, M. (1983) J. Biochem. Tokyo, in press.

6. West, S.B., Huang, M.-T., Miwa, G.T. and Lu, A.Y.H. (1979) Arch. Biochem. Biophys. 193, 42.

7. Harada, N. and Omura, T. (1981) J. Biochem. Tokyo, 89, 237.

8. Guengerich, F.P., Wang, P., Mitchell, M.B. and Mason, P.S. (1979) J. Biol. Chem., 254, 12248.

9. Watanabe, M., Sagami, I., Abe, T. and Ohmachi, T. (1982) in: Hietanen, E., Laitinen, M. and Hänninen, O. (Ed.), Cytochrome P-450, Biochemistry, Biophysics and Environmental Implications, Elsevier Biomedical Press, Amsterdam, p. 649.

10. Jernström, B., Capdevila, J., Jakobsson, S. and Orrenius, S. (1975) Biochem. Biophys. Res. Commun., 64, 814.

11. Thakker, D.R., Yagi, H., Akagi, H., Koreeda, M., Lu, A.Y.H., Levin, W., Wood, A.W., Conney, A.H. and Jerina, D.M. (1977) Chem.-Biol. Interactions, 16, 281.

12. Gozukara, E.M., Guengerich, F.P., Miller, H. and Gelboin, H.V. (1982) Carcinogenesis, 3, 129.

© 1983 Elsevier Science Publishers B.V.
Extrahepatic Drug Metabolism and Chemical Carcinogenesis,
J. Rydström, J. Montelius and M. Bengtsson eds.

EVIDENCE FOR THE PRESENCE AND REACTIVITY OF MULTIPLE FORMS OF CYTOCHROME
P-450 IN COLONIC MICROSOMES FROM RATS AND HUMANS

HENRY W. STROBEL, S. N. NEWAZ, WAN-FEN FANG, PAUL P. LAU, R. J. OSHINSKY,
DANIEL J. STRALKA AND FRED F. SALLEY
The University of Texas Medical School, P. O. Box 20708, Houston, Texas
77225 (U.S.A.)

INTRODUCTION

Although microsomal cytochrome P-450 dependent drug metabolizing activities have been demonstrated in many animal tissues and organs (1,2), as
well as in various species (3), the great majority of the work of definition and characterization of the cytochrome P-450 system has focused on
the liver. The liver system has been shown in various laboratories to
catalyze the metabolism of a broad range of structurally diverse compounds ranging from simple alkanes and fatty acids to polycyclic hydrocarbons and carcinogens (1,4). Multiple forms of cytochrome P-450 have
been purified to homogeneity by a number of investigators (5-18). Our
laboratory has previously purified five forms of cytochrome P-450 from
liver microsomes of β-naphthoflavone-pretreated rats (19). Each of these
forms is a distinct form since each form was shown to have a unique subunit molecular weight, substrate reactivity profile, immunological identity and peptide map (19).

Various laboratories have shown that the cytochrome P-450 system is
functional in extrahepatic tissues (20). For example, Philpot and coworkers have defined and described the cytochrome P-450 system of rabbit
lung (21). Our laboratory has reported the presence and activity of a
cytochrome P-450 dependent drug metabolism system capable of catalyzing
the hydroxylation of drugs and activation of carcinogens in rat colon mucosal microsomes (22,23). We also have shown that the rat colon system
is responsive to induction with gastrointestinal hormones such as secre-
tin, cholecystokinin octapeptide and pentagastrin, as well as with the
known inducers phenobarbital and β-naphthoflavone (24). This present
paper reports the identification of particular forms of cytochrome P-450
in rat and human colon and describes the presence of drug metabolism activities in human colon.

METHODS

Preparation of Microsomes from Human Colon and Human Colon Tumor Cells

Colons were obtained at autopsy between 3 and 7 hours *post mortem* and chilled in ice immediately. The colon was washed three times with cold 1.14% (w/v) KCl solution. The mucosal layer was scraped separately from the ascending, transverse and descending segments of colon into cold Tris-HCl buffer (20 mM, pH 7.4) containing 0.14 M KCl, 10 mM EDTA, 1 mM dithio-threitol, 0.25 mM phenylmethylsulfonyl fluoride and 0.25 M sucrose. The cells were homogenized in a Potter-Elvehjem homogenizer, microsomes were isolated by differential centrifugation and stored in the buffer medium containing 20% glycerol.

Human colon adenocarcinoma LS174T cells (25) were obtained from Dr. Lynne Rutzky of the Department of Surgery and maintained in Eagle's minimal essential medium (MEM) with 10% fetal bovine serum (FBS). Cells were induced by adding either 75 µg/ml phenobarbital, 50 µg/ml hydrocortisone, a combination of these two agents, or 10 µM benz[α]anthracene as a supplement to the culture medium. The medium was exchanged each day for 4 days. The cells were collected with a rubber policeman at the end of 4 days, suspended in the Tris buffer described above, but with the sucrose, and disrupted with a Sonifier cell disruptor using a micro tip at 80 watts for 1 min at 4°C. Microsomes were prepared as previously described.

Assays

The rate of benzo[α]pyrene hydroxylation was determined spectrofluori-metrically using the procedure of Nebert and Gelboin (26). The metabolism of benzo[α]pyrene hydroxylation was determined by estimation of formalde-hyde by the chromatropic acid method (27-29). Protein was measured by the method of Lowry *et al.* (30). Immunoquantitation by radial diffusion or immunoelectrophoresis was performed as described (31) using antibodies to purified rat cytochrome P-450 raised in rabbits (19). Electroblotting of proteins resolved by SDS gel electrophoresis onto nitrocellulose paper followed by immunochemical identification using a second antibody directed against the rabbit IgG linked to peroxidase (Western blots) was performed essentially according to the method of Bowen (32).

RESULTS AND DISCUSSION

The possibility that the cytochrome P-450 system might be present in human colon and play a role in the metabolism of drugs and carcinogens was suggested by the direct demonstration of the cytochrome P-450 system in rat colon microsomes by our laboratory (22,23) and the dramatic demonstration of others that human colon explants catalyzed the formation of covalent adducts of benzo[α]pyrene and dimethylhydrazine to cellular macromolecules (33). Interest was intensified by the possible significance of the system in colon carcinogenesis and chemotherapy. Thus, our pursuit of the human colon drug metabolism system has focused on the demonstration of the presence, composition and regulation of the system.

Presence and Activities of the Drug Metabolism System in Human Colon

Microsomes prepared from the ascending, transverse and descending segments of the colon obtained at autopsy of trauma victims were assayed for the ability to catalyze the hydroxylation of the putative organ-specific colon carcinogen dimethylhydrazine. As shown in Table I, all colonic segments from all cases showed good activity for dimethylhydrazine. Each segment from each case was treated separately and not pooled with any similar sample. Therefore, no range is given although each sample was assayed in triplicate. The data of Table I indicate a gradient of activity through the colon with the lowest activities occurring in the ascending segment and the highest activities for each sample in the descending segment. Activity in general seems to increase with age in the cases examined. Although these correlations must be taken cautiously in view of the low number of cases examined, they are nevertheless, consistent with the clinical observations that most cases of colonic cancer have lesions in the descending portion of the colon and that the incidence of colonic cancer increases with age.

TABLE I

METABOLISM OF DIMETHYLHYDRAZINE BY HUMAN COLON MICROSOMES

Case	Age	Colonic Segment		
		Ascending	Transverse	Descending
			nmol HCHO/min/mg	
1	48	74.1	74.5	95.3
2	25	18.0	19.3	21.5
3	60	40.8	56.0	64.6
4	22	13.1	14.3	24.3
5	29	21.9	35.7	55.4

In order to determine whether the human colon microsomes also catalyzed the metabolism of other substrates, each of the microsomal preparations was assayed for benzo[α]pyrene hydroxylation activity. As shown in Table II, all samples showed measurable activity, although no general gradient of activity was apparent with benzo[α]pyrene as substrate.

TABLE II

HYDROXYLATION OF BENZO[α]PYRENE BY HUMAN COLON MICROSOMES

Case	Ascending	Colonic Segment Transverse	Descending
	pmol	3-OH benzo[α]pyrene/min/mg	
1	2.9	3.8	4.1
2	3.5	3.4	6.4
3	6.3	5.3	6.4
4	3.7	5.6	6.7
5	2.0	8.4	12.1

The putative role of cytochrome P-450 in colonic hydroxylation activities was evaluated by determining the effects of known inhibitors of cytochrome P-450 mediated reactions on the colonic microsomal hydroxylation of dimethylhydrazine. As shown in Table III, SKF525A (2-diethylaminoethyl-2,2-diphenylvalerate hydrochloride) markedly inhibited the hydroxylation of dimethylhydrazine by microsomal preparations from all three segments of the colon. Carbon monoxide and disulfuram also inhibited the metabolism though at lower levels. The moderate inhibitory effect of carbon monoxide can be attributed to the viscous nature of the colon microsomal preparation used in this series of experiments. Thus, all these data are consistent with the postulate that a cytochrome P-450 system in human colon catalyzes these activities.

In addition to inhibition studies, the use of inducers is often employed to demonstrate the presence of cytochrome P-450. Since the use of human material rules out the possibility of induction data, we have utilized a cultured cell line of human colon tumor cells (LS147T) as a model to examine response of colonic tissues to inducers. As shown in Table IV, the hydroxylation rates of both dimethylhydrazine and benzo[α]pyrene respond dramatically to induction. The combination of phenobarbital and hydro-cortisone increases the rate of hydroxylation of dimethylhydrazine about 3-fold and benzo[α]pyrene 10-fold. Benz[α]anthracene (10 μM) on the other hand, increases the rate of benzo[α]pyrene hydroxylation 30-fold. Thus, as judged in the tissue culture system, colonic tissue microsomal hydrox-ylation rates can be markedly increased by the known specific inducers of cytochrome P-450.

TABLE III

EFFECT OF INHIBITORS ON DIMETHYLHYDRAZINE METABOLISM

| | Percent of Control Colonic Segment | | |
Additions	Ascending	Transverse	Descending
None	100	100	100
SKF525A (0.53 mM)	75	73	49
Disulfuram (1 mM)	81	81	84
CO:Air (10:1)	88	78	80

TABLE IV

HYDROXYLATION OF DIMETHYLHYDRAZINE AND BENZO[α]PYRENE BY HUMAN COLON TUMOR CELLS (LS174T) IN CULTURE

Pretreatment	Dimethylhydrazine Hydroxylation nmol HCHO/min/mg	Benzo[α]pyrene Hydroxylation pmol 3-hydroxy-benzo[α]pyrene/min/mg
None	15.2	3.7
Phenobarbital	32.4	-
Hydrocortisone	22.0	-
Phenobarbital + Hydrocortisone	42.8	34.1
Benz[α]anthracene	-	92.1

Presence and Quantitation of Cytochromes in Rat and Human Colon Microsomes

The availability of 6 purified hepatic cytochromes P-450 and antibodies makes possible the quantitation in colon of forms of cytochrome P-450 cross-reacting with antibodies raised to the pure liver antigens. Polyethyleneglycol (0%-16%) fractions of colonic microsomes prepared from rats treated with phenobarbital or β-naphthoflavone were quantitated by the radial immunodiffusion technique for their content of cytochromes P-450. As shown in Table V, the β-naphthoflavone pretreated colonic microsomes contained three forms of cytochrome P-450 immunologically identical with forms in the liver. That these three forms add up to more than the total spectrally detectable cytochrome P-450 reflects the fact that the spectral method accounts only for intact holocytochrome P-450, whereas, the immunochemical technique identifies both apo- and holocytochrome P-450 and P-420. This discrepancy is partially relieved by including the spectrally-detectable cytochrome P-420 in the calculation (numbers in parenthesis). Similarly, colonic microsomes from phenobarbital-treated rats contain two forms of cytochrome P-450 also present in liver. The immunoquantitation procedure is limited to those forms cross-reacting with available antibodies. It does not address forms of cytochrome P-450 unique to the colon.

TABLE V

QUANTITATION OF COLONIC CYTOCHROMES BY RADIAL IMMUNODIFFUSION

Cytochrome Forms			Percent of Spectrally Detectable Cytochrome in PEG Fraction of Colonic Microsomes	
			β-naphthoflavone treated	phenobarbital treated
β-Naphthoflavone	1	$(21.0)^a$	18.5 $(10.7)^b$	N.D.
	2*	(11.5)	N.D.	N.D.
	3	(9.6)	N.D.	N.D.
	4	(46.0)	40.0 $(23.0)^b$	13.6 $(6.0)^b$
	5	(70.0)	64.1 $(37.0)^b$	N.D.
Phenobarbital - Major				127.0 $(56.2)^b$
- Minor*			N.D.	N.D.

[a] Content of cytochromes in liver microsomes of β-naphthoflavone-treated rats.

[b] Percent composition based on cytochrome P-450 + cytochrome P-420.

* Immunochemically identical   N.D. - Not Detectable

The presence of reductase and cytochromes P-450 in human colon is indicated in the SDS gel electrophoresis patterns of microsomes from the ascending, transverse and descending segments of human colon shown in Fig. 1.
A sharp band migrating at the same level as cytochrome P-450 reductase
(lane b) can be observed in microsomes from all three segments of the
colon. The cytochrome P-450 region, defined by standards in lanes a, c
and d, shows multiple bands in each of the segments. A band comigrating
with the major phenobarbital-inducible form is observed in all three segments, while the band comigrating with Form 1 appears most clearly in the
ascending and transverse segments and is less evident in descending colon
microsomes. These data indicate the presence of various forms of cytochrome P-450 throughout the length of the human colon.

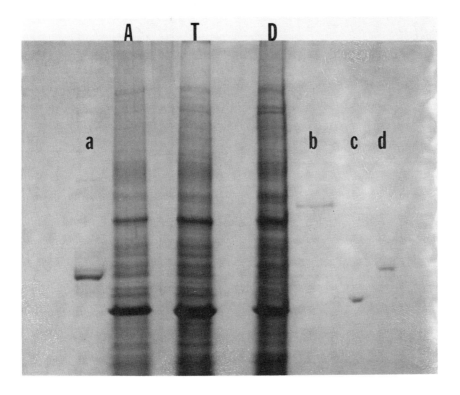

Fig. 1. SDS gel electrophoresis of microsomes from human colon. Lane A
contained microsomes from the ascending segment; Lane T, transverse segment; Lane D, descending segment; a, major phenobarbital inducible form
(52,000); b, cytochrome P-450 reductase (78,000); c, cytochrome P-450
Form 1 (47,000); d, cytochrome P-450 Form 4 (53,500).

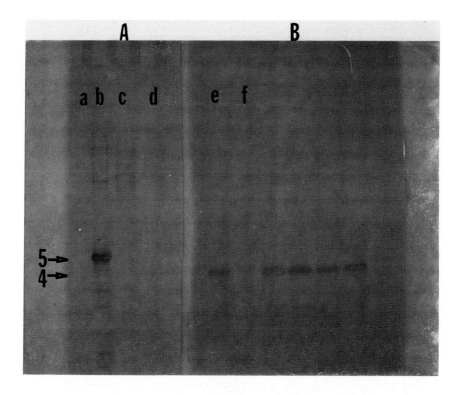

Fig. 2. Detection of cytochromes P-450 in human colon segments by electroblotting technique. Panel A: nitrocellulose blot was developed with
antibody to Form 5. Panel B: nitrocellulose blot was developed with antibody to Form 4. Lane a contained microsomes from descending segment; b,
Form 5 standard; c, microsomes from transverse segment; d, microsomes from
ascending segment; e, Form 4 standard; f, microsomes from descending segment. Lanes beyond lane f contain additional Form 4 standards added to
microsomes from ascending, transverse and descending segments.

Although the appearance of comigrating bands indicate the presence of
particular forms of cytochrome P-450 in human colon, a more definitive approach is required to demonstrate those forms present. The Western blot
(electroblotting) technique was used to provide a clearer definition. An
example of this approach is shown in Fig. 2. Nitrocellulose blots of
colon microsomal electrophoretic patterns were developed with antibody to
Form 5 (Fig. 2, A) and with antibody to Form 4 (Fig. 2, B). As shown in

Fig. 2, A, no colonic segment appeared to contain a band which cross-reacts with antibody to Form 5. On the other hand, crossreacting bands migrating with Form 4 are seen. Since antibody to pure Form 5 does recognize some determinants on Form 4, we tested for the presence of Form 4 crossreacting bands in human microsomes. As shown in Fig. 2, B, descending colon microsomes contain a band which crossreacts with antibody to Form 4 (lane f). Thus, Form 4, but not Form 5, can be detected in colon microsomes from this case. Similarly, we have been able to show the presence of the major phenobarbital inducible form in human colon. Other forms also are probably present. However, individual variation may complicate the quantitation of human colon cytochromes P-450. Nonetheless, these data show the presence and functionality of a cytochrome P-450 containing system in human colon. The role of this system in carcinogenesis and chemotherapy remains to be defined.

ACKNOWLEDGMENT

This research was supported by grants CA19105 and CA19621 from the National Cancer Institute and by grant Ag02081 from the National Institute on Aging, U.S. Public Health Service, DHHR.

REFERENCES

1. Gillette, J.R. (1966). Adv. Pharmacol. 4, 219-261.

2. Gram, T.E. (1980). Extrahepatic Metabolism of Drug and Other Foreign Compounds, Spectrum Press, New York.

3. Lu, A.Y.H. and West, S.B. (1980). Pharmacol. Rev. 31, 277-295.

4. Conney, A.H. (1967). Pharmacol. Rev. 19, 317-366.

5. Coon, M.J. and Vatsis, K.P. (1978). In: Polycyclic Hydrocarbons and Cancer, Vol. 1, Gelboin, H.V. and Tso, P.D.P. (eds), Academic Press, New York, pp. 335-360.

6. Guengerich, F.P. (1978). J. Biol. Chem. 253, 7931-7939.

7. Guengerich, F.P. (1979). Pharmacol. Ther. A 6, 99-121.

8. Thomas, P.E., Lu, A.Y.H., Ryan, D.E., West, S.B., Kawalek, J. and Levin, W. (1976). Mol. Pharmacol. 12, 746-758.

9. Johnson, E.F. (1979). Rev. Biochem. Toxicol. 1, 1-26.

10. Daniel, R.M. and Appleby, C.A. (1972). Biochem. Biophys. Acta 275, 347-352.

11. Wang, P., Mason, P.S. and Guengerich, F.P. (1980). Arch. Biochem. Biophys. 199, 206-219.

12. Ryan, D.E., Thomas, P.E., Korzeniowski, D. and Levin, W. (1979). J. Biol. Chem. 254, 1365-1374.

13. Elshourbagy, N.A. and Guzelian, P.S. (1980). J. Biol. Chem. 255, 1279-1285.

14. Saito, T. and Strobel, H.W. (1981). J. Biol. Chem. 256, 984-988.

15. Guengerich, F.P. and Martin, M.V. (1980). Arch. Biochem. Biophys. 205, 365-379.

16. Fisher, G.J., Fukushima, H. and Gaylor, J.L. (1981). J. Biol. Chem. 256, 4388-4394.

17. Ryan, D.E., Thomas, P.F. and Levin, W. (1980). J. Biol. Chem. 255, 7941-7955.

18. Hansson, R. and Wikvall, K. (1980). J. Biol. Chem. 255, 1643-1649.

19. Lau, P.P. and Strobel, H.W. (1982). J. Biol. Chem. 257, 5257-5262.

20. Lu, A.Y.H. and West, S.B. (1978). Pharmacol. Ther. A 2, 337-358.

21. Philpot, R.M. and Arinc, E. (1976). Mol. Pharmacol. 12, 483-493.

22. Fang, W.F. and Strobel, H.W. (1978). Arch. Biochem. Biophys. 186, 128-138.

23. Fang, W.F. and Strobel, H.W. (1978). Cancer Res. 38, 2939-2944.

24. Fang, W.F. and Strobel, H.W. (1981). Cancer Res. 41, 1407-1412.

25. Tom, B.H., Rutzky, L.P., Jakstys, M.M., Oyasu, R., Kaye, G.I. and Kahan, B.D. (1976). In Vitro 12, 180-190.

26. Nebert, D.W. and Gelboin, H.V. (1968). J. Biol. Chem. 243, 6242-6249.

27. McFayden, D.A. (1945). J. Biol. Chem. 158, 107-133.

28. Matsumoto, H. and Strong, F.V. (1963). Arch. Biochem. Biophys. 101, 199-210.

29. Newaz, S.N., Fang, W.F. and Strobel, H.W. (1983). Cancer (in press).

30. Lowry, A.H., Rosebrough, N.J., Farr, A.L. and Randall, R.J. (1951). J. Biol. Chem. 193, 265-275.

31. Strobel, H.W. and Lau, P.P. (1982). In: Cytochrome P-450, Biochemistry, Biophysics and Environmental Implications, Heitanen, E., Lautinen, M. and Hänninen (eds), Elsevier Biomedical Press, Amsterdam, pp. 321-328.

32. Bowen, B., Steinberg, J., Laemmli, U.K. and Weintraub, H. (1980). Nucleic Acid Res. 8, 1-20.

33. Autrup, H., Harris, C.C., Stoner, G.D., Jesudason, M.C. and Trump, B.F. (1977). J. Natl. Cancer Inst. 59, 351-354.

© 1983 Elsevier Science Publishers B.V.
Extrahepatic Drug Metabolism and Chemical Carcinogenesis,
J. Rydström, J. Montelius and M. Bengtsson eds.

CHARACTERIZATION OF CYTOCHROME P-450 IN THE RAT VENTRAL PROSTATE

TAPIO HAAPARANTA[1,2], JAMES HALPERT[1], LENA HAGLUND[1], HANS GLAUMANN[2] AND
JAN-ÅKE GUSTAFSSON[1]

[1]Department of Medical Nutrition and [2]Department of Pathology, Karolinska
Institute, Huddinge University Hospital F69, S-141 86 Huddinge, Sweden.

INTRODUCTION

Prostatic cancer is a common malignant disease in Europe and the United States,
yet its etiology is still largely unknown. The induction of prostatic cancer
appears to be dependent on androgens, and its occurrence is relatively restricted
to certain populations. Therefore, hormonal, genetic or environmental factors may
be involved. Recent epidemiological studies have shown a correlation between prostatic cancer and occupational exposure in rubber workers and those exposed to
cadmium (1,2).

To better understand a possible role of chemicals and environmental factors
in prostatic carcinoma we have studied the cytochrome P-450 (P-450) system in
the rat ventral prostate. The rat prostate is a commonly used animal model which
shares many common biochemical and morphological features with the human gland.

MATERIALS AND METHODS

Male rats of the Sprague-Dawley strain, weighing 350-400 g (200 g in case of
preparation of liver microsomes for cytochrome P-450 purification), were obtained
from Anticimex (Stockholm, Sweden). Phenobarbital (80 mg/kg in 0.5 ml saline) and
β-naphthoflavone (40 mg/kg in 0.5 ml corn oil) were injected intraperitoneally
once daily for 3 days, if not otherwise indicated. The animals were starved overnight after the last injection and then killed by decapitation. Prostatic microsomes were isolated as described earlier (3). The microsomal pellets were suspended in 0.3 M sucrose and, if not used immediately, stored at -80°C.

NADPH-cytochrome P-450 reductase and the major forms of cytochrome P-450 were
purified from liver microsomes of PB- and BNF-treated rats essentially according
to the method of Guengerich and Martin (4). Antibodies were raised against the
purified enzymes in rabbits. Immunoglobulin G (IgG) fractions were isolated by
affinity chromatography using a Protein A-Sepharose CL-4B column (Pharmacia Fine
Chemicals, Uppsala, Sweden). The eluted IgG fractions were dialyzed against PBS
(10 mM potassium phosphate buffer, pH 7.4 containing 0.15 M NaCl).

Proteins from SDS-polyacrylamide gels were transferred to nitrocellulose
filters essentially using the method of Towbin et al (5). The nitrocellulose
sheets were shaken in PBS, 3% (w/v) bovine serum albumin, 0.1% (w/v) Nonidet

P-40 and 0.01% (w/v) NaN_3 for 1 h. The sheets were then incubated with the appropriate antibody in the above solution (0.1 mg IgG/ml) for 2 h. The blots were washed in PBS, containing 0.1% Nonidet P-40 and 0.01% NaN_3, for 2 h with four changes. The blots were incubated with ^{125}I-labeled protein A (New England Nuclear, Dreieich, West Germany) in PBS (500,000 cpm/ml), 3% bovine serum albumin, 0.1% Nonidet P-40 and 0.01% NaN_3, for 1 h, and were then washed in PBS, 0.1% Nonidet P-40 and 0.01% NaN_3 for 1 h with three changes. The dried blots were exposed to LKB Ultrofilm, usually for 2-3 days. The radioactivity bound to the protein bands was proportional to the amount of antigen applied to the SDS-polyacrylamide gel, which allowed the quantitation of the proteins.

Localization of the antigens in tissue sections was performed essentially by the peroxidase-antiperoxidase method of Sternberger et al (6) using p-benzo-quinone (0.3%, w/v) as the fixative. Controls consisted of incubation of the tissue sections with preimmune IgG or with antigen-absorbed antibody.

RESULTS AND DISCUSSION

In the present investigation we have used antibodies against rat liver cyto-chromes P-450 PB-B_2 and P-450 BNF-B_2 and NADPH-cytochrome P-450 reductase to characterize the prostatic cytochrome P-450 dependent monooxygenase system. Anti-P-450 BNF-B_2 and anti-P-450 reductase were found to cross-react with pro-static proteins. Anti-P-450 reductase inhibited the prostatic NADPH-cytochrome c reductase activity by 60%, and the BNF induced prostatic AHH activity by 50%.

Table 1 Effects of Phenobarbital (PB) and β-Naphthoflavone (BNF) Treatment on Prostatic and Liver Microsomes.

	P-450 BNF-B_2	P-450 PB-B_2	NADPH-cytochrome P-450 reductase	NADPH-cytochrome c reductase (μmol/min/mg)	AHH (pmol/min/mg)	Amino-pyrine N-demethyl-ase (nmol/min/mg)
	(immunological content, n m o l / m g)					
Prostate						
Control	<0.0004[a]	<0.0004[a]	0.02	0.026	1.4	0.01
PB	<0.0004[a]	<0.0004[a]	0.02	0.023	n.m.[c]	0.20
BNF	0.05	<0.0004[a]	0.02	0.038	290	0.22
Liver						
Control	0.01	0.02[b]	0.20	0.27	54	1.7
PB	0.01	2.40[b]	0.35	0.42	n.m.[c]	6.0
BNF	1.31	0.02[b]	0.20	0.28	3400	1.3

The immunological content was measured using the immunoblotting method (see text).
[a] The content is below the detection limit, which was calculated to be 0.4 pmol/mg of microsomal protein.
[b] Represents the sum of P-450 PB-B_2 and P-450 PB-B_3.
[c] n.m., not measured.

Anti-P-450 BNF-B$_2$ inhibited prostatic AHH activity almost completely, whereas anti-P-450 PB-B$_2$ or preimmune IgG had no effect.

Table 1 summarizes the effects of PB and BNF on prostatic and liver microsomes with respect to cytochrome P-450 and NADPH-cytochrome P-450 reductase content in comparison with the activities of AHH, NADPH-cytochrome c reductase and amino-pyrine N-demethylase.

As judged by immunoblotting (Fig. 1), the anti-P-450 reductase recognized only a single protein in either liver or prostatic microsomes, which had the same

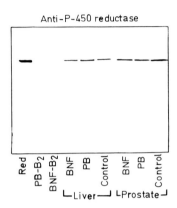

Fig. 1 Autoradiogram of an immunoblot incubated with antibodies against rat liver P-450 reductase. The SDS-gel was run with the following samples, from left to right in the Fig.: P-450 reductase, P-450 PB-B$_2$, 0.5 μg protein each. Liver and prostatic microsomes from animals pretreated with BNF, PB and from untreated animals. Five μg of liver and 100 μg of prostatic microsomal protein were applied to the gel.

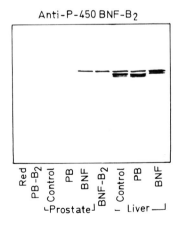

Fig. 2 Autoradiogram of an immunoblot incubated with antibodies against rat liver P-450 BNF-B$_2$. The following amounts of protein were applied: 0.5 μg of the purified enzymes, 400 μg of prostatic microsomes from untreated, PB- or BNF-treated rats; 50 μg of liver microsomes from untreated and PB-treated rats, and 1 μg of liver microsomes from BNF-treated rats.

molecular weight as the purified liver P-450 reductase. The prostatic microsomes were found to contain only one-tenth as much P-450 reductase as liver microsomes measured either by quantitative immunoblotting or by assay of NADPH-cytochrome c reductase activity. Neither PB nor BNF treatment affected the amount of the P-450 reductase in the prostate, whereas PB gave a 2-fold induction in the liver. The AHH and 7-ethoxyresorufin O-deethylase activities were induced by BNF about 500-fold in the prostate and about 100-fold in the liver.

Fig. 2 shows that anti-P-450 BNF-B$_2$ recognized only a single protein (Mw = 54,000) in prostatic microsomes from BNF-treated animals. In microsomes from control rats the level of this protein was below the limit of detection (0.4 pmol/mg) of the immunoblotting method, whereas 24 h after a single i.p. injection of BNF, prostatic microsomes contained 50 pmol/mg, which represents at least a 125-fold induction. In liver microsomes several bands with smaller molecular weight were recognized by anti-P-450 BNF-B$_2$ IgG (Fig. 2). No attempts were made to elucidate the identity of these bands. However, none of the unidentified bands were identical with P-450 PB-B$_2$. In a similar experiment with antibodies against

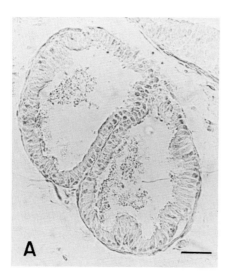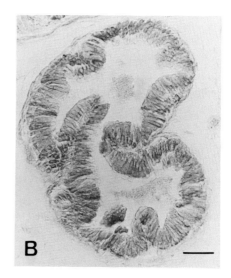

Fig. 3 Immunohistochemical localization of cytochrome P-450 BNF-B$_2$ in the ventral prostate of an untreated (A) and BNF-treated rat. The tissue sections were exposed to anti-P-450 BNF-B$_2$ in the unlabeled antibody peroxidase-antiperoxidase immunohistochemical staining procedure. Sections exposed to preimmune IgG or antigen absorbed antibody were similarly stained as the section in panel A. Panel B shows the localization of the antigen in the epithelial cells of the gland with no staining in muscle cells or in the lumen. Tissue sections exposed to anti-P-450 reductase showed a similar staining pattern as shown in panel B in untreated, PB- or BNF-treated rats. Bar, 15 μm.

P-450 PB-B$_2$ no immunoreactive protein bands were detected in prostatic microsomes regardless of treatment (not shown). The immunological cross-reactivity of liver and prostatic cytochrome P-450 BNF-B$_2$ and NADPH-cytochrome P-450 reductase enabled us to detect the antigens immunohistochemically in the prostatic gland. Both the reductase (not shown) and cytochrome P-450 BNF-B$_2$ (Fig. 3 A,B) were localized to the epithelial cells of the gland. The reductase was constitutively present in the epithelial cells, whereas cytochrome P-450 BNF-B$_2$ was only detected after BNF treatment of the animals.

In conclusion, this study shows that a cytochrome P-450 system is present in the epithelial cells of the rat ventral prostate and that this enzyme system is markedly responsive to P-450 inducers of the polycyclic hydrocarbon group. Whether or not the human prostate also contains highly inducible cytochrome P-450 isozymes remains to be established. If so, it may have important consequences for the understanding of the etiology of human prostatic cancer.

ACKNOWLEDGEMENTS

We thank Dr. F. Peter Guengerich for kindly providing a preprint of his manuscript and Dr. Maria Norgård for performing immunohistochemical experiments. This study was supported by grants from the Swedish Cancer Society and from the Swedish Board for Planning and Coordination of Research.

REFERENCES

1. Lemen, R.A., Lee, J.S., Wagoner, J.K. and Bleijer, H.P. Ann. N.Y. Acad. Sci., 271:273-279, 1976.

2. Goldsmith, D.F., Smith, A.H. and McMichael, A.J. J. Occup. Med., 22:533-541, 1980.

3. Haaparanta, T., Gustafsson, J.-Å. and Glaumann, H. Arch. Biochem. Biophys. In press, 1983.

4. Guengerich, F.P. and Martin, M.V. Arch. Biochem. Biophys., 205:365-379, 1980.

5. Towbin, H., Staehelin, T. and Gordon, J. Proc. Natl. Acad. Sci. U.S.A., 76: 4350-4354, 1979.

6. Sternberger, L.A., Hardy, P.H., Cuculis, J.J. and Meyer, H.G. J. Histochem. Cytochem. 18:315-333, 1970.

© 1983 Elsevier Science Publishers B.V.
Extrahepatic Drug Metabolism and Chemical Carcinogenesis,
J. Rydström, J. Montelius and M. Bengtsson eds.

LOCALIZATION OF CARCINOGEN-METABOLIZING ENZYMES IN HUMAN AND ANIMAL TISSUES

JEFFREY BARON[1], THOMAS T. KAWABATA[1], JAN A. REDICK[1], SHIRLEY A. KNAPP[1], DONALD
G. WICK[1], ROBERT B. WALLACE[2], WILLIAM B. JAKOBY[3], AND F. PETER GUENGERICH[4]

Departments of [1]Pharmacology and [2]Preventive Medicine, The University of Iowa
College of Medicine, Iowa City, IA 52242; [3]Section on Enzymes and Cellular
Biochemistry, National Institute of Arthritis, Diabetes, and Digestive and
Kidney Diseases, Bethesda, MD 20205; and [4]Department of Biochemistry,
Vanderbilt University School of Medicine, Nashville, TN 37232

INTRODUCTION

While all cancers must ultimately be a product of environmental and genetic
mechanisms, there is a growing appreciation that many human cancers are caused,
mediated, or modified by environmental factors (1,2). Among environmental
factors associated with cancer etiology are chemicals, including those found in
tobacco smoke, the diet, and the workplace. Chemical carcinogens may exert
their effects through genetic or epigenetic mechanisms, may act in concert with
other agents as co-carcinogens or promoters, and may either work unaltered or
require prior activation. The realization that most chemicals that are associated with human cancers and that induce neoplasia in laboratory animals are
not carcinogenic per se but, rather, must undergo prior bioactivation (3,4),
has led to intensive investigations on those enzymes that participate in the
activation and detoxication of chemical carcinogens. Thus, cytochromes P-450,
NADPH-cytochrome P-450 reductase, epoxide hydrolase, and glutathione S-transferases, enzymes that play pivotal roles in the metabolism of chemical carcinogens (3,4), are the subjects of a number of chapters in these proceedings.

While the exposure of laboratory animals to chemical carcinogens leads to the
induction of neoplasia in many tissues, not all cell types found within complex
tissues are susceptible to the carcinogenic actions of chemicals. Similarly,
human cancers do not involve all cell types within the diseased tissues. In an
attempt to determine the biochemical basis for this phenomenon, many studies
have been conducted to evaluate the abilities of different types of isolated or
cultured cells to metabolize chemical carcinogens (5-7). However, because of
the complex nature of mammalian tissues, this information is currently
available for only a limited number of different cell types. Moreover, the
capabilities of freshly isolated or cultured cells to metabolize chemical
carcinogens in vitro may not clearly reflect their metabolic functions in situ.
In order to gain more direct insight into the potential of all different cell

types found within complex tissues to enzymatically activate and detoxicate chemical carcinogens, this laboratory has employed exquisitely sensitive immunohistochemical techniques to localize several carcinogen-metabolizing enzymes at the light microscopic level within a number of tissues (8-15). In the present investigation, carcinogen-metabolizing enzymes were localized in human, rat, and mouse skin, human and rat breast, human prostate, rat and hamster pancreas, rat lung, and rat kidney.

MATERIALS AND METHODS

Enzymes

Antigens were localized at the light microscopic level employing antibodies raised against the hepatic enzymes listed in Table 1. While antibodies to the rat enzymes cross-reacted with antigens in human, mouse, and hamster tissues, the antigens detected in these species are most likely immunochemically similar, rather than identical, to the rat enzymes. In addition, since glutathione S-transferase C shares a common subunit with (16) and is immunochemically similar to glutathione S-transferase A (17), results obtained with this antibody must be interpreted as indicating the presence of transferases C and/or A.

TABLE 1

CARCINOGEN-METABOLIZING ENZYMES LOCALIZED IN HUMAN AND ANIMAL TISSUES

Enzyme	Source	References
Cytochrome P-450	Human liver microsomes	18
Cytochrome P-450 BNF-B[a]	Hepatic microsomes of BNF-treated rats	19
Cytochrome P-450 MC-B	Hepatic microsomes of MC-treated rats	20
Cytochrome P-450 PB-B	Hepatic microsomes of PB-treated rats	19,20
Cytochrome P-450 PCN-E	Hepatic microsomes of PCN-treated rats	19
NADPH-cytochrome P-450 reductase	Human liver microsomes	21
	Hepatic microsomes of PB-treated rats	8
Epoxide hydrolase	Human liver microsomes	22
	Hepatic microsomes of PB-treated rats	22
Glutathione S-transferase B	Rat liver	17
Glutathione S-transferase C	Rat liver	17
Glutathione S-transferase E	Rat liver	23

[a]Cytochromes P-450 BNF-B, MC-B, PB-B, and PCN-E represent the major isozymes of the hemeprotein isolated from hepatic microsomes of rats pretreated with β-naphthoflavone, 3-methylcholanthrene, phenobarbital, and pregnenolone-16α-carbonitrile, respectively (19,20).

Tissue preparation

Skin. Three-mm punch biopsy specimens obtained from the forearms of healthy male volunteers were fixed at 4°C by immersion in a solution of 1% acetic acid in 95% ethanol and embedded in paraffin. Specimens, approximately 3 X 5 mm in size, obtained from the shaved backs of 56-day-old female CD-1 mice and 57-day-old female Holtzman rats during the telogen (resting) phase of the hair growth cycle were fixed in ethanol:acetic acid and embedded in paraffin.

Breast. Specimens of breast tissue, 10 X 8 X 5 mm in size and peripheral to an adenocarcinoma, were obtained from a 65-year-old patient undergoing a mastectomy and were cut into smaller blocks which were fixed in ethanol:acetic acid and embedded in paraffin. Breast tissue obtained from 300-350 g female Sprague-Dawley rats was fixed in ethanol:acetic acid and embedded in paraffin.

Prostate. Specimens of prostates surgically removed from 59- to 72-year-old patients with benign prostatic hyperplasia were cut into pieces approximately 6 mm long and 1.5 mm thick which were fixed in ethanol:acetic acid and embedded in paraffin.

Pancreas. The splenic-gastric pancreatic lobe of 180-230 g male Holtzman rats and of 90-110 g male Syrian golden hamsters was fixed at 4°C by immersion in a solution containing 0.35% p-benzoquinone and 0.02 M $CaCl_2$ in 0.2 M sodium cacodylate buffer, pH 7.4, and embedded in paraffin.

Lung. Lungs of 180-230 g male Holtzman rats were inflated under 30 cm Hg with ice-cold ethanol:acetic acid. After ligation of the trachea, the lungs were excised, and pieces were fixed by immersion in ethanol:acetic acid and embedded in paraffin.

Kidney. One- to 2-mm thick slices taken through the centers of kidneys of 180-230 g male Holtzman rats were fixed in p-benzoquinone and embedded in paraffin.

Immunohistochemistry

Enzymes were localized at the light microscopic level in 4- to 7-µm thick tissue sections employing the unlabeled antibody peroxidase-antiperoxidase staining technique as described previously (8-15). Control serial sections were exposed to equal concentrations of normal (nonimmune) serum from the appropriate species. To block endogenous peroxidase activity, sections were exposed for 60 min at 37°C to 0.05-0.1% phenylhydrazine in Tris-HCl buffer, pH 7.75, containing 0.154 M NaCl. Identification of different cell types in immunohistochemically-stained sections was confirmed by examination of adjacent sections stained with either hematoxylin and eosin or toluidine blue.

RESULTS

Skin

Exposure of sections of human skin to anti-human hepatic microsomal epoxide hydrolase produced staining within the epidermis, sebaceous glands, the outer root sheath of hair follicles, the secretory and duct portions of sweat glands, and fibroblasts (Fig. 1). As seen in Table 2, each of these cell types was also stained by anti-human hepatic microsomal cytochrome P-450 and anti-rat hepatic microsomal cytochrome P-450 MC-B. Anti-human hepatic microsomal NADPH-cytochrome P-450 reductase and each of the antibodies raised against the other rat hepatic enzymes, however, produced staining within only certain cell types, with fibroblasts not being noticeably stained by any of these antibodies.

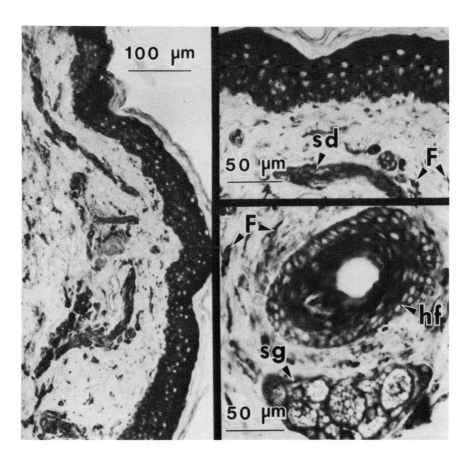

Fig. 1. Representative staining in a section of human skin exposed to anti-human hepatic microsomal epoxide hydrolase. Arrows point to a sweat gland duct (sd), a sebaceous gland (sg), a hair follicle (hf), and fibroblasts (F).

TABLE 2

IMMUNOHISTOCHEMICAL STAINING FOR CARCINOGEN-METABOLIZING ENZYMES IN HUMAN SKIN

Key: +, cells are stained; -, cells are not stained; ?, staining is not readily apparently; and *, insufficient observations.

Enzyme		Epidermis	Sweat Gland Secretory Cell	Duct Cell	Hair Follicle	Sebaceous Gland	Fibroblast
Cytochrome P-450:							
human		+	+	+	+	+	+
rat BNF-B		?	+	+	+	+	?
rat MC-B		+	+	+	+	+	+
rat PB-B		+	+	+	+	+	?
rat PCN-E		+	?	+	+	+	?
NADPH-cytochrome							
P-450 reductase		?	+	+	+	+	?
Epoxide hydrolase		+	+	+	+	+	+
Glutathione S-							
transferase:	B	?	?	?	*	*	-
	C	+	+	+	+	+	-
	E	+	+	+	+	+	?

In rat skin, cytochromes P-450 MC-B and PB-B, cytochrome P-450 reductase, and glutathione S-transferases were found in epidermis, sebaceous glands, and hair follicles (Table 3). Staining for cytochrome P-450 PCN-E and epoxide hydrolase was apparent only in sebaceous glands, while cytochrome P-450 BNF-B was not detected in any cell. None of the antibodies appreciably stained fibroblasts.

TABLE 3

IMMUNOHISTOCHEMICAL STAINING FOR CARCINOGEN-METABOLIZING ENZYMES IN RAT SKIN

Key: +, cells are stained; -, cells are not stained; and ?, staining is not readily apparent.

Enzyme		Epidermis	Hair Follicle	Sebaceous Gland	Fibroblast
Cytochrome P-450:					
rat BNF-B		-	-	-	-
rat MC-B		+	+	+	?
rat PB-B		+	+	+	?
rat PCN-E		?	?	+	?
NADPH-cytochrome					
P-450 reductase		+	+	+	?
Epoxide hydrolase		?	?	+	?
Glutathione S-					
transferase:	B	+	+	+	?
	C	+	+	+	?
	E	+	+	+	?

TABLE 4

IMMUNOHISTOCHEMICAL STAINING FOR CARCINOGEN-METABOLIZING ENZYMES IN MOUSE SKIN

Key: +, cells are stained; −, cells are not stained; and ?, staining is not readily apparent.

Enzyme	Epidermis	Hair Follicle	Sebaceous Gland	Fibroblast
Cytochrome P-450:				
rat BNF-B	+	+	+	−
rat MC-B	+	+	+	−
rat PB-B	+	+	+	?
NADPH-cytochrome P-450 reductase	+	+	+	+
Epoxide hydrolase	+	+	+	?
Glutathione S-transferase: B	+	+	+	+
C	+	+	+	+
E	+	+	+	+

Antibodies to rat liver enzymes also stained mouse cutaneous cells (Table 4). However, some species differences were readily apparent: in mouse skin, anti-cytochrome P-450 BNF-B stained the epidermis, sebaceous glands, and the outer root sheath of hair follicles, whereas it did not stain any of these cells in rat skin; anti-rat epoxide hydrolase also stained each of these cells in mouse skin, while it appeared to stain only sebaceous glands in rat skin; and antibodies to rat hepatic microsomal NADPH-cytochrome P-450 reductase and rat heptic glutathione S-transferases stained mouse fibroblasts, whereas fibroblasts were not noticeably stained for these enzymes in either rat or human skin.

Breast

Rabbit antiserum to human epoxide hydrolase stained human breast ductular epithelia (Fig. 2). The appearance of the fibromuscular stroma after exposure to the antiserum resulted from nonspecific staining, since these cells were stained similarly in serial sections exposed to normal rabbit serum. As seen in Table 5, ductular epithelia in human breast were also stained by each of the other antibodies employed. In contrast, staining of cells within the fibromuscular stroma of the human breast was noticeable only after exposure to the antibodies to rat liver cytochrome P-450 BNF-B and glutathione S-transferase E.

In rat breast, ductular epithelial cells were also stained by each of the antibodies to the rat hepatic enzymes, with the exception of anti-cytochrome P-450 BNF-B (Table 5). None of the antibodies, however, produced readily demonstrable staining of cells within the fibromuscular stroma of rat breast.

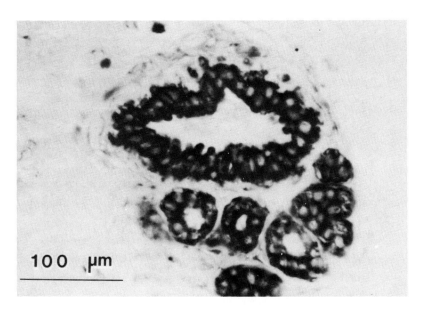

Fig. 2. Representative immunohistochemical staining of ductular epithelia in human breast exposed to rabbit anti-human hepatic microsomal epoxide hydrolase.

TABLE 5

IMMUNOHISTOCHEMICAL STAINING FOR CARCINOGEN-METABOLIZING ENZYMES IN HUMAN AND RAT BREAST

Key: +, cells are stained; -, cells are not stained; ?, staining is not readily apparent; and ND, not determined.

| | Human Breast | | Rat Breast | |
Enzyme	Ductular Epithelium	Fibromuscular Stroma	Ductular Epithelium	Fibromuscular Stroma
Cytochrome P-450:				
human	+	?	ND	ND
rat BNF-B	+	+	-	-
rat MC-B	+	?	+	?
rat PB-B	+	?	+	?
rat PCN-E	+	-	+	-
NADPH-cytochrome				
P-450 reductase	+	-	+	?
Epoxide hydrolase	+	-	+	-
Glutathione S-				
transferase: B	+	-	+	-
C	+	-	+	-
E	+	+	+	-

Human breast sections were exposed to anti-human reductase and epoxide hydrolase, and rat breast sections were exposed to anti-rat reductase and hydrolase.

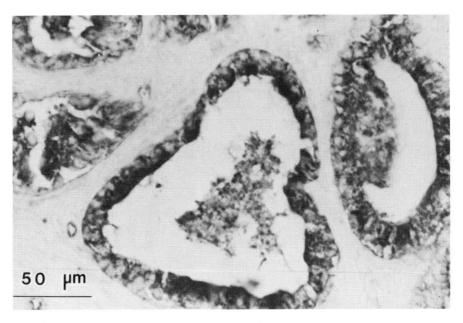

Fig. 3. Representative staining of glandular epithelia in sections of human prostate exposed to rabbit anti-human hepatic microsomal epoxide hydrolase.

Prostate

Anti-human epoxide hydrolase stained glandular epithelial cells in prostates of elderly patients with benign prostatic hyperplasia (Fig. 3). The appearance of the fibromuscular stroma and proteinaceous material in gland lumina is due to nonspecific staining: normal rabbit serum produced similar staining. Antibodies to human hepatic microsomal cytochrome P-450 and cytochrome P-450 reductase, rat hepatic microsomal cytochromes P-450, and rat hepatic glutathione S-transferases C and E also stained glandular epithelia (Table 6). In addition, prostatic ductular epithelial cells were stained by antibodies to human hepatic microsomal epoxide hydrolase, cytochrome P-450, and cytochrome P-450 reductase, rat hepatic microsomal cytochromes P-450, and rat hepatic glutathione S-transferase E. Stromal cells were appreciably stained only by antibodies to rat hepatic cytochromes P-450 PB-B and PCN-E and glutathione S-transferase B.

Pancreas

In rat pancreas, anti-rat epoxide hydrolase stained acinar cells, ductular epithelia, and A cells of islets (Fig. 4). Because of nonspecific staining, it was not possible to determine if islet B cells were also stained.

TABLE 6

IMMUNOHISTOCHEMICAL STAINING FOR CARCINOGEN-METABOLIZING ENZYMES IN HUMAN
PROSTATE

Key: +, cells are stained; -, cells are not stained; and ?, staining is not
readily apparent.

Enzyme	Glandular Epithelium	Ductular Epithelium	Fibromuscular Stroma
Cytochrome P-450:			
human	+	+	?
rat BNF-B	+	+	-
rat MC-B	+	+	?
rat PB-B	+	+	+
rat PCN-E	+	+	+
NADPH-cytochrome			
P-450 reductase	+	+	-
Epoxide hydrolase	+	+	?
Glutathione S-			
transferase: B	?	?	+
C	+	?	-
E	+	+	?

As seen from the information presented in Table 7, acinar cells in the rat
exocrine pancreas were also stained by antibodies to rat hepatic cytochromes
P-450 BNF-B and PB-B, NADPH-cytochrome P-450 reductase, and glutathione
S-transferases B, C, and E. Furthermore, rat pancreatic ductular epithelia
were also stained for each enzyme except cytochrome P-450 BNF-B and PB-B. In
pancreatic islets, A cells were appreciably stained for each enzyme except
cytochrome P-450 BNF-B and glutathione S-transferase E, while B cells appeared
to be stained only by antibodies to cytochrome P-450 PB-B, NADPH-cytochrome
P-450 reductase, and glutathione S-transferases B and E.

The results of immunohistochemical analyses summarized in Table 7 further
demonstrate that exocrine and endocrine cells in the hamster pancreas were also
stained by antibodies to the rat hepatic enzymes. However, in marked contrast
to findings in the rat pancreas, exposure of sections of hamster pancreas to
the anti-rat cytochrome P-450 BNF-B did not produce detectable staining within
any cell. In addition, two other potentially important differences were noted
between the rat and hamster pancreas: (a) ductular epithelial cells in the
hamster pancreas were readily observed to be stained by the antibody to
cytochrome P-450 PB-B, whereas this antibody did not noticeably stain ductular
epithelial cells in the rat pancreas; and (b) antibody to glutathione S-transferase E did not stain ductular epithelial cells in the hamster pancreas, while
it was found to stain these cells in the rat pancreas.

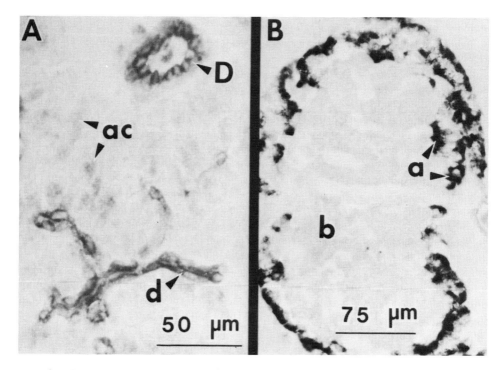

Fig. 4. Representative staining of rat pancreatic cells by anti-rat epoxide hydrolase. A, exocrine pancreas: ac = acinar cells; d = intralobular duct; D = interlobular duct. B, pancreatic islet: a = A cells and b = B cells.

TABLE 7

IMMUNOHISTOCHEMICAL STAINING FOR CARCINOGEN-METABOLIZING ENZYMES IN RAT AND HAMSTER PANCREAS

Key: +, cells are stained; -, cells are not stained; and ?, staining is not readily apparent.

Enzyme	Rat Pancreas				Hamster Pancreas			
	Acinar Cells	Ductular Epithelium	Islet Cells A	B	Acinar Cells	Ductular Epithelium	Islet Cells A	B
Cytochrome P-450:								
rat BNF-B	+	-	-	-	-	-	-	-
rat PB-B	+	?	+	+	+	+	+	+
NADPH-cytochrome								
P-450 reductase	+	+	+	+	+	+	+	+
Epoxide hydrolase	+	+	+	?	+	+	+	?
Glutathione S-								
transferase: B	+	+	+	+	+	+	+	+
C	+	+	+	?	+	+	+	?
E	+	+	?	+	+	-	-	+

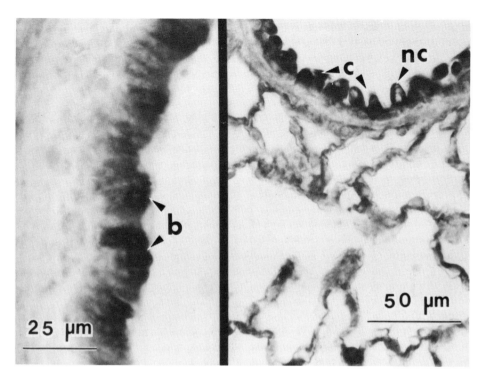

Fig. 5. Typical staining of bronchial (b), ciliated bronchiolar (c), and non-ciliated bronchiolar (nc) epithelial cells in rat lung by anti-rat P-450 PB-B.

TABLE 8

IMMUNOHISTOCHEMICAL STAINING FOR CARCINOGEN-METABOLIZING ENZYMES IN RAT LUNG

Key: +, cells are stained; and −, cells are not stained.

Enzyme	Bronchial Epithelium	Ciliated Bronchiolar Epithelium	Nonciliated Bronchiolar Epithelium	Alveolar Wall
Cytochrome P-450:				
rat BNF-B	+	+	+	+
rat MC-B	−	−	−	−
rat PB-B	+	+	+	+
rat PCN-E	+	+	+	+
NADPH-cytochrome P-450 reductase	+	+	+	+
Epoxide hydrolase	+	+	+	+
Glutathione S-transferase: B	+	+	+	+
C	+	+	+	+
E	+	+	+	+

Lung

Cytochrome P-450 PB-B was readily detected within bronchial epithelial cells, ciliated and nonciliated (Clara) bronchiolar epithelial cells, and the alveolar wall in sections of rat lung exposed to anti-rat hepatic microsomal cytochrome P-450 PB-B (Fig. 5). Although cytochrome P-450 MC-B could not be detected in lungs of untreated rats, bronchial and both ciliated and nonciliated bronchiolar epithelial cells, as well as cells within the alveolar wall, were stained for cytochromes P-450 BNF-B, PB-B, and PCN-E, NADPH-cytochrome P-450 reductase, epoxide hydrolase, and glutathione S-transferases B, C, and E (Table 8).

Kidney

In rat kidney, sheep antiserum to rat hepatic microsomal NADPH-cytochrome P-450 reductase stained proximal and distal convoluted tubules (Fig. 6A), thick loops of Henle (Fig. 6B), and collecting ducts (Fig. 6B). Thin loops of Henle, however, appeared to be stained equally by this antiserum and normal sheep serum. While each of the other antibodies also stained rat kidney cells, only collecting ducts were stained for all enzymes (Table 9). Other marked differences in staining for these enzymes were also obvious: (a) thin loops of Henle were stained only for cytochrome P-450 MC-B; (b) cytochrome P-450 PCN-E was detected only within collecting ducts; (c) all enzymes except cytochrome P-450 PCN-E were detected within proximal and distal convoluted tubules; and (d) thick loops of Henle were stained only by antibodies to cytochrome P-450 PB-B, NADPH-cytochrome P-450 reductase, and glutathione S-transferases B, C, and E.

TABLE 9

IMMUNOHISTOCHEMICAL STAINING FOR CARCINOGEN-METABOLIZING ENZYMES IN RAT KIDNEY

Key: +, cells are stained; and -, cells are not stained.

Enzyme	Proximal Convoluted Tubule	Distal Convoluted Tubule	Thick Loops of Henle	Thin Loops of Henle	Collecting Ducts
Cytochrome P-450:					
rat MC-B	+	+	-	+	+
rat PB-B	+	+	+	-	+
rat PCN-E	-	-	-	-	+
NADPH-cytochrome P-450 reductase	+	+	+	-	+
Epoxide hydrolase	+	+	-	-	+
Glutathione S-transferase: B	+	+	+	-	+
C	+	+	+	-	+
E	+	+	+	-	+

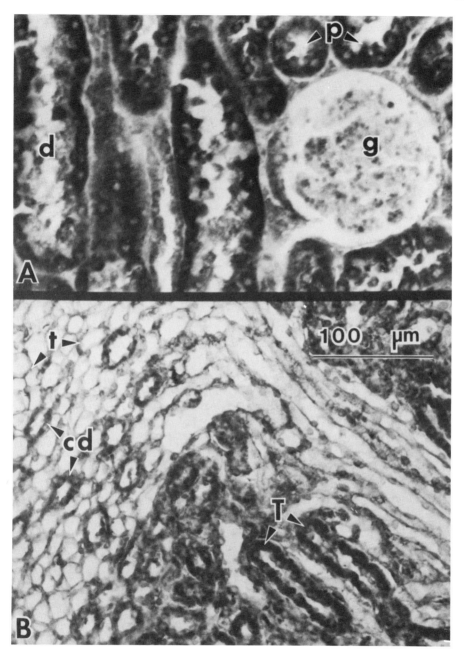

Fig. 6. Typical staining in rat kidney by anti-rat cytochrome P-450 reductase.
A, cortex: p = proximal and d = distal convoluted tubules; g = glomerulus.
B, medulla: T = thick and t = thin loops of Henle; cd = collecting ducts.

DISCUSSION

The results of this immunohistochemical investigation have unequivocally demonstrated that various cytochrome P-450 isozymes, NADPH-cytochrome P-450 reductase, epoxide hydrolase, and glutathione S-transferases B, C/A, and E, enzymes that participate in the metabolic activation and detoxication of most classes of chemical carcinogens (3,4), are present within the skin, breast, pancreas, lung, and kidney of untreated rats. Furthermore, human skin, breast, and prostate were also each found to contain cytochrome P-450 and NADPH-cytochrome P-450 reductase as well as antigens immunochemically related to rat hepatic microsomal cytochromes P-450 BNF-B, MC-B, PB-B, and PCN-E [the major isozymes of cytochrome P-450 that are induced in liver following pretreatment of rats with β-naphthoflavone, 3-methylcholanthrene, phenobarbital, and pregnenolone-16α-carbonitrile, respectively (19,20)] and rat hepatic glutathione S-transferases B, C/A, and E. Indeed, this communication contains the first description of the presence of these carcinogen-metabolizing enzymes in situ within cells in human breast, prostate, and skin, including cells of the secretory and duct portions of sweat glands. In addition to being present in these rat and human tissues, antigens that are immunochemically similar to rat hepatic microsomal cytochromes P-450 BNF-B, MC-B, PB-B, and PCN-E, NADPH-cytochrome P-450 reductase, and epoxide hydrolase and to rat hepatic glutathione S-transferases B, C/A, and E were also detected within the skin of untreated mice and pancreases of untreated hamsters. Thus, each of these tissues which is a target for chemically-induced carcinogenesis contains all of the carcinogen-metabolizing enzymes studied, thereby indicating that each possesses the enzymatic capability necessary for metabolically activating and detoxicating chemical carcinogens. It should be borne in mind, however, that the immunohistochemical staining technique employed in this investigation reveals only the presence of the antigens without providing any information regarding their catalytic functions within the cells in which they are found.

While the presence of carcinogen-metabolizing enzymes was immunohistochemically detected in each tissue examined, not all cell types within each tissue were found to be stained for these enzymes. These observed differences in the cellular localizations of carcinogen activating and detoxicating enzymes may be of potentially profound importance when attempting to understand the underlying biochemical bases for differences in susceptibilities to chemically-induced cancer and other toxicities among both morphologically similar and dissimilar cell types within a tissue, as well as among cells that originate from the same precursor cell.

In addition to differences observed in the intratissue distributions of these enzymes, a number of rather obvious species differences were apparent in the in situ localizations of certain enzymes within many of the tissues examined. Species differences in the intratissue localizations and distributions of carcinogen-metabolizing enzymes may provide an explanation for the numerous conflicting results that have been obtained employing different species as experimental models for investigations on carcinogenesis induced within a specific tissue by a given chemical or class of chemicals.

Finally, and perhaps of greatest importance, if one assumes that initiation of the neoplastic process occurs preferentially within those cells in which carcinogenic metabolites are generated and concentrated to the greatest extent, knowledge of differences in the intratissue localizations and distributions of enzymes that catalyze the activation and/or detoxication of chemical carcinogens may be critical for determining the cell(s) of origin of chemically-induced neoplasms in the skin, breast, prostate, pancreas, lung, and kidney.

ACKNOWLEDGMENTS

This investigation was supported in part by United States Public Health Service Grants GM 12675, CA 30140, CA 30907, ES 01590, and ES 02205. Dr. Guengerich is the recipient of Research Career Development Award number 00041 from the National Institute of Environmental Health Sciences, DHHS.

REFERENCES

1. Goldsmith, J.R. (1980) J. Environ. Pathol. Toxicol. 3, 205-217
2. Machine, R.M. and MacMahon, B. (1980) Epidemiol. Rev. 2, 18-48
3. Miller, E.C. (1978) Cancer Res. 38, 1479-1496
4. Wright, A.S. (1980) Mutat. Res. 75, 215-241
5. Greiner, J.W., Malan-Shibley, L.B. and Janss, D.H. (1980) Life Sci. 26, 313-319
6. Bartley, J., Bartholomew, J.C. and Stampfer, M.R. (1982) J. Cell. Biochem. 18, 135-148
7. Harris, C.C., Trump, B.F., Grafstrom, R. and Autrup, H. (1982) J. Cell. Biochem. 18, 285-294
8. Taira, Y., Redick, J.A., Greenspan, P. and Baron, J. (1979) Biochim. Biophys. Acta 583, 148-158
9. Taira, Y., Redick, J.A. and Baron, J. (1980) Mol. Pharmacol. 17, 374-381
10. Taira, Y., Greenspan, P., Kapke, G.F., Redick, J.A. and Baron, J. (1980) Mol. Pharmacol. 18, 304-312
11. Redick, J.A., Kawabata, T.T., Guengerich, F.P., Krieter, P.A., Shires, T.K. and Baron, J. (1980) Life Sci. 27, 2465-2470

12. Baron, J., Redick, J.A. and Guengerich, F.P. (1981) J. Biol. Chem. 256, 5831-5937

13. Kawabata, T.T., Guengerich, F.P. and Baron, J. (1981) Mol. Pharmacol. 20, 709-714

14. Baron, J., Redick, J.A. and Guengerich, F.P. (1982) J. Biol. Chem. 257, 953-957

15. Redick, J.A., Jakoby, W.B. and Baron, J. (1982) J. Biol. Chem. 257, 15200-15203

16. Mannervik, B. and Jensson, H. (1982) J. Biol. Chem. 257, 9909-9912

17. Habig, W.H., Pabst, M.J. and Jakoby, W.B. (1974) J. Biol. Chem. 249, 7130-7139

18. Wang, P., Mason, P.S. and Guengerich, F.P. (1980) Arch. Biochem. Biophys. 199, 206-219

19. Guengerich, F.P., Dannan, G.A., Wright, S.T., Martin, M.V. and Kaminsky, L.S. (1982) Biochemistry 21, 6019-6030

20. Guengerich, F.P. (1978) J. Biol. Chem. 253, 7931-7939

21. Guengerich, F.P., Wang, P. and Mason, P.S. (1981) Biochemistry 20, 2379-2385

22. Guengerich, F.P., Wang, P., Mitchell, M.B. and Mason, P.S. (1979) J. Biol. Chem. 254, 12248-12254

23. Fjellstedt, T.A., Allen, R.H., Duncan, B.K. and Jakoby, W.B. (1973) J. Biol. Chem. 248, 3702-3707

© 1983 Elsevier Science Publishers B.V.
Extrahepatic Drug Metabolism and Chemical Carcinogenesis,
J. Rydström, J. Montelius and M. Bengtsson eds.

IMMUNOHISTOCHEMICAL EVIDENCE FOR A HETEROGENEOUS DISTRIBUTION OF NADPH-CYTOCHROME P-450 REDUCTASE IN THE RAT AND MONKEY BRAIN

LENA HAGLUND[1], CHRISTER KÖHLER[2], TAPIO HAAPARANTA[1], MENEK GOLDSTEIN[3] AND JAN-ÅKE GUSTAFSSON[1]

[1]Department of Medical Nutrition, Karolinska Institute, Huddinge University Hospital F69, S-141 86 Huddinge, Sweden, [2]Department of Pharmacology, Astra Research Laboratories, ASTRA, S-151 85 Södertälje, Sweden and [3]Department of Neurochemistry, New York University Medical Center, New York, USA.

INTRODUCTION

The microsomal cytochrome P-450-dependent mixed function oxidases metabolize a variety of endogenous and exogenous compounds including drugs, carcinogens, fatty acids and steroids (1). The enzyme system consists of a lipid fraction, cytochrome P-450 and NADPH-cytochrome P-450 reductase. The latter enzyme supplies reducing equivalents from NADPH to cytochrome P-450 (2-5). Both cytochrome P-450 and NADPH-cytochrome P-450 reductase have been detected in brain tissue (6,7). Using specific antibodies against purified rat liver NADPH-cytochrome P-450 reductase in combination with immunohistochemical techniques we have now localized this enzyme, and possibly also indirectly identified cytochrome P-450, to defined neuronal structures in the rat and monkey brain.

METHODS

NADPH-cytochrome P-450 reductase was purified from rat liver microsomes according to the method of Guengerich and Martin (8) with minor modifications (9). The purified NADPH-cytochrome P-450 reductase was over 95% pure and the specific activity of the reductase was 44 μmoles cytochrome c reduced/min/mg protein as assayed in 300 mM potassium phosphate buffer, pH 7.7 at 25°C. Protein concentrations were determined by the method of Lowry et al (10), using bovine serum albumin as the standard. Antibodies were raised in rabbits and immunoglobulin G (IgG) fractions were isolated from the serum by affinity chromatography using a protein A-Sepharose CL-4B column (11) and concentrated to contain 25 mg protein/ml. IgG was isolated in a similar way from preimmune serum. The IgG fractions were dialyzed against potassium phosphate buffer (PBS, 10 mM, pH 7.4, containing 0.15 M NaCl). The antibodies were specific for the antigen by the following criteria: inhibition of NADPH-cytochrome c reductase activity with the purified antigen and with crude microsomes from rat liver, Ouchterlony immunodiffusion and immunoblotting. Brain microsomes were prepared according to the procedure described by Holtzman and Desautel (12). Immunoblotting was performed

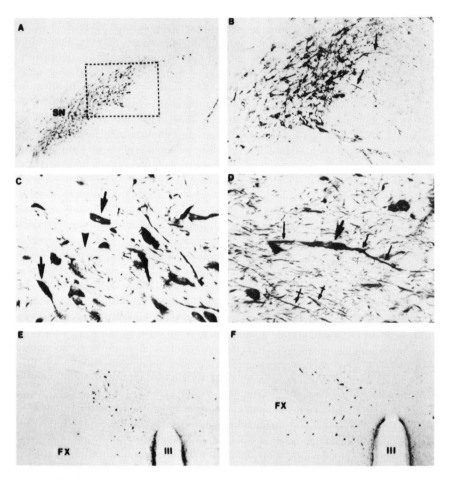

Fig. 1 (A-F)
Photomicrographs showing neurons in the substantia nigra (A-D) and hypothalamus
(E,F) containing strong NADPH-cytochrome P-450 reductase-LI. A large number of
NADPH-cytochrome P-450 reductase positive cell bodies are present throughout the
substantia nigra (SN) of the rat (A). Photomicrograph in B is an enlarged view
of the enclosed area in A. Photomicrographs in C and D shows NADPH-cytochrome
P-450 reductase positive neurons in pars compacta (arrows in C) and reticulata
(large arrow in D) of the monkey substantia nigra. Small arrows in D mark dendrites, crossed arrows point at dendrites of pars compacta cells that extend into
reticulata. Photomicrographs in E and F show NADPH-cytochrome P-450 reductase
positive neurons in the hypothalamus after incubation with the antibody alone
(E) and antibody preabsorbed with pure TH (150 μg/1000 μl diluted antibody at
+4°C for 24 hrs) (F). Peroxidase method. Nomarski phase interference contrast
for A-D. Magn. 80x(A,E,F), 325x(B), 520x(C,D). Abbreviations: Fx = fornix, SN =
substantia nigra, 111 = third ventricle.

essentially by the method of Towbin et al (13) with minor modifications (9).

For the immunohistochemical studies 15 rats (Sprague-Dawley, Anticimex, Stockholm, 180 g) of both sexes and two female monkeys (Talapoin, 1 kg) were sacrificed by transcardial perfusion. The rats were perfused with 600 ml, the monkeys with 1000 ml of a 0.1 M phosphate-buffer solution containing 4% para-formaldehyde (w/v, pH 7.4). Their brains were removed and cut in a cryostat (at 10 μm thickness) or on a Vibratome (at 70 μm). The sections were incubated with anti-NADPH-cytochrome P-450 reductase antibody (diluted 1:300 to 1:1500 in PBS containing 0.3% Triton X-100) for one to six days and the antigen-antibody com-plex visualized using either the immunofluorescence method of Coon (14) or the avidin-biotin-complex method of Hsu et al (15).

Two control experiments were performed to test the specific binding of the antibody: incubation of the sections with (a) preimmune serum or (b) anti-NADPH-cytochrome P-450 reductase IgG preabsorbed with the pure antigen. In neither of these experiments was immuno-reactivity detected in any of the brain areas examined. In double labelling experiments, to study the possible coexistence of NADPH-cytochrome P-450 reductase and tyrosine hydroxylase (TH) within the same neuron the method described by Nakane (16) and Gu (17) was used with elution pro-cedure according to the method of Tramu et al (18).

As control experiment against cross-reactivity between the anti-NADPH-cytochrome P-450 reductase antibody and TH, the antibody was preabsorbed with pure TH. This preabsorption did not block the neuronal staining with NADPH-cytochrome P-450 reductase antibody (Fig. 1; E, F).

RESULTS AND DISCUSSION

Neurons containing a strong NADPH-cytochrome P-450 reductase-like immuno-reactivity (-LI) are present within neuronal cell bodies of the following brain areas: the substantia nigra (SN) (Fig. 1; A-D), the ventral tegmental area of Tsai, the rostral part of dorsal raphe, the nucleus locus coeruleus and the ventrolateral medulla region of both rats and monkeys. NADPH-cytochrome P-450 reductase positive neurons are present also in the periventricular nucleus of the hypothalamus, the nucleus arcuatus (including the tanycytes of this nucleus) and the medial aspect of the zona incerta. No immunoreactivity could be seen in glia cells or in major myelinated fiber bundles.

All the brain areas listed above are known to harbour neurons containing the catecholamines dopamine (DA), noradrenaline (NA) or adrenaline (A) (19). Since the catecholamines (CA) are dependent on tyrosine hydroxylase (TH) for their syn-thesis (20), alternating sections were incubated with a well characterized anti-TH antibody (21,22). Analysis of these sections revealed an over-lapping distribution of cell bodies containing TH- and NADPH-cytochrome P-450 reductase -LI in the mes- and diencephalon and nerve terminals in several forebrain regions. These experiments strongly suggest that NADPH-cytochrome P-450 reductase and TH occur in the same populations of neurons. This hypothesis was confirmed in direct double labelling experiment where the same neuron in the SN and the hypothalamus was found to contain both NADPH-cytochrome P-450 reductase and TH-LI.

While most, if not all TH-positive cells contained NADPH-cytochrome P-450 reductase, many reductase-positive neurons did not contain tyrosine hydroxylase immunoreactivity.

The present study represents the first histochemical demonstration of NADPH-cytochrome P-450 reductase in the brain. The presence of NADPH-cytochrome P-450 reductase-LI in central neurons supports earlier biochemical findings of this enzyme in brain microsomal preparations (7).

Our immunohistochemical observation further extends the biochemical findings by identifying those neurons in the brains of the rat and monkey that contain the NADPH-cytochrome P-450 reductase.

The presence of NADPH-cytochrome P-450 reductase immunoreactivity in TH positive cells most likely indicates the existence of a cytochrome P-450 system within these neurons. This is of particular interest since cytochrome P-450 has been implied in the formation of catecholoestrogens. The conversion of oestradiol and oestrone to catecholoestrogens has been demonstrated in the CNS of rat (23) and good evidence has been provided (24) that the enzyme responsible for this conversion in the brain is identical to the cytochrome P-450 found in peripheral tissue. The presence of NADPH-cytochrome P-450 reductase in central CA neurons is of particular interest since the action of the catecholoestrogens in the CNS has been linked to their interaction with biogenic amines as competitive inhibitors of catechol-O-methyl-transferase (COMT) (25) and as possible inhibitors of TH (26) although it could also imply that CA's are being synthesized through an alternative pathway involving cytochrome P-450.

ACKNOWLEDGEMENTS

We thank Dr. James Halpert for providing the purified NADPH-cytochrome P-450 reductase. This study was supported by grants from the Swedish Medical Research Council (13X-2819).

REFERENCES
1.   Conney, A.H. (1982) Cancer Res. 42, 4875-4917.
2.   Lu, A.Y.H., Junk, K.W. & Coon, M.J. (1969) J. Biol. Chem. 244, 3714-3721.
3.   Dignam, J.D. & Strobel, H.W. (1977) Biochemistry 16, 1116-1123.

4. Yasukochi, Y. & Masters, B.S.S. (1976) J. Biol. Chem. 251, 5337–5344.

5. Vermilion, J.L. & Coon, M.J. (1978) J. Biol. Chem. 253, 2694–2704.

6. Cohn, J.A., Alvares, A.P. & Kappas, A. (1977) J. Exp. Med. 145, 1607–1611.

7. Sasame, H.A., Ames, M.M. & Nelson, S.D. (1977) Biochem. Biophys. Res. Commun. 78, 919–926.

8. Guengerich, F.P. & Martin, M.V. (1980) Arch. Biochem. Biophys. 205, 365–379.

9. Haaparanta, T., Halpert, J., Glaumann, H. & Gustafsson, J.-Å. (1983) Cancer Res. Submitted for publication.

10. Lowry, O.H., Rosebrough, N.J., Farr, A.L. & Randall, R.J. (1951) J. Biol. Chem. 193, 265–275.

11. Goding, J.W. (1976) J. Immunol. Meth. 13, 215–226.

12. Holtzman, D. & Desautel, M. (1980) J. Neurochem. 14, 1535–1537.

13. Towbin, H., Staehelin, T. & Gordon, J. (1979) Proc. Natl. Acad. Sci. USA 76, 4350–4354.

14. Coon, A.H. (1958) in: General Cytochemical Methods (Ed. Danielli, J.F.), Academic Press, New York, pp. 399–422.

15. Hsu, S.-M., Raine, L. & Fanger, H. (1981) J. Histochem. Cytochem. 29, 577–580.

16. Nakane, P.K. (1968) J. Histochem. Cytochem. 16, 557–560.

17. Gu, J., de Mey, J., Moeremans, M. & Polak, J.M. (1981) Regul. Peptides 1, 365–374.

18. Tramu, G., Pillez, A. & Leonardelli, J. (1978) J. Histochem. Cytochem. 26, 322–324.

19. Dahlström, A. & Fuxe, K. (1964) Acta Physiol. Scand. 62, Suppl. 232, 1–55.

20. Patrick, R.L. (1976) in: Neuroregulators and psychiatric disorders (eds. Usdin, E. et al), Oxford University Press, New York, pp. 88–94.

21. Hökfelt, T., Johansson, O., Fuxe, K. et al (1976) Medical Biol. 54, 427–453.

22. Markey, K.A., Kondo, H., Shenkman, L. & Goldstein, M. (1980) Molec. Pharm. 17, 79–85.

23. Fishman, J. & Norton, B. (1975) Endocrinology 96, 1054–1058.

24. Paul, S.M., Axelrod, J. & Diliberto, E.J.Jr. (1977) Endocrinology 101, 1604–1610.

25. Ball, P., Knuppen, R., Haupt, M. et al (1972) J. Clin. Endocrinol. Metab. 34, 736–746.

26. Lloyd, T. & Weisz, J. (1978) J. Biol. Chem. 253, 4841–4843.

© 1983 Elsevier Science Publishers B.V.
Extrahepatic Drug Metabolism and Chemical Carcinogenesis,
J. Rydström, J. Montelius and M. Bengtsson eds.

MICROSOMAL AND CYTOSOLIC EPOXIDE HYDROLASES: TOTAL ACTIVITIES, SUBCELLULAR
DISTRIBUTION AND INDUCTION IN THE LIVER AND EXTRAHEPATIC TISSUES

JOSEPH W. DePIERRE[1], JOHAN MEIJER[1], WINNIE BIRBERG[2], ÅKE PILOTTI[2],
LENNART BALK[2] AND JANERIC SEIDEGÅRD[3]

[1]Department of Biochemistry and [2]Department of Organic Chemistry, Arrhenius
Laboratory, University of Stockholm, S-106 91 Stockholm, Sweden and
[3]Wallenberg Laboratory, University of Lund, S-220 07 Lund, Sweden

INTRODUCTION

A large number of the xenobiotics to which we are exposed in increasing
amounts - including polycylic hydrocarbons, aflatoxins, vinyl chloride, and
many other compounds containing aromatic rings and/or unsaturated alkyl chains
- can be metabolized via the cytochrome P-450 system to epoxide intermediates.
It is also becoming clear that a number of endobiotics - including certain
steroids and vitamin K - are metabolized to epoxides as well.

Many of these intermediate epoxides are reactive enough to bind covalently
to cellular macromolecules, in particular protein, RNA and DNA. Such binding
is now thought to be responsible for many of the toxic and genotoxic (e.g.,
chemical carcinogenesis) effects of xenobiotics.

Epoxide hydrolases, localized both on the endoplasmic reticulum and in the
cytosol, can metabolize many reactive epoxides to non-reactive dihydrodiols.
These enzymes thus constitute an important cellular defense mechanism in
connection with the metabolism of numerous xenobiotics and even, it appears,
of certain endobiotics. Consequently, it is of great interest to characterize
the distribution, properties, and induction of these enzymes in different
tissues.

We have been studying the microsomal epoxide hydrolase for a number of
years (e.g., 1-5) and have recently begun investigating the cytosolic enzyme
as well (e.g., 6, 7). In the present communication we summarize our findings
concerning the total activities, certain properties, subcellular distribution
and induction of these enzymes in the liver and extrahepatic tissues.

MATERIALS AND METHODS

The tissues investigated here include the liver and lung from 180-200 g male
Sprague-Dawley rats (ALAB, Sollentuna, Sweden); the liver, lung, kidney and
testis from 20 g male C57 Bl mice (ALAB, Sollentuna, Sweden); the liver,
trunk kidney (homologous to the mammalian kidney) and the head kidney (homo-

logous to the mammalian adrenal gland) of 1-3 kg Northern pike (*Esox lucius*) of both sexes (local fishermen); and circulating lymphocytes prepared from healthy human volunteers using the Isopaque-Ficoll gradient technique. The experimental animals were starved before sacrifice. After homogenization of the different tissues in 0.25 M sucrose, nuclear, mitochondrial, microsomal, and cytosol fractions were prepared by differential centrifugation.

Epoxide hydrolase activity towards ^{3}H-styrene oxide (Radiochemical Centre, Amersham, England) and ^{3}H-*cis*- and -*trans*-stilbene oxide (synthesized by a modification of a published procedure (8)) was assayed using an extraction procedure to separate remaining substrate from the product (1, 8). The inducers phenobarbital (80 mg/kg body weight in 0.9% saline), 3-methylcholanthrene (20 mg/kg body weight in corn oil) and *trans*-stilbene oxide (400 mg/kg body weight in corn oil) were administered by intraperitoneal injection once daily for 5 days. Other inducers were administered at various doses in the same manner. Controls received the appropriate vehicle alone.

RESULTS

Total epoxide hydrolase activity in different tissues. In Table 1 the total epoxide hydrolase activities in different tissues of the rat, mouse and pike and in human lymphocytes are given. It can be seen that, as expected, the hepatic activity is considerably greater than that observed in other organs, but significant epoxide hydrolase activity can also be measured in the kidney, testis and lung (in order of decreasing activity) of rats and mice. Rat brain, pike head kidney (homologous to the mammalian adrenal gland) and human lymphocytes also demonstrate easily dectectable levels of this enzyme.

Properties of epoxide hydrolase in different tissues. Table 2 lists certain properties of the microsomal epoxide hydrolase activity in rat liver and lung and in human lymphocytes and of the cytosolic enzyme in human lymphocytes. The apparent K_m's for styrene oxide lie between 100 and 250 μM, whereas the apparent K_m values for *cis*- and *trans*-stilbene oxide are considerably lower. The microsomal enzyme demonstrates a pH optimum between 9 and 10, a value which is unusually high and for which no explanation has yet been offered. However, at pH 7.5, which is presumably the pH at which this enzyme operates *in vivo*, the microsomal epoxide hydrolase is about 70% as active as at its optimal pH. Another peculiar property of the soluble epoxide hydrolase in human lymphocytes is its unusually high optimal temperature. The epoxide hydrolase activity of pike liver microsomes also demonstrates an optimal temperature of about 50°C (9). Again, no explanation for this behaviour is available at present.

TABLE 1

TOTAL ACTIVITIES OF EPOXIDE HYDROLASE IN DIFFERENT TISSUES[a]

Organ	Activity (nmol/min-g wet weight) with		
	styrene oxide	*cis*-stilbene oxide	*trans*-stilbene oxide
Rat liver	306	910	–
lung	4.75	–	–
kidney	42.4	–	–
testis	26.6	–	–
brain	2.77	–	–
Mouse liver	–	27.9	384
lung	–	7.01	6.24
kidney	–	16.2	156
testis	–	17.2	4.24
Pike liver	51	–	–
trunk kidney[b]	–	24.8	–
head kidney[c]	–	4.37	–
Human lymphocytes	–	4.3	5.3

[a] Some of these data are from references 1 and 9
[b] homologous with the mammalian kidney
[c] homologous with the mammalian adrenal gland

Subcellular distribution of epoxide hydrolase activity. In Table 3 the
subcellular distributions of epoxide hydrolase activity towards styrene oxide
and *cis*- and *trans*-stilbene oxide in different tissues are illustrated. A
number of interesting conclusions can be drawn from these data. In the first
place, as originally reported by Oesch and coworkers (10), epoxide hydrolase
activity towards styrene oxide in rat tissues is located primarily in the
microsomal fraction. However, the rat is a special case in this respect,
since this animal demonstrates much lower cytosolic epoxide hydrolase
activity than is found in the organs of other rodents (11, 12). The distribution of epoxide hydrolase activity towards styrene oxide in pike liver is
probably more typical. In this case the specific activities in the mitochondrial, microsomal and cytosolic fractions are approximately equal. Since
both the microsomal and cytosolic epoxide hydrolases can metabolize styrene oxide
(6, 13) and since mitochondria have also been shown to contain these two

enzymes (14), the subcellular distribution of styrene oxide hydrolase activity seen with pike liver is what would be expected for a tissue containing both microsomal and cytosolic epoxide hydrolases.

TABLE 2

SELECTED PROPERTIES OF EPOXIDE HYDROLASES IN RAT LIVER AND LUNG AND IN HUMAN LYMPHOCYTES

The rat liver and lung microsomal enzymes were measured with styrene oxide as substrate (1). The lymphocyte enzymes were measured both with *cis*-stilbene oxide (microsomal) and *trans*-stilbene oxide (cytosolic) as substrates.

Property	Rat liver[a]	Rat lung[a]	Human lymphocytes	
			microsomal	cytosolic
Specific activity[b]	8	0.5	7.26	8.26
Apparent K_m (mM)	0.25	0.11-0.25	0.010	0.0016
pH optimum	8.7-9	9.7	9.8	6.8
Subcellular localization	endoplasmic reticulum	endoplasmic reticulum	membrane fraction	soluble fraction
Inducibility with Methylcholanthrene	none	none	?	?
Phenobarbital	300%	none	?	?
Styrene oxide	none	none	?	?
trans-stilbene oxide	720%	none	?	?
Inhibition with[c] 1,1,1-Trichloropropene 2,3-oxide	Uncomp.	Uncomp.		
Cyclohexane oxide	Noncomp.	Noncomp.		
Temperature maximum	?	?	40	60

[a] From reference 1
[b] nmols product/min-mg protein or 10^7 cells
[c] comp. = competitive

We have found the substrates *cis*- and *trans*-stilbene oxide to be useful in distinguishing between microsomal and cytosolic epoixde hydrolase activities. As can be seen in Table 3, *cis*-stilbene oxide hydrolase activity is distributed in subcellular fractions from the liver, lung, kidney and testis of mice and from the trunk and head kidneys of the pike in a manner typical of a component of the endoplasmic reticlum. Indeed, we feel that epoxide hydrolase activity

TABLE 3

SUBCELLULAR DISTRIBUTION OF EPOXIDE HYDROLASE ACTIVITIES IN RAT LIVER AND LUNG; MOUSE LIVER, LUNG, TESTIS AND KIDNEY; AND PIKE LIVER, TRUNK KIDNEY AND HEAD KIDNEY

The nuclear, mitochondrial, microsomal and cytosolic fractions were prepared using a traditional procedure of differential centrifugation (for further details, see references 1 and 9).

Tissue	Substrate	Specific activity (nmol product/min-mg protein)			
		Nuclear	Mitochondrial	Microsomal	Cytosolic
Rat liver	styrene oxide	0.62	0.98	3.53	0.15
lung	styrene oxide	0.11	0.31	0.51	0.070
Mouse liver	*cis*-stilbene oxide	0.12	0.25	1.55	0.075
	trans-stilbene oxide	1.26	6.83	0.38	6.91
lung	*cis*-stilbene oxide	0.060	0.16	0.86	0.007
	trans-stilbene oxide	0.067	0.067	0.100	0.050
kidney	*cis*-stilbene oxide	0.036	0.053	0.31	0.0081
	trans-stilbene oxide	0.79	3.17	0.35	2.44
testis	*cis*-stilbene oxide	0.36	0.50	2.41	0.034
	trans-stilbene oxide	0.144	0.132	0.075	0.060
Pike liver	styrene oxide	0.30	0.74	0.92	0.81
trunk kidney	*cis*-stilbene oxide	0.30	0.31	1.20	0.023
head kidney	*cis*-stilbene oxide	0.068	0.085	0.30	0.0098

towards *cis*-stilbene oxide is an excellent marker for the endoplasmic reticulum in all tissues which we have examined to date. On the one hand, the relative ease with which substrate of high specific radioactivity can be synthesized provides a sensitive assay procedure. On the other hand, microsomal epoxide hydrolase is quite resistant to attack by proteases (2) and would thus be expected to survive the relatively high protease activities present in homogenates from many extrahepatic tissues intact. For instance, in our attempts to prepare subcellular fractions suitable for studies of drug metabolism from the trunk and head kidneys of the pike we originally used NADPH-cytochrome *c* reductase as a marker for the endoplasmic reticulum. However, we soon found that 30-40% of this enzyme is solubilized in an active form from the microsomal membranes by endogenous proteases. This observation is consistent with earlier reports (e.g., 15) that NADPH-cytochrome *c* reductase activity can be solubilized from rat liver microsomes with proteases such as trypsin. In homogenates from the trunk and head kidneys of the pike epoxide hydrolase activity towards *cis*-stilbene oxide is not solubilized at all and could thus serve as a marker.

In contrast epoxide hydrolase activity towards *trans*-stilbene oxide is distributed in subcellular fractions from the liver and kidney of mice in a manner indicating that the enzyme responsible is present both in the cytosol and in mitochondria (Table 3). As mentioned above, Hammock and his coworkers (14) have demonstrated that the epoxide hydrolase enzyme which they originally discovered in the cytosol is also present in mitochondria. Most of the total *trans*-stilbene oxide hydrolase activity in mouser liver and kidney is localized in the cytosol, however, since this fraction contains 37% and 31%, respectively, of the total protein in these organs, whereas only 7% and 5%, respectively, of the total protein is recovered in the mitochondrial fraction.

The distribution of epoxide hydrolase activity towards *trans*-stilbene oxide in subcellular fractions from mouse lung and testis shown in Table 3 is somewhat unexpected. All of the fractions have approximately equal specific activities, a distribution pattern which cannot be satisfactorily explained at present. However, there is much more of the total *trans*-stilbene oxide hydrolase activity in the cytosol than in the mitochondrial and microsomal fractions in these organs as well, since the cytosol contains much more protein.

This presentation of results has assumed the existence of two major epoxide hydrolases, namely, a microsomal and a cytosolic enzyme. Recently, good evidence has been presented for the presence of a second epoxide hydrolase specific for cholesterol-5,6α-oxide on the endoplasmic reticulum (16, 17). The existence of this and of other as yet unidentified forms of epoxide hydrolase might effect the interpretations made here, i.e., such additional enzymes might clarify why the *trans*-stilbene oxide hydrolase activity is distributed among subcellular fractions from mouse lung and testis in the manner documented in Table 3.

TABLE 4

INDUCTION OF MICROSOMAL EPOXIDE HYDROLASE IN DIFFERENT ORGANS OF THE RAT

Styrene oxide was used as substrate.

	Percentage induction by		
Organ	3-Methylcholanthrene	Phenobarbital	*trans*-Stilbene oxide
Liver	35[a]	445[c]	521[c]
Intestine	17	78[b]	0
Kidney	0	0	77[b]
Lung	72	75	60
Testicles	0	31	23
Brain	0	0	0

[a] greater than the control value at the level of $P < 0.05$
[b] greater than the control value at the level of $P < 0.01$
[c] greater than the control value at the level of $P < 0.001$

Induction of epoxide hydrolase. It has been known for some time that pheno-barbital and *trans*-stilbene oxide both effectively induce the epoxide hydrolase activity of rat liver microsomes towards styrene oxide; whereas treatment of rats with the other classical inducer 3-methylcholanthrene or with the sub-strate styrene oxide has little or no effect on this enzyme (Table 2). In Table 4 we present the effects of administration of 3-methylcholanthrene, phenobarbital, or *trans*-stilbene oxide on epoxide hydrolase activity in different organs of the rat. (No significant epoxide hydrolase activity could be detected in the adrenal gland, spleen, or heart with styrene oxide, possibly because of the high background which characterizes use of this substrate).

The expected changes were observed in the liver after treatment with each of these inducers. In addition a 78% increase in the small intestinal activity was seen after phenobarbital treatment and a 77% increase in the kidney activity occurred during induction with *trans*-stilbene oxide. No other signi-ficant changes were seen. Other workers (18, 19) have also reported that administration of *trans*-stilbene oxide increases the activity of microsomal epoxide hydrolase in the rat kidney.

Recently, we have invested much effort in attempting to obtain induction of the cytosolic epoxide hydrolase with different chemicals (Table 5).

TABLE 5

SOME SUBSTANCES TESTED UNSUCCESSFULLY AS INDUCERS OF CYTOSOLIC EPOXIDE HYDRO-
LASE ACTIVITY IN MOUSE LIVER

phenobarbital	diethylnitrosamine
3-methylcholanthrene	ethionine
trans-stilbene oxide	ellipticine
cis-stilbene oxide	chalcone epoxide
2-acetylaminofluorene	3'-methyl-4-dimethyldiaminoazobenzene
dibenzoylmethane	aflatoxin B_1
cholesterol 5,6α-oxide	quercetin
cis-9,10-epoxystearate	5-pregnen-16α,17α-epoxy-3β-ol-20-one

A number of epoxides, including naturally occurring epoxides, were tested
as potential inducers in hopes of obtaining clues concerning possible endogenous functions of the cytosolic epoxide hydrolase. No induction was obtained with any of the substances which we have tried to date, with the
exception of phthalate, which gives an approximately 71% induction of the
specific activity. Hammock and his coworkers (personal communication) have
achieved substantial induction of the cytosolic epoxide hydrolase in mouse
liver with clofibrate and other hypolipidemic drugs. This finding raises
the interesting possibility that the cytosolic epoxide hydrolase may be mainly
responsible for the metabolism of lipid epoxides. Both the microsomal (20)
and cytosolic (21) enzymes are known to hydrolyze fatty acid oxides.

Future studies. We are in the process of isolating the cytosolic epoxide
hydrolase from the livers of rabbits and mice, a process which requires at
least 5 chromatographic steps with an overall yield of about 0.4%. Subsequently, we plan to characterize this enzyme using standard techniques of
protein chemistry and to obtain antibodies, which will be used, among other
things, to quantitate the enzyme in different subcellular fractions and organs.

ACKNOWLEDGEMENTS

The different studies reported here were supported by several different
grants - NIH grant 1RO1 CA 26261-04 and grants from the Swedish Natural
Science Research Council and Swedish Natural Environment Protection Board.

REFERENCES

1. Seidegård, J., DePierre, J.W., Moron, M.S., Johannesen, K.A.M. and Ernster, L. (1977) Cancer Res., 37, 1075-1082.

2. Seidegård, J., Moron, M.S., Eriksson, L.C. and DePierre, J.W. (1978) Biochim. Biophys. Acta, 543, 29-40.

3. Seidegård, J., Morgenstern, R., DePierre, J.W. and Ernster, L. (1979) Biochim. Biophys. Acta, 586, 10-21.

4. Seidegård, J., DePierre, J.W., Morgenstern, R., Pilotti, Å. and Ernster, L. (1981) Biochim. Biophys. Acta, 672, 65-78.

5. Seidegård, J. and DePierre, J.W. (1981) Eur. J. Biochem., 112, 643-648.

6. Meijer, J., Månér, S., Birberg, W., Pilotti, Å. and DePierre, J.W. (1982) Acta Chem. Scand., B36, 549-551.

7. Meijer, J., Birberg, W., Pilotti, Å. and DePierre, J.W., this volume.

8. Gill, S.S. and Hammock, B.D., Anal. Biochem., in press.

9. Balk, L., Meijer, J., Seidegård, J., Morgenstern, R. and DePierre, J.W. (1980) Drug Metab. Dispos., 8, 98-103.

10. Oesch, F., Jerina, D.M. and Daley, J. (1971) Biochim. Biophys. Acta, 227, 685.

11. Gill, S.S. and Hammock, B.D. (1980) Biochem. Pharmacol., 29, 389.

12. Ota, K. and Hammock, B.D. (1980) Science, 207, 1479.

13. Waechter, F., Merdes, M., Bieri, F., Stäubli, W. and Bentley, P. (1982) Eur. J. Biochem., 125, 457.

14. Gill, S.S. and Hammock, B.D. (1981) Biochem. Pharmacol., 30, 2111.

15. Orrenius, S., Berg, A. and Ernster, L. (1969) Eur. J. Biochem., 11, 193.

16. Watabe, T., Kanai, M., Isobe, M. and Ozawa, H. (1981) J. Biol. Chem., 256, 2900.

17. Levin, W., Michaud, D.P., Thomas, P.E. and Jerina, D.M. (1983) Arch. Biochem. Biophys., 220, 485.

18. Oesch, F. and Schamssmann, H. (1979) Biochem. Pharmacol, 28, 171.

19. Kuo, C.-H., Hook, J.B. and Bernstein, J. (1981) Toxicol., 22, 149.

20. Sevanian, A., Stein, R.A. and Mead, J.F. (1981) Lipids, 16, 78.

21. Gill, S.S. and Hammock, B.D. (1979) Biochem. Biophys. Res. Commun, 89, 965.

METABOLISM OF CHEMICAL CARCINOGENS BY PROSTAGLANDIN H SYNTHASE

T. E. ELING, G. A. REED, J. A. BOYD, R. S. KRAUSS AND K. SIVARAJAH

National Institute of Environmental Health Sciences, Laboratory of
Pulmonary Function and Toxicology, Prostaglandin Group, P.O. Box 12233,
Research Triangle Park, N.C. 27709

The ubiquitous enzyme prostaglandin H synthase (PHS) catalyzes the conversion of arachidonic acid (AA) to the endoperoxide PGH_2. PGH_2 is a pivotal point from which prostaglandins, thromboxane and prostacyclin arise. A unique aspect of PHS is that a single protein possesses two enzymatic activities. The fatty acid cyclooxygenase activity of PHS catalyzes the formation of the hydroperoxy endoperoxide PGG_2, while the hydroperoxidase activity reduces the hydroperoxide moiety of PGG_2 to the alcohol, yielding PGH_2 (Fig. 1).

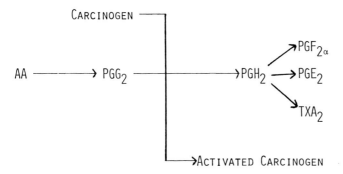

Fig. 1. Scheme for the conversion of chemicals to carcinogens by PHS.

A wide variety of chemicals are oxidized during this reduction of PGG_2 to PGH_2. This has been termed co-oxidation. In addition to PGG_2, other lipid hydroperoxides and hydrogen peroxide can support the oxidation of various chemicals. Non-steroidal anti-inflammatory drugs (i.e., indomethacin) inhibit the fatty acid cyclo-oxygenase activity but not the peroxidase activity. This can inhibit AA-dependent PHS-catalyzed oxidation of chemicals by inhibiting the formation of PGG_2. (For review see Ref. 1).

Metabolism of chemicals, particularly oxidation, is of importance in determining the carcinogenic activity of the chemical. It is generally accepted that many chemicals are not themselves carcinogenic but must be metabolized or activated to electrophilic metabolite(s) which are the ultimate carcinogens (2,3). Considerable literature testifies to the importance of mixed-function oxidases in chemical metabolism. However, it is possible that PHS could serve as an alternate system for carcinogen metabolism, particular in extra-hepatic tissues which are low in mixed-function oxidase activity and, in many cases, rich in PHS activity. To investigate this possibility, we have examined the metabolism of two classes of carcinogens by PHS and the possible role of PHS-dependent metabolism in the initiation of tumors in extra-hepatic tissues.

Polycyclic aromatic hydrocarbons (PAH)

Extensive studies show that the ultimate carcinogenic metabolite of the polycyclic aromatic hydrocarbon benzo(a)pyrene (BP) is the anti-diol epoxide (anti-BPDE) formed by oxidation of trans-7,8-dihydroxy-7,8-dihydro-benzo(a)pyrene (BP-7,8-diol) (4,5). Ram seminal vesicle microsomal fractions and the microsomal fractions (6,7) from a variety of pulmonary tissues including human tissue (8), catalyzed the PHS dependent conversion of (±)-BP-7,8-diol to (±)-anti-BPDE. In contrast, the mixed function oxidase system converted (±)-BP-7,8-diol to a mixture of syn- and anti-BPDE (Fig. 2) (9,10). BP-7,8-diol became covalently bound to poly G added to incubations containing AA, BP-7,8-diol, and PHS (11). Furthermore, PHS converted BP-7,8-diol to a mutagen(s) as measured in a modified Ames test (12,13). Studies with C3H 10T1/2 fibroblasts and BP-7,8-diol demonstrated that stimulation of PHS activity leads to increased cell transformation (14). These in vitro studies suggested a role for PHS in the initiation of tumors by PAH.

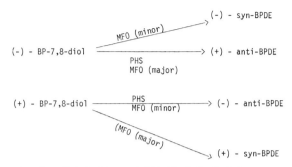

Fig. 2. Metabolism of (±) BP-7,8-diol by PHS and Mixed Function Oxidases.

From these studies a question arises: Can the co-oxidation of BP-7,8-diol by PHS occur in intact cells which are targets for the tumorigenic action of BP. To answer this question we have studied the metabolism of (±)-BP-7,8-diol in hamster trachea, which has been used as a model for studying BP-induced carcinogenesis. (±)-BP-7,8-diol was metabolized by the hamster trachea to a mixture of tetrols derived from the anti- and syn-BPDE (15). The ratio of anti- to syn-BPDE was approximately 2:1, as seen in Fig. 3.

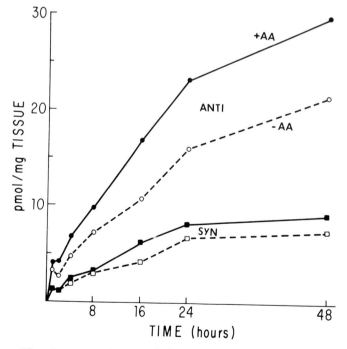

Fig. 3. Metabolism of (±)-BP-7,8-diol to BPDE's by hamster trachea explants.

The addition of AA (100 μM) produced a 50% increase in the formation of
anti-BPDE. The ratio of anti- to syn-BPDE increased to approximately 3:1.
Indomethacin did not inhibit basal metabolism but did inhibit the AA-induced
increase in metabolism (data not shown). The stimulation of anti-BPDE formation by AA and the sensitivity of the stimulation to indomethacin
suggested that the increased anti-BPDE formation was catalyzed by PHS.
These findings indicate a possible role for the co-oxidation of BP-7,8-diol in
the induction of neoplasia in hamster trachea by BP.

Aromatic Amines:

Aromatic amines, in general, are excellent subtrates for PHS hydroperoxidase. We have previously shown that a number of N-methyl substituted aromatic
amines are extensively N-demethylated by PHS via a free radical mechanism
(16). We have recently demonstrated that PHS and horseradish peroxidase
metabolize the aromatic amine bladder carcinogen benzidine and its noncarcinogenic congener tetramethylbenzidine, converting each to a free

radical cation and a diimine (17,18,19). We have also recently studied
the metabolism of the liver and bladder carcinogen 2-aminofluorene (2-AF)
by PHS and characterized the metabolites formed (20). The metabolites isolated by HPLC and characterized by UV-visible spectrophotometry and mass
spectrometry were 2-nitrofluorene and azofluorene (Table 1). In addition
to the formation of organic extractable metabolites, AA-dependent co-oxidation of 2-AF resulted in products which were water soluble and covalently
bound to the microsomal protein. The metabolism was dependent on AA, inhibited by the addition of indomethacin and also supported by H_2O_2 or
15-hydroperoxy-AA rather than AA. The addition of glutathione depressed
the overall metabolism of 2-AF by PHS and significantly increased the percentage of water soluble metabolite(s). These data suggest that 2-AF is
metabolized by PHS to an electrophilic metabolite. The electrophiles could

be N-hydroxy-2-AF and/or 2-nitrosoflourene, since both of these oxygenated

metabolites are rapidly converted to 2-nitrofluorene by PHS. However we were

unable to detect either of these metabolites. Other data suggest that 2-AF

is oxidized to a free radical intermediate in a manner similar to the oxi-

dation of benzidine by PHS (20). These free radicals could be the

electrophilic metabolites that bind to protein and are mutagenic (see below).

TABLE 1   ARACHIDONIC ACID - DEPENDENT CO-OXIDATION OF 2-AF BY PHS[a]

Incubation	2-Nitro-fluorene	Azo-fluorene	Water Soluble	Covalently Bound
Complete system[b]	5.0 ± 1.8	7.3 ± 1.1	3.0 ± 0.2	7.9 ± 0.6
-Arachidonic acid	0.9 ± 0.2	2.2 ± 0.3	0.2 ± 0.0	0.5 ± 0.0
+Indomethacin[c]	1.2 ± 0.6	2.4 ± 0.5	0.2 ± 0.1	0.9 ± 0.1
+Gluthathione[d]	1.1 ± 0.4	1.9 ± 0.8	4.1 ± 0.3	3.4 ± 0.3
-Arachidonic acid +NADPH[e]	0.8 ± 0.1	1.3 ± 0.6	0.3 ± 0.6	0.6 ± 0.1

[a]All values are (nmol/incubation) mean ± standard deviation, n=4. [b]The
complete systems contains: 0.025 M potassium phosphate buffer, pH 7.8,
0.8 mg ram seminal vesicle microsomal protein, 50 μM (^{3}H)-2-AF, 100 μM
arachidonic acid, and water to make 2 ml. [c]Indomethacin = 100 μM.
[d]Gluthathione =500μM. [e]NADPH = 1 mM.

Formation of mutagens

Ample evidence exists for the formation of electrophilic metabolites

from aromatic amines and polycyclic aromatic hydrocarbons by PHS. PHS, used

in place of the mixed-function oxidase of rat liver microsomes, will metabolize

chemicals to mutagens as measured in strains of Salmonella typhimurium. As

seen in Table 2, PHS selectively activates dihydrodiol metabolites of PHS

which contain an isolated bay-region double bond, to mutagens (12,13). The

parent hydrocarbons and other diol metabolites are not activated. Thus, the

proximate carcinogenic metabolites of PHS can be activated by PHS to their

ultimate carcinogenic forms.

TABLE 2   CHEMICALS TESTED FOR MUTAGENICITY USING PHS AS THE ACTIVATING
ENZYME

Chemical	Relative Mutagenicity	Strain
Polycyclic Aromatic Hydrocarbons:		
Benzo[a]pyrene	–	TA98, TA100
Benzo[a]pyrene-7,8-diol	++++	TA98, TA100
Benzo[a]pyrene-4,5-diol	–	TA98
Benzo[a]pyrene-9,10-diol	–	TA98
Benzo[a]pyrene,7,8-dihydro-	+++++	TA98
Benzo[a]pyrene,9,10-dihydro-	–	TA98
Benzo[a]anthracene	–	TA100
Benzo[a]anthracene-3,4-diol	+++	TA100
Benzo[a]anthracene-1,2-diol	–	TA100
Benzo[a]anthracene-8,9-diol	–	TA100
Benzo[a]anthracene-10,11-diol	–	TA100
Chrysene	–	TA100
Chrysene trans-1,2-diol	+++	TA100
Chrysene trans-3,4-diol	–	TA100
Chrysene trans-5,6-diol	–	TA100
Chrysene cis-5,6-diol	–	TA100
Aromatic Amines		
2-Aminofluorene	+++	TA98
2-Acetylaminofluorene	+	TA98
Benzidine	++	TA98
2,4,-Diaminoanisole	+	TA1538
2,5,-Diaminoanisole	++	TA1538
α-Naphthylamine	–	TA1538
β-Naphthylamine	++	TA1538
Aniline	–	TA98
2-Aminoanthracene	–	TA98

Aromatic amines are also oxidized by PHS to derivatives mutagenic to
S. typhimurium. 2-Aminofluorene, benzidine and β-naphthylamine are activated
to mutagens by PHS, whereas 2-acetylaminofluorene and α-napthylamine are not
(Table 2) (21). 2-aminofluorene was also activated by PHS to a species
mutagenic toward a bacterial strain (TR-98) deficient in nitroreducase.
The mutagen thus appears to be an intermediate in the conversion of 2-AF to
2-nitrofluorene and azofluorene (22), and does not result from the activation of 2-nitrofluorene by bacterial reductases. These results suggest
that PHS is capable of activating a wide range of chemicals and may serve
as an additional activating system to the mixed-function oxidases for use in
the study and screening of chemicals as potential mutagens.

SUMMARY

Co-oxidation of chemicals during prostaglandin biosynthesis are hydroperoxide-dependent oxidations catalyzed by the hydroperoxidase component of PHS. Electrophilic derivatives of polycyclic aromatic hydrocarbons and aromatic amines are generated which bind to protein and DNA and, in certain cases, are mutagenic. Mechanisms of oxidations by PHS appear to be distinct from those of cytochrome P-450. Consequently, PHS may provide a complementary enzyme for the metabolic activation of toxins, mutagens, and carcinogens.

Most of the research on co-oxidation has employed in vitro studies designed to determine whether PHS can catalyze the formation of toxic and/or carcinogenic derivatives of xenobiotics. Such studies have shown that it can. The focus of future investigations will shift to determine if this pathway of metabolism can play a role in chemically-induced toxicity in vivo.

REFERENCES

1.   Marnett, L. J., and Eling, T. (1982) in: Hodgson, E., Bend, J. R. and Philpot, R. M. (Eds.), Review of Biochemical Toxicology, Elsevier Press.

2.   Miller, E. C. and Miller, J. A. (1966) Pharmacol. Rev., 18, 805.

3.   Miller, E. C. and Miller, J. A. (1981) Cancer 47, 2327.

4.   Sims, P. and Grover, P. L. (1974) Adv. Cancer Res. 20, 165-274.

5.   Huberman, E., Sach, L., Yang, S. K. and Gelboin, H. V. (1976) Proc. Natl. Acad. Sci. USA 73, 607-611.

6.   Marnett, L. J., Johnson, J. T., and Bienkowski, M. J. (1979) FEBS Letts., 106, 13.

7.   Sivarajah, K., Mukhtar, H., and Eling, T. E. (1979) FEBS Letts., 106, 17.

8.   Sivarajah, K., Lasker, J. M., and Eling, T. E. (1981) Cancer Res., 41, 1834.

9.   Thakker, D. R., Yagi, H., Akagi, H., Koreeda, M., Lu, A. Y. H., Levin, W. Wood, A. W., Conney, A. H., and Jerina, D. M. (1977) Chem. Biol. Interactions, 16, 281.

10. Deutsch, J., Vatsis, K. P., Coon, M. J., Leutz, J. C., and Gelboin, H. V. (1979) Mol. Pharmacol., 16, 1011.

11. Panthananickal, A., and Marnett, L. J. (1981) Chem. Biol. Interactions, 33, 239.

12. Marnett, L. J., Reed, G. A., and Dennison, D. J. (1978) Biochem. Biophys. Res. Comm., 82, 210.

13. Guthrie, J., Robertson, I. G. C., Zeiger, E., Boyd, J. A., and Eling, T. E. (1982) Cancer Res., 42, 1620.

14. Boyd, J. A., Barrett, J. C., and Eling, T. E. (1982) Cancer Res., 42, 2628.

15. Reed, G., Grafstrom, R., Krauss, R., Harris, C., Autrup H., and Eling T. E. (1983), submitted.

16. Sivarajah, K., Lasker, J. M., Eling, T. E., and Abou-Donia, M. B. (1982) Mol. Pharmacol., 21, 133.

17. Josephy, P. D., Mason, R. P., and Eling, T. E. (1982) Cancer Res., 42, 2567.

18. Josephy, P. D., Eling, T. E., and Mason, R. P. (1982) J. Biol. Chem., 257, 3669.

19. Josephy, P. D., Eling, T. E., and Mason, R. P. (1983) J. Biol. Chem., in press.

20. Boyd, J. A., Harvan, D. J., and Eling, T. E. (1983) J. Biol. Chem., in press.

21. Robertson, I. G. C., Sivarajah, K., Eling, T. E., and Zeiger, E. (1983) Cancer Res., 43, 476.

22. Boyd, J. A., Zeiger, E., and Eling, T. E. Unpublished observations.

© 1983 Elsevier Science Publishers B.V.
Extrahepatic Drug Metabolism and Chemical Carcinogenesis,
J. Rydström, J. Montelius and M. Bengtsson eds.

PROSTAGLANDIN SYNTHASE CATALYZED METABOLISM OF p-PHENETIDINE TO REACTIVE PRODUCTS

PETER MOLDÉUS[1], ROGER LARSSON[1], DAVID ROSS[1], BO ANDERSSON[1], MAGNUS NORDENSKJÖLD[2], ANVER RAHIMTULA[3] AND BJÖRN LINDEKE[4]
[1]Department of Forensic Medicine, Karolinska Institutet,
[2]Department of Clinical Genetics, Karolinska Hospital,
S-104 01 Stockholm (Sweden), [3]Department of Biochemistry,
Memorial University of New Foundland, New Foundland (Canada)
and [4]Department of Organic Pharmaceutical Chemistry, University
of Uppsala, S-751 23 Uppsala (Sweden).

INTRODUCTION

There are now several examples of xenobiotics which are metabolized in peroxidase-type reactions catalyzed by enzyme systems such as prostaglandin synthase (PGS) and horse radish peroxidase (HRP) (1,2). With certain compounds these reactions may result in the formation of reactive metabolites which can bind to protein and nucleic acids (3-5), and induce bacterial mutations (6). Since the PGS activity is relatively high in certain extrahepatic tissues, such as the lung, kidney and gastrointestinal tract (7), this enzyme system has been suggested to catalyze the metabolic activation of compounds exhibiting extrahepatic toxicity and carcinogenicity.

Even though a peroxidase-type reaction implies the formation of substrate free radicals the existence of a radical intermediate has been firmly established in only a few cases. Formation of free radical intermediates of acetaminophen (8), aminopyrine (9), 1-phenyl-3-pyrazolidone (10) and 3,5,3',5'-tetramethylbenzidine (11,12) have been demonstrated directly by electron spin resonance spectroscopy.

The stable products which are ultimately formed in free radical reactions are bound to be numerous, and are frequently complex. When aromatic structures are involved, free radical reactions tend to give rise to intensely colored products, indicating the formation of extended conjugated systems (1,11).

Phenacetin is an analgesic and antipyretic drug which is recognized to be responsible for several toxic effects in the kidney and lower urinary tract including both renal necrosis and tumours after long-term exposure. The mechanism of this nephrotoxicity is not well understood but since PGS activity is high in the kidney a PGS catalyzing deactivation has been suggested to be involved. Phenacetin itself is not a substrate for PGS but p-phenetidine, a major *in vitro* metabolite of phenacetin, is (13,14). The present manuscript summarizes recent findings regarding the PGS dependent metabolism of p-phenetidine to reactive and stable products. The relevance of this metabolism for phenacetin-induced toxicity is discussed.

METHODS

Microsomes from ram seminal vesicles (RSV) were isolated as described previously (15).

Incubations with RSV microsomes and horse radish peroxidase were performed in a 0.1 M phosphate buffer, pH 8.0, supplemented with 1.0 mM EDTA.

Experiments involving irreversible binding to protein and DNA, and DNA single strand breaks in cultured human fibroblasts were performed as described elsewhere (14,16,13).

Oxidized glutathione was determined using the method by Reed *et al.* (17). Glutathione conjugates of p-phenetidine were determined in the water phase after extraction with ether.

Thin layer chromatography was performed using silica plates and a mobile phase of chloroform 19, methanol 1.

RESULTS AND DISCUSSION

Microsomes from RSV contain high PGS activity. In the presence of arachidonic acid (AA) RSV microsomes catalyzed the irreversible binding of p-phenetidine to protein and a calf thymus DNA (Table I; 14,16). The reactions which had high affinity for p-phenetidine, were linear only for a few seconds and levelled off after one minute of incubation (14,16) probably due to the selfdeactivation of PGS known to occur during PG synthesis from AA.

TABLE I

PROSTAGLANDIN SYNTHASE DEPENDENT BINDING OF (^{14}C) p-PHENETIDINE
TO PROTEIN AND DNA

Incubation conditions	p-Phenetidine bound	
	nmol/mg protein /30 sec	pmol/mg DNA /30 sec
Complete system	15.2±1.2	17.0±1.2
Boiled microsomes	0	0
- Arachidonic acid	0	1.0±0.9
+ Indomethacin, 100 μM	0.5±0.2	1.7±0.1
+ BHA, 0.5 mM	0.1	1.7±0.5
- Arachidonic acid		
+ Hydrogen peroxide, 1 mM	16.6±0.2	14.5±0.9

Complete system: RSV microsomes (1 mg/ml); p-phenetidine,
50 μM; EDTA, 1 mM; Phosphate buffer pH 8, 100 mM and arachidonic acid, 100 μM. Reactions were started by the addition
of arachidonic acid.

The metabolism of p-phenetidine to species which bind to both
DNA and protein was dependent on AA and inhibited by indomethacin,
an inhibitor of the cyclooxygenase activity of PGS. PGS contain
two activities, a cyclooxygenase activity catalyzing the oxygenation of AA to the hydroperoxy endoperoxide (PGG_2) and a hydroperoxidase activity catalyzing the reduction of PGG_2 to the hydroxy
endoperoxide PGH_2. It is the latter activity which is responsible
for the metabolism of p-phenetidine since organic hydroperoxides
like linolenic hydroperoxide as well as hydrogen peroxide were
able to support the reaction (Table I; 14,16). The hydroperoxide
supported reaction was thus not inhibited by cyclooxygenase inhibitors like indomethacin.

In the presence of RSV microsomes and AA p-phenetidine is
metabolized to reactive product(s) that not only bind to protein
and exogenous DNA but also induce single strand breaks in DNA of
cultured human fibroblasts (Table II; 13). When RSV microsomes
were coincubated with cultured human fibroblasts the fraction

TABLE II

EFFECT OF p-PHENETIDINE ON THE INDUCTION OF DNA STRAND BREAKS
IN HUMAN FIBROBLASTS

Incubation conditions	Fraction of single-stranded DNA (%)
Solvent control	24.3±7.3
p-Phenetidine, 50 μM	41.5±9.8
+ Indomethacin, 0.1 mM	20.8±2.8
+ Acetyl salicylic acid, 1 mM	24.7±2.3

Incubations were performed as described in (13)

single stranded DNA was doubled in the presence of p-phenetidine.
The reaction was catalyzed by PGS since indomethacin and acetyl-
salicylic acid prevented the p-phenetidine induced increase in
the fraction single stranded DNA.

It is generally agreed that peroxidase catalyzed reactions such
as PGS dependent cooxidation, involve the formation of free radical intermediates from the substrate undergoing oxidation. Radical intermediates have been positively identified by ESR spectroscopy during PGS dependent cooxidation of several substrates. As
yet we have been unable to detect any radical intermediate produced during the peroxidase catalyzed metabolism of p-phenetidine
using ESR spectroscopy. This may be due to the inherent instabil-
ity of such a species and indeed several other lines of experimental data indicate that the PGS dependent metabolism of p-phenetidine involvs the formation of a free radical intermediate. For
instance glutathione (GSH) is rapidly oxidized if included in a
reaction containing RSV microsomes, AA and p-phenetidine (Fig. 1;
13). The oxidation of GSH is considerably higher than the formation of glutathione conjugates (Fig. 1). GSH thus probably serve
as an electron donor to a p-phenetidine radical, resulting in the
formation of a glutathione thiyl radical which yields GSSG after
dimerization (See Fig. 3). Other radicals such as chlorpromazine
radicals have been shown to be reduced by GSH in a similar manner

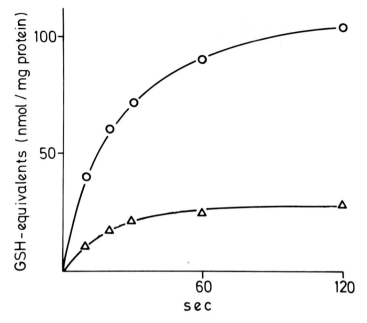

Fig. 1. Phenetidine GSH conjugate formation and p-phenetidine
dependent oxidation of GSH in an incubation with RSV microsomes
(1 mg/ml) AA (100 µM) and GSH (1 mM). GSSG, o; p-phenetidine
glutathione conjugate, Δ.

(18). Furthermore, a stoichiometry of 2 between AA and p-phenetidine metabolism has been observed indicating a radical reaction
(19). If GSH is present in the incubation much less p-phenetidine
is consumed due to the GSH dependent reduction of the radical
back to p-phenetidine.

The structure of the p-phenetidine radical is not known but
initially a cation radical localized on the nitrogen is probably
formed which may subsequently rearrange to a carbon centered
radical (see Fig. 3).

Further support for a radical mechanism in the PGS catalyzed
oxidation of p-phenetidine lies is the broad spectrum of coloured
products formed (Table III;19). Seven coloured bands could be
separated on thin layer chromatography, two of which consisted
of more than one metabolite. The yellow band (RF = 0.70) contained
two metabolites and the one at the origin four metabolites.

TABLE III

CHARACTERISTICS OF p-PHENETIDINE METABOLITES FORMED IN PROSTA-
GLANDIN SYNTHASE AND HORSERADISH PEROXIDASE CATALYZED REACTIONS

Metabolite	RSVM/AA[1]		HRP/H_2O_2[2]	
	Rf	Colour	Rf	Colour
7	0.74	Pink	–	–
6[+]	0.70	Yellow	0.70	Yellow
5	0.65	Orange	0.65	Orange
4	0.56	Purple	0.56	Purple
3	0.25	Brown	0.25	Brown
2	0.10	Red	0.10	Red
1[†]	0	Origin	0	Origin

[1]- 100 μM phenetidine, 100 μM AA, solubilized PGS prep.
[2]- 500 μM phenetidine, 1 mM H_2O_2, 0.2 μg/ml HRP
[+]- A mixture of two yellow metabolites
[†]- A mixture of four metabolites

The metabolite pattern was almost identical when horseradish
peroxidase (HRP) and hydrogen peroxide (H_2O_2) was used in place
of RSV microsomes and AA (Table III). This clearly indicate that
the mechanism of metabolism of p-phenetidine by the two peroxidases are very similar. The HRP/H_2O_2 system could therefore be used
in place of PGS for studies on the mechanism of formation and
structural identification of the secondary products.

So far reliable structural identification of only two products
has been achieved. Using electron impact (EI) mass spectrometry
the red metabolite (Rf = 0.40) has been identified as a p-phenetidine trimer and the yellow band (Rf = 0.70) has been shown to
contain two diazo phenetidine derivatives. These metabolites are
stable and do not react with GSH and protein.

Thus, it seems probable that the peroxidase catalyzed metabolism
of p-phenetidine yields a radical intermediate and several secondary oligmeric products. Whether the radical intermediate or the
secondary product(s) are responsible for the binding and DNA

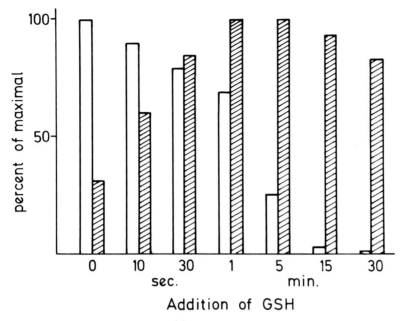

Fig. 2. GSH oxidation (□) and GSH conjugate formation (▨) in incubations with HRP/H_2O_2 and p-phenetidine. Reactions were run for 30 min and GSH added at the times indicated. Data from ref. 20.

damage was investigated in an experiment where GSH was added after various times after initiation of HRP/H_2O_2 catalyzed metabolism of p-phenetidine (Fig. 2). The reactions were run for 30 min and the fraction of GSSG versus GSH conjugate formed was followed, the amount of GSSG thus indicating the amount of p-phenetidine radical.

From the results presented in Fig. 2 it is evident that the fraction of GSH oxidized decreases rapidly if GSH is added after the start of incubation. This result was expected since HRP/H_2O_2 catalyzed metabolism of p-phenetidine during these conditions levelled off after a few minutes and all p-phenetidine metabolized after 5 min. On the contrary the amount of GSH conjugate(s) formed increased if GSH was added after the incubation had started and was maximal after 5 min of incubation. These results thus suggest that a reactive product secondary to a radical intermediate is to

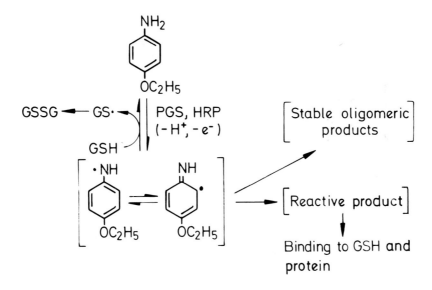

Fig. 3. Possible mechanism for peroxidase catalyzed oxidation of p-phenetidine.

a major extent responsible for the binding to GSH. Similar results have been obtained with protein added after incubation.

The nature of the reactive p-phenetidine product has not yet been firmly elucidated but preliminary evidence points to a dimeric product, probably the diimine formed by a head to tail coupling of two p-phenetidine radicals and loss of acetaldehyde. This is also supported by the fact that acetaldehyde is formed during p-phenetidine metabolism (20).

The relevance for the peroxidase dependent metabolic activation of p-phenetidine catalyzed by prostaglandin-synthase for the phenacetin induced nephrotoxicity in man remains to be established. Support for such an involvement comes from results using human kidney medulla. This tissue was shown to be able to catalyze the irreversible binding of p-phenetidine to protein in the presence of either AA or a hydroperoxide (21). If the same reactive metabolite is formed with this tissue as with RSV or HRP needs to be further investigated.

ACKNOWLEDGEMENTS

Supported by grants from the Medical Research Council of Sweden and Canada, Swedish Cancer Society, The Royal Society and Funds from Karolinska Institutet.

REFERENCES

1. Saunders, B.C. (1973) in: Inorganic Biochemistry (Eichhorn, G.L., ed) vol. 2, pp 988-1021, Elsevier, New York.

2. Marnett, L.J. (1981) Life Sci. 29, 531-546.

3. Moldéus, P., Andersson, B., Rahimtula, A. and Berggren, M. (1982) Biochem. Pharmacol. 31, 1363-1368.

4. Sivarajah, K., Lasker, J.M. and Eling, T.E. (1981) Cancer Res. 41, 1834-1839.

5. Zenser, T.V., Mattammal, M.B., Armbrecht, H.J. and Davis, B.B. (1980) Cancer Res. 40, 2839-2845.

6. Marnett, L.J., Reed, G.A. and Dennison, D.J. (1978) Biochem. Biophys. Res. Commun. 82, 210-216.

7. Christ, E.J. and Van Dorp, D.A. (1972) Biochim. Biophys. Acta, 270, 537-545.

8. Nelson, S.D., Dahlin, D.C., Rauckman, E.J. and Rosen, G.M. (1981) Mol. Pharmacol. 20, 195-199.

9. Griffin, B.W. and Ting, P.L. (1978) Biochemistry, 17, 2206-2211.

10. Marnett, L.J., Siedlik, P.H. and Fung, L.W.M. (1982) J. Biol. Chem. 257, 6957-6964.

11. Josephy, D.P., Eling, T. and Mason, R.P. (1982) J. Biol. Chem. 257, 3669-3675.

12. Josephy, D.P., Mason, R.P. and Eling, T. (1982) Cancer Res. 42, 2567-2570.

13. Andersson, B., Nordenskjöld, M., Rahimtula, A. and Moldéus, P. (1982) Mol. Pharmacol. 22, 479-485.

14. Andersson, B., Larsson, R., Rahimtula, A. and Moldéus, P. (1983) Biochem. Pharmacol. 32, 1045-1050.

15. Egan, R.W., Paxton, J. and Kuehl,Jr., F.A. (1976) J. Biol. Chem. 251, 7329-7335.

16. Andersson, B., Larsson, R., Rahimtula, A. and Moldéus, P. (1983) Submitted to Carcinogenesis.

17. Reed, D.J., Babson, J.R., Beatty, P.W., Brodie, A.E., Ellis, W. and Potter, D.W. (1980) Anal. Biochem. 106, 55-62.

18. Ohniski, K., Yamazaki, H., Iyanagi, T., Nakamura, T. and Yamazaki, I. (1969) Biochim. Biophys. Acta, 172, 357-369.

19. Andersson, B., Larsson, R., Ross, D., Moldéus, P. and Lindeke, B. (1983) Submitted to Eur. J. Biochem.

20. Ross, D., Larsson, R., Andersson, B., Rahimtula, A. and Moldéus, P. (1983) Submitted to J. Biol. Chem.

21. Larsson, R., Andersson, B., von Bahr, C. and Moldéus, P. (1983) Submitted to Biochem. Pharmacol.

© 1983 Elsevier Science Publishers B.V.
Extrahepatic Drug Metabolism and Chemical Carcinogenesis,
J. Rydström, J. Montelius and M. Bengtsson eds.

PEROXIDASE-DEPENDENT COVALENT BINDING OF 7,12-DIMETHYLBENZ(A)-ANTHRACENE METABOLITES TO RAT ADRENAL MICROSOMES

JOHAN MONTELIUS AND JAN RYDSTRÖM
Department of Biochemistry, University of Stockholm, Sweden

INTRODUCTION

The adrenal cortex is a steroidogenic organ and thus contains a high level of cytochrome P-450 (P-450) in the microsomal and mito-chondrial fractions (0.3-0.4 and 0.7-0.9 nmol/mg protein, respect-ively). In addition to steroid hydroxylases rat adrenal microsomes contain a high aryl hydrocarbon hydroxylase (AHH) activity.

The two polycyclic aromatic hydrocarbons benzo(a)pyrene (BP) and 7,12-dimethylbenz(a)anthracene (DMBA) are metabolized by rat adre-nal microsomes at rates three to five times greater than those ob-tained with liver microsomes from untreated rats. The activity with DMBA as substrate in male and female rat adrenal microsomes are 90-150 and 200-300 pmol/min,mg protein, respectively, and 2-5% of the metabolites are covalently bound to protein. The activity with BP as substrate is slightly higher (1), whilst the mitochondrial frac-tion, in spite of the high P-450 content, is virtually inactive (2). Although both hydrocarbons are highly potent carcinogens, only DMBA causes necrosis in the rat adrenal cortex and the adrenocorticoly-tic metabolite has been proposed to be 7-hydroxymethyl-12-methyl--benz(a)anthracene and/or reactive products of this substance for-med after further metabolism (3).

Ethanol oxidation by P-450 has been proposed to proceed by a free radical mechanism (4) and it has been claimed (5) that the carcinogenic potency of DMBA is related to the ionisation poten-tial and the tendency of this compound to undergo one-electron oxidation. In order to elucidate whether a free activated oxygen species in some way is involved in the metabolism and activation of DMBA and BP in rat adrenal microsomes, the metabolism and cova-lent binding of metabolites to protein were assayed simultaneously in the absence and in the presence of enzymes metabolizing oxygen-reduction products, i.e., horseradish peroxidase (peroxidase), su-peroxide dismutase (SOD) and catalase, and various radical scaven-gers, i.e., dimethyl sulfoxide (DMSO), mannitol, butylated hydroxy-toluene (BHT) and DL-α-tocopherol (tocopherol).

MATERIALS AND METHODS

Rat adrenal microsomes were isolated and stored as described previously (6). Control incubations for estimating DMBA and BP metabolism and covalent binding in the presence of various additions were carried out in a medium composed of 2 mM isocitrate, 1 mM MgCl$_2$, 30 µg isocitrate dehydrogenase and 20 mM Tris-HCl (pH 7.3). Microsomal protein concentration was 0.4 to 1.0 mg/ml. DMBA and BP were added dissolved in acetone (5 µl/incubation) and the reaction was started by the addition of 600 µM NADPH (final concentration); final volume was 0.5 ml. After incubation for 60 min at 30°C, aliquots of 2 x 50 µl were withdrawn for measuring covalently bound metabolites by a filter assay (7); the remainder of the incubation was used for AHH assay by the distribution method (8) and/or HPLC analysis (2), and for SDS-polyacrylamide gel elctrophoresis. The sum of water soluble metabolites and covalently bound metabolites was taken as a measure of the total activity (metabolism).

[14C]-DMBA (97.4 mCi/mmol) and [14C]-BP (21.7 mCi/mmol) were obtained from NEN chemicals (D-6072 Dreireich W. Germany). Peroxidase, SOD, catalase and other biochemicals were obtained from Sigma Chem. Co. (St. Louis, Mo., USA).

RESULTS AND DISCUSSION

As shown in Fig. 1 the HPLC profile of DMBA metabolites obtained with female and male rat adrenal microsomes were identical whereas the activity in the female microsomes was about twice that found in the male microsomes. The main metabolites were phenols (fraction 74-76) and dihydrodiols (fraction 49-50), (1,2). These results indicate that the sexual difference in rat adrenal AHH is a quantitative rather than a qualitative difference.

Table 1 shows the effect on metabolism and covalent binding of DMBA metabolites by different enzymes metabolizing oxygen-reduction products and various radical scavengers. Except for BHT which caused about 20% inhibition and peroxidase which slightly increased the metabolism none of the added compounds significantly affected the metabolism. The covalent binding was drastically increased, 6- to 8-fold, by the addition of peroxidase while the other additions were virtually without effect except for BHT which caused a decrease in covalent binding corresponding to the inhibition of metabolism. With BP as substrate similar results were obtained although the increase in covalent binding was less pronounced in the presence of peroxidase. However, the covalent binding in the control incubation with BP as substrate was about twice that obtained with DMBA as substrate, i.e., the total rate of covalent binding was about the same for the two substrates.

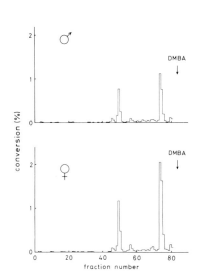

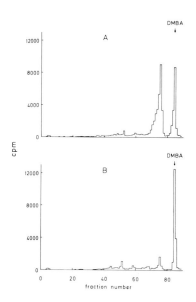

Fig. 1 Metabolism of DMBA (50μM) catalyzed by male and female rat adrenal microsomes. The total conversion was 4.8% and 8.1%, respectively.

Fig. 2 Metabolism of DMBA (10μM) by male rat adrenal microsomes; control (A), control plus peroxidase (B). The total conversion was 75%.

Fig. 2 shows the HPLC pattern of DMBA-metabolites in the absence (A) and in the presence (B) of peroxidase. A large portion of the phenols was removed by the addition of peroxidase with little or no change in the dihydrodiol fractions, indicating that peroxidase-dependent activation of DMBA primarely involves phenols. The relative difference in phenol and dihydrodiol formation between the experiments in fig. 1 and 2 was due to the low substrate concentration and therefore the higher total conversion in the latter case.

Addition of catalase inhibited the peroxidase-mediated covalent binding (Table 2) suggesting the involvement of endogeneously formed hydrogen peroxide. The complete inhibition of peroxidase-dependent covalent binding by BHT is probably an effect of competition between BHT, being a phenol, and DMBA-phenols for the peroxidase. The lack of effect by SOD, mannitol and DMSO indicates that superoxide anion and hydroxyl radicals do not participate in the peroxidase-mediated covalent binding, while the lack of effect by tocopherol, a more general radical scavenger, could be due to the hydrophobicity of this compound.

TABLE 1

EFFECT OF PEROXIDASE, SOD, CATALASE, MANNITOL, DMSO, BHT AND
TOCOPHEROL ON THE METABOLISM AND COVALENT BINDING OF DMBA AND BP
IN MALE RAT ADRENAL MICROSOMES

Conditions	Total activity[a] (% of control)		Covalent binding[a] (% of control)	
Substrate DMBA[b]				
Control	100		100	
+Peroxidase, 2U/ml	106.2	$\pm$5.8	728.8	$\pm$132.0
+SOD, 20µg/ml	97.5	$\pm$7.4	102.9	$\pm$ 10.5
+Mannitol, 100 mM	98.9	$\pm$0.5	96.5	$\pm$ 4.1
+DMSO, 10mM	99.8	$\pm$0.9	92.2	$\pm$ 2.2
+Catalase, 40µg/ml	96.5	$\pm$6.4	99.2	$\pm$ 4.3
+Catalase, 200µg/ml	97.1	$\pm$5.4	103.8	$\pm$ 2.9
+BHT, 1mM	80.7	$\pm$4.0	86.1	$\pm$ 3.3
+Tocopherol, 500µM	93.8	$\pm$8.1	91.8	$\pm$ 3.8
Substrate BP[c]				
Control	100		100	
+Peroxidase, 2U/ml	100.7	$\pm$2.5	266.5	$\pm$ 11.5
+SOD, 20µg/ml	96.9	$\pm$1.0	92.3	$\pm$ 2.4
+Mannitol, 100 mM	100.9	$\pm$3.1	106.3	$\pm$ 4.1
+DMSO, 10 mM	99.6	$\pm$1.3	99.6	$\pm$ 10.6

[a]Mean $\pm$SD. All values have been corrected for the activity obtained where NADPH was omitted.
[b]Control values for the total activity and covalent binding were
142,4 and 6,61 pmol/min,mg protein, respectively. The concentration of DMBA was 10 µM.
[c]Control values for the total activity and covalent binding were
197,3 and 12,31 pmol/min,mg protein, respectively. The concentration of BP was 10 µM.

Fig. 3 shows the time course of total metabolism and covalent
binding in the absence and in the presence of peroxidase. The
slight increase in total metabolism by the addition of peroxidase
was probably due to the fact that peroxidase itself is able to metabolize DMBA in the presence of hydrogen peroxide (not shown).
The possibility that this increased peroxidase-dependent metabolism
accounts for the increased covalent binding is unlikely because
the increased metabolism was less than half the resulting increase
in covalent binding (Fig. 3). Also, the preferential disappearance
of phenolic metabolites favours covalent binding of these metabolites rather than DMBA itself (cf. fig. 2). In addition, adrenal
microsomes metabolized DMBA in the presence of added hydrogen peroxide and gave rise to reactive metabolites that bound covalently

TABLE 2

EFFECT OF SOD, CATALASE, MANNITOL, DMSO, BHT AND TOCOPHEROL ON
METABOLISM AND PEROXIDASE MEDIATED COVALENT BINDING OF DMBA
METABOLITES IN MALE RAT ADRENAL MICROSOMES

Conditions[a]	Total activity[b] (% of control)	Covalent binding[c] (% of control)
Control[c]	100	100
Control, peroxidase, 2U/ml	104.4 ±4.3	689.6 ±101.2
+Catalase, 40µg/ml	93.0 ±2.3	499.5 ±112.3
+Catalase, 20µg/ml	98.0 ±1.5	377.4 ± 25.9
+BHT, lmM	77.3 ±3.5	94.9 ± 3.6

[a] SOD (20µg/ml), mannitol (100mM), DMSO (10mM) and tocopherol
(500µM) did not significantly affect the total activity or the
peroxidase dependent covalent binding. The concentration of DMBA
was 10µM.
[b] Mean ±SD. All values have been corrected for the activity obtained where NADPH was omitted.
[c] Control values for the total activity and covalent binding were
128,4 and 5,86 pmol/min, mg protein, respectively. The concentration of DMBA was 10µM.

to protein (not shown).

Analysis by SDS-slab gel electrophoresis of the protein - DMBA
adducts revealed that addition of peroxidase increased the covalent
binding to the same proteins that also bound DMBA metabolites in
the absence of peroxidase (Fig. 4). No detectable binding to peroxidase was observed.

With uninduced rat liver microsomes, peroxidase only marginally
increased the extent of covalent binding. This difference between
liver and adrenal microsomes may be due to the difference in product patterns for DMBA in these organs, i.e. in untreated liver the
7-hydroxymethyl derivative is the main metabolite and only small
amounts of phenolic metabolites are formed. Alternatively, liver
microsomes may generate a lower steady-state level of hydrogen peroxide.

CONCLUSIONS

The AHH activity of male and female rat adrenal appears to be
catalyzed by the same type of P-450 as judged by metabolite patterns. No difference in the activation of DMBA and BP could be demonstrated, which may explain the selective adrenocorticolytic
effect of DMBA. Endogeneously formed peroxide, probably hydrogen
peroxide, can be utilized in the presence of a peroxidase to activate aromatic hydrocarbons, preferentially phenolic metabolites,

128

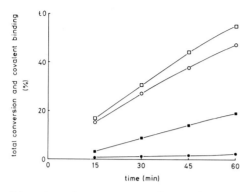

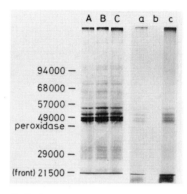

Fig. 3 Time course of total metabolism of DMBA in the absence (o)
and in the presence (□) of peroxidase and of the covalent binding
in the absence (●) and in the presence (■) of peroxidase, in male
rat adrenal microsomes.

Fig. 4. 8.5% SDS-polyacrylamide
gel electrophoresis of male rat
adrenal microsomal incubations;
control (A), control minus NADPH
(B), control plus peroxidase (C),
and the corresponding autoradio-
graph (a,b and c, respectively).
Each lane contained 400μg protein. The NADPH regenerating
system was omitted.

functioning as hydrogen donors to the peroxidase. This provides an
additional pathway, besides the epoxidation pathway, for the activation of DMBA and related compounds, suggesting that the peroxidase-dependent pathway may be important in the subcellular com-
partments where the peroxide production is high and/or the activities of the enzymes metabolizing oxygen-reduction products are low.

ACKNOWLEDGEMENTS

Supported by the Swedish Cancer Society and Swedish Council for
Planning and Coordination of Research.

REFERENCES

1. Bengtsson, M., Montelius, J., Mankowitz, L. and Rydström, J.
   (1983) Biochem. Pharmacol. 32, 129.

2. Montelius, J., Papadopoulos, D., Bengtsson, M. and Rydström, J.
   (1982) Cancer Res. 42, 1479.

3. Huggins, C.B. (1979) Experimental Leukemia and Mammary Cancer.
   Induction, Prevention, Cure. The University of Chicago Press,
   Chicago and London.

4. Ingelman-Sundberg, M. and Johansson, I. (1981) J. Biol. Chem.
   256, 6321.

5. Cavalieri, E., Rogan, E. and Roth, R. (1982) in Free Radicals and Cancer (R.A. Floyd, ed.) Marcel Dekker, New York, pp. 117.

6. Ogle, T.F. (1977) J. Steroid Biochem. 8, 1033.

7. Wallin, H., Schelin, C., Tunek, A. and Jergil, B. (1982) Chem.-Biol. Interact. 38, 109.

8. van Cantfort, J., De Grave, J. and Gielen, J.E. (1977) Biochem. Biophys. Res. Commun. 79, 505.

© 1983 Elsevier Science Publishers B.V.
Extrahepatic Drug Metabolism and Chemical Carcinogenesis,
J. Rydström, J. Montelius and M. Bengtsson eds.

ACTIVATION OF THE ORGANOSPECIFIC CARCINOGEN, METHYLAZOXYMETHANOL,
VIA DEHYDROGENASE ENZYMES: PREVENTION OF COLON TUMORIGENESIS
IN RATS AND HUMAN STUDIES

MORRIS S. ZEDECK, MARTIN LIPKIN AND QUENG HUI TAN

Memorial Sloan-Kettering Cancer Center, 1275 York Avenue,

New York, N.Y. 10021 (U.S.A.)

INTRODUCTION

The interaction of carcinogenic compounds with cellular components often involves prior metabolic conversion of the substance
to a highly reactive molecule with a very short half-life. Though
the original substance may undergo several metabolic conversions,
the production of the ultimate carcinogen usually occurs within
the affected cell. Most carcinogens are activated via the microsomal mixed-function oxygenase system, and there are numerous studies of this metabolic pathway in different organs and of its significance in carcinogenesis. We have been studying the mechanism
of activation of a potent organospecific carcinogen, methylazoxymethanol (MAM), and the data indicate that, unlike other carcinogens, it is activated by alcohol dehydrogenase and other dehydrogenases within the organs sensitive to its carcinogenic action.

Studies of MAM, a hydrazine derivative, began in 1965 when Laqueur (1) reported on the carcinogenicity of MAM and cycasin,
methylazoxymethanol-ß-D-glucoside, found naturally in Cycad
plants. The intestinal flora are required to cleave the gluco-
side moiety of cycasin and liberate MAM; the aglycone, MAM, can
induce tumors by any route of administration (2). The induction
of tumors by cycasin or MAM in various species (monkeys, rats,
mice, hamsters, guinea pigs and fish), in conventional and germ-

suggest that in kidney and liver MAM is substrate for the enzyme, choline dehydrogenase (15). Choline is converted to betaine aldehyde by choline dehydrogenase, and it could be expected that MAM is converted by choline dehydrogenase to its aldehydic derivative. Thus, there would be at least 2 mechanisms for the generation of an active carcinogenic form of MAM.

It is conceivable that pyrazole inhibits MAM metabolism via alcohol dehydrogenase in rat colon and more MAM is shunted to the kidney where it can be metabolized by choline dehydrogenase. This would account for the enhanced incidence of renal tumors noted above in MAM-treated rats that had been pretreated with pyrazole.

Chemical reactivity of MAM metabolite

We investigated whether the proposed aldehydic metabolite of MAM is reactive without further decomposition or whether it gives rise to carbonium ions at a rate faster than that occurring spontaneously from MAM. MAM was incubated with ^{14}C-sodium acetate and NAD^+ with and without horse liver alcohol dehydrogenase enzyme, and the formation of ^{14}C-methyl acetate (MeAc) was measured (16). Incubation of MAM with NAD^+ and enzyme gave rise to significantly more MeAc than did incubation of MAM with only NAD^+. The amount of NADH formed in the enzyme reaction correlated with the additional amount of MeAc obtained relative to incubation of MAM alone. The data indicate that the enzyme-derived metabolite gives rise to carbonium ions at a rate faster than does MAM itself and that the organospecificity is probably due to the ability of certain tissue to metabolize MAM to reactive metabolite(s).

Human studies

Numerous epidemiological studies have concluded that environmental factors play a key role in the induction of human colon cancer (17). MAM is a hydrazine derivative and, since some of the hydrazines that are carcinogenic in laboratory animals (18) are found throughout our environment (various classes of medicinals, foods, herbicides, propellants, dyes), it is possible that man is exposed to a hydrazine that can be converted to a compound similar to MAM.

We are studying whether human colon can utilize MAM as a substrate and whether, as in rats, alcohol dehydrogenase is the activating enzyme. There are 3 gene loci in humans responsible for synthesis of alcohol dehydrogenase, ADH_1, ADH_2 and ADH_3, with polymorphism at ADH_2 and ADH_3. The enzyme is dimeric, and the number of combinations, therefore, that could arise from these 3 genes number 15 (19). Other forms of alcohol dehydrogenase have been found recently, and now the number of isozymes that can occur in liver is 19 (20-22). Smith et al. (23) have reported that ADH_3 (γ) is the active gene locus in human stomach. Since the gene is polymorphic, individuals can be either $\gamma_1\gamma_1$ or $\gamma_2\gamma_2$ or $\gamma_1\gamma_1$, $\gamma_2\gamma_2$ and $\gamma_1\gamma_2$. We hope to determine the isozyme pattern in human colon and which, if any, of the many isozymes of human alcohol dehydrogenase can activate MAM.

The subjects participating in these studies are normal volunteers; individuals with the autosomal dominant disease, familial polyposis, and asymptomatic members of their families; subjects from strongly colon cancer-prone families without polyposis; cancer-prone families manifesting a variety of malignancies; and individuals from familial aggregations who have been cancer-free for two or more generations. We are seeking to determine whether a particular isozyme is characteristic for a particular group and whether there is a correlation between the sensitivity of some groups to develop colon cancer and their isozyme pattern and their ability to activate MAM.

MATERIALS AND METHODS

The tissue is obtained from the operating room or as biopsy material and frozen until needed. For spectrophotometric analysis of alcohol dehydrogenase activity, the tissue is homogenized in 2 volumes of 0.1 M sodium phosphate buffer, pH 7.4. The homogenate is centrifuged at 12,000 x g for 15 min, and the supernatant (S-12) is frozen until analyzed. The supernatant is analyzed spectrophotometrically at 340 mμ (reduction of NAD) for total alcohol dehydrogenase activity, using ethanol, pentanol or MAM as substrates. The reaction mixture contains: 80 mM glycine buffer, pH 9.4, 2.4 mM NAD, 10-50 μl S-12 supernatant, and various concentrations of substrate. Endogenous activity of S-12 is determined and subtracted from the activity with substrate. Protein concentration is determined, using the protein-dye binding procedure of Bradford (24). The free MAM is prepared from commercially available MAM acetate as previously described (12). The kinetics of the reactions are plotted, and the K_m is determined for each substrate. The isozyme pattern of each patient is determined by separating the isozymes of alcohol dehydrogenase by starch gel electrophoresis. For these studies, the colon and stomach is homogenized without addition of buffer. For liver, the S-12 fraction is used. Small strips of filter paper are used to absorb homogenate or supernatant and then applied to the starch gel (10.5% starch in 25 mM Tris buffer, pH 8.6, containing 4 mM NAD) and electrophoresis is conducted at 12 V/cm for 5 hr. The electrode reservoirs contain 300 mM Tris buffer, pH 8.6. Activity of the isozymes on the gel is determined by histochemical techniques. The gel is incubated for 1 hour at 37° in media containing 0.1 M glycine buffer, pH 9.4, 2 mM NAD, 0.45 mM nitro blue tetrazolium chloride monohydrate, 0.13 mM phenazine methosulfate and 170 mM 2-hexene-1-ol, pentanol, or ethanol. After incubation, the gel is washed with fixing solutions and photographed.

RESULTS

The data in Table 1 show the K_m values for pentanol, ethanol and MAM, using S-12 fractions from human liver and colon. The results indicate that pentanol has a much lower K_m than ethanol for liver alcohol dehydrogenase. Others have reported that increasing the primary alcohol chain length results in a decrease in K_m (19). In colon, however, this marked difference was not always observed. The V_{max} for each of the 3 substrates was 20-fold higher in liver than in colon. Though these findings are preliminary, the data do indicate that human liver and colon can utilize MAM as substrate.

Also, we have found that the isozyme pattern of alcohol dehydrogenase in human colon is similar to what has been reported for human stomach (23), namely, proteins corresponding to dimers of either $\gamma_1\gamma_1$, $\gamma_2\gamma_2$ or $\gamma_1\gamma_2$ (Fig. 1). Samples of human liver (A), stomach (B) and colon (C, D) were applied to starch gels and analyzed for enzyme activity as described under Materials and Methods. The liver sample (A) shows the presence of many isozymes, as has been reported by others (19). The stomach sample (B) has one prominant band corresponding to $\gamma_1\gamma_1$ and one unidentified area of staining near the origin, as reported by others (23). The colon samples show either a single isozyme (C) corresponding to $\gamma_1\gamma_1$ or the presence of all 3 isozymes (D), corresponding to $\gamma_1\gamma_1$, $\gamma_2\gamma_2$ and $\gamma_1\gamma_2$. The band furthest from the origin in D and higher than the $\gamma_1\gamma_1$ isozyme in stomach might be the "cathodic band" previously described in human liver (20). Also, the bands of activity seen below the origin, towards the anode, might correspond to the X_1-ADH and X_2-ADH isozymes described by Parés and Vallee (21). They reported finding these isozymes in liver, using pentanol as substrate. We have seen such activity in colon, using either pentanol or 2-hexene-1-ol as substrates. We have analyzed colon samples from 12 patients and found that 58.3% have the dimer $\gamma_1\gamma_1$, 33.3% have alleles γ_1 and γ_2 (dimers $\gamma_1\gamma_1$, $\gamma_1\gamma_2$, $\gamma_2\gamma_2$) and 8.3% have the dimer $\gamma_2\gamma_2$. Using many samples of human stomach, the results are 36%, $\gamma_1\gamma_1$; 48%, γ_1 and γ_2; and 16%, $\gamma_2\gamma_2$ (23).

TABLE 1
HUMAN LIVER AND COLON ALCOHOL DEHYDROGENASE ACTIVITY

Pat.	Diagnosis	Isozyme(s)	K_m		
			Pentanol	Ethanol	MAM
A.	Normal Liver	Heterogenous	35.7μM	413μM	N.D.
B.	Normal Liver	Heterogenous	26.4μM	935μM	20.8mM
C.	F.P.	$\gamma_1\gamma_1$, $\gamma_1\gamma_2$, $\gamma_2\gamma_2$	29.9mM	58.8mM	N.D.
D.	F.P.	$\gamma_1\gamma_1$	14.8mM	45.2mM	17.3mM
E.	F.P.	$\gamma_1\gamma_1$	38.7mM	Inactive[a]	Inactive[b]
F.	F.P.	$\gamma_2\gamma_2$	45.5mM	371.6mM	43.9mM
G.	F.P.	$\gamma_1\gamma_1$, $\gamma_1\gamma_2$, $\gamma_2\gamma_2$	56.0mM	Inactive[c]	N.D.

F.P., Familial Polyposis; N.D., not determined; [a] No activity up to 400mM; [b] No activity up to 23.3mM; [c] No activity up to 250mM.

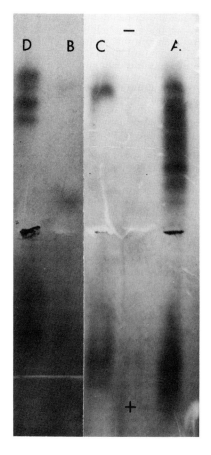

Fig. 1. Alcohol dehydrogenase isozyme activity of human liver, stomach and colon following electrophoresis on starch gel.

DISCUSSION

This report summarizes the studies which led to the conclusion that MAM is activated by dehydrogenase enzymes and that the organospecificity exhibited by this carcinogen is related to the presence of such dehydrogenase(s) in select tissues. The tumor prevention study with pyrazole, in which tumors were prevented in one tissue while tumorigenesis was exaggerated in others, serves as a clear example of the caution one must exercise in the area of chemoprevention. Other studies have illustrated the same point. Clinical investigators interested in chemoprevention should be fully aware of the possibility that such treatment might alter the site of tumor development. A total understanding of the metabolism of the carcinogen in all tissues must be known before chemoprevention can be initiated.

Our preliminary studies of human tissue dehydrogenase enzyme activity indicate that human liver and colon can utilize MAM as substrate. Also, as part of the study to determine whether any correlation exists between an individual's genetic susceptibility to develop colon cancer, activation of MAM and alcohol dehydrogenase isozyme pattern in colon, we have found that the isozyme pattern in human colon is like that in human stomach, namely, the proteins are products of gene locus ADH3. These experiments are part of an overall study to understand what mechanism is responsible for individual susceptibility to the development of colon cancer, and it is hoped that the findings can be of value in programs aimed at prevention of colon cancer.

ACKNOWLEDGEMENTS

The work was supported, in part, by USPHS Grants CA 08748 from the National Cancer Institute, CA 15637 from the National Cancer Institute through the National Large Bowel Cancer Project, and by American Cancer Society Grant, SIG-7.

REFERENCES

1. Laqueur, G.L. (1965) Virchows Arch. Pathol. Anat. 340, 151.

2. Laqueur, G.L., McDaniel, E.G. and Matsumoto, H. (1967)
    J. Nat. Cancer Inst. 39, 355.

3. Laqueur, G.L. and Spatz, M. (1975) Gann Monograph on
    Cancer Research 17, 189.

4. Magee, P.N., Montesano, R. and Preussmann, R. (1976) in:
    Searle, C.E. (Ed.), Chemical Carcinogens - ACS Monograph
    173, American Chemical Society, Washington, D.C., pp. 491-
    625.

5. Sieber, S.M., Correa, P., Dalgard, D.W., McIntire, K.R.
    and Adamson, R.H. (1980) J. Nat. Cancer Inst. 65, 177.

6. Zedeck, M.S. and Sternberg, S.S. (1974) J. Nat. Cancer
    Inst. 53, 1419.

7. Zedeck, M.S. and Sternberg, S.S. (1977) Chem.-Biol.
    Interactions 17, 291.

8. Notman, J., Tan, Q.H. and Zedeck, M.S. (1982) Cancer
    Res. 42, 1774.

9. Nagasawa, H.T., Shirota, F.N. and Matsumoto, H. (1972)
    Nature 236, 234.

10. Gennaro, A.R., Villaneuva, R., Sukonthaman, Y., Vathanophas,
    V. and Rosemond, G.P. (1973) Cancer Res. 33, 536.

11. Schoental, R. (1973) Brit. J. Cancer 28, 436.

12. Grab, D.J. and Zedeck, M.S. (1977) Cancer Res. 37, 4182.

13. Fiala, E.S., Kulakis, C. and Weisburger, J.H. (1979)
    Proc. Amer. Assoc. Cancer Res. 20, 20.

14. Wattenberg, L.W. and Sparnins, V.L. (1979) J. Nat. Cancer
    Inst. 63, 219.

15. Tan, Q.H., Penkovsky, L. and Zedeck, M.S. (1981)
    Carcinogenesis 2, 1135.

16. Feinberg, A. and Zedeck, M.S. (1980) Cancer Res. 40, 4446.

17. Correa, P. and Haenszel, W. (1978) Adv. Cancer Res. 26, 1.

18. Toth, B. (1975) Cancer Res. 35, 3693.

19. Bosron, W.F. and Li, T.-K. (1980) in: Jakoby, W.B. (Ed.),
    Enzymatic Basis of Detoxication, Academic Press, New
    York, pp. 231-248.

142

20. Bosron, W.F., Li, T.-K. and Vallee, B.L. (1979) Biochem. Biophys. Res. Comm. 91, 1549.

21. Parés, X. and Vallee, B.L. (1981) Biochem. Biophys. Res. Comm. 98, 122.

22. Bosron, W.F., Li, T.-K. and Vallee, B.L. (1980) Proc. Nat. Acad. Sci. U.S.A. 77, 5784.

23. Smith, M., Hopkinson, D.A. and Harris. H. (1972) Ann. Human Genet., London 35, 243.

24. Bradford, M.M. (1976) Anal. Biochem. 72, 248.

© 1983 Elsevier Science Publishers B.V.
Extrahepatic Drug Metabolism and Chemical Carcinogenesis,
J. Rydström, J. Montelius and M. Bengtsson eds.

THE ROLE OF EXTRAHEPATIC AND HEPATIC SULFATION AND GLUCURONIDATION IN CHEMICAL CARCINOGENESIS: AN OVERVIEW

GERARD J. MULDER AND JOHN H.N. MEERMAN

Department of Pharmacology, State University of Groningen, Bloemsingel 1, Groningen (The Netherlands)

INTRODUCTION

Glucuronidation and sulfation are conjugation reactions that, in general, convert their substrates into toxicologically inert metabolites: the majority of the substrates investigated so far, mostly phenols (1), are more toxic than the corresponding conjugates. However, in recent years several conjugates have been discovered that were very toxic, both because of their chemical reactivity, and their pharmacological properties. Some have been implicated in the carcinogenic action of the parent compound (2). In this chapter a brief overview will be given of the role that hepatic and extrahepatic conjugation may play in the generation of such conjugates. Furthermore, the importance of pharmacokinetics in the metabolism of the substrate and the site of tumor formation, will be discussed.

REACTIVE SULFATE AND GLUCURONIDE CONJUGATES

Several sulfate conjugates have been suggested to be proximate or ultimate carcinogens (see 2 and 3 for reviews and complete lists of references). The first sulfate conjugate recognized as being chemically reactive and possibly involved in tumor formation was the *O*-sulfonate of *N*-hydroxy-2-acetylamino-fluorene (N-hydroxy-AAF; Fig. 1). Since N-hydroxy-AAF itself was found not to react with DNA and RNA *in vitro*, it was apparent that chemical activation had

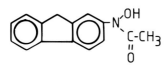

to occur *in vivo*; esters of N-hydroxy-AAF did react with DNA *in vitro*, and thus the *O*-sulfonate ester became a candidate for the ultimate carcinogenic metabolite of 2AAF *in vivo*. Because the *O*-sulfonate of N-hydroxy-AAF is too labile to be detected in aqueous media at pH 7.4, the evidence for its involvement in carcinogenesis was

Fig. 1. N-hydroxy-2-acetylamino-fluorene.

unavoidably indirect, as had been discussed elsewhere (2,3). It is unclear yet, whether sulfation of N-hydroxy-AAF is involved in initiation or promotion of tumor formation in the liver and other organs (5,6).

O-sulfonation generates reactive intermediates from many other hydroxamic acids, such as N-hydroxy-2-acetylaminophenanthrene and N-hydroxy-phenacetin (2,3,7). Further, from the hydroxylamine N-hydroxy-N-methyl-4-aminoazobenzene (8), the benzylic alcohols 7-hydroxy-12-methyl-benzo[a]anthracene (9), o- and p-chlorobenzylalcohol (10) and from 1'-hydroxy-saffrole (2).

Glucuronide conjugates, in general, are more chemically stable than the sulfate conjugates (2). Thus, the N,O-glucuronide conjugate of N-hydroxy-AAF is only reactive at alkaline pH, but scarcely binds to DNA *in vitro* at pH 7.4. Also, at neutral pH the glucuronide conjugate of N-hydroxy-phenacetin breaks down only slowly (11). Such conjugates might leave the cells where they are synthesized, and cause tumors elsewhere in the body. The N,O-glucuronides of hydroxylamines, on the other hand, are more reactive, like that of N-hydroxy-2-aminofluorene (12), which can be generated by deacetylation of the glucuronide conjugate of N-hydroxy-AAF. An alternative route for hydroxylamines is the formation of an N-glucuronide, as with N-hydroxy-2-naphthylamine (13). Although this and similar conjugates are stable at pH 7.4, they rapidly break down at pH 5 to generate the more reactive hydroxylamine.

The glucuronide of 3-hydroxy-benzo[a]pyrene is a reactive conjugate, even though it is a phenolic glucuronide (14,15). Recently, a reactive ester-type glucuronide of clofibrate has been identified that spontaneously reacts with glutathione in an S_N2 reaction (16). A further evaluation of the role of such ester-glucuronides still has to be made.

TRANSFERASE ACTIVITIES IN THE LIVER AND IN EXTRAHEPATIC TISSUES

Generation of reactive conjugates in a tissue requires the presence of the tools of conjugation in the cells of that tissue; for sulfation the sulfotransferases and the cosubstrate adenosine 3'-phosphate 5'-sulfato-phosphate (PAPS) (17), and for glucuronidation UDP-glucuronosyltransferase and UDP-glucuronate (UDPGA) (18).

Relatively little data is available concerning the tissue distribution of the transferase activities specific for potentially carcinogenic substrates. For sulfation of N-hydroxy-AAF a high activity is present in male rat liver, but other tissues, especially in female rats, had low or no activity (2,3). The pronounced sex-difference (happens to?) correlate(s) with a higher liver tumor incidence in males. Some tissues that yield a high number of tumors after exposure of rats to N-hydroxy-AAF, like mammary gland and a sebaceous gland (Zymbal's gland), are devoid of sulfotransferase activity for N-hydroxy-AAF, indicating that other activating steps play a role in those tissues.

A similar high sulfotransferase activity in rat liver was found for N-hydroxy-N-methyl-4-aminoazobenzene (8), with low activity outside the liver. For other substrates little data is available. The sulfotransferase that converts N-hydroxy-AAF is most likely the same which also sulfates 4-nitrophenol; it has been purified from rat liver (19). Platelets contain reasonable activities of sulfotransferases (20); so far, they have not been tested for the ability to sulfate N-hydroxy-2AAF.

In general, sulfotransferases have a much lower capacity (V_{max}) than UDP-glucuronosyltransferases (UDPGT's), but a much higher affinity (i.e. a lower K_m), so that sulfation is saturated at a lower dose than glucuronidation. UDPGT's are ubiquitously present in the tissues. Again, little is known about the UDPGT's that are involved in the conversion of proximate carcinogenic substrates. The most studied activity, so far, is the glucuronidation of N-hydroxy-2-naphthylamine (13); it is a 3-methylcholanthrene-inducible, 'GT-1' or 'late-foetal' activity (21). Activities towards various benzo[a]pyrene derivatives are highest in the liver, but are present in several other tissues as well (13,15,21).

In preneoplastic nodules in the liver the glucuronidation of the 'late foetal' UDPGT substrates is increased over the normal level (22-24). A similar finding was reported in the lung: in several human periferal lung tumors, especially squamous cell carcinomas, 1-naphthol and 3-hydroxy-benzo-[a]pyrene were primarily glucuronidated, while in comparable tissues from healthy lungs the substrates were mainly sulfated (25,26). The same was found in various carcinoma cell lines *in vitro* by this group, and in the rat *in vivo* with a hepatoma (Reuber M-35) with the substrate 4-nitrophenol (27). The implications of these findings are as yet unclear, but, obviously, for some reason a shift from sulfation to glucuronidation can take place in tumors.

CO-SUBSTRATE AVAILABILITY

The concentration of PAPS in the liver and other organs is rather low, of the order of 5 - 30 nmol/g tissue; however, if required, large amounts can be rapidly synthesized (1,28). Therefore, a low concentration of PAPS need not indicate a low sulfation potential. Most likely, every tissue possesses the enzymes required for PAPS synthesis; however genetic defects in PAPS generation have been identified (1,17). In some tissues the rate limiting step in PAPS generation may be the uptake of inorganic sulfate. In isolated lung cells, cysteine seemed to be a better precursor for PAPS than inorganic sulfate (29); this was, however, not confirmed in the isolated perfused rat lung (30).

UDPGA is an intermediate in the glucaric acid pathway: it is generated from UDP-glucose by reduction of NAD^+ to NADH (18). This offers one way of reducing the generation of UDPGA: when the NAD^+/NADH ratio is decreased by administration of e.g. ethanol glucuronidation is inhibited due to a shortage of UDPGA (31). The rate at which (under normal conditions) UDPGA can be generated, at least in the liver, is very high. No data is available in this respect from other tissues (although the concentration of UDPGA in a number of organs has been determined). The liver has a large store of glycogen which can be used for UDPGA generation. This, however, is not available in extrahepatic tissues and, thus, extrahepatic glucuronidation could be limited by UDPGA availability. In the liver the availability of UDPGA can be decreased by treatment with galactosamine; however, the effect is either rapidly reversible, or (at only slightly higher doses) causes pronounced liver-damage (18).

UPTAKE OF THE SUBSTRATES BY VARIOUS ORGANS

An important factor in tumor formation in a tissue is the ease with which cells in an organ take up the substrate from the blood. Within an organ this may, obviously, be very different for different cell types. Autoradiography will give an indication of organ and even cell distribution, but does not tell whether the unchanged compound, or a metabolite is taken up and stored. The alternative approach uses isolated organs or cells. Thus, with the isolated perfused liver it can be shown that hepatic uptake of many drugs is very effective. However, the contribution of the liver to the total elimination of a drug may be overestimated, especially when only low doses of a substrate are used *in vivo*: in the rat, phenol at low level seems to be mainly conjugated in the lung, rather than in the liver (32). The isolated lung indeed effectively conjugates phenol with sulfate and glucuronate (33). The location of the lungs in the circulation gives them a distinct advantage over other organs in that the total cardiac output passes the lung during each circulation.

The results with phenol have been confirmed with the phenolic compound harmol: at low infusion rate of harmol up to 67% of sulfation (which is the major reaction) seems to take place outside the liver, while glucuronidation is mainly confined to the liver (34). These findings were obtained in a study in which harmol was infused either in the portal vein, or in the jugular vein. Since in the isolated perfused rat lung the conjugation of harmol is very slow (30), this seems to imply that extrahepatic sulfation of this compound

TABLE 1

THE ROLE OF SULFATION IN THE ACTIVATION OF N-HYDROXY-4'-FLUORO-4-ACETYL-
AMINOBIPHENYL TO REACTIVE INTERMEDIATES IN VARIOUS ORGANS IN THE RAT

Rats were given 60 μmol/kg of [^{3}H]N-hydroxy-FAAB intravenously, and covalent binding of [^{3}H]-radioactivity to the total macromolecular fraction
was determined in various organs, 4 hours after injection. In another group,
sulfation was inhibited by the prior injection (45 min before the substrate)
of pentachlorophenol (40 μmol/kg, i.p.). Data taken from ref. 38.

| Organ | Covalently bound [^{3}H]N-hydroxy-FAAB | |
| | (pmole per mg protein to the total macromolecular fraction) | |
	Control	Pentachlorophenol-pretreated
Liver	530 + 31	290 + 29[a]
Kidney	897 + 28	561 + 67[a]
Spleen	179 + 48	202 + 21

[a]Significantly different from control (P < 0.05).

must take place elsewhere, for instance in the kidneys. In similar experiments
with 4-nitrophenol also over 50% extrahepatic conjugation was found (35), when
intravenous and intraportal injections were compared; the conclusion (35) that
sulfation occurred exclusively in the liver was based solely on *in vitro* data,
and may be inaccurate.

In the isolated perfused kidney appreciable sulfation and glucuronidation
occurs (17,36,37). Sulfation of N-hydroxy-4'-fluoro-4-acetylaminobiphenyl
(N-hydroxy-FAAB) leads to the formation of reactive intermediates that bind
covalently to macromolecules. Covalent binding of N-hydroxy-FAAB in the kidney
was inhibited by the selective sulfation inhibitor pentachlorophenol (PCP),
indicating that in the kidney sulfation plays a role in the activation; however, PCP had no effect on the low level of covalent binding in the spleen
indicating, that either PCP is not taken up in the spleen, or that in the
spleen sulfation does not play a role in the covalent binding of this compound (38) (Table 1).

The intestines have a relatively high capacity to conjugate orally administered drugs, e.g. benzo[a]pyrene (39), during their absorption from the
gut lumen (40). Pronounced species differences are known in this first pass
conjugation, and may be the cause of species differences in carcinogenic
response to orally administered compounds which will not be observed when the

compounds are given by a parenteral route. Moreover, the supply of sulfate (or cysteine) in the food may strongly affect the extent of sulfation during first pass uptake in the gut (17). Even when the substrate is given intravenously it may be conjugated in the gut, such as lorazepam in the dog (41).

Since tumors occur in many other tissues, such as mammary gland, testis, Zymbal's gland and bladder, uptake and activation of carcinogens must occur in all these tissues; or, they must take up proximate carcinogens that have been made in other organs. In most of these tissues, only the presence or apparent absence of the 'tools' of conjugation has been investigated, which tells only a little about the activity of conjugation *in situ*. Perfusion, to measure uptake of the substrate and 'overall' activity of conjugation in the intact organ often is not possible, so that direct evidence is hard to obtain. Isolated cell experiments (if the cell suspension is representative for the whole organ) may be useful in those cases.

PHARMACOKINETICS OF CONJUGATION: ANOMALITIES RESULTING FROM COMPETITION FOR METABOLISM *IN VIVO*

In most cases more than one pathway is available for metabolism of a xenobiotic. Thus, sulfation and glucuronidation often compete for the same substrate. Due to this competition, the pharmacokinetics of conjugation may show deviations from the normal pattern, and that may have important consequences for toxicity. In general, sulfation has a higher affinity for the substrates, but a much lower capacity for conversion (V_{max}). Thus, under conditions of limited substrate supply, sulfation will be the predominant conjugation reaction. But when the substrate supply increases and sulfation becomes saturated, glucuronidation may, 'all of a sudden' increase more than proportional with the increase in substrate concentration in e.g. plasma or blood. Fig. 2 illustrates this for a substrate of both sulfation and glucuronidation, where the K_m for glucuronidation is 100-fold higher than the K_m for sulfation, and the V_{max} values for both conjugations are equal. Above a certain extracellular substrate concentration sulfation becomes saturated and, suddenly, glucuronidation increases much faster than anticipated (42). In fact, below a certain concentration, the product of the pathway with the lower affinity is hardly formed at all. The extent to which such a 'lag' occurs may be different for different organs, dependent on blood flow through that organ, and rate at which the substrate is taken up by the organ.

If a conjugate of which the formation is suddenly increased is an ultimate carcinogen, a threshold for carcinogenicity may be related to the saturation

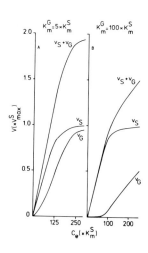

Fig. 2. Rates of sulfation (v_s) and glucuronidation (v_g) of a substrate for both conjugations when substrate supply for the intracellular conjugations is rate limiting. It should be realized that under these conditions the intracellular substrate concentration (C_i) is much lower than the extracellular substrate concentration in e.g. blood or plasma (C_e), plotted in this figure.
In A: $K_m^g = 5 \times K_m^S$; in B: $K_m^g = 100 \ K_m^S$
Data taken from ref. 42 where further details can be found for the model used for these calculations.

of an alternative, competing pathway with a higher affinity but a limited capacity. Such an increase in rate that is more than proportional to the substrate concentration is rather unexpected, but may be crucial in the apparently sudden appearance of a reactive intermediate.

INHIBITION OF SULFATION OF N-HYDROXY AROMATIC AMINES AND DERIVATIVES

Pentachlorophenol (PCP) has recently been introduced to inhibit selectively the sulfation of hydroxamic acids and similar substrates *in vivo* and *in vitro* (6,43-45); glucuronidation is unaffected and is able to compensate for the loss of sulfation (46). Towards sulfation of hydroxamic acids, PCP is more effective than 2,6-dichloro-4-nitrophenol (DCNP), another selective inhibitor of sulfation (46). Thus, the covalent binding of ^{3}H-N-hydroxy-FAAB to total macromolecules through sulfation in the kidney was inhibited by 35% by PCP, but not at all by DCNP (38). The same was observed in the liver also, with the substrate N-hydroxy-AAF.

PHARMACOKINETICS OF REACTIVE INTERMEDIATES AND EXTRAHEPATIC TUMOR FORMATION

If a reactive intermediate is relatively stable, it may get a chance to 'escape' from the cell where it is formed. In general, most likely, the reactive intermediates will be too labile. Thus, the sulfate ester of N-hydroxy-AAF is not mutagenic in the Ames test, probably because it does not reach the Salmonella DNA (47). On the other hand, clofibrate forms a glucuronide conjugate that reacts non-enzymatically with glutathione through an

S_N2 mechanism (16). Since the glucuronide is relatively stable under physiological conditions, it might bind covalently to other nucleophilic groups outside the cells where it is formed.

The N-glucuronide of N-hydroxy-2-naphthylamine is stable at pH 7.4, but breaks down rapidly at slightly acidic pH, such as may occur in urine. It is probably formed mainly in the liver, and is eliminated in urine in most species. When the urine is acidic (pH 5 to 6) it slowly hydrolyses in the bladder, and the carcinogenic hydroxylamine N-hydroxy-2-naphthylamine is released. Young and Kadlubar (48) have given a kinetic model in which the urine pH and bladder voiding intervals are correlated with bladder cancer incidence in several species. It is tempting to speculate that acid-labile glucuronide or sulfate conjugates can be hydrolysed inside the cell if they are taken up by lysosomes, which have an acidic pH.

Another site of carcinogenesis that may depend on pharmacokinetics is the gut lumen. Glucuronides are eliminated mainly through biliary excretion, especially in the rat; further metabolism by the gut flora, e.g. after hydrolysis by bacterial β-glucuronidase, may locally yield ultimate carcinogens, causing bowel cancer (49). In this respect the rat is expected to be more sensitive to such 'indirect' gut carcinogens than humans, because humans excrete drugs and their metabolites to a lesser extent in bile than rats.

ACKNOWLEDGEMENTS

We are indebted to Dr. Janet R. Dawson for a critical reading of the manuscript.

REFERENCES

1. Mulder, G.J. (1982) in: Jakoby, W.B., Bend, J.R. and Caldwell, J. (Eds.), Metabolic Basis of Detoxication, Academic Press, New York, N.Y. (USA), pp. 247-269.

2. Irving, C.C. (1970) in: Fishman, W.H. (Ed.), Metabolic Conjugation and Metabolic Hydrolysis, Academic Press, N.Y. (USA), pp. 53-120.

3. Mulder, G.J. (1981) in: Mulder, G.J. (Ed.), Sulfation of Drugs and Related Compounds, CRC Press, Boca Raton, FL (USA), pp. 213-226.

4. DeBaun, J.R., Miller, E.C. and Miller, J.A. (1970) Cancer Res., 30, 577-595.

5. Wirth, P.J. and Thorgeirsson, S.S. (1981) Molec. Pharmacol., 19, 337-344.

6. Meerman, J.H.N. and Mulder, G.J. (1982) in: Mulder, G.J., Caldwell, J., Van Kempen, G.M.J. and Vonk, R.J. (Eds.), Sulfate Metabolism and Sulfate Conjugation, Taylor & Francis Ltd, London (UK), pp. 145-153.

7. Vaught, J.B., McGarvey, P.B., Lee, M.S., Garner, C.D., Wang, C.Y., Linsmaier-Bednar, E.M. and King, C.M. (1981) Cancer Res., 41, 3424-3429.

8. Kadlubar, F.F., Miller, J.A., Miller, E.C. (1976) Cancer Res., 36, 2350-2359.

9. Watabe, T., Ishizuka, T., Isobe, M. and Ozawa, N. (1982) Science, 215, 403-405.

10. Rietveld, E.C., Plate, R. and Seutter-Berlage, F. (1983) Archs. Tox., 52, 199-207.

11. Mulder, G.J., Hinson, J.A. and Gillette, J.R. (1977) Biochem. Pharmacol., 27, 1641-1649.

12. Cardona, R.A. and King, C.M. (1976) Biochem. Pharmacol., 25, 1051-1056.

13. Kadlubar, F.F., Miller, J.A. and Miller, E.C. (1977) Cancer Res., 37, 805-814.

14. Kinoshita, N. and Gelboin, H.V. (1977) Science, 199, 307-309.

15. Nemoto, N. (1981) in: Polycyclic Hydrocarbons and Cancer, Academic Press, New York, N.Y. (USA) vol. 3, pp. 213-258.

16. Stogniew, M. and Fenselau, C. (1982) Drug Metabol. Disposit., 10, 609-613.

17. Mulder, G.J. (Ed.) Sulfation of Drugs and Related Compounds, CRC Press, Boca Raton, FL (1981).

18. Dutton, G.J. (Ed.) Glucuronidation of Drugs and Other Compounds, CRC Press, Boca Raton, FL (USA) (1980).

19. Wu, S.G. and Straub, K.D. (1976) J. Biol. Chem. 251, 6529-6536.

20. Sandler, M. and Usdin, E. (Eds.) Phenolsulfotransferase in Mental Health Research, MacMillan Publ. Ltd, London, U.K.

21. Bock, K.W., Von Clausbruch, U.C., Kaufmann, R., Lilienblum, W., Oesch, F., Pfeil, H. and Platt, K.L. (1980) Biochem. Pharmacol. 29, 495-500.

22. Bock, K.W., Lilienblum, W., Pfeil, H. and Eriksson, L.C. (1982) Cancer Res., 42, 3747-3752.

23. Yin, Z., Sato, K., Tsuda, H. and Ito, N. (1982) Gann 73, 239-248.

24. Shirai, T. and King, C.M. (1982) Carcinogenesis, 3, 1385-1391.

25. Cohen, G.M., Gibby, E.M. and Mehta, R. (1981) Nature, 291, 662-664.

26. Gibby, E.M., Mehta, R., Ellison, M. and Cohen, G.M. (1981) Biochem. Pharmacol., 30, 3333-3336.

27. Gessner, T. (1974) Biochem. Pharmacol., 23, 1809-1816.

28. Wong, K.P. (1982) in: Mulder, G.J., Caldwell, J., Van Kempen, G.M.J. and Vonk, R.J. (Eds.), Sulfate Metabolism and Sulfate Conjugation, Taylor & Francis Ltd, London (UK), pp. 85-92.

29. Dawson, J.R., Norbeck, K. and Moldeus, P. (1983) Biochem. Pharmacol., 32, in press.

30. Dawson, J.R. et al. in preparation.

31. Aw, T.Y. and Jones, D.P. (1983) Chem. Biol. Interact., 43, 283-290.

32. Cassidy, M.K. and Houston, J.B. (1980) Biochem. Pharmacol., 29, 471-474.

33. Hogg, S.I., Curtiss, C.G., Upshall, D.G. and Powell, G.M. (1981) Biochem. Pharmacol., 30, 1551-1555.

34. Mulder et al., in preparation.

35. Machida, M., Morita, Y., Hayashi, M. and Awazu, S. (1982) Biochem. Pharmacol., 31, 787-791.

36. Emslie, K.R., Smail, M.C., Calder, I.C., Hart, S.J. and Tange, J.D. (1981) Xenobiotica, 11, 43-50.

37. Elbers, R., Kampffmeyer, H.G. and Rabes, H. (1980) Xenobiotica, 10, 621.

38. Meerman, J.H.N. et al. (1983) in preparation.

39. Bock, K.W., Von Clausbruch, U.C. and Winne, D. (1979) Med. Biol., 57, 262.

40. George, C.F. (1981) Clin. Pharmacokin., 6, 259-274.

41. Gerkens, J.F., Desmond, P.V., Schenker, S. and Branch, R.A. (1981) Hepatology, 1, 329-335.

42. Koster, H. and Mulder, G.J. (1982) Drug Metabol. Disposit., 10, 330-335.

43. Meerman, J.H.N., Van Doorn, A.B.D. and Mulder, G.J. (1980) Cancer Res., 40, 3772-3779.

44. Meerman, J.H.N. and Mulder, G.J. (1981) Life Sci., 28, 2361-2365.

45. Meerman, J.H.N., Beland, F.A. and Mulder, G.J. (1981) Carcinogenesis, 2, 413-416.

46. Koster, H., Halsema, I., Scholtens, E., Meerman, J.H.N., Pang, K.S. and Mulder, G.J. (1982) Biochem. Pharmacol., 31, 1919-1924.

47. Mulder, G.J., Hinson, J.A., Nelson, W.L. and Thorgeirsson, S.S. (1977) Biochem. Pharmacol., 26, 1356-1358.

48. Young, J.F. and Kadlubar, F.F. (1982) Drug Metabol. Disposit., 10, 641-644.

49. Chipman, J.K. (1982) Toxicology, 25, 99-111.

© 1983 Elsevier Science Publishers B.V.
Extrahepatic Drug Metabolism and Chemical Carcinogenesis,
J. Rydström, J. Montelius and M. Bengtsson eds.

SPECIES AND TISSUE DIFFERENCES IN THE OCCURRENCE OF MULTIPLE FORMS OF RAT AND HUMAN GLUTATHIONE TRANSFERASES

BENGT MANNERVIK, CLAES GUTHENBERG, HELGI JENSSON, MARGARETA WARHOLM AND
PER ALIN
Department of Biochemistry, Arrhenius Laboratory, University of Stockholm,
S-106 91 Stockholm, Sweden

Conjugation reactions with glutathione (GSH) are important chemical processes in the biotransformation of xenobiotics in mammalian tissues (1). Such reactions are catalyzed by GSH transferases, which are abundant proteins, especially in the liver (2). Boyland and coworkers demonstrated that GSH transferase activity with several classes of organic substances is present in a single tissue, and concluded that different enzymes are responsible for the reactions studied (3). It was suggested that the transferases have specificities directed towards organic groups such as alkyl, aryl, and epoxy in the electrophilic substrates. The enzymes were consequently named GSH S-alkyltransferase, GSH S-aryltransferase, GSH S-epoxide transferase etc. In a symposium on GSH in 1973 we reported that GSH S-aryltransferase in rat liver cytosol could be resolved into two non-interconvertible isozymes (4). The two forms of the enzyme were purified and characterized and the only significant differences between them were found in their chromatographic and electrophoretic properties (5). The explanation for the similarities between the two isozymes were recently found in the discovery that they have a subunit in common (6).

Jakoby and coworkers demonstrated that the substrate specificities of the various forms of GSH transferase in rat liver cytosol are overlapping, and that the enzymes cannot accurately be distinguished on the basis of organic functional groups of the substrate, such as alkyl, aryl etc. (7). A nomenclature simply based on the chromatographic properties of the different enzyme forms was introduced. Recent studies show that Jakoby's nomenclature does not account for all GSH transferases and that some of the enzyme forms are heterodimeric proteins, the subunits of which can also occur as homodimers (6). Six basic isozymes have therefore been renamed to account for their respective subunit composition (6).

This paper consists of a status report of our work on identifying various isozymes of GSH transferase in rat and human tissues. The approach has been to characterize the hepatic enzymes and subsequently identify the extrahepatic isozymes that are identical with the enzyme forms in liver. Since most hepatic

GSH transferases are present in relatively large amounts, it is generally more convenient to study these enzymes in liver. The investigation of extra-hepatic isozymes can then be restricted to those that do not occur in liver.

GSH TRANSFERASES IN RAT TISSUES

Rat liver cytosol contains large amounts of 4 different protein subunits that are combined into 6 dimeric proteins with GSH transferase activity (6). Our analyses by quantitative immunoelectrophoresis of hepatic cytosol fractions from 200 g male Sprague Dawley rats show that approximately 5% of the cytosolic protein are accounted for by the GSH transferases (8). After treatment with inducers this percentage of cytosolic GSH transferases increased 3-4 fold (8). The 6 quantitatively dominating isozymes have been purified by affinity chromatography on S-hexylglutathione bound to epoxy-activated Sepharose 6B, followed by chromatofocusing in the pH range of pH 11 to 8 (9). These 6 basic proteins have been named GSH transferases L_2, BL, B_2, A_2, AC, and C_2, in the order of decreasing isoelectric points and in accordance with their respective subunit composition (6). Four of the transferases have earlier been named by Jakoby and coworkers (7, cf. Table 1), but the discovery of additional isozymes and the establishment of the relationships in subunit structure called for a new nomenclature. It is foreseen that similar names will be given to the remaining GSH transferases once their subunit structures have been clarified.

The identity of the 4 major subunits L, B, A, and C can be accurately established by the combined use of antibodies directed against the homodimeric proteins (Table 1) and specific substrates and inhibitors (Table 2). Thus, we possess a set of criteria for identification of GSH transferases containing these subunits, which includes isoelectric point, subunit M_r, reactions with antisera, substrate and inhibitor specificity.

In addition to the 6 hepatic GSH transferases discussed above, 4 different isozymes appear to exist in the cytosol fraction. Preliminary data (H. Jensson and B. Mannervik, unpublished work) suggest that 3 isozymes with isoelectric points at pH < 8 are formed as binary combinations of 2 subunits. At present, these enzyme forms are shown to differ from the more basic proteins by negative evidence, such as lack of reaction with antibodies or the characteristic substrates for the basic isozymes. An additional cytosolic GSH transferase is distinguished from the above 9 enzyme forms by not being bound to the affinity matrix containing immobilized S-hexylglutathione. This enzyme has been purified by isoelectric focusing of the fraction of

TABLE 1

CHARACTERISTICS OF BASIC GSH TRANSFERASES IN RAT LIVER CYTOSOL

Property	GSH transferase					
	L_2	BL	B_2	A_2	AC	C_2
Previous nomenclature (2)	–	B	AA	A	C	–
Isoelectric point	Decreasing ⟶ (pH interval 10-8)					
Subunit M_r	22K	22K +25K	25K	23.5K	23.5K	23.5K
Precipitin reaction with antiserum against GSH transferase						
L_2	+	+	–	–	–	–
B_2	–	+	+	–	–	–
A_2	–	–	–	+	+	–

TABLE 2

DISCRIMINATING SUBSTRATES AND INHIBITORS FOR IDENTIFICATION OF GSH TRANS-
FERASE SUBUNITS L, B, A, AND C IN RAT TISSUES

Characteristic	Subunit			
	L	B	A	C
Good substrate	Δ^5-andro-stene-3,17-dione	cumene hydro-peroxide	bromosulfo-phthalein	*trans*-4-phenyl-3-buten-2-one
Poor substrate	ethacrynic acid	*p*-nitro-phenyl-acetate	*trans*-4-phenyl-3-buten-2-one	bromosulfo-phthalein
Strong inhibitor	hematin	tributyl-tin acetate	triethyltin bromide	bromosulfo-phthalein
Poor inhibitor	triethyltin bromide	hematin	bromosulfo-phthalein	triethyltin bromide

TABLE 3

CHARACTERISTICS OF THE THREE TYPES OF HUMAN GSH TRANSFERASE

Characteristic	Transferase		
	$\alpha-\epsilon$	μ	π
M_r	51K	53K	47K
Isoelectric point	approx. 8-9	6.6	4.8
Precipitin reaction with antiserum against GSH transferase			
$\alpha-\epsilon$	+	-	-
μ	-	+	-
π	-	-	+
Good substrates	cumene hydroperoxide, Δ^5-androstene-3,17-dione	*trans*-4-phenyl-3-buten-2-one, benzo(a)pyrene 4,5-oxide, styren 7,8-oxide	ethacrynic acid

TABLE 4

OCCURRENCE OF THE THREE TYPES OF HUMAN GSH TRANSFERASE

Tissue	Transferase		
	basic ($\alpha-\epsilon$)	near-neutral (μ)	acidic (π/ρ)
Adult liver	+	+/-[a]	?
adrenal gland	+	+[b]	?
brain			+
lung			+
placenta			+
erythrocytes			+
Fetal liver	+		+
adrenal gland	+		+

[a] Some individuals (approx. 60% of the 23 livers tested) contain and some lack this isozyme (17, 18)
[b] Only few samples tested (*cf.* adult liver)

the cytosol that is not bound to the affinity column and is presumably identical with GSH transferase E (7). The purified enzyme reacts with antibodies raised against GSH transferase E (kindly provided by Dr. W.B. Jakoby), has an isoelectric point at approximately pH 7.5, and displays high relative activity with the substrate 1,2-epoxy-3-(p-nitrophenoxy)propane.

Furthermore, rat liver microsomes contain a protein with GSH transferase activity that is not present in the hepatic cytosol fraction. This enzyme is distinguished from the cytosolic transferases by being activatable by thiol-blocking agents, by analysis with specific antibodies, and by the smaller size of its polypeptide chain (M_r = 14000) (10).

GSH transferases in organs other than liver have not yet been studied in such detail as the enzymes in liver. Only in the case of rat testis (11, 12) have the isozymes been resolved and characterized by the methods discussed above. Rat testis cytosol has a specific activity of GSH transferase, measured with 1-chloro-2,4-dinitrobenzene as electrophilic substrate, that is similar to the value for liver cytosol. It has been found that the basic GSH transferases B_2, A_2, AC, and C_2, described in liver, also occur in testis (11, 12). However, no significant amount of GSH transferases L_2 and BL could be demonstrated in the testicular cytosol. The explanation for the absence of these isozymes in testis is presumably that the gene for subunit L is not expressed in this organ. Support for this interpretation is derived from the finding that 3-methylcholanthrene, which causes significant increase of the concentration of GSH transferases L_2 and BL (but not of B_2) in liver, does not induce GSH transferase activity (measured in the cytosol with 1-chloro-2,4-dinitrobenzene) in testis (13). Lack of induction of the same activity in kidney suggests the absence of protein subunit L also in this organ (13).

Significantly, rat testis cytosol differs from liver cytosol in having several GSH transferase isozymes with acidic isoelectric points (11-13). Approximately 50% of the activity with 1-chloro-2,4-dinitrobenzene is carried by a protein with an isoelectric point at pH 5.8. This acidic transferase, which is not detectable in liver, has been purified and has the highest specific activity (130 µmol/min per mg protein) noted for any GSH transferase in rat tissues (12).

The spectrum of GSH transferase isozymes in the cytosol of various rat tissues has been determined by isoelectric focusing (13). Even though the resolution is much inferior to that obtainable by chromatofocusing, certain general features become apparent. Kidney, adrenal gland, and ovary are similar to liver in having the major fraction of the GSH transferase activity

associated with proteins having isoelectric points at pH > 7. Proteins with
an acidic isoelectric point displayed small or negligible activity. Thus,
the testis stands out as special in having an acidic protein bearing a major
fraction of the activity. The lung is another organ, which, by other separation methods, has been found to contain a major GSH transferase that is not
detectable in liver (14). The contribution of this enzyme form to the total
transferase activity is of the same magnitude as the contributions of the
major basic isozymes. In the same study, a distinct isozyme originating from
blood was demonstrated (14). We believe that this enzyme is similar to the
acidic GSH transferase previously demonstrated in human erythrocytes (15).

In conclusion, our studies show the existence of a variety of GSH transferases and distinctly different isozyme distributions in different rat
tissues. The separation techniques and the set of identification criteria used
to identify hepatic isozymes should prove valuable in the further study of
extrahepatic enzyme forms.

GSH TRANSFERASES IN HUMAN TISSUES

In general, the isozyme pattern of GSH transferase is simpler in human
tissues than in rat tissues. It has not been demonstrated so far that different
subunits can generate hybrid enzyme forms such as GSH transferases BL and AC
in rat liver. However, such binary combinations may exist also in human tissues
and would provide a simple and reasonable explanation for the occurrence of
several basic GSH transferases in liver cytosol (16). So far, the multiple
forms studied in human tissues can be divided into 3 groups of proteins:
acidic, near-neutral, and basic GSH transferases (13, 17). Within the group
of basic transferases, 5 forms have been purified from the same liver and been
named GSH transferases α, β, γ, δ, and ϵ (16). No significant differences in
physical or catalytic properties between these 5 basic isozymes were detected,
and it was suggested that post-translational modification (such as, $e.g.$, de-
amidation) of a single gene product was the origin of the multiple forms.
However, studies in our laboratory demonstrated distinctly different isoelectric focusing patterns, including 1 to several basic isozymes for different individuals, suggesting a genetic basis for the multiplicity (18).
Multiple forms of the near-neutral transferase μ (17, 19) have not been found,
and also in the case of acidic GSH transferase is multiplicity less well
demonstrated, even though 2 acidic forms have been described in liver (20).
Nevertheless, the functional properties of any form within each of the 3
groups of human GSH transferases do not appear to differ significantly, and

for lack of evidence to the contrary, we will assume for the present discussion that the human enzymes can be dealt with as 3 different types of protein. The basic isozymes, first described in liver (16), will be called GSH transferase α-ε. The near-neutral isozyme is GSH transferase μ (17, 19). The acidic isozyme will be referred to as GSH transferase π, because this form, isolated from placenta, has been characterized in greatest detail (21). It appears as if transferase π is identical with transferase ρ, previously purified from erythrocytes (15, 21).

Detailed studies of GSH transferases α-ε, μ, and π show convincingly that the three types of enzyme are distinct proteins encoded by different genes (13, 17). Table 3 summarizes some of the characteristic properties that can be used to distinguish between the 3 forms. Like the rat enzymes, the human GSH transferases are dimeric proteins, but in no case has any of the human enzymes been shown to consist of two subunits of unequal size. Amino acid analyses provide one piece of evidence that the different isozymes do not arise post-translationally, *e.g.*, by partial proteolysis: the largest protein, transferase μ (M_r = 53000) has a lower content of, for example, valine (12.6 residues per molecule) than has transferase α-ε (M_r = 51000, 19.3 valine residues) or transferase π (M_r = 47000, 28.1 valine residues) (17). Other pieces of evidence, including analyses with specific antisera, characteristic substrates, circular dichroism spectra in the near ultraviolet region, and differences in occurrence, support the classification of the isozymes as three distinct groups (17).

In human liver cytosol basic GSH transferases (α-ε) are always found. In 13 of a total of 23 livers analyzed in our laboratory, the near-neutral transferase μ is present in addition to one or several basic isozymes (17, 18). The occurrence of transferase μ in some individuals is evidently genetically determined, but whether in other individuals the gene is present and silent or absent is unknown. The importance of GSH transferase μ in the protection against toxic, mutagenic, and carcinogenic substances is suggested by the finding that the enzyme has a specific activity with epoxide substrates such as benzo(α)pyrene 4,5-oxide and styrene 7,8-oxide that is one order of magnitude higher than the corresponding specific activities of transferases α-ε and π with these substrates (17). It would appear that individuals possessing transferase μ have a better protection against chemical challenges by certain electrophilic substances.

Small amounts of acidic GSH transferases have also been detected in adult human liver (18, 20, 22), but its possible origin from contaminating blood has

not been rigorously excluded. It should be added that human liver microsomes
have low but significant GSH transferase activity with 1-chloro-2,4-dinitro-
benzene (unpublished experiments).

Adrenal glands contain both basic and near-neutral GSH transferases in the
cytosol. All of the few samples tested contained transferase μ, but it is
possible that, as in the case of liver, some individuals lack this isozyme.
It has not yet been possible to obtain samples of liver and adrenal gland
from the same individual in order to investigate differential expression of
the gene in these two organs.

Other human tissues investigated in our laboratory include brain (cortex)
(23), lung (13), and placenta (21). These tissues display significant GSH
transferase activity only of the acidic type and judging from identical precipitin reactions with antiserum against transferase π from placenta the same isozyme is present in all cases. High relative activity with ethacrynic acid and
the molecular size support the identification of the enzyme in brain with
transferase π (23). A detailed comparison of transferase ρ from erythrocytes
with transferase π from placenta also points to identity or close similarity
of these enzyme forms (21). The acidic GSH transferase found in a 20 weeks old
placenta obtained at abortion appears identical with the isozyme of full-term
placenta. In the liver of 18 to 25 weeks old fetuses the cytosol contains two
major isozymes, one basic and one acidic (24). In the samples examined only
one basic isozyme was detected; it has not been proven that this isozyme is
identical with any of the several basic forms in adult liver. More noteworthy
than the sparsity of basic isozymes in fetal liver is the occurrence of a
major acidic GSH transferase (isoelectric point at pH 4.8). A quantitatively
significant acidic transferase has never been found in adult liver. The acidic
fetal isozyme gives a reaction of identity when tested with antiserum against
transferase π.

SIGNIFICANCE OF DIFFERENCES IN THE ISOZYME PATTERN

The significance of the differences in the occurrence of isozymes of GSH
transferase in different species and in different organs in the same organism
is not fully understood. It is generally assumed that the transferases serve
both as detoxication enzymes and as intracellular binding proteins (1, 2). In
both capacities the proteins interact with xenobiotics of a wide variety and
affect their biotransformation. Whether or not chemical compounds endogenous
to the organism are "natural" ligands and substrates of the GSH transferases
is unknown at present. Nevertheless, it seems evident that qualitative and

quantitative differences in occurrence of the various isozymes in different organs will cause differential susceptibility of the tissues to toxic, mutagenic, and carcinogenic effects of certain chemical substances. Further studies of the differences in isozyme patterns and the correlation of the presence or absence of certain enzyme forms to the occurrence of noxious effects of chemicals may give clues to the understanding of the origins of harmful effects and their prevention.

ACKNOWLEDGEMENTS

This work was supported by grants (to B.M.) from the Swedish Council for Planning and Coordination of Research, the Swedish Natural Science Research Council, and the Swedish Cancer Society.

REFERENCES

1. Chasseuad, L.F. (1979) Adv. Cancer Res. 29, 175-274.

2. Jakoby, W.B. and Habig, W.H. (1980) in: Jakoby, W.B. (Ed.), Enzymatic Basis of Detoxication, Vol. 2, Academic Press, New York, pp. 63-94.

3. Boyland, E. and Chasseaud, L.F. (1969) Adv. Enzymol. 32, 173-219.

4. Mannervik, B. and Eriksson, S.A. (1974) in: Flohé, L., Benöhr, H.C., Sies, H., Waller, H.D. and Wendel, A. (Eds.), Glutathione, Thieme Publishers, Stuttgart, pp. 120-131.

5. Askelöf, P., Guthenberg, C., Jakobson, I. and Mannervik, B. (1975) Biochem. J. 147, 513-522.

6. Mannervik, B. and Jensson, H. (1982) J. Biol. Chem. 257, 9909-9912.

7. Habig, W.H., Pabst, M.J. and Jakoby, W.B. (1974) J. Biol. Chem. 249, 7130-7139.

8. Guthenberg, C., Morgenstern, R., DePierre, J.W. and Mannervik, B. (1980) Biochim. Biophys. Acta 631, 1-10.

9. Jensson, H., Älin, P. and Mannervik, B. (1982) Acta Chem. Scand. B36, 205-206.

10. Morgenstern, R., Guthenberg, C. and DePierre, J.W. (1982) Eur. J. Biochem. 128, 243-248.

11. Guthenberg, C., Åstrand, I.-M., Älin, P. and Mannervik, B. (1983) Acta Chem. Scand. B37, in press.

12. Guthenberg, C., Älin, P., Åstrand, I.-M., Yalçin, S. and Mannervik, B., this volume.

13. Mannervik, B., Guthenberg, C., Jensson, H., Warholm, M. and Älin, P. (1983) in: Larsson, A., Orrenius, S., Holmgren, A. and Mannervik, B. (Eds.), Functions of Glutathione - Biochemical, Physiological, Toxicological, and Clinical Aspects, Raven Press, New York, pp. 75-88.

14. Guthenberg, C. and Mannervik, B. (1979) Biochem. Biophys. Res. Commun. 86, 1304-1310.

15. Marcus, C.J., Habig, W.H. and Jakoby, W.B. (1978) Arch. Biochem. Biophys. 188, 287-293.

16. Kamisaka, K., Habig, W.H., Ketley, J.N., Arias, I.M. and Jakoby, W.B. (1975) Eur. J. Biochem. 60, 153-161.

17. Warholm, M., Guthenberg, C. and Mannervik, B. (1983) Biochemistry 22, in press.

18. Warholm, M., Guthenberg, C., Mannervik, B., von Bahr, C. and Glaumann, H. (1980) Acta Chem. Scand. B34, 607-610.

19. Warholm, M., Guthenberg, C., Mannervik, B. and von Bahr, C. (1981) Biochem. Biophys. Res. Commun. 98, 512-519.

20. Awasti, Y.C., Dao, D.D. and Saneto, R.P. (1980) Biochem. J. 191, 1-10.

21. Guthenberg, C. and Mannervik, B. (1981) Biochim. Biophys. Acta 661, 255-260.

22. Koskelo, K. and Valmet, E. (1980) Scand. J. Clin. Lab. Invest. 40, 179-184.

23. Olsson, M., Guthenberg, C. and Mannervik, B., this volume.

24. Warholm, M., Guthenberg, C., Mannervik, B., Pacifici, G.M. and Rane, A. (1981) Acta Chem. Scand. B35, 225-227.

© 1983 Elsevier Science Publishers B.V.
Extrahepatic Drug Metabolism and Chemical Carcinogenesis,
J. Rydström, J. Montelius and M. Bengtsson eds.

IDENTIFICATION OF NOVEL GLUTATHIONE S-TRANSFERASES IN KIDNEY AND LUNG AND THE INDUCIBILITY OF VARIOUS ISOZYMES IN LIVER AND OTHER ORGANS

F. OESCH[1], U. MILBERT[1], T. FRIEDBERG[1] and C.R. WOLF[2]

[1]Institute of Pharmacology, University of Mainz (FRG) and [2]Imperial Cancer Research Fund., Medical Oncology Unit, Western General Hospital, Edinburgh (UK)

INTRODUCTION

The glutathione S-transferases (GST's) comprise a family of proteins with a major role in the deactivation of toxic or carcinogenic metabolites produced from foreign compounds (1,2). In contrast to this function they also appear to be involved in the activation of certain chemicals, particularly halogenated compounds, to toxic, mutagenic and therefore potentially carcinogenic products (3).

It is now clear that drug metabolizing enzymes are distributed through all the organs of the body. The multiplicity of drug metabolizing enzymes and the relative roles of the different isozymes in the above reactions is a fascinating and intensivly studied research area. It has now been demonstrated that there are multiple forms of cytochrome P-450 in extrahepatic tissues such as lung and kidney (4-6) with different specificities in the metabolism (4-8) and activation of foreign compounds (7).

Similar knowledge of the glutathione S-transferases in extrahepatic tissues is still relatively sparse, not only in the relative amounts of different forms but also in the inducibility of these forms. On the basis of immuno-chemical reactivity the hepatic enzymes can be split into two major categories: forms B, AA and ligandin, and forms A, C and X (9-11). Antibodies to B react with AA and ligandin and antibodies to C react with A and X. Other forms, M and E, do not appear to belong to either group and have very different substrate specificities to the above (9). In this paper we have separated GST forms from rat liver, lung and kidney. The substrate specificities, immuno-chemical cross-reactivity and inducibility of the lung and kidney forms have been investigated and compared to the hepatic enzymes. The data presented demonstrate many significant and potentially important differences in GST populations between these organs.

MATERIALS AND METHODS

Hepatic cytosolic fractions were prepared from Male Sprague Dawley rats (200 g) as described previously. Animals treated with Aroclor 1254 received one injection (500 mg/kg) i.p. one weak before use. Glutathione S-transferases

TABLE 1

GLUTATHIONE S-TRANSFERASE ACTIVITIES IN VARIOUS ORGANS OF THE RAT AND THE EFFECT OF AROCLOR 1254 TREATMENT

		GST activity (nmol per min per protein)					
		2,4-DNCB	1,2-DCNB	TPB	ENP	MS	AD
Liver	Control	964 $\pm$ 9.7	35.8 $\pm$ 9.6	11.3 $\pm$ 1.4	78 $\pm$ 7.9	11.9 $\pm$ 0.9	48 $\pm$ 1.1
	Aroclor 1254	3865 $\pm$ 263 (401)*	76.3 $\pm$ 6.6 (213)*	22.5 $\pm$ 2.2 (219)*	128 $\pm$ 7.8 (164)*	12.3 $\pm$ 1.5 (103)	148 $\pm$ 13 (308)*
Kidney	Control	86 $\pm$ 28	0.84 $\pm$ 0.2	1.4 $\pm$ 0.07	30.3 $\pm$ 1.2	7.8 $\pm$ 2.5	3.24 $\pm$ 0.2
	Aroclor 1254	180 $\pm$ 12 (209)*	1.01 $\pm$ 0.2 (120)*	1.4 $\pm$ 0.2 (100)	30 $\pm$ 1.2 (99)	7.2 $\pm$ 0.8 (92)	4.08 $\pm$ 0.7 (125)*
Lung	Control	51 $\pm$ 3.2	1.05 $\pm$ 0.3	0.82 $\pm$ 0.03	42 $\pm$ 5.9	5.2 $\pm$ 1.0	0.87 $\pm$ 0.09
	Aroclor 1254	76.2 $\pm$ 16.6 (149)*	1.74 $\pm$ 6.6 (166)*	1.12 $\pm$ 0.2 (136)*	58.1 $\pm$ 1.4 (138)*	8.9 $\pm$ 2.5 (171)*	1.08 $\pm$ 0.1 (124)*

* = significantly different from control. p = < 0.01. Values in parenthesis are percentages of the control value.
2,4-DNCB = 2,4-Dinitrochlorobenzene; 1,2-DCNB = 1,2-dichloronitrobenzene; TPB = trans-4-phenyl-3-butene-2-one;
ENP = 1,2-epoxy-3-p(nitrophenoxy)propane; MS = menaphthylsulphate; AD = androstene-3,17-dione.

A, B, C and X were separated by the method of Pabst et al. (13) and purified by the method of Friedberg et al. (14). These proteins were apparently homogeneous as judged by polyacrylamide gel electrophoresis. Antisera to the glutathione S-transferases B and C were raised in rabbits. Antigen (250 µg in 1 ml Freunds complete adjuvant; diluted 1:1 with water) was injected s.c. at several sites. Two further injections of 100 µg in 1 ml incomplete adjuvant, diluted 1:1 with water were carried out at 4 week intervals. Sera were obtained two weeks following the final injections.

Glutathione S-transferase activities were determined with the following substrates (13,14,15,16) 2,4-dinitrochlorobenzene (DNCB), 1,2-dichloronitrobenzene (DCNB), 1,2-epoxy-3-p(nitrophenoxy)propane (ENP), trans-4-phenyl-3-butene-2-one (TPB), androstene-3,17-dione (AD) and menaphthylsulphate (MS). Preparative isoelectric focusing of the cytosolic fractions was carried out on Ultrodex gels (LKB Ltd.) using an LKB multiphore apparatus (12). Following focusing of 30 mg cytosol the gel was divided into 30 fractions and the proteins eluted as described previously (12). Samples were assayed for GST activity and for immunochemical reactivity. In the latter case samples containing peak activities (2 ml) were concentrated to 100 µl by ultrafiltration (Amicon Ltd.). SDS electrophoresis and protein determinations were as described previously (12). Enzyme linked immunosorbent assays (ELISA) and immunodiffusion analysis were carried out by the methods of Burger et al. (17) and Ouchterlony (18).

RESULTS AND DISCUSSION

Glutathione S-transferase activities in rat liver, lung and kidney using various substrates and the effect of Aroclor 1254 on these activities are shown in Table 1. In control cytosol DNCB, activities were approximately 10 to 20 fold higher in the liver than in the kidney or lungs. The reaction of extrahepatic cytosol with DCNB and TPB was very weak. Since GST's A, C and X have highest activities towards these substrates these results demonstrate the low amounts of these proteins in kidney and lung. On the other hand extrahepatic ENP activity was relatively high compared to liver. The kidney had 39% and the lung 54% of the hepatic control value indicating a high concentration of GST E or the presence of a new transferase form. The substrate specificity of GST E is at present poorly defined and it would therefore be extremely interesting to determine its activity towards carcinogens and cytotoxic compounds. Similarly menaphthylsulphate activity associated with GST M was comparatively high in lung and kidney (Table 1).

The low activity towards AD suggests that GST B is present in the kidney at 10% or less of the hepatic level and at less than 3% of this level in the lungs. This is in contrast to the related protein ligandin which has been reported to be present in the kidney cytosol at 50% of the hepatic value (19).

The data in Table 1 also demonstrate the complexity of glutathione S-transferases' regulation in different organs, with respect to the relative proportions of different forms and their inducibility. For example MS activity (GST M) was significantly induced in the lungs but not in the other organs by Aroclor 1254. DNCB and DCNB activities for example were increased in all tissues whereas the percentage increase varied. Activity towards TPB, which is high with GST C and X, was not increased substantially in the kidney or the lungs. The data show differences in the inducibility between organs, but also in a particular organ the GST forms would appear to be induced to different extents which suggests that the various forms are regulated differently. This is potentially a very important factor in the sequestration of toxic metabolites. Different GST forms have been shown to exhibit significantly different activities in the deactivation of carcinogenic compounds (20).

Two questions are raised by the above findings 1) are the low GST activities of lung and kidney due to the presence of low concentrations of enzymes found in the liver or to new transferase forms? and 2) does the change in activity on induction reflect an increase in synthesis of forms already present or of new proteins?

In an attempt to answer these questions the GST's present in cytosolic fractions from rat liver, lung and kidney were separated by isoelectric focusing from control animals and after treatment of the animals with Aroclor 1254. Figure 1 shows the peaks of activity obtained with control samples. In no case did pretreatment with Aroclor 1254 result in the appearance or disappearance of peaks indicating that changes in activity in all organs are changes in forms of the GST's already present. A striking difference in the GST forms between the various organs was observed. In the liver all the peaks observed could be accounted for by known GST's. However, in the kidney forms with I.P. values of 9.3, 7.4 and 6.0 were observed. The values of 7.4 and 6.0 do not correspond to well characterized GST forms in the liver. The peak with I.P. 9.3 would be in agreement with GST B. Pure GST B focused at this pH under the conditions used here. Hales et al. (21) have reported three peaks of activity in the kidney with I.P. values of 9.0, 8.5 and 7.0 with activity towards DNCB, p-nitrobenzyl-chloride and TPB. It is not clear how these peaks relate to those observed in the present study. The difference in I.P. values may be attributed to the different experimental procedure used.

Only the peak at 9.3 reacted with antibodies to GST B on immunodiffusion and none of the GST's reacted with anti GST C. However the more sensitive ELISA

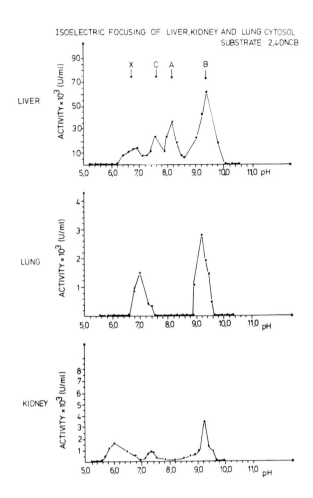

Fig. 1. Isoelectric focusing of cytosol samples from rat liver, lung and kidney. 30 mg of cytosolic protein were focused in an Ultrodex bed, using LKB ampholites pH 7-11, for 16 h. Following this period the gels were divided into 30 segments and the proteins contained in each segment were eluted with distilled water (2 ml). pH was measured and the samples were assayed for DNCB activity.

showed that all the kidney peaks had structural similarities to GST B and essentially none with GST C (Table 2).

On the basis of these data the GST form at I.P. 9.3 could be GST B or ligandin. SDS electrophoresis of this peak gave bands which correspond to molecular weights of 23000 and 25000. Fleischer et al. (19) using an immuno-assay reported that ligandin is present in the kidney at approx. 50% of

TABLE 2

IMMUNOCHEMICAL REACTIVITY OF GLUTATHIONE S-TRANSFERASE FORMS FROM RAT LUNG
AND KIDNEY IN THE ELISA

| | Peak at I.P. | units at 423 nm | |
		Anti GST B	Anti GST C
Lung	7.0	0.13	0
	9.3	0.99	0
Kidney	6.0	0.97	0.03
	7.4	0.77	0
	9.3	1.31	0

the hepatic level. Kidney cytosol activity towards AD, a good substrate for
GST B, was less than 8% of the hepatic value. Thus, the peak at 9.3 has immunochemical similarities to GST B and ligandin, whilst the relatively low activity towards AD argues against its identity with GST B.

The GST's at I.P. 6.0 and 7.4 appear unique to the kidney although they bear
immunological similarities to GST B. They did not metabolise AD at a measurable level. None of the three kidney peaks showed activity towards MS (GST M)
or ENP (GST E), whilst these activities were relatively high in kidney cytosol.
These findings taken together indicate that the kidney contains at least five
glutathione S-transferase forms. The hepatic forms A,C and X appear to be
essentially absent in kidney cytosol.

In the lungs only two peaks of GST activity were obtained on isoelectric
focusing (I.P. 7.0 and 9.3). Both these fractions reacted with anti GST B
(Table 2), neither reacted with anti GST C, which is in agreement with the low
activities towards DCNB and TPB (Table 1). This indicates that, similar to the
kidney, GST's A, C and X are essentially absent. The exact identity of the two
peaks remains to be clarified but the peak at 9.3 could be GST B. Guthenberg
et al. (22) have reported the isolation of five GST forms from the rat lung
including GST B. They also identified GST's A and C which would be in contrast
to the findings here, but our data also indicate that at least four GST's are
present in rat lung i.e. GST's M and E, or analogous enzymes (Table 1), possibly GST B and an as yet unreported form with an I.P. of 7.0.

In addition to the various forms of GST's found in the liver other forms
exist in extrahepatic tissues. The poor response of extrahepatic enzymes to
compounds which induce GST's in the liver substantiates the general finding

that GST's in different organs are regulated by different mechanisms. These control mechanisms represent a challenging aspect of this enzyme system. It would appear that there are at least twelve hepatic and extrahepatic GST's whose subunits possibly originate from 12 different genes under very different control. The above facts raise the questions of the primary role of these proteins in extrahepatic tissues and whether it is related to foreign compound metabolism.

ACKNOWLEDGEMENTS

The authors would like to thank the Deutsche Forschungsgemeinschaft for financial support and Ms. I. Böhm for typing this manuscript.

REFERENCES

1. Chasseaud, L.F. (1979) Adv. Canc. Res. 29, 175-274.

2. Jakoby, W.B., Habig, W.H. (1980) in: Enzymatic Basis of Detoxication. Vol. II. (W.B. Jakoby ed.), Academic Press, New York, pp. 63-94.

3. Rannug, U. (1980) Mutation Res. 76, 269-295.

4. Philpot, R.M. and Wolf, C.R. (1981) in: Review in Biochemical Toxicology. Vol. III (Hodgson E. Bend, J.R. and Philpot, R.M. eds.), Elsevier: North Holland, pp. 51-76.

5. Wolf, C.R., Hook, J.B., Lock, E.A. (1983) Mol. Pharmacol. 23, 206-212.

6. Dees, J.H., Masters, B.S.S., Muller Eberhard, U. and Johnson, G.F. (1982) Cancer Res. 42, 1423-1432.

7. Robertson, I.G.C., Philpot, R.M., Zeiger, E. and Wolf, C.R. (1981) Mol. Pharmacol. 20, 662-668.

8. Wolf, C.R., Statham, C.N., McMenamin, M.G., Bend, J.R., Boyd, M.R. and Philpot, R.M. (1982) Mol. Pharmacol. 22, 738-744.

9. Jakoby, W.B., Habig, W.H., Keen, J.H., Kettey, J.N. and Pabst, M.J. (1976) in: Glutathione: Metabolism and Functions (Jakoby, W.B. and Arias, J.M. eds.), Raven Press, New York, pp. 189-211.

10. Tu, C-P, Weiss, M.J. and Reddy, C.C. (1982) Biochem. Biophys. Res. Commun. 108, 461-467.

11. Frey, A.B., Friedberg, T., Oesch, F. and Kreibich, G. (1983) Biol. Chem., in press.

12. Friedberg, T., Bentley, P., Stasiecki, P., Glatt, H.R., Raphael, D. and Oesch, F. (1979) J. Biol. Chem. 254, 12028-12033.

13. Pabst, M.J., Habig, W.B. and Jakoby, W.B. (1974) J. Biol. Chem. 249, 7140-7150.

14. Friedberg, T., Bentley, P., Guenthner, T.M. and Oesch, F. (1983) Biochem. J., submitted.

15. Benson, A.H., Talalay, P., Heen, J.H., Jakoby, W.B. (1977) Proc. Natl. Acad. Sci. USA 74, 158-162.

16. Gilham, B. (1971) Biochem. J. 121, 667-672.

17. Burger, R., Deubel, U., Hadding, U. and Bitter-Suermann, D. (1982) J. Immunol. 129, 2042-2050.

18. Ouchterlony, O. (1958) Progr. Allergy 5, 1-78.

19. Fleischer, G., Kamisaka, K., Gatmaitan, F. and Arias, I.M. (1976) in: Glutathione Metabolism and Functions (Arias, I.M. and Jakoby, W.B. eds.), Raven Press, New York, pp. 259-265.

20. Glatt, H.R., Friedberg, T., Grover, P.L., Sims, P. and Oesch, F., Cancer Res., submitted.

21. Hales, B.F., Jaeger, J. and Neims, A.H. (1978) Biochem. J. 175, 937-943.

22. Guthenberg, C. and Mannervik, B. (1979) Biochem. Biophys. Res. Commun. 86, 1304-1310.

© 1983 Elsevier Science Publishers B.V.
Extrahepatic Drug Metabolism and Chemical Carcinogenesis,
J. Rydström, J. Montelius and M. Bengtsson eds.

ISOZYMES OF GLUTATHIONE TRANSFERASE IN RAT TESTIS

CLAES GUTHENBERG, PER ÅLIN, ING-MARI ÅSTRAND, SÜHA YALÇIN AND BENGT MANNERVIK
Department of Biochemistry, Arrhenius Laboratory, University of Stockholm,
S-106 91 Stockholm, Sweden

INTRODUCTION

   Conjugation of reduced glutathione with a large number of electrophilic
substances, including chemical carcinogens and mutagens, constitutes an
important detoxication mechanism (1). Many of these conjugation reactions are
catalyzed by glutathione transferases (EC 2.5.1.18). In addition to their
enzymatic function many of the transferases are able to bind chemical compounds such as steroids, steroid metabolites, carcinogens and other substances (2). The occurrence of glutathione transferase in animal species is
widespread. Several transferase isozymes have been purified from both human
liver and rat liver (3). Six basic transferases in rat liver have now been
characterized as binary combinations of four protein subunits: A, B, C and L
(4). The presence of glutathione transferases is not restricted to the liver
but has also been demonstrated in extrahepatic organs. Most transferases
studied are basic proteins, but acidic or neutral isozymes have been isolated
from rat liver (5), human liver (6-8), erythrocytes (9), placenta (10, 11) and
lung (12). In vertebrates, the liver is one of the most important organs for
biotransformation of xenobiotics. However, in view of the differences in
susceptibility of different organs to toxic effects of foreign compounds, it is
of importance to study detoxication systems in extrahepatic organs as well. In
comparison with the liver, most other organs show considerably lower glutathione
transferase activity; one exception is rat testis, which also shows high transferase activity. In evaluating the significance of glutathione transferase in
protection of an organ against reactive substances, not only the total enzymatic activity is of interest, but also the properties of the different isozymes present are of importance. In the present study isozymes of glutathione
transferase in rat testis were isolated and characterized.

RESULTS

   The cytosol fraction of rat testis was found to have a glutathione transferase activity with 1-chloro-2,4-dinitrobenzene of 1.6 μmol per min per mg
protein. This specific cytosolic activity is considerably higher than that
determined for other extrahepatic organs such as kidney, ovary, intestine,

adrenals, brain, and lung. It was also sligthly higher than the specific activity of rat liver cytosol. When the cytosol fraction of rat liver, adrenal gland, ovary, and testis was analyzed by means of isoelectric focusing, it was found that the major part of the activity in all tissues except the testis was localized to the basic pH range of the gradient. In testis the major form was found to have an isoelectric point at pH 5.8.

A procedure for the separation of the glutathione transferases in rat testis has been worked out in our laboratory (13). The transferase activity was separated from contaminating cytosolic proteins by use of affinity chromatography on S-hexylglutathione coupled to epoxy-activated Sepharose 6B, and the various isozymes of glutathione transferase were subsequently resolved by chromatofocusing. Chromatofocusing in the pH interval of 10.8-8 of the pooled fractions from the affinity chromatography clearly resolved 5 separate peaks of activity towards the substrate 1-chloro-2,4-dinitrobenzene. The isozymes were eluted with a pH gradient, and the peaks were labeled I-V according to the order of elution as the pH of the chromatographic gradient decreases. Further elution with 1 M NaCl released approximately 50% of the activity that had been applied to the column. This result is clearly different from that of rat liver for which the fraction released by NaCl is approximately 5%. The five basic transferases were identified with the corresponding liver enzymes, by use of the positions of the peaks in the elution profile, subunit size, substrate specificity, reactivity with antibodies, and inhibition pattern. Analysis by sodium dodecyl sulfate polyacrylamide electrophoresis showed that peak I consists of a subunit with a molecular weight of 25000. Peaks II, III, IV, and V gave bands corresponding to a molecular weight of 23500. The double diffusion method of Ouchterlony with antibodies raised against glutathione transferases B_2, L_2, and A_2 revealed that peak I reacted with antibodies to subunit B, whereas peaks II, III, and IV gave precipitates with antibodies to subunit A (but not vice versa). Peak V did not give a precipitin reaction with any of the two antisera, and none of the 5 peaks gave a precipitate with antibodies to transferase L_2.

Table 1 gives ratios of catalytical activities with different substrates for the 5 basic transferase isozymes in rat testis as well as for the previously characterized basic rat liver transferases. These ratios of activities were determined in order to identify the testis transferases with the corresponding rat liver enzymes. The I_{50} values (the concentration of an inhibitor giving 50% inhibition of the enzymatic activity) obtained with hematin, triethyltin bromide and bromosulfophthalein as inhibitors have recently been found to

TABLE 1

COMPARISON OF ACTIVITY RATIOS ($\times 10^3$) OF BASIC GLUTATHIONE TRANSFERASE ISOZYMES FROM TESTIS AND LIVER[a]

Substrate ratio	Peak no. of basic testis isozymes (liver isozyme)[b]					
			I	II	III	IV	V
	(L_2)	(BL)	(B_2)	(A_2)	(AC)		(C_2)
DCNB/CDNB			2.1	84	46	100	7.0
	(1.5)	(1.0)	(2.6)	(100)	(70)		(10)
tPBO/CDNB			0	2.0	22	4.2	100
	(0)	(0)	(0)	(1.3)	(18)		(81)
ethacrynic acid/ CDNB			84	3.3	18	14	42
	(4.8)	(2.3)	(69)	(6.5)	(15)		(46)

[a] DCNB = 1,2-dichloro-4-nitrobenzene; CDNB = 1-chloro-2,4-dinitrobenzene; tPBO = *trans*-4-phenyl-3-buten-2-one
[b] Isozymes were separated by chromatofocusing (4)

TABLE 2

COMPARISON OF I_{50} VALUES (μM) FOR BASIC GLUTATHIONE TRANSFERASE ISOZYMES FROM TESTIS AND RAT LIVER[a]

Inhibitor	Peak no. of basic testis isozymes (liver isozyme)[b]					
			I	II	III	IV	V
	(L_2)	(BL)	(B_2)	(A_2)	(AC)		(C_2)
Hematin			>10	2.0	1.0	2.0	0.7
	(0.1)	(10)	(>10)	(2.0)	(2.0)		(1.0)
Triethyltin bromide			0.5	0.5	1.0	50	100
	(500)	(100)	(3.0)	(1.0)	(1.5)		(100)
Bromosulfophthalein			200	10	6.0	20	0.5
	(2.0)	(10)	(200)	(10)	(6.0)		(0.5)

[a] Transferase activity was determined using 1-chloro-2,4-dinitrobenzene as electrophilic substrate
[b] Isozymes were separated by chromatofocusing (4)

serve as important characteristics for discrimination between the four subunits constituting the six basic rat liver transferases (14). Table 2 shows
the I_{50} values found with the basic testis isozymes, together with the corresponding values for the liver transferases.

By putting all the above results together, peak I of the testis isozymes
obtained after chromatofocusing was identified as transferase B_2, peak II as
transferase A_2, peak III as transferase AC, and peak V as transferase C_2. The
identification of the isozyme in peak IV has not been completed, but its properties suggest a relationship to protein subunit A. The pattern of basic
transferases in rat testis differs from that of rat liver in that no significant amounts of glutathione transferases L_2 and BL are detectable in the
testis. The absence of the small subunit of glutathione transferase "B" (subunit L in the new nomenclature) in rat testis has earlier been reported (15).

The glutathione transferase eluted from the chromatofocusing column with 1 M
NaCl was further separated after a second chromatofocusing in the pH interval
of 8-5. One major and 5 minor peaks were found. The existence of acidic transferases has earlier been reported (16) but the resolution of these enzymes
into several isozymes has only recently been obtained in our group (13). The
acidic transferases are all active with 1-chloro-2,4-dinitrobenzene, but have
low or very low activity with all other substrates tested. The substrates used
include ethacrynic acid, 1,2-dichloro-4-nitrobenzene, *trans*-4-phenyl-3-buten-
2-one, bromosulfophthalein, 1,2-epoxy-3-(p-nitrophenoxy)propane, and p-nitro-
benzylchloride.

The dominating acidic transferase has been purified in a separate experiment
by use of a modified procedure in which the first chromatofocusing step is
omitted. After affinity chromatography on S-hexylglutathione Sepharose 6B the
active fractions were chromatofocused directly in the pH interval of 8-5. The
enzyme was purified 80-fold and this procedure is an efficient method to obtain highly purified enzyme in good yield. The isoelectric point of the purified enzyme was at pH 5.8. The subunit molecular weight was determined as
22000 by use of sodium dodecyl sulfate slab gel electrophoresis. The non-
identity of the acidic testicular transferase with any of the basic hepatic
transferases was confirmed by Ouchterlony immunodiffusion. No precipitin reaction was found with antibodies raised against rat liver transferases B_2, L_2 or
A_2.

The most conspicuous finding was the high activity found with 1-chloro-2,4-
dinitrobenzene (130 μmol/min per mg protein). This activity is higher than that
for any other rat glutathione transferase. However, somewhat higher specific

activity has been determined with transferase μ, isolated from human liver (8). In addition to the substrates mentioned above some compounds of physiological interest were tested. No activity was detectable in catalyzing the isomerization of Δ^5-androstene-3,17-dione to Δ^4-androstene-3,17-dione. This reaction, which is catalyzed by some of the glutathione transferases, constitutes a step in the biosynthesis of testosterone. However, the enzyme showed significant activity with styrene-7,8-oxide and with benzo(a)pyrene-4,5-oxide. The following steroids were tested as inhibitors (in 0.2 mM concentration) of the activity with 1-chloro-2,4-dinitrobenzene: hydrocortisone, corticosterone, progesterone, estriol, testosterone, Δ^4-androstene-3,17-dione, betamethasone, and dexamethasone. No inhibitory effect was found with any of these steroids.

CONCLUSION

The isozyme pattern of glutathione transferase in rat testis differs markedly from that of rat liver in that no significant amounts of glutathione transferases L_2 and BL are detectable in the testis. However, the most conspicuous difference was that a major part of the activity is borne by a protein with an acidic isoelectric point. The possible significance of this dominating acidic testicular transferase in the protection of the testis against toxic effects of electrophilic substances such as mutagens, as well as its possible role in transport and metabolism of steroids needs to be further investigated.

ACKNOWLEDGEMENT

This work was supported by grants (to B.M.) from the Swedish Council for Planning and Coordination of Research.

REFERENCES

1. Chasseaud, L.F. (1979) Adv. Cancer Res. 29, 175-274.
2. Smith, G.J. and Litwack, G. (1980) Rev. Biochem. Toxicol. 2, 1-47.
3. Jakoby, W.B. and Habig, W.H. (1980) in: Jakoby, W.B. (Ed.), Enzymatic Basis of Detoxication, Vol. 2, Academic Press, New York, pp. 63-94.
4. Mannervik, B. and Jensson, H. (1982) J. Biol. Chem. 257, 9909-9912.
5. Gillham, B. (1973) Biochem. J. 135, 797-804.
6. Koskelo, K. and Valmet, E. (1980) Scand. J. Clin. Lab. Invest. 40, 179-184.
7. Awasthi, Y.C., Dao, D.D. and Saneto, R.P. (1980) Biochem. J. 191, 1-10.
8. Warholm, M., Guthenberg, C., Mannervik, B. and von Bahr, C. (1981) Biochem. Biophys. Res. Commun. 98, 512-519.
9. Marcus, C.J., Habig, W.H. and Jakoby, W.B. (1978) Arch. Biochem. Biophys. 188, 287-293.

10. Polidoro, G., Di Ilio, C., Del Boccio, G., Zulli, P. and Federici, G. (1980) Biochem. Pharmacol. 29, 1677-1680.

11. Mannervik, B. and Guthenberg, C. (1981) Meth. Enzymol. 77, 231-235.

12. Koskelo, K., Valmet, E. and Tenhunen, R. (1981) Scand. J. Clin. Lab. Invest. 41, 683-689.

13. Guthenberg, C., Åstrand, I.-M., Ålin, P. and Mannervik, B. (1983) Acta Chem. Scand. B37, in press.

14. Yalçin, S., Jensson, H. and Mannervik, B., this volume.

15. Bhargava, M.M., Ohmi, N., Listowski, I. and Arias, I.M. (1980) J. Biol. Chem. 255, 724-727.

16. Dierickx, P.J. and De Beer, J.O. (1981) Biochemistry Internat. 3, 565-571.

© 1983 Elsevier Science Publishers B.V.
Extrahepatic Drug Metabolism and Chemical Carcinogenesis,
J. Rydström, J. Montelius and M. Bengtsson eds.

PEROXISOME PROLIFERATION, FATTY ACID β-OXIDATION AND CANCER INITIATION BY PHENOXYACETIC ACID HERBICIDES

H. VAINIO[1,3], E. HIETANEN[2,3], K. LINNAINMAA[1] AND E. MANTYLA[2]

[1]Institute of Occupational Health, Helsinki 29 (Finland) and [2]Department of Physiology, University of Turku, Turku 52 (Finland)

INTRODUCTION

Epidemiological studies suggest an increased risk of soft-tissue sarcomas and malignant lymphomas among persons occupationally exposed to the phenoxyacetic acid herbicides 2,4,5-T (2,4,5-trichlorophenoxyacetic acid), 2,4-D (2,-4-dichlorophenoxyacetic acid) and MCPA (4-chloro-2-methylphenoxyacetic acid) (1,2). These findings have aroused a great deal of discussion, since available animal studies provide no convincing evidence for the carcinogenicity of phenoxyacetic acid herbicides. Furthermore, these chemicals have shown no DNA reactivity and give negative results in point mutation assays (3).

2,4-D and MCPA are close structural analogues of clofibrate, a hypolipidaemic drug that is hepatocarcinogenic to rodents. It has been suggested that peroxisome proliferation is a key feature of clofibrate-induced carcinogenesis (4). It was threrefore our aim to study whether phenoxyacetic acid herbicides (2,4-D and MCPA) and a non-phenoxyacetic acid herbicide, glyphosate, also act as hypolipidaemic agents and cause peroxisome proliferation in rats.

MATERIALS AND METHODS

Six-week-old male Wistar rats given free access to food and drinking-water received 1 mmol/kg body weight of solutions containing 550 g/l 2,4-D (as amine salt) or 500 g/l MCPA (as isooctyl ester) (obtained from Kemira Company, Helsinki, Finland) intragastrically every morning for 1, 3, 7 or 14 days; the last dose was given 24 h before sacrifice. After 4 days the dose of MCPA was lowered to 0.5 mmol/kg because of excessive toxicity. Doses of 1 mmol/kg body weight of a solution containing 360 g/l glyphosate (Roundup, Monsanto) (N-phosphonomethylglycine) were given intragastrically as the isopropylamine salt. Positive controls received 1 mmol/kg body weight clofibrate (ethyl-2-[p-chlorophenoxy]-2-methylpropionate, Klofiran[R], Remeda, Kuopio, Finland) intragastrically; negative controls received equivalent volumes of saline (5,6).

---

[3]Present address: International Agency for Research on Cancer, 69372 Lyon (France)

Methods used for counting the number and surface area of peroxisomes have been described previously (5). Liver mitochondria were prepared for determination of catalase and carnitine acetyltransferase activities and peroxisomes for β-oxidative activity; postmicrosomal supernatant (105 000 x $\underline{g}$, 60 min) was used to assay glutathione peroxidase and reductase activities. Subcellular fractions were isolated essentially as described previously (7,8), with some modifications (5,6). Serum triglyceride concentration was measured using a method described by Wahlefeld (9). Carnitine acetyltransferase was measured by following the release of coenzyeme A (CoA)-SH from acetyl-CoA in the presence or absence of carnitine (10). Catalase was measured by following the disappearance of hydrogen peroxide (11). β-Oxidation of fatty acids was estimated on the basis of the degree of oxidation of palmitoyl CoA in the presence of NAD, which was reduced to NADH (12). The content of reduced glutathione was measured according to the method of Ellman (13), and glutathione reductase activity was recorded by monitoring the rate of NADPH oxidation at 340 nm (14). The glutathione peroxidase catalysing the reduction of hydroperoxides was measured as described by Tappel (15) using glutathione as a reductant. Protein content was determined according to Lowry et al. (16) or Gornall (17), depending on the subcellular fraction.

RESULTS AND DISCUSSION

A significant increase in relative liver weights was observed after administration of clofibrate or of MCPA or 2,4-D for seven days. Both 2,4-D and MCPA, but not glyphosate, induced proliferation of hepatic peroxisomes.

β-Oxidation, with palmitoyl Co-A as the substrate, was measured in isolated peroxisomes after the herbicides or clofibrate had been administered for two weeks (Table 1); it was increased about six-fold in rats treated with clofibrate, two-fold in rats given MCPA, and three-fold in rats receiving 2,4-D when compared with controls. Glyphosate caused no increase in β-oxidation.

2,4-D and MCPA had several effects similar to those of clofibrate: all three compounds decreased serum lipid levels and increased hepatic carnitine acetyltransferase and catalase activities (Table 1). The specific catalase activity was less than doubled and the total cellular proportion of peroxisomes quadrupled, resulting in peroxisomes with decreased catalase activity. A similar, disproportionately small increase in catalase activity has been observed with other hypolipidaemic peroxisome proliferations (18).

TABLE 1

SERUM TRIGLYCERIDE (TRIGLY), HEPATIC CATALASE (C-ASE), CARNITINE ACETYLTRANS-
FERASE (CATF), β-OXIDATION (β-OX), GLUTATHIONE PEROXIDASE (GSH-Px) AND GLUTA-
THIONE REDUCTASE (GSH-RED) ACTIVITIES AFTER EXPOSURE TO HERBICIDES OR CLOFIB-
RATE FOR 2 WEEKS[a]

Treatment group	Trigly (mmol/l)	C-ASE (μmol x min^{-1}	CATF x mg protein^{-1})	β-OX	GSH-Px (μmol x min^{-1}	GSH-RED x g(wwt)$^{-1}$)
Controls	1.82	0.330	5.0	2.2	22	2.1
Clofibrate	1.11*	0.366	113.5***	14.1***	24	1.7
Glyphosate	2.18	0.507*	9.0	1.6	23	2.6
2,4-D	0.89	0.572*	66.1**	6.4**	35**	3.3*
MCPA	0.88*	0.493*	43.1**	4.4*	26	3.2*

[a]Means are given. Statistical differences from controls are shown by the
following symbols: *, $p < 0.05$; **, $p < 0.01$; ***, $p < 0.001$.

Since peroxisomal β-oxidation associated with lowered catalase activity may
result in increased production of intracellular peroxides and radicals, the
content of intracellular glutathione and the activities of glutathione metabolizing enzymes were measured. A 30% increase in the activity of glutathione
peroxidase was observed after administration of MCPA for two weeks, and an
approximately 40% increase in the activity of glutathione reductase was seen
after two weeks' treatment with either 2,4-D or MCPA (Table 1). No change was
found in the reduced glutathione content.

Potent hepatic peroxisome proliferators have been shown to induce hepatocellular carcinomas in rodents (4). Our results support further the hypothesis
that phenoxyacetic acid herbicides belong to a class of carcinogens which exert their action indirectly via peroxisome proliferation. However, there is
as yet little direct evidence to link peroxisome proliferation with the development of neoplasia. The observation of an accumulation of lipofuscin in
liver represents almost the only evidence for a sustained increase in the in-
trahepatic production of oxygen radicals in animals treated with peroxisome
proliferators (19).

REFERENCES
1. Hardell, L. and Sandström, A. (1979) Br. J. Cancer, 39, 711.

2. Hardell, L. (1981) Scand. J. Work environ. Health, 7, 119.

3. IARC (1983) IARC Monographs on the Evaluation of the Carcinogenic Risk of Chemicals to Humans, Vol. 30, Miscellaneous Pesticides, International Agency for Research on Cancer, Lyon, p. 137.

4. Reddy, J.K., Azarnoff, D.L. and Hignite, E.E. (1980) Nature, 283, 397.

5. Vainio, H., Linnainmaa, K., Kähönen, M., Nickels, J., Hietanen, E., Marniemi, J. and Peltonen, P. (1983) Biochem. Pharmacol. (in press)

6. Hietanen, E., Ahotupa, M., Heinonen, T., Hämäläinen, H., Kunnas, T., Linnainmaa, K., Mäntylä, E. and Vainio, H. (1983) (Submitted)

7. Myers, P.K. and Slater, E.C. (1957) Biochem. J., 67, 558.

8. Neat, C.E., Thomassen, M.S. and Osmundsen, J. (1980) Biochem. J., 196, 369.

9. Wahlefeld, A.W. (1974) in: Bergmayer, H.V. (Ed.), Methods of Enzymatic Analysis, 2nd ed., Verlag Chemie and Academic Press, New York and London, pp. 1831-1835.

10. Bieber, L.L., Abraham, T. and Helmrath, T. (1972) Anal. Biochem., 50, 509.

11. Aebi, H. (1970) in: Bergmayer, H.V. (Ed.), Methoden der Enzymatischen Analyse, Verlag Chemie, Weinheim, p. 636.

12. Lazarow, P.B., Shio, H. and Leroy-Houyet, M.A. (1982) J. Lipid Res., 23, 317.

13. Ellman, G.L. (1959) Arch. Biochem. Biophys., 82, 70.

14. Heinonen, T. and Vainio, H. (1981) Eur. J. Drug Metab. Pharmacokin., 6, 275.

15. Tappel, A.L. (1978) in: Fleischer, S. and Packer, L. (Eds), Methods in Enzymology, Academic Press, New York, p. 506.

16. Lowry, O.H., Rosebrough, N.J., Farr, A.L. and Randall, R.J. (1951) Biol. Chem., 193, 265.

17. Gornall, A.G., Bardawill, C.J. and David, M.M. (1949) J. Biol. Chem., 177, 751.

18. Warren, J.R., Lalwani, N.D. and Reddy, J.K. (1983) Environ. Health Perspect., 45, 35.

19. Reddy, J.K., Lalwani, N.D., Reddy, M.K. and Qureshi, S.A. (1982) Cancer Res., 42, 259.

© 1983 Elsevier Science Publishers B.V.
Extrahepatic Drug Metabolism and Chemical Carcinogenesis,
J. Rydström, J. Montelius and M. Bengtsson eds.

INDUCTION OF EXTRAHEPATIC GLUTATHIONE S-TRANSFERASES AND NAD(P)H:QUINONE REDUCTASE BY ANTICARCINOGENIC HINDERED PHENOLS, LACTONES AND SUDAN III

MARY J. DE LONG, HANS J. PROCHASKA AND PAUL TALALAY
Department of Pharmacology and Experimental Therapeutics, The Johns
Hopkins University School of Medicine, Baltimore, MD, 21205 (U.S.A.)

The induction of detoxification enzymes appears to be a major mechanism whereby 2(3)-tert-butyl-4-hydroxyanisole (BHA) and other phenolic dietary antioxidants protect rodents against the carcinogenic, mutagenic, and toxic effects of various chemical entities. Administration of BHA under experimental conditions similar to those which protect against mutagenesis and carcinogenesis, results in marked elevations of the specific activities of glutathione S-transferases and NAD(P)H:quinone acceptor reductase (DT-diaphorase, menadione reductase) in the cytosols of liver and many peripheral tissues of rodents (1-3). Tissue glutathione concentrations are also elevated, as are some of the enzymes concerned with the generation of reduced glutathione.

These elevations of the specific activities of nonoxygenative enzymes may be important mechanisms for the detoxification of usually short-lived and highly reactive electrophilic metabolites of procarcinogens and pro-mutagens. Evidence in support of this view is based in part on the finding that compounds which protect against neoplasia are also enzyme inducers (4).

Studies on the tissue and chemical specificity of enzyme induction have now been extended to additional phenolic derivatives, including the two isomers of BHA (3-BHA, the major isomer; and 2-BHA, the minor isomer), the methyl ether of BHA (methyl-BHA), tert-butylhydroquinone, and 4-hydroxy-anisole. Other types of compounds which protect against chemical carcinogens, including lactones (coumarin and α-angelicalactone) (4) and Sudan III (an azo dye) (5,6) have also been examined for their ability to induce glutathione S-transferases and quinone reductase in a number of tissues.

Female CD-1 mice received daily gavage feedings of 100 μmol of each compound except coumarin (20 μmol) and Sudan III (0.5 μmol), for 5 days before enzyme specific activities were measured in tissue cytosols. Methyl-BHA resembled 3-BHA in being an efficient enzyme inducer in liver and upper small intestine, but had little effect on forestomach or gland-ular stomach. In contrast, 2-BHA is a much less effective enzyme inducer

182

in liver than 3-BHA or methyl-BHA, and is essentially inactive as an inducer in the upper small intestine and glandular stomach. However, 2-BHA and 4-hydroxyanisole are enzyme inducers in the forestomach where these compounds also protect against benzo(a)pyrene neoplasia (7). Coumarin and α-angelicalactone are also efficient inducers of glutathione S-trans-ferases in the forestomach. These compounds protect against benzo(a)pyrene-induced forestomach tumors in mice and DMBA-induced mammary tumors in rats (4). Sudan III is a potent protector against hydrocarbon-induced mammary cancer, leukemia and adrenal necrosis (6). It is unusual in that it appears to induce quinone reductase (as first shown by Huggins) in liver and forestomach but has only minor effects on the glutathione S-transfer-ases in these tissues. (These studies were supported by a Special Institu-tional Grant of the American Cancer Society).

REFERENCES

1. Benson, A.M., Batzinger, R.P., Ou, S.-Y.L., Bueding, E., Cha, Y.-N. and Talalay, P. (1978) Cancer Res. 38, 4486-4495.

2. Benson, A.M., Cha, Y.-N., Bueding, E., Heine, H.S. and Talalay, P. (1979) Cancer Res., 39, 2971-2977.

3. Benson, A.M., Hunkeler, M.J. and Talalay, P. (1980) Proc. Natl. Acad. Sci. U.S.A., 77, 5216-5220.

4. Wattenberg, L.W., Lam, L.K.T. and Fladmoe, A.V. (1979) Cancer Res., 39, 1651-1654.

5. Huggins, C.B., Ueda, N. and Russo, A. (1978) Proc. Natl. Acad. Sci. U.S.A., 75, 4524-4527.

6. Huggins, C.B. (1979) Experimental Leukemia and Mammary Cancer, University of Chicago Press, Chicago.

7. Sparnins, V.L. and Wattenberg, L.W. (1981) J. Natl. Cancer Inst., 68, 769-771.

© 1983 Elsevier Science Publishers B.V.
Extrahepatic Drug Metabolism and Chemical Carcinogenesis,
J. Rydström, J. Montelius and M. Bengtsson eds.

GLUTATHIONE AND GSH-DEPENDENT ENZYMES IN THE HUMAN GASTRIC MUCOSA

CLAUS-PETER SIEGERS[1], RENATE HOPPENKAMPS[1], ERNST THIES[2] AND
MAGED YOUNES[1]

[1]Institut für Toxikologie and [2]Klinik für Chirurgie der Medizinischen
Hochschule Lübeck, Ratzeburger Allee 160, D-2400 Lübeck (FRG)

INTRODUCTION

Boyd and coworkers (1,2) found high glutathione concentrations in the
glandular stomach of different rodent species which even exceeded those found
in the liver. This might point at the importance of the GSH-conjugating enzyme
system in the cellular defense against toxic compounds entering the body via
the gastrointestinal tract. There is, however, no information available concerning the glutathione contents and GSH-dependent enzyme activities of human
gastric tissue. Therefore we were interested to estimate glutathione levels
and dependent enzyme activities in human gastric tissue specimens with normal
and pathological morphology.

MATERIALS AND METHODS

The stomach biopsy specimens obtained during gastroscopy were transferred
into ice-cold sucrose-buffer (0.25 mol/l) and frozen until use. Protein contents were determined by the method of Lowry et al. (3). Total glutathione
was estimated according to Sedlack and Lindsay (4) after preincubation with
6 U of GSH-reductase at 37^{0} C for 20 min. The cytosolic GSH S-transferase
(CDNB) was estimated according to Habig et al. (5); GSH peroxidase was measured
according to Günzler et al. (6).

RESULTS

As shown in the table in specimens of normal gastric mucosa a remarkably high
GSH level of 47 $\pm$ 5 nmol/mg protein was found; the mean GSH peroxidase activity
amounted to 4.42 $\pm$ 0.58 mU/mg protein and the GSH S-aryltransferase activity
to 156 $\pm$ 22 mU/mg protein. Tissue specimens of acute and chronic atrophic
gastritis showed no significant alterations in GSH and enzyme activities.
Specimens of gastric ulcer had significantly lower enzyme activities and
carcinoma specimens a 50 % lower GSH level; the latter finding was confirmed
by intraindividual comparison of tumorous and non-tumorous tissue specimens.

TABLE

Total glutathione (GSH), GSH peroxidase (GSH-PO) and GSH S-aryltransferase
(GSH-AT) in the S9-fraction of biopsy specimens from human gastric mucosa
($\bar{x} \pm$ S.E.M.; *p< 0.05, Scheffé-test).

Group	n	Total GSH (nmol/mg prot.)	GSH-PO (mU/mg prot.)	GSH-AT (mU/mg prot. · min)
Normal mucosa	24	47 $\pm$ 5	4.42 $\pm$ 0.58	156 $\pm$ 22
Acute gastritis	15	42 $\pm$ 7	3.43 $\pm$ 0.48	149 $\pm$ 17
Chron.atr.gastritis	10	61 $\pm$ 11	4.28 $\pm$ 0.73	143 $\pm$ 31
Gastric ulcer	9	50 $\pm$ 13	2.26 $\pm$ 0.40*	57 $\pm$ 13*
Carcinoma	12	26 $\pm$ 6*	3.41 $\pm$ 0.50	143 $\pm$ 37

DISCUSSION

The glutathione content of human gastric mucosa was found to be remarkably
higher than that of human liver (7,8), whereas the GSH peroxidase activity was
only 10 % (9) and the aryltransferase activity about 5 % of that in human liver
(8). The decreased GSH content of gastric carcinomas correspond to the hypothesis of Calcutt (10) that an elevation in the target tissue SH-level is an
essential feature of tumor induction, whilst in the tumor itself there is a
lowered SH-level. The decreased activity of the GSH-peroxidase in gastric
ulcer might lead to lower prostaglandin tissue levels (11) which are thought
to be involved in ulcerogenesis (12).

REFERENCES

1. Boyd,S.C.,Sasame,H.A. and Boyd,M.R. (1979) Science 205,1010.
2. Boyd,S.C.,Sasame,H.A. and Boyd,M.R. (1981) Physiol. Behav. 27,377.
3. Lowry,O.H.,Rosebrough,N.J.,Farr,A.L. and Randall,R.J. (1951)
   J. Biol. Chem. 193,265.
4. Sedlack,J. and Lindsay,R.H. (1968) Analyt. Biochem. 25,192.
5. Habig,W.H.,Pabst,M.J. and Jacoby,W.B. (1974) J. Biol. Chem. 249,7130.
6. Günzler,W.A.,Kremers,H. and Flohé,L. (1974) Z.Klin.Chem.Klin.Biochem.12,444.
7. Poulsen,H.E.,Ranek,L. and Andreasen,P.B. (1981) Scand. J. clin. Lab.
   Invest. 41, 573.
8. Siegers,C.-P.,Bossen,K.-H.,Younes,M.,Mahlke,R. and Oltmanns,D. (1982)
   Pharmacol. Res. Commun. 14,61.
9. Konz,K.H. (1979) Z. Klin. Chem. Klin. Biochem. 17,353.
10. Calcutt,G. (1961) Brit. J. Cancer 15,683.
11. Kuehl,F.A. and Eagan,R.W. (1980) Science 210,978.
12. Vane,J.R. (1971) Nature new Biol. 231,232.

© 1983 Elsevier Science Publishers B.V.
Extrahepatic Drug Metabolism and Chemical Carcinogenesis,
J. Rydström, J. Montelius and M. Bengtsson eds.

EXTRAHEPATIC DISTRIBUTION OF MICROSOMAL GLUTATHIONE TRANSFERASE IN THE RAT

RALF MORGENSTERN AND JOSEPH W. DePIERRE

Department of Biochemistry, Arrhenius Laboratory, University of Stockholm,
S-106 91 Stockholm, Sweden

INTRODUCTION

Microsomal glutathione transferase has been purified and characterized
from rat liver (1,2). This enzyme is distinct from the cytosolic glutathione
transferases with respect to a number of different properties, including minimum molecular weight, substrate specificity, activatibility with sulfhydryl
reagents and immunological characteristics. In order to gain clues into the
possible function(s) of this enzyme in addition to its role in the conjugation
of xenobiotics and/or their metabolites with glutathione, we have examined its
distribution in different organs of the rat, using both activity measurements
and quantitation by immunoblotting.

MATERIALS AND METHODS

250 g male Sprague-Dawley rats were starved overnight and sacrificed by
decapitation. Microsomes were prepared from the various organs as described
previously (4) and subsequently washed twice in 0.15 M Tris-Cl, pH 8.0. Activity with 1-chloro-2,4-dinitrobenzene as the second substrate (5) and the activation of this activity by N-ethylmaleimide (3) were assayed by published
procedures. Microsomal glutathione transferase was also quantitated by immunoblotting   using radioiodinated protein A after SDS-PAGE (15%) according
to Laemmli.

RESULTS

As seen in Table 1, the activity of microsomal glutathione transferase
is greatest in the liver, testis, adrenal, and intestine and low in other organs. The distribution of the corresponding cytosolic activity is somewhat
similar and is included in the table for comparison. It has been shown (4)
that microsomal glutathione transferase can be activated by N-ethylmaleimide
only in the liver. Similar treatment of extrahepatic microsomes is without
effect or even inhibitory in some cases.

Immunoblotting revealed that 3% of the total protein of liver microsomes
consists of the microsomal glutathione transferase and significant amounts of
this enzyme were also detected in microsomes from the intestine, adrenal,

TABLE 1

DISTRIBUTION OF MICROSOMAL AND CYTOSOLIC GLUTATHIONE TRANSFERASES IN DIFFERENT ORGANS OF THE RAT

Extrahepatic values are the means $\pm$ S.E.M. (in the case of immunoblotting) of 2 determinations. The limit of 0.3 μg/mg for immunoblotting is 50% above the background. N.D. = not detectable.

Organ	Activity[a] (nmol conjugate formed/min-mg protein)		Amount in microsomes (μg/mg protein)
	microsomal	cytosolic	
Liver	130	1400	31±6
Kidney	8.5	336	≤ 0.3
Lung	15	79	0.9±0.2
Intestine	60	429	4.0±2
Adrenal	52	253	3.2±0.5
Testis	130	3850	2.5±0.7
Spleen	9.0	56	0.5±0.1
Brain	8.0	190	≤ 0.3
Heart	7.2	93	N.D.
Thymus	4.4	46	1.1±0.3

[a]from reference 4

testis and thymus (0.1-0.4% of the total protein). The measurements of activity and amount are thus comparable, even though the activity measurement also includes cytosolic glutathione transferases which contaminate the microsomal fraction.

ACKNOWLEDGEMENTS

These studies were supported by NIH grant 1 R01 CA 26261-04 and by a grant from the Swedish Natural Science Research Council.

REFERENCES

1. Morgenstern, R., Guthenberg, C. and DePierre, J.W. (1982) Europ.J. Biochem., 128, 243-248.

2. Morgenstern, R. and DePierre, J.W. Europ.J.Biochem., in press.

3. Morgenstern, R., DePierre, J.W. and Ernster, L. (1979) Biochem. Biophys. Res.Commun., 87, 657-663.

4. DePierre, J.W. and Morgenstern, R. (1983)Biochem.Pharmacol., 32, 721-723.

5. Habig, W.H., Pabst,M.J. and Jakoby,W.B.(1974)J.Biol.Chem., 249, 7130-7139.

© 1983 Elsevier Science Publishers B.V.
Extrahepatic Drug Metabolism and Chemical Carcinogenesis,
J. Rydström, J. Montelius and M. Bengtsson eds.

INHIBITORS FOR IDENTIFICATION OF GLUTATHIONE TRANSFERASE SUBUNITS IN THE RAT

SÜHA YALÇIN, HELGI JENSSON AND BENGT MANNERVIK
Department of Biochemistry, Arrhenius Laboratory, University of Stockholm,
S-106 91 Stockholm, Sweden

Glutathione transferases exist in many organs, although in general the
levels are lower than that of the liver (1). Isozymes of glutathione transferase have been demonstrated in liver as well as in extrahepatic tissues.
Some of the extrahepatic isozymes appear identical with the isozymes in liver,
but others are not demonstrable in this organ. In spite of differences between
the various isozymes in substrate specificities, reactions with antibodies, or
physical properties, it has proved difficult to identify transferases in liver
with those found in other tissues. In this study a set of inhibitors has been
used to facilitate discrimination between the multiple forms of glutathione
transferase.

Six homogeneous well-characterized basic glutathione transferases from rat
liver cytosol were used to design the set of inhibitors. These isozymes are
dimeric proteins, each composed of two of the four most abundant transferase
subunits. The enzymes have been named glutathione transferases L_2, BL, B_2, A_2,
AC, and C_2 (2), according to their subunit compositions. The effect of inhibitors on the catalytic activity with 1-chloro-2,4-dinitrobenzene was evaluated and the inhibitor concentration giving rise to 50% inhibition (I_{50}) was
determined for each isozyme. The most potent inhibitor for each homodimeric
transferase was as follows: transferase L_2: hematin (I_{50} = 0.1 μM); transferase B_2: tributyltin acetate (I_{50} = 0.5 μM); transferase A_2: triethyltin
bromide (I_{50} = 1 μM); transferase C_2: bromosulfophthalein (I_{50} = 0.5 μM). In
many cases a 100-fold difference between the I_{50} values of two isozymes was
found with a given inhibitor.

The most difficult discrimination among the four basic subunits is between
subunits A and C, which have similar sizes. It was found that these two subunits can clearly be differentiated by use of bromosulfophthalein and triethyltin bromide as inhibitors.

The heterodimeric transferases BL and AC show the expected intermediate I_{50}
values. By use of a substrate specific for one of the subunit in a heterodimer,
it was demonstrated that the I_{50} value for the subunit was the same in the
heterodimer as in the corresponding homodimer. It was also found that the
shape of the graph of activity versus inhibitor concentration could reveal the

presence of two nonidentical subunits in an unknown sample.

The application of the inhibitors for identification of glutathione transferases in extrahepatic tissues have proved the usefulness of the approach.
For example, the results of the inhibition studies were instrumental in the
identification of the basic isozymes in rat testis.

ACKNOWLEDGEMENTS

This work was supported by the Swedish Council for Planning and Coordination
of Research and the Swedish Natural Science Research Council. S.Y. is a
recipient of a fellowship from the Swedish Institute.

REFERENCES

1. Mannervik, B., Guthenberg, C., Jensson, H., Warholm, M. and Ålin, P.
   (1983) in: Larsson, A., Orrenius, S., Holmgren, A. and Mannervik, B.
   (Eds.), Functions of Glutathione: Biochemical, Physiological, Toxicological,
   and Clinical Aspects, Raven Press, New York, pp. 75-88.

2. Mannervik, B. and Jensson, H. (1982) J. Biol. Chem. 257, 9909-9912.

© 1983 Elsevier Science Publishers B.V.
Extrahepatic Drug Metabolism and Chemical Carcinogenesis,
J. Rydström, J. Montelius and M. Bengtsson eds.

A COMPARISON OF THE GLUTATHIONE TRANSFERASES (GST) OF THREE EXTRAHEPATIC ORGANS WITH DIFFERENT FUNCTIONS – THE ADRENAL, THE LACTATING MAMMARY GLAND AND THE MALE REPRODUCTIVE SYSTEM.

D.J. MEYER, L.G. CHRISTODOULIDES, O. NYAN, R. SCHUSTER BRUCE AND B. KETTERER.

Courtauld Institute of Biochemistry, Middlesex Hospital Medical School, London W1P 7PN, UK.

INTRODUCTION
To determine to what extent tissues with different specializations vary in their GST isoenzymes a preliminary study has been made of the adrenal (which produces steroids), the lactating mammary glands (which synthesizes nutrients including proteins, lipids, lactose etc.) and the male reproductive tract (which not only produces steroids but also forms and stores sperm which may need protection from genotoxic agents).

RESULTS AND DISCUSSION
Table 1 lists the various tissues and fluids examined in order of decreasing GST activity.

TABLE 1
GSH Transferase (GST)[1] activities in various tissue fractions

Source	GST	Source	GST
liver	0.95	epididymus	0.15
testis	0.64	epididymal fluid	0.06
seminiferous tubules	0.48	seminal vesicles	0.03
male adrenal	0.40	lactating mammary gland	0.03
female adrenal	0.25	epididymal sperm	0.02
Leydig cells tubular		ejaculated sperm[2]	0.03
and contents etc.	0.16	seminal fluid[2]	0.01

[1] GST is expressed as μmol 1-chloro-2,4-dinitrobenzene (CDNB) conjugated with GSH per min per mg protein.
[2] refers to human samples (all others are derived from the rat).

The male genital system is of particular interest because it contains among its elements the most and least active sources of GST in this study. The seminiferous tubules where the biogenesis of sperm occurs in the protective environment of Sertoli cells is the richest in GST, while the maturing and mature sperm, together with the fluid which bathes them contain, the least. If GST are required to protect sperm from electrophiles they seem to be most vulnerable when during spermatogenesis in the tubules. The next most active source of GST is the adrenal, which, like the liver, is rich in cytochome P_{450} and a potential site of the conversion of xenobiotics to electrophiles. Activity found in the testicular fraction containing Leydig cells may be comparable. It is interesting to note that lactating mammary gland, though a metabolically active tissue, is low in GST activity. The same applies to the seminal vesicles which not only synthesize protein but also prostaglandins.

TABLE 2. Enzymic Activities Associated with the GSH Transferases
Separated from 18 g Rat Testis by Sephadex G100 Chromatography Followed
by Isoelectric Focusing.
The following substrates were used. CDNB, 1,2-dichloro-4-nitrobenzene
(DCNB), cumene hydroperoxide (CuOH), ethacrynic acid (ETH) trans-4-
phenyl-3-buten-2-one (T4), Δ 5-androsten-3,17-dione (ANDR) and 1,2-
epoxy-3-(p-nitrophenoxy)propane (EPX).

Fraction	pI	CDNB	DCNB	CuOH	ETH	T4	ANDR	EPX
1	10	20.5	0.11	3.1	0.55	0	0.19	–
2	8.7	17.1	0.7	0.1	0.02	0.04	0	–
3	8.1	34.3	6.3	0.07	0.17	0.48	0	–
4	7.7	14.0	1.3	0	0.20	0.11	0	–
5	7.5	–	–	–	–	–	0	1.26
6	7.2	10.1	0.7	0.19	0.15	0.68	0	–
7	6.8	24.5	0.7	0.07	0.11	0.25	0	–
8	6.0	45.9	0.4	0.04	0.55	0.05	0	–
9	5.8	112.7	1.5	0.04	0.50	0.05	0	–

Having established quantitative differences in total GST. It becomes of
interest to study qualitative relationships. Table 2 shows the
characterization of testicular GST by pI and substrate specificity.
Fractions 1, 2, 4, 5 and 6 appear to correspond to hepatic GSH transferases B & AA, A, C, E and D respectively. Fractions 4, 6 and 7 are
not so readily related to hepatic GST. isoelectric focusing of the tubular

Fig. 1
Separation of GST in tubular and
non-tubular fraction of the testis by
isoelectric focusing.

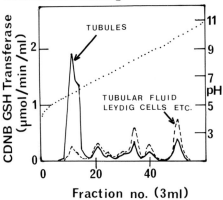

Fraction no. (3ml)

Fig. 1 shows the separation by
and non-tubular fractions of
the testis. Both fractions have
all the components seen in whole
testis, but the tubule fraction
is remarkable for its high content
of anionic GST's. The same
enzymes are seen in epididymus
and its fluid and with the
exception of the anionic GST's
in the seminal vesicles. The
lactating mammary gland also
has a number of GST's, but as
much as 90% of the activity is
due to a form which resembles
hepatic GST AA. The adrenals
have a wide range of GST's
including anionic forms. The
differences between the male
and female adrenal are almost
entirely due to the absence of
a form resembling hepatic GST
B from the female gland. Even
when present, GST B or the Ya
subunit is much less important
in the tissues examined here than in the liver. On the other hand
apparent GST AA and the Yc subunit is always present and account for:
70% (epididymus), 50% (testis), 30% (adrenal and lactating mammary
gland) and 15% (seminal vesicle) of the total GSH peroxidase activity.

© 1983 Elsevier Science Publishers B.V.
Extrahepatic Drug Metabolism and Chemical Carcinogenesis,
J. Rydström, J. Montelius and M. Bengtsson eds.

GLUTATHIONE TRANSFERASE IN HUMAN BRAIN

MARIA OLSSON, CLAES GUTHENBERG AND BENGT MANNERVIK
Department of Biochemistry, Arrhenius Laboratory, University of Stockholm,
S-106 91 Stockholm, Sweden

Glutathione transferases play an important role in the biotransformation and detoxication of electrophilic xenobiotics (1). It has been reported that neurotoxins such as acrylamide and styrene oxide, a metabolite of styrene, are conjugated with glutathione through reactions catalyzed by glutathione transferase in rat brain (cf. Ref. 2). Although the highest activity of glutathione transferase is found in liver, these enzymes are also present in many other organs. In human tissues three groups of transferases have been distinguished, based on widely different isoelectric points, amino acid compositions, substrate specificities, reactions with antibodies, and CD spectra (3). The different enzyme forms are not all present in every tissue. All the individuals appear to have at least one basic hepatic transferase, but only the livers of some contain acidic or neutral transferases. Only small amounts of acidic glutathione transferase have been found in adult liver. In all fetal tissues tested, as well as in erythrocytes, placenta, and lung from adults, a major form of glutathione transferase with an acidic isoelectric point (at pH 4.8) has been demonstrated (3). In the present investigation it is shown that also adult human brain contains a dominating transferase with an acidic isoelectric point.

The glutathione transferase activity in a $100000\,g$ supernatant fraction from human brain cortex was determined with 1-chloro-2,4-dinitrobenzene and was found to be considerably lower (approx. 10%) than the corresponding activity in human liver. The brain transferase was separated from contaminating proteins by affinity chromatography. The affinity matrix consisted of S-hexylglutathione linked to epoxy-activated Sepharose 6B (4). After application of the sample and washing with 10 mM Tris buffer (pH 7.8) containing 0.2 M NaCl, the glutathione transferase activity was eluted with 5 mM S-hexylglutathione in the same buffer. Gel filtration on Sephadex G-25 of the active fractions preceded isoelectric focusing in the pH interval of 3.5-10. One major peak containing glutathione transferase activity was found after isoelectric focusing. The brain transferase, in resemblance to the enzyme isolated from erythrocytes (transferase ρ) and from placenta (transferase π) (5), has an isoelectric point at about pH 4.8. The substrate specificity was analyzed and the activity with 1,2-dichloro-4-nitrobenzene, bromosulfophthalein and p-nitrophenylacetate

was low or very low. However, in accordance to the results found with transferases π and ρ, ethacrynic acid is the second best substrate. The molecular
size of the subunits (23400 dalton), as determined by SDS polyacrylamide gel
electrophoresis, is identical with that found for transferases ρ and π. When
the placental enzyme and the brain enzyme were tested in parallel by the
Ouchterlony double-diffusion technique against antibodies raised against
transferase π, a continuous precipitin line without spurs was obtained indicating immunological identity between the two transferases.

In conclusion, the dominating form of glutathione transferase in human brain
is an acidic enzyme which is closely related to, and may be identical with,
glutathione transferase π from human placenta.

ACKNOWLEDGEMENT

This work was supported by the Swedish Council for Planning and Coordination
of Research.

REFERENCES

1. Jakoby, W.B. and Habig, W.H. (1980) in: Jakoby, W.B. (Ed.), Enzymatic Basis
   of Detoxication, Vol. 2, Academic Press, New York, pp. 63-94.
2. Das, M., Seth, P.K. and Mukhtar, H. (1981) Res. Commun. Chem. Pathol.
   Pharmacol. 33, 377-380.
3. Mannervik, B., Guthenberg, C., Jensson, H., Warholm, M. and Ålin, P. (1983)
   in: Larsson, A., Orrenius, S., Holmgren, A. and Mannervik, B. (Eds.),
   Functions of Glutathione: Biochemical, Physiological, Toxicological, and
   Clinical Aspects, Raven Press, New York, pp. 75-88.
4. Mannervik, B. and Guthenberg, C. (1981) Meth. Enzymol. 77, 231-235.
5. Guthenberg, C. and Mannervik, B. (1981) Biochim. Biophys. Acta 661, 255-260.

© 1983 Elsevier Science Publishers B.V.
Extrahepatic Drug Metabolism and Chemical Carcinogenesis,
J. Rydström, J. Montelius and M. Bengtsson eds.

NON-MICROSOMAL ACTIVATION OF STYRENE TO STYRENE OXIDE

GIORGIO BELVEDERE[1,2], FRANCESCO TURSI[1] AND HARRI VAINIO[3]

[1]Istituto di Ricerche Farmacolgiche 'Mario Negri', Via Eritrea, 62 - 20157 Milan (Italy), [2]Supported by an EEC fellowship and [3]Institute of Occupational Health, Haartmaninkatu 1, SF-00290 Helsinki 29 (Finland)

INTRODUCTION

Styrene is oxidized in liver microsomes to styrene oxide which has been found to be a mutagenic metabolite in bacterial and mammalian cell systems (1,2). Oxidation of styrene like several xenobiotics, is catalyzed by reactive oxygen species formed by an enzyme system dependent on cytochrome P-450 (3,4). However, other enzyme systems such as xanthine oxidase in the presence of xanthine and ferredoxin reductase with NADPH can produce reactive oxygen intermediates such as the superoxide ion ($O_2^{-\cdot}$) and H_2O_2 (5,6).

It is also known that oxyhemoglobin can support metabolic reactions typically catalyzed by cytochrome P-450, such as lipid peroxidation (7), the dealkylation of aromatic N,N-dimethylaniline-N-oxides (8) and the hydroxylation of aniline (9,10). These reactions could be attributed to the presence of the oxygen in a partially activated form in the oxyhemoglobin molecule (11).

We investigated the oxidation of styrene to styrene oxide catalyzed by oxyhemoglobin and non-microsomal enzymes such as xanthine oxidase and ferredoxin reductase.

MATERIALS AND METHODS

Human venous blood suitable for transfusion was obtained from AVIS (Associazione Volontari Italiani del Sangue); PBS (phosphate buffered saline without Ca^{++} and Mg^{++}) was purchased from Eurobio (Paris, France). Superoxide dismutase type I, xanthine oxidase, ferrodoxin reductase, catalase, methylene blue, NADPH, NADH,nicotinamide, tryptophane, mannitol and dimethylsulfoxide were obtained from Sigma (St. Louis, Mo., U.S.A.)

NADPH dependent cytochrome c (P-450) reductase was purified from rat liver according to a previously published procedure (12). Erythrocytes were isolated as described (13); the cells were deoxygenated at 37°C in small, tightly sealed Pyrex flasks (14), previously washed with N_2 when full deoxygenation was required. Partial deoxygenation was carried out in a tonometer (Instrumentation Laboratories, Paderno Dugano, Italy) under a continuous flow at an appropriate N_2/O_2 ratio. The concentration of oxyhemoglobin was determined at the end of tonometry (25 min) by a micromethod (15). Incubations were in PBS pH 7.4, reactions were started by the addition of styrene, disolved in acetonitrile for erythrocytes, and of the enzymes for xanthine oxidase and ferredoxin reductase. The reactions were stopped with 0.4 ml of 0.6 N H_2SO_4, and styrene oxide formation was evaluated according to a previously described method (16,17). At the end of incubation the styrene oxide formed is quantitatively chemically hydrated by overnight incubation with H_2SO_4 to the glycol, which is more suitable for gas chromatographic analysis. Styrene glycol is quantitatively determined by a sensitive gas chromatographic procedure using an electron capture detector (18).

RESULTS AND DISCUSSION

It has been shown that hemoglobin can replace cytochrome P-450 in a reconstituted aniline hydroxylase system composed of human methemoglobin, NADPH, cytochrome P-450 reductase and oxygen (9). In this system hemoglobin was formed by enzymatic reduction of methemoglobin by the purified reductase (9). Aniline was also oxidized in intact erythrocytes and a reaction mechanism has been worked out involving oxidation of aniline by oxyhemoglobin with formation of methemoglobin, that is then reduced by reductase endogenous to the erythrocytes or by the purified liver reductase in the reconstituted system (9,10). Methemoglobin reduction in erythrocytes was stimulated by the presence of methylene blue (10,19).

A similar reaction mechanism could be applied to the oxidation of styrene to styrene oxide in the same systems. However, stimulation of the reaction by methylene blue was observed only in the reconstituted system containing methemoglobin and not in intact erythrocytes (Table 1), probably because styrene does not cause methemoglobin formation in intact cells (data not shown) as with aniline (20). In washed erythrocytes styrene oxidation was strongly inhibited by CO but not by superoxide dismutase, catalase and scavengers of $\cdot OH$ (Table 1). These results seem to indicate that free reactive oxygen intermediates are not responsible for styrene oxidation. The reaction occurred to the same extent in whole blood and washed erythrocytes and was not dependent on cofactors typically required for cytochrome P-450 catalyzed reactions (Table 1).

In erythrocytes, where hemoglobin was completely oxidized to methemoglobin with sodium nitrite, a correlation was found between methemoglobin disappearance (i.e. oxyhemoglobin formation) and styrene oxidation after washing and incubating the cells with glucose and methylene blue to reduce methemoglobin (10) (Fig. 1).The involvement of oxyhemoglobin in the oxidation of styrene was demonstrated more directly by the linear relationship between styrene oxide formation and the molar fraction of oxyhemoglobin in partially deoxygenated samples of erythrocytes (Fig. 2).

Although the Km of styrene oxide formation in erythrocytes is 80 times lower than in liver microsomes, the absence of epoxide inactivating enzyme systems and the ubiquitous nature of these cells might make this system suitable for activating styrene in the presence of other cells sensitive to the epoxide toxicity.

Styrene was also oxidized to styrene oxide in a system containing xanthine oxidase in the presence of xanthine, the reaction being stimulated by addition of Fe^{3+} (Table 2). It is known that xanthine oxidase produces $O_2^{-\cdot}$ and H_2O_2 in the presence of xanthine (5). in this system Fe^{3+} is reduced by $O_2^{-\cdot}$ to Fe^{2+}, that reacts with H_2O_2 producing $\cdot OH$ radicals (21). The inhibition of styrene oxide formation by catalase and partially by superoxide dismutase (Table 2) suggests that $\cdot OH$ radicals are the oxygen intermediates involved in styrene oxidation. Inhibition of the reaction on addition of OH scavengers such as mannitol, tryptophan and dimethyl-sulfoxide confirmed this hypothesis (Fig. 3). Ferredoxin reductase, an enzyme present in plant chloroplasts, oxidizes NADPH with production of $O_2^{-\cdot}$ and H_2O_2 (6). In this system

TABLE 1

STYRENE OXIDATION TO STYRENE OXIDE IN HUMAN ERYTHROCYTES AND A RECONSTITUTED HEMOGLOBIN SYSTEM

System	Styrene glycol[a] nmol/30 min/ml
A) Erythrocytes	
Erythrocytes[b]	130.0+ 6.0
+ Cofactors[c]	203.2∓13.0
+ CO[d]	29.2∓ 1.0
+ Superoxide dismutase	117.2∓ 1.4
+ Catalase	158.3∓16.2
+ Tryptophan (2 mM)	104.0∓ 5.2
+ Mannitol (20 mM)	126.0∓ 6.3
+ Dimethyl sulfoxide (280 mM)	150.0∓ 8.0
+ Glucose (120 mM)+	
Methylene blue (10 µM)	113.0+ 5.2
membranes + Cofactors	n.d.[e]
Blood	163.3+ 6.5
+ Cofactors	171.8∓ 5.5

	Styrene glycol nmol/30 min
B) Reconstituted system	
Methemoglobin[f] + NADPH (0.87 mM)	n.d.
+ NADPH + Reductase[g] (0.38 nmol)	4.5+ 0.1
+ NADPH + " + Methylene blue (1 µM)	14.3∓ 0.9

Styrene concentration in 1 ml of incubation mixture was 50 mM. The data represent the mean + S.E.

[a] The enzymatically formed styrene oxide was chemically converted to styrene glycol (see Materials and Methods).

[b] Eryhtrocytes were isolated and washed, the original blood volume was reconstituted with phosphate buffered saline (PBS) pH 7.4, 0.114 ml was used for incubation.

[c] The cofactor mixture consisted of NADPH 0.87 mM, NADH 0.25 mM, nicotinamide 2.7 mM and $MgCl_2$ 5 mM.

[d] CO was bubbled into the incubation mixture for 1 min with a flow of 50 ml/min before addition of styrene.

[e] Styrene glycol values, after styrene incubation with erythrocyte membrane (1 mg protein/ml) were the same as for blank samples consisting of PBS, styrene and cofactors. n.d. not detectable

[f] The concentration of purified human methemoglobin was 1 µM.

[g] Cytochrome c reductase was purified from rat liver.

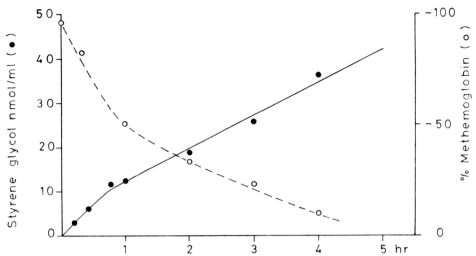

Fig. 1. Time course of styrene oxide formation and methemoglobin reduction in erythrocytes. The amount of styrene oxide formed is reported as styrene glycol (see Materials and Methods). Methemoglobin was formed by treatment of erythrocytes with 1 % sodium nitrite (w/v); after extensive washing with 0.9 % (w/v) saline solution containing 6 mM glucose, cells were incubated with 1 mM styrene in the presence of 120 mM glucose and 10 μM methylene blue, Disappearance of methemoglobin was monitored spectrally by the decrease in absorbance at 494 nm.

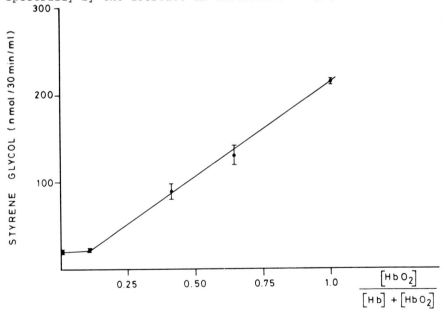

Fig. 2. Relationship between the molar fraction of oxyhemoglobin and styrene oxidation to styrene oxide in human erythrocytes. Styrene concentration was 50 mM.

TABLE 2

STYRENE OXIDATION TO STYRENE OXIDE DURING REACTION OF XANTHINE
(X) WITH XANTHINE OXIDASE (XO) IN THE PRESENCE OF Fe^{3+}

Additions[a]	Styrene glycol	Control
	nmol	%
$X + XO + Fe^{3+}$	12.80+0.74	100
$-Fe^{3+}$	4.33+0.65*	33
+ Superoxide dismutase 0.93 µg/ml	9.33+0.65*	73
+ Superoxide dismutase 93.0 µg/ml	6.50+0.46*	51
+ Catalase 6.6 µg/ml	2.40+ 0.24*	23
$XO + H_2O_2$ (0.1 mM)	n.d.[d]	-

Reaction mixtures contained 50 mM styrene (disolved in
acetonitrile), 50 µM xanthine, 0.50 µM xanthine oxidase, 0.15
mM EDTA, 50 µM $Fe_2(SO_4)_3$, 50 mM potassium phosphate,
and the indicated additions at pH 7.4 and at 37°C. The data
are the mean + S.E. Styrene glycol values were the same as for
blank samples consisting of buffer and styrene. n.d. not
detectable. *p < 0.01

TABLE 3
STYRENE OXIDATION TO STYRENE OXIDE CATALYZED BY FERREDOXIN
REDUCTASE

System	Styrene glycol
	nmol/nmol of protein
Ferredoxin reductase + NADPH	15.7+0.5
- NADPH	n.d.
+ Ferredoxin (4.1 µM)	4.9+0.5
+ Catalase (6.6 µg/ml)	0.7+0.1
+ Superoxide dismutase (93 µg/ml)	1.9+0.2
- NADPH + H_2O_2 (0.1 mM)	28.1+2.8
Ferredoxin reductase (boiled) + NADPH	n.d.

Incubation mixtures consisted of 0.2 M Na^+-phosphate buffer
pH 7.4, ferredoxin reductase (0.49 µM) and NADPH (5.3 µM).
Samples were incubated with styrene (0.8 mM) at 37°C for 10
min. Styrene glycol formed in control samples consisting of
buffer and NADPH or H_2O_2 was substrated.

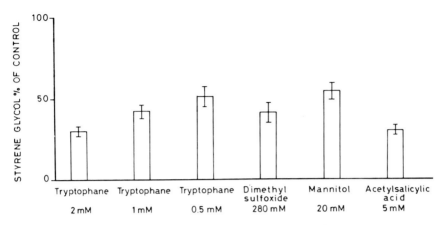

Fig. 3. Effect of scavengers of hydroxyl radicals on styrene oxide formation catalyzed by xanthine oxidase in the presence of xanthine and Fe^{3+}.

too styrene was oxidized to styrene oxide, the reaction being inhibited by addition of catalase and superoxide dismutase (Table 3). inhibition of styrene oxidation after addition of ferredoxin is explained by the depression of NADPH oxidation caused by the formation of a complex between ferredoxin reductase and ferredoxin (22). Unlike xanthine oxidase, ferredoxin reductase was also able to oxidize styrene only by addition of H_2O_2 to the enzyme (Table 2,3). Thus a different reaction mechanism might be involved.

These examples show that different reactive oxygen intermediates, either enzyme bound as in the case of oxyhemoglobin, or free as for xanthine oxidase and ferredoxin reductase, could be responsible for the oxidation of styrene to styrene oxide. The relevance of these activation pathways in the onset of styrene toxicity in vitro and in vivo is how being evaluated.

ACKNOWLEDGEMENTS

This work was partially founded by tha CNR (National Research Council, Rome, Italy) program on Clinical Pharmacology and Rare Diseases. We thank Dr. M. Lang (Eflab Oy, Helsinki, Finland) for providing the purified reductase.

REFERENCES

1. Linnainmaa, K., Meretoja, T., Sorsa, M. and Vainio, H. (1978) Mutat. Res. 58, 277.

2. Conner, M.K.., Alarie, Y. and Dombroske, R.L. (1980) Toxicol. Appl. Pharmacol. 55, 37

3. White, R.E. and Coon, M.J. (1980) Ann. Rev. Biochem. 49, 315.

4. Salmona, M., Pachecka, J., Cantoni, L., Belvedere, G., Mussini, E. and Garattini, S. (1976) Xenobiotica 6, 585.

5. Beauchamp, C. and Fridovich, I. (1970) J. Biol. Chem. 245, 4641.

6. Ballou, D., Palmer, G. and Massey, V. (1969) Biochem. Biophys. Res. Commun. 36, 898.

7. Tappel, A.L. (1953) Arch. Biochem. Biophys. 44, 378.

8. Kiese, M., Renner, G. and Schlaeger, R. (1971) Naunyn-Schmiedeberg's Arch. Pharmakol. 268, 247

9. Mieyal, J.J., Ackerman, R.S., Blumer, J.L. and Freeman, L.S. (1976) J. Biol. Chem. 251, 3436.

10. Blisard, K.S. and Mieyal, J.J. (1979) J. Biol. Chem. 254, 5104.

11. Piesach, J., Blunberg, W.E.,Wittemberg, B.A. and Wittemberg, J.B. (1968) J. Biol. Chem. 243, 1871,

12. Vermilon, J.L. and Coon, M.J. (1974) Biochem. Biophys. Res. Commun. 60, 1315.

13. McCall, C.E., Bass, D.A., Cousart, S. and DeChatelet, L.R. (1979) Proc. Nat. Acad. Sci. USA 76, 5896.

14. Samaja, M., Mosca, A., Luzzana, M., Rossi-Bernardi, L. and Winslow, R.M. (1981) Clin. Chem. 27, 1856.

15. Rossi-Bernardi, L., Perella, M., Luzzana, M., Samaja, M. and Raffaele, I. (1977) Clin. Chem. 23, 1215.

16. Belvedere, G., Pachecka, J., Cantoni, L., Mussini, E. and Salmona, M. (1976) J. Chromatogr. 118, 387.

17. Cantoni, R., Vignazia, F., Belvedere, G., Cantoni, L. and Salmona, M. (1980) Experientia 36, 640.

18. Gazzotti, G., Garattini, E. and Salmona, M. (1980) J. Chromatogr. 188, 400.

19. Blisard, K.S. and Mieyal, J.J. (1981) Arch. Biochem. Biophys. 210, 762.

20. Warburg, O. and Christian, W. (1931) Biochem. Z. 242, 206

21. McCord, J.J. and Day, E.D. Jr. (1978). FEBS Lett. 86, 139.

22. Nakamura, S. and Kimura, T. (1972) J. Biol. Chem. 247, 6462

© 1983 Elsevier Science Publishers B.V.
Extrahepatic Drug Metabolism and Chemical Carcinogenesis,
J. Rydström, J. Montelius and M. Bengtsson eds.

BIOTRANSFORMATION OF ETHYLLOFLAZEPATE (VICTAN[®]) IN PLASMA AND RAT TISSUES

HORACE DAVI , ERIC MARTI , ANDREE BONDON , WERNER CAUTREELS
SANOFI - Centre de Recherches CLIN-MIDY, rue du Prof. J.
Blayac, 34082, Montpellier, FRANCE.

INTRODUCTION

Double blind controlled studies in patients revealed for Ethyl-loflazepate potent anxiolytic properties at daily dosage of 4 mg/day with a lack of undesirable side effects. The compound is presently marketed in France (Victan[®]) and commonly used by general practitionners as an anxiolytic drug.

The drug was found to be stable in the lumen of the gastrointestinal tract after its oral administration to the rat and the baboon and further *in vivo* experiments in man and several animal species revealed that a major and early step in the biotransformation of the drug was the hydrolysis of the ester bond. Accordingly *in vitro* studies were performed to look for the presence of esterases acting on Ethylloflazepate as substrate in biological media.

MATERIALS AND METHODS

Chemicals. Ethylloflazepate, 7-chloro-5-(2'-fluorophenyl)-3-carboxethyl-2,3-dihydro-1H-1,4-benzodiazepine-2-one, (EL), Dese-thylloflazepate, 7-chloro-5-(2'-fluorophenyl)-3-carboxy-2,3-dihy-dro-1H-1,4-benzodiazepine-2-one, (DEL) and Descarbethoxyloflazepa-te, 7-chloro-5-(2'-fluorophenyl)-2,3-dihydro-1H-1,4-benzodiazepine-2-one, (DCL) were synthesized at the CLIN-MIDY Research Center.

Preparation of rat tissue homogenate fractions and plasma. Liver, small intestine and plasma were obtained from adult Sprague Dawley, male rats. Tissues were washed in ice-cold 0.25 M potassium phosphate buffer (pH 7.4) and then homogenized in 4 volumes of the same ice-cold buffer.

The 9000 g liver supernatent and the 27000 g small intestine supernatent were prepared from the corresponding homogenate by centrifugation for 20 min at 4°C.

Standard incubation procedure. Incubations were carried out under air at 37°C. The incubation medium consisted of 20 ml of enzyme preparation and 1.5 micromole of substrate in solution.

A study of the chemical stability of the 3 substrates in 0.25 M
phosphate buffer (pH 7.4) and a blank in the absence of substrate
were carried out under the same conditions.

A 2 ml aliquot of each incubation medium was removed at selected
time intervals.

Extraction procedure. Aliquots removed from incubation media
were transferred into 4 ml of 0.1 M borate buffer (pH 9) and immediately extracted 4 times with 4 ml of diisopropyl ether. Under
these experimental conditions EL and DCL were quantitatively extracted and DEL quantitatively remained in the water phase. These
latter were acidified to pH 2 in order to decarboxylate the anionic derivative readjusted to pH 9 and quantitatively formed DCL
derivative extracted again with diisopropyl ether.

Thin-Layer chromatography. Organic extracts were spotted on silica gel plates (Merck GF 254) and chromatographed along with authentic standards in chloroform-diisopropyl ether-ethanol (70 : 25
: 5 by vol.). Compounds detected under U.V. light at 254 nm by
quenching of fluorescence were elucidated by comparison with homologous extracts from blank incubation mixtures and with synthetic
reference samples, EL (Rf 0.7) and DCL (Rf 0.5).

Quantitative analysis. Quantitative data were obtained by ultraviolet spectrophotometry of eluates obtained after scraping and
elution of the analyte zone and centrifugation of the methanolic
layer.

RESULTS AND DISCUSSION

In all biological media used, EL was very rapidly converted to
DEL and to DCL. Values reported on figure 1 and table 1 represented the evolution in time of the amounts of each constituent in
the medium studied. These values were those determined in the 2
ml aliquot of samples analysed. Since EL was found to be stable
in the buffer under the same incubation conditions it could be indicated that hydrolysis of the ester bond was obviously enzymic.

With regard to decarboxylation, kinetic profiles obtained from
biological media were different from those obtained by spontaneous
decarboxylation of DEL in the buffer.

In the buffer, DCL was found in trace amounts over the entire period of incubation. In contrast, amounts of DCL obtained from biological media increased as function of time and were notably higher than those determined from spontaneous break down of DEL in the buffer. This would imply an enzymic origin of DCL from DEL in biological media.

Kinetics obtained from incubation of DEL used as substrate were not reported. Results were virtually identical to those of DEL formed *de novo* from EL.

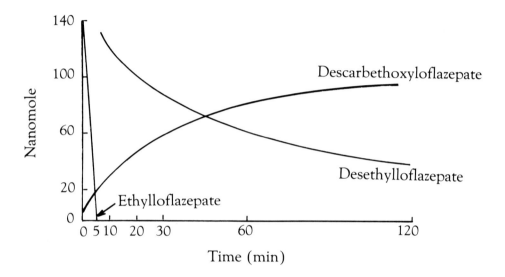

Fig. 1. Kinetics of bioconversion of EL in the plasma.

In all of the media studied, DCL used as a substrate underwent no conversion and extraction and elution yields were 100%. This result validate all measurements involving DCL.

In other respects, it is of interest to note the relative stability of DEL in the small intestine fraction. This observation would be suggestive of a phenomenon of protection of the carboxyl moiety in this medium, by a biological or chemical micro-environment.

TABLE 1 KINETICS OF BIOCONVERSION OF EL IN LIVER AND SMALL INTES-
TINE HOMOGENATE FRACTIONS

Time of incubation (min)	Liver			Small intestine		
	EL	DEL	DCL	EL	DEL	DCL
	(nanomole)					
0	140	0	0	140	0	0
10	0	120	20	0	130	10
20		75	65		130	10
30		75	65		120	20
60		65	75		90	50

CONCLUSION

In vitro studies revealed the existence of high levels of esterase
activity towards EL as a substrate in the plasma, the liver and the
intestinal mucosa of the rat. So it can be concluded that EL after
oral administration is very rapidly biotransformed first during the
crossing of the intestinal wall, then in the blood and the liver.
Thus, the presence of intact drug at significant levels in circulating blood or in excreta is unlikely.

From the standpoint of the formation of DCL by an enzyme process,
data obtained with the *in vitro* and *in vivo* experiments gave discordant results. The significant excretion of DEL in the urine of a-
nimals treated with EL and DEL was in contradiction with the decarboxylase activity determined *in vitro* in the various biological
media. Furthermore, DEL was found to be the major plasma circulating metabolite following oral administration of ^{14}C-EL to the baboon, using direct injection of plasma samples on HPLC with on line radioactivity detection technique. These observations would be
correlated to the phenomenon of protection of the carboxyl moiety
previously suggested.

© 1983 Elsevier Science Publishers B.V.
Extrahepatic Drug Metabolism and Chemical Carcinogenesis,
J. Rydström, J. Montelius and M. Bengtsson eds.

METABOLISM OF PROMUTAGENS TO ULTIMATE MUTAGENS BY THE RAT VENTRAL PROSTATE AND
COVALENT BINDING OF BENZO(A)PYRENE TO PROSTATIC MICROSOMAL PROTEINS.

PETER SÖDERKVIST[1], LEIF BUSK[2], RUNE TOFTGÅRD[1] AND JAN-ÅKE GUSTAFSSON[1]

[1]Department of Medical Nutrition, Huddinge University Hospital F69, S-141 86
Huddinge and [2]Toxicology Laboratory, National Food Administration, Box 622,
S-751 26 Uppsala, Sweden

INTRODUCTION

The cytochrome P-450 enzyme system have been proposed to play a significant
role in environmentally related diseases. Prostatic carcinoma is a malignant
disease which, by epidemiological investigations, have been etiologically related
to several environmental factors as well as influenced by endogenous compounds.
Earlier we and others have shown that cytochrome P-450-depending activities are
present in the rat ventral prostate and that these activities are easily increased
by inducers of the polycyclic aromatic hydrocarbon (PAH)-type (1,2). To furhter
elucidate the toxicological significance of this induction, we studied the formation of mutagens in the Ames´ Salmonella assay.

RESULTS AND DISCUSSION

Rats were treated with β-naphthoflavone (BNF) and phenobarbital (PB), 80 mg/kg
for four days. PCB (Arochlor 1254) was given as a single i.p. injection five days
prior to decapitation. Microsomes and 5000 x g supernatants (S-5 fraction) were
prepared from rat ventral prostates. S-5 fractions were added as metabolic
activation system in the Ames´ test and the mutagenicity of 2-aminofluorene (2-AF)
and aflatoxin B_1 (AFB) were registered. The mutagenicity of 2-AF is primarily
mediated by cytochrome P-448, when liver is used as activation system. This isozyme is induced in the liver by pretreatment of BNF or PCB but not by PB, which
induces another isozyme. A dose-dependent increase in mutagenicity of 2-AF was
observed for all treatment groups including corn oil. BNF and PCB strongly
potentiated the activation of 2-AF while PB had no effect when compared to control
(Fig. 1). Similar results were obtained with benzo(a)pyrene (BP) as promutagen.
The activation of AFB to an ultimate mutagenic metabolite is catalysed by the
cytochrome P-450 isozyme inducible by PB while cytochrome P-448 metabolizes AFB
to a non-mutagenic compound. S-5 fractions from all groups gave a dose dependent
mutagenic response but this was not potentiated by BNF, PCB or PB (Fig. 2). BNF
and PCB induces cytochrome P-448 and do not enhance AFB-mutagenicity. The inability
of PB to increase AFB-mutagenicity in the rat ventral prostate contrasts to what

is known for rat liver and supports the contention that PB has no effect on the metabolism of xenobiotics in the rat ventral prostate.

A time dependent covalent binding of BP to microsomal proteins was observed after incubation of BP with prostatic microsomal proteins (Fig. 3). This shows that the ventral prostate after induction with BNF is capable of generating metabolites with electrophilic properties which reacts with nucleophilic proteins.

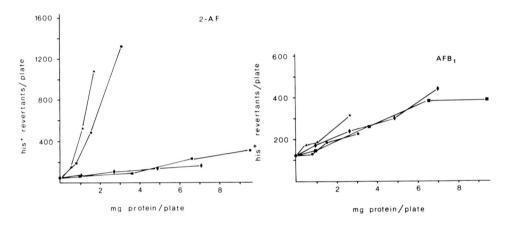

Figs. 1 and 2. Dose-response relationship for formation of mutagenic metabolites (S. typhimurium TA 98 and TA 100, 60 μg 2-AF and 0.75 μg AFB per plate respectively) versus the amount of S-5 fraction added. The symbols used are ▲ BNF, ● PCB, ◆ PB and ■ corn oil.

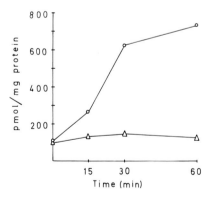

Fig. 3. Quantitative determination of covalent binding of BP to prostatic microsomal proteins (o) and boiled microsomes (Δ) from BNF treated animals.

The findings presented shows that prostatic tissue is very sensitive to certain inducers and possess capacity to produce metabolites that interacts with DNA (mutations) and binds covalently to proteins. This might be of importance for initiation of prostatic cancer by environmental factors.

© 1983 Elsevier Science Publishers B.V.
Extrahepatic Drug Metabolism and Chemical Carcinogenesis,
J. Rydström, J. Montelius and M. Bengtsson eds.

THE METABOLIC ACTIVATION OF AFB₁ IN RAT AND MAN

SIMON PLUMMER, ALAN R BOOBIS, CLARE KAHN AND DONALD S DAVIES

Department of Clinical Pharmacology, Royal Postgraduate Medical School,
London W12 0HS, UK.

Aflatoxin B_1 (AFB_1) is metabolically activated by cytochrome P-450 to a highly
reactive epoxide which is believed to initiate liver cancer in man. Recent
epidemiological evidence has suggested a significant association between
susceptibility to aflatoxin induced cancer and capacity to oxidize the anti-
hypertensive drug debrisoquine (1). One explanation for these results is that
the same form of cytochrome P-450 catalyses the oxidation of debrisoquine and
metabolic "activation" of AFB_1. This hypothesis has been investigated in two
ways. i) Strain differences in the "activation" of AFB_1 in DA (AFB_1 resistant)
and Fischer (AFB_1 sensitive) rats which show an 8-fold difference in their
oxidation of debrisoquine (2). ii) The effects of debrisoquine on the
"activation" of AFB_1 by human and rat liver microsomes.

The "activation" of AFB_1 by cytochrome P-450 was measured in 3 ways. (i) The
Ames Test (ii) Covalent binding of ^3H AFB_1 to microsomal protein (iii) Covalent
binding of ^3H AFB_1 to DNA in vitro and in vivo. In the Ames Test, liver
microsomes from the 2 strains of rat were equipotent in the activation of
AFB_1 and 10 times more active than human liver microsomes. The addition of
debrisoquine (2.5 mM) produced only a 25% inhibition of AFB_1 activation in
both strains of rat microsomes compared with a 75% inhibition with metyrapone
(3.0 mM). Debrisoquine did not inhibit AFB_1 "activation" by human liver
microsomes (Figure 1). There was no difference in the covalent binding of
^3H AFB_1 (20 μM) to microsomal protein from DA (0.71 ± 0.08 nmol/mg) and
Fischer (0.53 ± 0.09 nmoles/mg) rats. Debrisoquine (2.5 mM) produced only
a 10% inhibition. At 20 μM AFB_1 binding to human microsomal protein
(0.98 nmoles/mg) was greater than rat (0.63 nmoles/mg) and debrisoquine
(2.5 mM) caused only a small (25%) non-competetive inhibition. There was
no strain difference in the binding of ^3H AFB_1 to DNA in vitro (Fischer
183 ± 8.8 pmoles/mg DNA, DA 180 ± 41.6 moles/mg DNA). However, the binding
of ^3H AFB_1 to rat liver DNA in vivo was 2-fold higher in Fischer (37.5 ± 5.9
pmoles/mg) than DA (18.0 ± 7.8 pmoles/mg DNA) rats.

These results show that i) there is no difference in the metabolic "activation"
of AFB_1 in DA and Fischer rats, despite an 8-fold difference in debrisoquine

208

oxidation and ii) debrisoquine had little or no effect on the metabolic "activation" of AFB$_1$ which suggest that the same form of P-450 does not catalyse the oxidation of debrisoquine and "activation" of AFB$_1$. A significant difference in covalent binding of ^{3}H AFB$_1$ to DA and Fischer rat liver DNA in vivo suggest that other mechanisms apart from metabolic activation by P-450 are important in DNA adduct formation with AFB$_1$. The metabolic inactivation of AFB$_1$ by glutathione transferase has been studied in DA and Fischer rats using a modified tri-layer Ames Test and there is no difference between the 2 strains of rats in the activity of this enzyme.

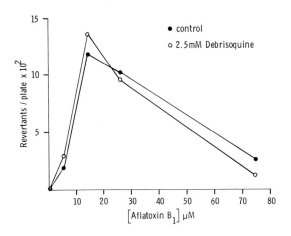

Fig.1. Activation of AFB$_1$ by human liver microsomes (0.75 mg/plate)
in the Ames test in the absence and presence of debrisoquine (2.5 mM)

REFERENCES
1. Idle, J.R. (1981). In: Davis, M, Tredger, J M and Williams, R (eds), Drug Reactions and the Liver, Pitman Medical Publishers, London, pp.313-320.
2. Dabbagh-Al, S.G., Idle, J.R. and Smith, R.L. (1981). J. Pharm. Pharmacol., 33, 161-164.

S.P. is supported by a Medical Research Council Studentship.

© 1983 Elsevier Science Publishers B.V.
Extrahepatic Drug Metabolism and Chemical Carcinogenesis,
J. Rydström, J. Montelius and M. Bengtsson eds.

DRUG METABOLIZING ENZYMES IN RESTING HUMAN LYMPHOCYTES

JANERIC SEIDEGÅRD[1] AND JOSEPH W. DEPIERRE[2]

[1]Wallenberg Laboratory, University of Lund, S-220 07 Lund and [2]Department of
Biochemistry, Arrhenius Laboratory, University of Stockholm, S-106 91 Stockholm,
Sweden.

INTRODUCTION

Because of the central importance of metabolizing systems to the toxic and
genotoxic effects of many xenobiotics, there is at present a rapidly growing
interest in increasing our understanding of drug metabolism in human cells. Such
increased knowledge will probably prove to be useful in a number of different
respects, including determining the dosage of a medicine which a patient should
receive; monitoring the exposure of a given population to xenobiotics in the
work or general environment; predicting the susceptibility of an individual to
the toxic and genotoxic effects of different chemicals; etc. Since circulating
lymphocytes can be obtained without undue stress or damage to the individual,
these cells have received much attention in this respect. In our opinion an
extensive, thorough characterization of drug-metabolizing systems in human
lymphocytes from individuals in various life situations would provide highly
valuable information which would complement and facilitate the understanding of
data obtained by other approaches (e.g., studies of chromosome breakage, sister
chromatid exchange, single strand breaks in DNA, binding of xenobiotics and/or
their metabolites to DNA, DNA repair).

MATERIALS AND METHODS

Human lymphocytes were isolated from whole blood by the standard procedure
of Isopaque-Ficoll gradient centrifugation. Resting human lymphocytes from
normal indivduals were sonicated and the resulting preparation centrifuged at
105,000g for 60 min to obtain membrane and a soluble fraction. Subsequently, a
wide spectrum of drug-metabolizing activities was measured using assay procedures and conditions developed for rat liver preparations.

RESULTS

As can be seen from table 1, a number of drug-metabolizing and related enzymes - including NADPH-cytochrome P-450 and NADH-cytochrome c reductase, microsomal and cytosolic epoxide hydrolases and glutathione transferases, and DT-
diaphorase - can easily be measured in resting human lymphocytes.

TABLE 1

LEVELS OF DRUG-METABOLIZING AND RELATED ENZYMES IN RESTING HUMAN LYMPHOCYTES

Enzyme	Substrate	Level/min-10^7 cells
NADPH-cytochrome P-450 reductase	cytochrome c	0.70 nmol
cytochrome P-450	-	n.d.[a]
cytochrome P-450 catalyzed metabolism	2-acetylaminofluorene	n.d.
NADH-cytochrome c reductase	cytochrome c	27 nmol
cytochrome b_5	-	n.d.
microsomal epoxide hydrolase	cis-stilbene oxide	6.5 pmol
	trans-stilbene oxide	n.d.
	androstene oxide	190 pmol
	estroxide	16 pmol
cytosolic epoxide hydrolase	cis-stilbene oxide	n.d.
	trans-stilbene oxide	8.0 pmol
microsomal glutathione transferase	1-chloro-2.4-dinitro-benzene	3 nmol
	cis-stilbene oxide	n.d.
	trans-stilbene oxide	n.d.
cytosolic glutathione transferase	1-chloro-2.4-dinitro-benzene	51 nmol
	cis-stilbene oxide	n.d.
	trans-stilbene oxide	63 pmol
DT-diaphorase	2.6-dichlorophenol-indophenol	2.1 nmol
UDP-glucose dehydrogenase	UDP-glucose	n.d.
glucose-6-phosphate dehydrogenase	glucose-6-phosphate	44 μmol

[a]n.d. = not detectable

We are continuing these investigations of drug-metabolizing enzymes in resting human lymphocytes and will subsequently examine their possible induction by different xenobiotics.

© 1983 Elsevier Science Publishers B.V.
Extrahepatic Drug Metabolism and Chemical Carcinogenesis,
J. Rydström, J. Montelius and M. Bengtsson eds.

COVALENT BINDING OF BENZO(a)PYRENE TO CYTOCHROME P-448 AND OTHER PROTEINS
IN RECONSTITUTED MIXED FUNCTION OXIDASE SYSTEMS

CECILIA SCHELIN[1], BENGT JERGIL[1] AND JAMES HALPERT[2]

[1]Biochemistry, Chemical Centre, University of Lund, P.O.B. 740, S-220 07 Lund,
Sweden and [2]Department of Medical Nutrition, Karolinska Institute, Huddinge
Hospital, S-141 86 Huddinge, Sweden

INTRODUCTION

Many carcinogenic and mutagenic polycyclic hydrocarbons, including benzo(a)-
pyrene, may bind covalently to DNA, RNA and proteins after metabolic activation. Such binding has been implicated in the toxic, mutagenic and carcinogenic properties of these compounds.

The metabolically activated compounds will bind specifically rather than
randomly to cellular proteins as shown earlier with benzo(a)pyrene (1). The
aim of this study has been to identify microsomal target proteins for activated benzo(a)pyrene.

MATERIALS AND METHODS

Microsomes from male Sprague-Dawley rats, pretreated with phenobarbital or
β-naphtoflavone, were prepared as described earlier (2). The following enzymes
involved in the metabolism of polycyclic aromatic hydrocarbons were isolated:
NADPH-cytochrome P-450-reductase and the major forms of cytochrome P-450 from
phenobarbital- and β-naphtoflavone pretreated animals (2).

Quantitative determination of covalently bound ^{14}C-benzo(a)pyrene was performed as described by Wallin et al. (3). The amount of enzymes are indicated
under the figure, and the incubation time was 30 min. Analysis of protein
binding patterns and fluorography were analyzed as described elsewhere (2).

RESULTS AND DISCUSSION

The possibility that benzo(a)pyrene would bind covalently to components of
a reconstituted mixed function oxidase system containing cytochrome P-450,
NADPH-cytochrome P-450-reductase and phosphatidylcholine was examined. Binding
was seen in systems containing cytochrome P-450 from β-naphtoflavone pretreated rats (Fig. 1). The binding was proportional to the amount of cytochrome
added up to 0.05 nmol. No binding was seen using the phenobarbital-induced
form of cytochrome P-450. NADPH and NADPH-cytochrome P-450-reductase were

212

required for binding, indicating
that metabolic activation preceded
binding.

The identity of the targets for
the metabolically activated ben-
zo(a)pyrene was examined by SDS-
polyacrylamide gel electrophoresis
and fluorography. In a reconstituted
system radioactivity incorporated
into β-naphtoflavone-induced cytochrome P-450, but not into NADPH-
cytochrome P-450 reductase. No
adducts were formed in incubations
with phenobarbital-induced cytochrome P-450. If both forms of cytochrome P-450 were incubated together, and with reductase, radio-
label was found in both of them.
This shows that both forms have
target groups but that only one
form catalyzes the formation of
benzo(a)pyrene metabolites that
can react with these groups.

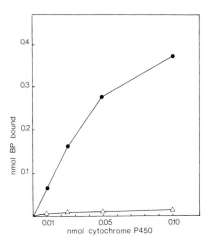

Fig. 1. Effect of the amount of cytochrome
P-450 on the covalent binding of benzo(a)-
pyrene to proteins in reconstituted systems containing NADPH-cytochrome P-450-
reductase in a molar excess of 8 to the
cytochrome, 10 µg phosphatidylcholine and
the amount of phenobarbital-(△) or β-
naphtoflavone-(●) induced forms as indicated of cytochrome P-450.

Activated chloramphenicol has previously been shown to form adducts with
mainly lysine residues of the phenobarbital-induced form of cytochrome P-450
(4) causing an inactivation of the enzyme. The target amino acids for benzo(a)-
pyrene metabolites and the effect of their binding on cytochrome activity is
presently under investigation.

REFERENCES
1. Tunek, A., Schelin, C. and Jergil, B. (1979) Chem.-Biol. Interact., 27, 133.
2. Schelin, C., Wallin, H., Halpert, J. and Jergil, B. (1983) Eur.J. Biochem.
   (Submitted for publication).
3. Wallin, H., Schelin, C., Tunek, A. and Jergil, B. (1981) Chem.-Biol. Interact., 88, 109.
4. Halpert, J. (1982) Mol. Pharmacol., 21, 166.

© 1983 Elsevier Science Publishers B.V.
Extrahepatic Drug Metabolism and Chemical Carcinogenesis,
J. Rydström, J. Montelius and M. Bengtsson eds.

THE DOSE DEPENDENT METABOLISM OF ANETHOLE, ESTRAGOLE AND p-PROPYLANISOLE IN RELATION TO THEIR SAFETY EVALUATION.

SUSAN A. SANGSTER, JOHN CALDWELL, ANDREW ANTHONY, ANDREW J. HUTT AND
ROBERT L. SMITH.
Department of Pharmacology, St. Mary's Hospital Medical School, Norfolk Place,
London W2 1PG, England.

The anisole derivatives anethole (A; 4-methoxypropenylbenzene), estragole
(E; 4-methoxyallylbenzene) and p-propylanisole (PPA) are all structurally
related food flavours. A and E are naturally occurring in the oils of many
herbs, while PPA is of synthetic origin. All three compounds have been
reported as being hepatotoxic in rodents at high doses (0.5-1g/kg/day) (1,2).
However, it is important to consider how far these findings can be extrapolated
to man. Of the many relevant factors, two of the most important are
differences in the sizes of the doses received by test animals and man, and
in the rates and routes of metabolism of the compound. These are of particular
concern in the case of these anisole derivatives as (i) the doses used to
show adverse effects in animals are vastly greater than the human exposure
from the diet (1-70µg/day) and (ii) the toxicity of the allylic compound
estragole apparently arises from metabolites produced subsequent to 1'-hydroxy-
lation of the side chain (3).

[^{14}C-methoxy] labelled A, E and PPA were administered to female Wistar rats
p.o. and male CD-1 mice i.p. in the range 0.05-1500 mg/kg. After administration of all three compounds to both species, ^{14}C was excreted in the expired
air (as $^{14}CO_2$), urine and to a small extent the faeces.

In each case, with increasing dose, the excretion of $^{14}CO_2$ (arising from
O-demethylation) falls (from ca. 60% to ca. 40% of dose) and urinary excretion
rises (from ca. 20% to ca. 50% of dose). The urinary metabolites of all three
compounds in both species arise from various oxidations of the side chain
giving both alcohols and acids.

With E, oxidation of the side chain at C-1 giving the proximate carcinogen
1'-hydroxy E occurs, this becoming more important with increasing dose
(1% of dose at 0.05mg/kg and 10% at 1000mg/kg). Other metabolites, apparently
not involved in toxicity, arise from epoxidation of the allylic double bond.
A is principally oxidised at the propenyl double bond, leading via the
epoxide to 2 isomers of 1'-(4-methoxyphenyl)-propane-1',2'-diol, and at the
ω-carbon giving 4-methoxycinnamyl alcohol and 4-methoxycinnamic acid and via

β-oxidation to 4-methoxybenzoic acid, mainly excreted as its glycine conjugate. Epoxidation of A increases greatly with dose yielding more of the diols. PPA is metabolised by α and (ω-1)-hydroxylation, and by side chain cleavage to 4-methoxybenzoic acid.

The fates of all these compounds in man (oral doses of 100μg-1mg) resemble the metabolic patterns in rodents. 0.25% of the dose of E is excreted as 1'-hydroxyE in man which is representative of a low dose rodent experiment. The excretion routes and metabolic pattern of PPA in man resemble those seen in a low/medium dose rodent experiment, with 60% of the dose being 0-demethylated. A is rapidly metabolised by man and excreted with 12h of dosing, mainly as 4-methoxy-hippuric acid (45% of dose), the other major metabolites being the diols (total 9% of the dose).

It is thus clear that animal toxicity tests using very high doses are not representative of the situation obtaining in man at normal (low) levels of exposure to these food flavours. The alteration in disposition of each compound at very high doses in rodents compared with the low dose animal or human situation leads to the tissues being exposed to different metabolites for longer periods of time. It would be thus expected that the effects seen at high doses would be qualitatively different from those seen at low doses. These data thus contribute to the interpretation of the significance of rodent toxicity tests for the human safety of these three food flavours.

ACKNOWLEDGEMENTS

Supported by grants from F.E.M.A., Washington. AJH is a post-doctoral fellow of the Sir Halley Stewart Trust.

REFERENCES

1. Hagen, E.C., Hansen, W.H., Fitzhugh, O.G. Jenner, P.M., Jones, W.T., Taylor, J.M., Long, E.L., Nelson, A.A. and Brouwer, J.B. (1967). Fd. Cosmet. Toxicol. 5, 141-157.

2. Taylor, J.M., Jenner, P.M. and Jones, W.I. (1964). Toxic. appl. Pharmac. 6, 378-387.

3. Drinkwater, N.R., Miller, E.C., Miller, J.A. and Pitot, H.C. (1976). J. Natl. Cancer Inst. 57, 1323-1331.

© 1983 Elsevier Science Publishers B.V.
Extrahepatic Drug Metabolism and Chemical Carcinogenesis,
J. Rydström, J. Montelius and M. Bengtsson eds.

DT-DIAPHORASE IN MOUSE EPIDERMIS, INDUCTION OF THE ENZYME BY
METHYLCHOLANTHRENE.

OLVE RØMYHR, VEMUND DIGERNES, OLAV HILMAR IVERSEN
Inst. of Pathology, University of Oslo, Rikshospitalet,
Oslo 1, Norway.

INTRODUCTION

The cytosole enzyme DT-diaphorase has previously been demonstrated in the liver and in several other tissues (1,2). The
exact physiological function of the enzyme is not yet established,
but the enzyme may serve as a quinon-reductase in connection with
conjugation of hydroquinones during e.g. detoxification of polycyclic hydrocarbons (3). The DT-diaphorase is present in the epidermis of hairless mice, and induction of the enzyme by topical
application of methylcholanthrene (MCA) is here demonstrated.

MATERIALS AND METHODS

Hairless mice of the hr/hr Oslo strain of both sexes were used.
MCA disolved in 100 µl acetone was applied topically. The enzyme-
activity in the cytosole-fraction (105 000 g, 60 min) of homogenized epidermal cells was measured spectrophotometrically
(530 nm) as reduction of nitroblue tetrazolium (NBT) in a medium
supplied with NADH (76 µM), NADPH (76 µM), and menadion (10 µM).

RESULTS

Characterization of the method

The reaction was linear with cytosole protein-concentrations
between 15-100 µg in the medium. NADH and NADPH served equally
well as substrates for the enzyme. The activity of the enzyme
could be 90-95% inhibited with 10 µM dicumarol in the medium.

Induction with MCA

Enzyme-activity following one application of MCA is shown in
fig. 1. Maximum activity (10 x control values) was obtained
36 hours after treatment. The induction was dose-dependent.

216

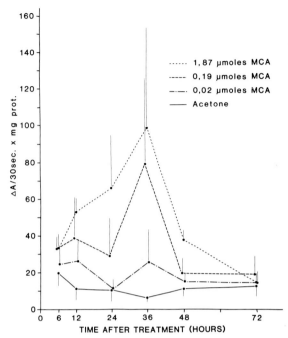

Fig.1. Time course of the DT-diaphorase-activity, MCA was given in 3 different doses: 1,87 µmol, 0,19 µmol, 0,02 µmol, in 100 µl acetone. Control animals received 100 µl acetone. Each time point represents the average of the measurements from 6 animals, 3 males and 3 females. The rather high SD at some of the points is probably a result of sex-variations in the responsiveness. (The male mice responded with enzyme-induction earlier than the females).

DISCUSSION

DT-diaphorase has been thoroughly investigated in the liver of experimental animals, and its possible roles in the carcinogenic process have been suggested.

Both the existence of the enzyme in the epidermis and its inducibility by MCA indicate possible physiological functions also in this organ. As discussed in ref. (4) the DT-diaphorase may be part of the tetrazolium-test for skin carcinogens which is based on an increased ability of the epidermis to reduce tetrazolium-salt after application of skin carcinogens.

REFERENCES

1. Ernster, L., Ljunggren, M., Danielson, L. (1960) Biochem. biophys. Research Comm. 2:88-92.

2. Benson, A.M., Hunkeler, M.J. and Talaley, P. (1980) Proc. Natl. Acad. Sci. 77:5216-5220.

3. Lind, C., Vadi, H. and Ernster, L. (1978) Arch. Biochem. Biophys. 190:97-108.

4. Iversen, O.H. and Digernes, V. (1981) Virchows Arch. (Cell Pathol.) 36:133-138.

© 1983 Elsevier Science Publishers B.V.
Extrahepatic Drug Metabolism and Chemical Carcinogenesis,
J. Rydström, J. Montelius and M. Bengtsson eds.

INHIBITION OF XENOBIOTIC AND STEROID METABOLISM BY AMINOGLUTETH-
IMIDE IN HUMAN PLACENTAS FROM SMOKING AND NON-SMOKING MOTHERS

MARKKU PASANEN AND OLAVI PELKONEN
Department of Pharmacology, University of Oulu, SF-90220 Oulu 22,
Finland

INTRODUCTION

Ever since Welch and coworkers (1) showed a striking association
between cigarette smoking and metabolism of benzo(a)pyrene in
human placentas, several investigators have tried to elucidate the
effects of cigarette smoking on the placental enzymology of
steroid and xenobiotic metabolism.

In this work we studied the inhibitory effects of a specific inhibitor of steroid metabolism, aminoglutethimide (AG), on aryl
hydrocarbon hydroxylase (AHH), 7-ethoxycoumarin O-deethylase and
aromatase activities, in order to further characterize cytochrome
P-450 form(s) involved in these activities and also the effect of
cigarette smoking.

EXPERIMENTAL DESIGN, RESULTS AND DISCUSSION

Human placentas obtained after normal delivery at term were
excised free of connective tissue and coagulated blood and then
stored at $-20^{\circ}C$ until examined.

Placental microsomal fractions were prepared as described previously (2) and enzymatic activities were determined as follows:
AHH according to Nebert and Gelboin (3), 7-ethoxycoumarin O-
deethylase according to Greenlee and Poland (4) and aromatase
according to Pasanen (5). Comparative inhibition experiments were
done at an AG concentration of 400 µM.

AG inhibition studies showed that AHH activity ($\bar{x}=111.4 \pm 207$
(SD) pmol/min/mg, variation from 5.6 to 619.5) was decreased by
$37 \pm 14.4\%$ (SD, n=8) in the group of smokers. Percent inhibition
was of similar degree in all cases although the actual extent of
induction varied greatly. AHH activity was very low or undetectable in the placentas of non-smokers and consequently AG
inhibition could not be measured.

7-ethoxycoumarin O-deethylase activity was inhibited by $97 \pm$
1.4% (SD, n=11) in placentas from non-smoking mothers (basal

activity x̄=5.3 ± 2.3 (SD) pmol/min/mg) and by 54 ± 15% (SD,n=9) in placentas from smoking mothers (23.1 ± 35 SD pmol/min/mg, variation from 2.7 to 114.4).

Aromatase and AHH activities exhibited a correlation coefficient of 0.858 in placentas from smoking mothers, while no correlation was found in the group of non-smokers. Although aromatase activity was slightly increased (about 30%) in the placentas from smoking mothers, the effect of cigarette smoking appeared to be complex and could not be definitely characterized. The inhibition caused by AG was at the same level (39%) in both smokers and non-smokers.

The results of these studies suggest that 1) aromatase and the two xenobiotic-oxidizing activities are catalyzed by different forms of placental cytochrome P-450; 2) maternal cigarette smoking seems to affect both biotransformations although the effect on aromatase seems to be complex; 3) maternal cigarette smoking probably induces a novel enzyme metabolizing benzo(a)pyrene and 7-ethoxycoumarin which is not present in uninduced placentas, and 4) aromatase is probably similar in placentas both from smokers and non-smokers, at least as judged by inhibition studies.

ACKNOWLEDGEMENTS

The technical assistance of Ms Ritva Saarikoski and Ms Päivi Kylli is gratefully acknowledged. This work was supported by grants from The Finnish Foundation for Cancer Research, The Emil Aaltonen Foundation and The Academy of Finland (Medical Reseach Council).

REFERENCES
1. Welch, R.M., Harrison, Y.E., Conney, A.H., Poppers, P.J. and Finster, M. (1968) Science, 160 541-542.
2. Pasanen, M. and Pelkonen, O. (1981) Biochem. Biophys. Res. Commun. 103, 1310-1317.
3. Nebert, D.W. and Gelboin, H.V. (1968) J. Biol. Chem., 243, 6242-6249.
4. Greenlee, W.F. and Poland, A.A. (1978) J. Pharmacol. Exp. Ther. 205, 596-605.
5. Pasanen, M. (submitted) Anal. Biochem.

© 1983 Elsevier Science Publishers B.V.
Extrahepatic Drug Metabolism and Chemical Carcinogenesis,
J. Rydström, J. Montelius and M. Bengtsson eds.

METABOLIC CONVERSION OF STYRENE TO STYRENE GLYCOL IN THE MOUSE. OCCURRENCE OF THE INTERMEDIATE STYRENE-7,8-OXIDE

MARIANNE NORDQVIST, ELISABETH LJUNGQUIST AND AGNETA LÖF

Research Department, National Board of Occupational Safety and Health, S-171 84 Solna Sweden

INTRODUCTION

Styrene is known to be metabolized to the weak carcinogen styrene-7,8-oxide (SO) by rat liver microsomes (1). Recently it was detected in vivo in trace amounts in lungs and liver of mice pretreated with an inhibitor of epoxide hydrolase (2). Studies on the enzyme activities in different mouse tissues have indicated that the rate of formation of SO exceeds its rate of detoxification only in the lungs (3). Consequently an accumulation of SO could be suspected to occur in this tissue. On the basis of this the present investigation was initiated.

| styrene | styrene-7,8-oxide (SO) | styrene glycol (SG) |

MATERIALS AND METHODS

To determine the occurrence in time of the styrene metabolites SO and styrene glycol (SG), (7-14C)-styrene (3.95 MBq/mmol) was given i.p. (3.8 mmol/kg) to groups of four male mice which were sacrificed after 0.5, 1, 2, and 5 h, respectively. To study the influence of the dose groups of four mice were killed 2 h after a dose of 1.1, 2.3, 3.4 and 5.1 mmol/kg, respectively. Blood, liver, kidneys, lungs, brain and subc. adip. tissue were isolated and extracted first with hexane to remove styrene and SO, secondly with ethyl acetate to remove SG. ß-glucuronidase type H-1 was used to liberate conjugated SG. A gas chromatographic method based on electron capture detector (GC-EC) was used to quantify SG as well as SO after hydrolysis to SG. In a complementary study the epoxide hydrolase inhibitor trichloropropene oxide was added to the removed tissues and the hexane extract was analyzed both by GC-EC and mass fragmentography (GC-MID).

RESULTS

SO and SG reached a maximal concentration within 2 h. The highest levels of SO were detected in the kidneys, subc. adip. tissue and blood (Fig 1) . The SO contents in liver and lungs increased considerably when the homogenisation was performed in the presence of the epoxide hydrolase inhibitor (GC-EC, GC-MID) indicating that the level of SO in vivo may be higher in the liver than in the kidneys. SG was found in the highest concentrations in the kidneys, liver, blood and lungs. Styrene increased exponentially at higher doses in all the tissues but the relative formation of SG was mainly unaffected by the dose. The SO concentration increased with the dose in the kidneys and adip. tissue but leveled off in the blood (Fig 2). The accumulation of SO in the kidneys and the profound increase of the pulmonary concentration when the inhibitor was added could not be predicted from the previous in vitro findings on enzyme activities (3).

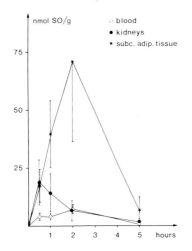 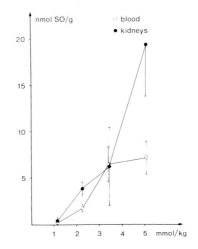

Fig 1. Tissue conc. of SO at different times.

Fig 2. Tissue conc. of SO after different doses of styrene.

REFERENCES

1. Leibman, K.C. and Ortiz, E. (1970) J. Pharmacol. Exp. Ther., 173, 242.

2. Pantarotto, C., Salmona, M., Szczawinska, K. and Bidoli, F. (1980) in: A'lbaiges, J. (Ed.), Analytical Techniques in Environmental Chemistry, Pergamon Press, Oxford, pp. 245-279.

3. Cantoni, L., Salmona, M., Facchinetti, T., Pantarotto, C. and Belvedere, G. (1978) Toxicol. lett., 2, 179.

© 1983 Elsevier Science Publishers B.V.
Extrahepatic Drug Metabolism and Chemical Carcinogenesis,
J. Rydström, J. Montelius and M. Bengtsson eds.

SUBCELLULAR DISTRIBUTION OF EPOXIDE HYDROLASE ACTIVITY IN THE LIVER, LUNG, KIDNEY AND TESTIS OF THE C57 Bl MALE MOUSE

JOHAN MEIJER, WINNIE BIRBERG[*], ÅKE PILOTTI[*] AND JOSEPH W. DePIERRE
Department of Biochemistry and [*]Department of Organic Chemistry, Arrhenius Laboratory, University of Stockholm, S-106 91 Stockholm, Sweden

INTRODUCTION

Many epoxide intermediates formed during the metabolism of both endogenous compounds and xenobiotics have been shown to be toxic and geno-toxic. The major enzymatic routes for the conversion of epoxides to less reactive products are hydrolysis by epoxide hydrolases (giving rise to dihydro-diols) and conjugation with glutathione via the glutathione transferases (1). In contrast to earlier beliefs, it is now known that both of these enzymes occur in several different parts of the cell, both in membrane-bound and in soluble forms. Here we have examined the subcellular distribution of epoxide hydrolase activity towards cis- and trans-stilbene oxide in the liver, lung, kidney and testis of the male mouse.

MATERIALS AND METHODS

20 g male C57 Bl mice (ALAB, Sollentuna, Sweden) were starved overnight before sacrifice by cervical dislocation. After homogenization of the different organs in 0.25 M sucrose, nuclear (600 g_{av} pellet), mitochondrial (10,000 g_{av} pellet), microsomal (105,000g_{av} pellet) and cytosol (105,000g_{av} supernatant) fractions were prepared by differential centrifugation. Epoxide hydrolase activity towards (^{3}H)-cis- and trans-stilbene oxide (synthesized by a published procedure (2)) was measured in 0.1 M glycine, pH 9, and 0.1 M potassium phosphate, pH 7, respectively, according to Hammock and coworkers (2).

RESULTS

In Figure 1 the total capacities of the liver, lung, kidney and testis to metabolize cis- and trans-stilbene oxide are compared. In all organs the capacity for metabolizing trans-stilbene oxide is considerably greater than the total activity towards the cis-isomer. This may explain why trans-stilbene oxide, which is an efficient inducer of drug-metabolizing enzymes in the rat (3), does not induce these enzymes in the mouse.

In mouse liver epoxide hydrolase activity towards cis-stilbene oxide appears to be specifically catalyzed by the microsomal enzyme. This is also

222

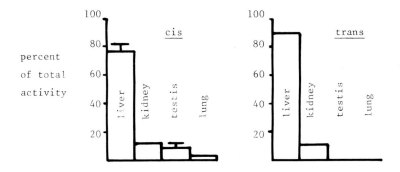

Fig. 1. The relative contribution of liver, kidney, testis and lung to the total metabolism of cis- and trans-stilbene oxide in these four organs (35.2 ±
5.2 nmol/mouse-min and 398 ± 56 nmol/mouse-min, respectively). The results
shown are means ± SD of 4 experiments.

the case for the lung, kidney and testis. These findings, together with others
in our laboratory, lead us to suggest that the epoxide hydrolase activity towards cis-stilbene oxide may be a better marker for the endoplasmic reticulum
than traditional markers such as NADPH cytochrome c reductase.

trans-Stilbene oxide, on the other hand, seems to be much more efficiently
metabolized by the cytosolic enzyme in mouse liver and kidney. The specific
activity of the mitochondrial fraction in these organs is of the same order of
magnitude as that of the cytosol, but the latter has a much higher total activity due to its higher protein content. In the testis, however, the relative
specific activity in both the mitochondrial and the microsomal fractions is
higher than that of the cytosol. Nonetheless, for both lung and testis the
total activity is highest in the cytosol.

ACKNOWLEDGEMENTS
      These studies were supported by NIH grant 1R01 CA 26261-04 and by a grant
from the Swedish Natural Science Research Council.

REFERENCES
1. DePierre,J.W. and Ernster,L. (1978) Biochim.Biophys.Acta.,473, 149
2. Gill,S.S. and Hammock,B.D. Anal.Biochem., in press.
3. Seidegård,J-E.,Morgenstern,R.,DePierre,J.W. and Ernster,L. (1979) Biochim.
   Biophys.Acta., 586, 10

© 1983 Elsevier Science Publishers B.V.
Extrahepatic Drug Metabolism and Chemical Carcinogenesis,
J. Rydström, J. Montelius and M. Bengtsson eds.

EFFECT OF POLYCHLORINATED NAPHTHALENES AND BIPHENYLS ON POLYSUBSTRATE MONOOXY-
GENASE AND UDPGLUCURONOSYLTRANSFERASE ACTIVITIES IN RAT LUNG

EERO MÄNTYLÄ[1], ANTERO AITIO[2] AND MARKKU AHOTUPA[1]
[1]Department of Physiology, University of Turku, SF-20520 Turku 52 (Finland) and
[2]Institute of Occupational Health, SF-00290 Helsinki 29 (Finland)

INTRODUCTION

Polychlorinated biphenyls (PCBs) are widespread and persistent environmental
contaminants having many harmful biological effects (1). Polychlorinated naphthalenes (PCNs) have been used to replace PCBs and they are suspected environmental pollutants. Both PCBs and PCNs enhance the activities of polysubstrate
monooxygenases and UDPglucuronosyltransferase in rat liver (2-5). The increase
in hepatic enzyme activities is maximal 1-2 weeks after a single i.p. dose
(100 mg/kg) of the chemicals (3, 4). PCBs elevate monooxygenase activity in rat
lung (2) and kidney (2, 5), and PCNs in rat kidney (5) but either chemicals
have no effect on intestinal monooxygenases. Renal and intestinal transferase
activity remains unchanged after treatment with PCBs or PCNs (5). As lungs may
be an important entry of PCBs and PCNs into the body we studied the effects of
these compounds on monooxygenase and transferase activities in rat lung.

MATERIALS AND METHODS

Adult male Wistar rats were treated i.p. (100 mg/kg) with a PCB-mixture
(Clophen A50-, 54% chlorine, Bayer AG, F.R.G.) or a PCN-mixture (either Halowax
1051, 70% chlorine, Koppers Co, U.S.A., or Nibren D130, 50-60% chlorine, Bayer).
Control animals received mere vehicle (corn oil). Ca^{2+}-aggregated microsomes
(6) were prepared from the lung 7 days after the treatment. From the Halowax-
trated animals also alveolar macrophages were isolated by lavage. The activities of arylhydrocarbon hydroxylase (7)(AHH), 7-ethoxycoumarin O-deethylase (8)
(ECDE) and UDPglucuronosyltransferase (4-methylumbelliferone as the aglycone)
(9) (UDPGT) were determined.

RESULTS AND DISCUSSION

Seven days after a single i.p. dose Halowax 1051 had increased pulmonary AHH-
activity 1.9-fold, ECDE-activity 3.8-fold and UDPGT-activity 2.0-fold (Table 1).
Nibren D130 enhanced ECDE-activity 2.7-fold. Clophen A50 had no effect on the
enzyme activities. Halowax 1051 did not change UDPGT-activity in alveolar macrophages.

224

TABLE 1.

MONOOXYGENASE AND UDPGLUCURONOSYLTRANSFERASE ACTIVITIES IN RAT LUNG ($x \pm$ S.E.)

Treatment	Lung microsomes			Alv. macrophages
	AHH[a]	ECDE[a]	UDPGT[a]	UDPGT[b]
Control	0.199+0.040	0.296+0.117	11.9+1.3	0.268+0.033
Halowax 1051	0.384+0.058[+]	1.12 +0.21[++]	24.0+1.4[++]	0.309+0.136
Nibren D130	0.325+0.082	0.789+0.165[+]	15.7+1.8	–
Clophen A50	0.405+0.090	0.383+0.148	11.9+1.8	–

[a] nmol/min/g wet weight, n = 4
[b] nmol/min/10^6 cells (homogenate), n = 3
+ = $2p < 0.05$, ++ = $2p < 0.01$ (Student´s t-test)

These data indicate that PCNs are more effective than PCBs in enhancing the activities of monooxygenases and UDPglucuronosyltransferase in rat lung. Vainio (2) has reported 5-fold increase in rat pulmonary AHH-activity by Clophen A50 but the dosing was different (15 mg/kg x 3). The increase in the monooxygenase activities caused by PCNs was small when compared to the 24-53-fold increase in kidney (5). In contrast to results from kidney (5), pulmonary UDPGT-activity was increased by PCN-treatment.

ACKNOWLEDGEMENTS

This study was supported by grants from The Academy of Finland and NIH R01 ES-01684.

REFERENCES

1. Wassermann, M., Wassermann, S., Cucos, S. and Miller, H.J. (1979) Ann. N.Y. Acad. Sci., 320, 69-124.

2. Vainio, H. (1974) Chem.-Biol. Interact., 9, 379-387.

3. Parkki, M.G., Marniemi, J. and Vainio, H. (1977) J. Toxicol. Environ. Health, 3, 903-911.

4. Ahotupa, M. and Aitio, A. (1980) Biochem. Biophys. Res. Commun., 93, 250-256.

5. Ahotupa, M., Hietanen, E., Mäntylä, E. and Vainio, H. (1982) J. Appl. Toxicol., 2, 47-53.

6. Aitio, A. and Vainio, H. (1976) Acta Pharmacol. Toxicol., 39, 555-561.

7. DePierre, J.W., Moron, M.S., Johannesen, K.A.M. and Ernster, L. (1975) Anal. Biochem., 63, 470-484.

8. Aitio, A. (1978) Anal. Biochem., 85, 488-491.

9. Aitio, A. (1974) Int. J. Biochem., 5, 617-621.

© 1983 Elsevier Science Publishers B.V.
Extrahepatic Drug Metabolism and Chemical Carcinogenesis,
J. Rydström, J. Montelius and M. Bengtsson eds.

COMPARISON OF THE PATTERNS OF BENZO(A)PYRENE CONJUGATES FORMED IN VIVO IN THE
LIVER AND KIDNEY OF THE NORTHERN PIKE (ESOX LUCIUS)

LENNART BALK, SUSANNE MÅNÉR AND JOSEPH W. DePIERRE
Department of Biochemistry, Arrhenius Laboratory, University of Stockholm,
S-106 91 Stockholm, Sweden

INTRODUCTION

The fact that all pollutants sooner or later reach our aquatic environment has lead in recent years to a growing interest in the fate and effects
of these xenobiotics on this portion of the biosphere. We have begun a series
of investigations on the metabolism of xenobiotics in the Northern pike (e.g.,
1, 2), a teleost fish which is a top predator, has a stationary habitat and
demonstrates high tumor frequencies in certain waters. Here we have characterized the conjugates produced in the liver and kidney of Northern pike
after exposure to benzo(a)pyrene in the water.

MATERIALS AND METHODS

The pike used in this study were purchased from a local hatchery and were
1-1.5 years old, approximately 10 cm long, 19-32 g in weight and of both sexes.
These animals were exposed to 68 ng ^{3}H-benzo(a)pyrene (the Radiochemical Centre,
Amersham, England)/l water for 4.5 days. The liver and kidney were then removed and extracted 3 times with 70% ethanol. Part of this extract was subjected to a simple extraction procedure with hexane to separate remaining benz-
o(a)pyrene from metabolites. The remaining portion was used to separate different classes of benzo(a)pyrene metabolites by chromatography on alumina oxide
essentially according to Autrup (3): Benzo(a)pyrene + unconjugated metabolites
were eluted with absolute ethanol, presumptive sulfate esters with water, presumptive glucuronides with 0.05 M ammonium phosphate, pH 3.0, and presumptive
glutathione conjugates with 25% formic acid (see Figure 1).

RESULTS

The metabolite pattern obtained with the trunk kidney from the Northern
pike (homologous to the mammalian kidney) contained all the different types
of benzo(a)pyrene metabolites, as well as unmetabolized benzo(a)pyrene. However, the distribution of radioactivity between these different groups was
quite different from that seen in the liver. The total amount of benzo(a)pyrene
+ metabolites recovered in the trunk kidney was 40% of that found in the liver.

226

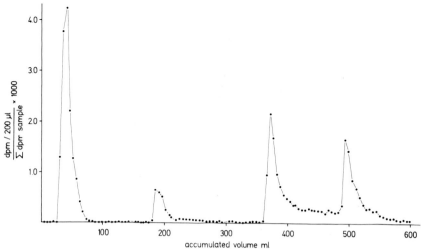

Fig. 1. Elution (from left to right) of benzo(a)pyrene + unconjugated metabolites, presumptive sulfate esters, presumptive glucuronides, and presumptive glutathione conjugates from the trunk kidney on an alumina oxide column.
Both organs contained essentially the same amount of unmetabolized benzo(a)-
pyrene (3-7%), whereas the recovery of unconjugated metabolites (37% of the
total radioactivity in the trunk kidney and 5% in the liver), presumptive
sulfate esters (9% and 2%, respectively), presumptive glucuronides (29% and
18%, respectively), and presumptive glutathione derivatives (25% and 46%,
respectively)were quite different in the two organs. We are now in the process of definitively identifying the different peaks obtained from the alumina
oxide column and determining why the patterns of benzo(a)pyrene metabolites
obtained in the trunk kidney and liver of the Northern pike differ as they do.

ACKNOWLEDGEMENTS

This study was supported by a grant from the National Swedish Environmental
Protection Board.

REFERENCES

1. Balk, L., Meijer, J., Seidegård, J., Morgenstern, R. and DePierre, J.W.
   (1980) Drug Metab. Dispos., 8, 98.

2. Balk, L., Meijer, J., Bergstrand, A., Åström, A., Morgenstern, R., Seidegård, J. and DePierre, J.W. (1982) Biochem. Pharmacol., 31, 1491.

3. Autrup, H. (1979) Biochem. Pharmacol., 28, 1727.

© 1983 Elsevier Science Publishers B.V.
Extrahepatic Drug Metabolism and Chemical Carcinogenesis,
J. Rydström, J. Montelius and M. Bengtsson eds.

DOES HUMAN PLACENTAL PAH METABOLISM PROTECT THE CONCEPTUS?

David K. Manchester, Natalie B. Parker, Karen Gottlieb and C. Michael Bowman,
Department of Pediatrics and Pharmacology, University of Colorado School of
Medicine, Denver, CO 80262, USA.

Activities of detoxication enzymes in human placentas vary greatly in
response to environmental exposures such as maternal cigarette smoking, but
the consequences of these placental responses for the conceptus are unkown
(1). We hypothesized that the ability of placental xenobiotic metabolism to
respond to environmental stimuli might protect the conceptus from chemical
toxicity. Our studies of monooxygenase activities in placentas from smoking
and nonsmoking women support this premise.

We have found that monooxygenase activities toward 7-ethoxyresorufin (ERR)
and benzo(a)pyrene (BP) are 10 to 100 fold higher in placentas from smokers
than from nonsmokers (2). The first step in metabolism of polycyclic aromatic
hydrocarbons (PAHs) present in cigarette smoke is their oxidation by inducible
cytochrome P-450 monooxygenase systems. Elevated levels of these enzymes
indicate both exposures to PAHs and placental responses. The intermediates
produced by oxidation of PAHs can be further metabolized by epoxide hydrolase
and the glutathione S-transferases. Placental activiaties of these enzymes,
however, do not increase when mothers smoke which indicates that variability
in monooxygenase activities is more likely to control the effects of placental
PAH metabolism (3,4).

We have shown that placental activity toward ERR that is inhibited by 7,8-
benzoflavone (BF) is sensitive even to passive smoking (5). Our studies of
monooxygenase activities in twin placentas from smoking women have also demonstrated high intraclass correlation coefficients in dichorionic placentas from
monozygotic twins (r_I(BP)=0.924, r_I(ERR)=0.916, N=5 pairs) and in placentas
from same sex (r_I(BP)=0.845, r_I(ERR)=0.863, N=11 pairs) and opposite sex
(r_I(BP)=0.907, r_I(ERR)=0.880, N=10 pairs) dizygotic twins. These results
indicate that the placenta is very sensitive to maternal PAH exposures and
that environmental factors contribute most to variability in placental monooxygenase activities in vivo.

Since placentation preceeds organogenesis in humans, failure of placental detoxication systems might contribute to birth defects. In a study of 82 placentas from women who smoked we found that while 10% of placentas from normal infants could be catagorized as having failed to respond to maternal smoking according to previously established criteria (2), 44% of placentas from infants with major structural abnormalities lacked response (p<0.01) when monooxygenase activities toward BP and ERR and effects of BF were compared.

In order to determine whether increased placental monooxygenase activity acts through first pass metabolism to diminish toxic exposure to the concenptus, we measured monooxygenase activities in placentas and umbilical vein endothelium from 20 pregnancies. We found that while monooxygenase activity toward BP was significantly increased in placentas from 10 smoking women as compared with activities in placentas from 10 nonsmoking women (15.5±4.4 vs 0.09±0.02 pmoles/mg protein min, p 0.01), activity in umbilical in endothelium from these same pregnancies was unaffected (0.445±.32, smokers vs 0.717±.20 pmoles/ g DNA in 16 hrs, nonsmokers, p=ns). In order to show that monooxygenases present in endothelium were inducible if exposed to PAHs, we demonstrated dose dependent increases in activity toward BP (2 to 10 fold) in primary cultures of human umbilical vein endothelial cells exposed to 3-methylcholanthrene and 5,6-benzoflavone.

Our studies indicate that human placental monooxygenase activities that increase when mothers smoke are very sensitive to the environment. Further, placental PAH metabolism may provide necessary protection for the conceptus.

REFERENCES

1. Juchau, M.R. (1982) in: Snell, K. (Ed.), Developmental Toxicology, Praeger Publishers, New York, pp. 187-210.

2. Manchester, D.K. (1981) Biochem. Pharmacol., 30, 757.

3. Manchester, D.K.and Jacoby, E.H. (1982) Xenobiotica, 12, 543.

4. Knight, J.B., Gurtoo, H.L., Parker, N.B., Le Boueuf, R., Doctor, G., Cancer Res., 39, 3177.

5. Manchester, D.K. and Jacoby, E.H. (1981) Clin. Pharmacol. Therap., 30, 187.

© 1983 Elsevier Science Publishers B.V.
Extrahepatic Drug Metabolism and Chemical Carcinogenesis,
J. Rydström, J. Montelius and M. Bengtsson eds.

SEPARATION OF MULTIPLE FORMS OF CYTOCHROME P-450 FROM RABBIT KIDNEY CORTEX MICROSOMES

MASAMICHI KUSUNOSE[1], KIYOKAZU OGITA[1], EMI KUSUNOSE[1], SATORU YAMAMOTO[1], AND KOSUKE ICHIHARA[2]

[1]Toneyama Institute, Osaka City University Medical School, Toyonaka 560 (Japan) and [2]Department of Biochemistry, Kawasaki Medical School, Kurashiki 701-01 (Japan)

Limited information is available on the multiplicity of cytochrome P-450 in the microsomes of extrahepatic tissues. In the present report, we provide evidence for the occurrence of multiple forms of P-450 in rabbit kidney cortex microsomes.

An inducible form of P-450 from kidney cortex microsomes of rabbits treated with 3-methylcholanthrene (MC) has been puri- fied to a specific content of 15 nmol of P-450/mg of protein (referred to as P-448) (1). This form had a monomeric molecular weight of 58,000, based on SDS-PAGE. Its CO-reduced difference spectral peak was at 448 nm. The absolute spectrum of the oxi- dized form had low-spin characteristics. It catalyzed benzo(a)- pyrene hydroxylation with a turnover rate of 8.5 nmol/min/nmol of P-450. This activity was strongly inhibited by α-naphtho- flavone. This form had the most resemblance to rabbit hepatic P-450 Form 6, the major form induced by 2,3,7,8-tetrachloro-$\underline{p}$- dioxin (TCDD).

Two other forms (referred to as P-450a and P-450b) have been purified to specific contents of 16 and 12 nmol of P-450/mg of protein, respectively, from kidney cortex microsomes of rabbits treated with phenobarbital (2). P-450a was also purified from MC-treated kidney microsomes, indicating that it was a constitutive form. This cytochrome had a monomeric molecular weight of 53,000 and its CO-reduced difference spectral peak was at 450 nm. It catalyzed the ω-hydroxylation of prostaglandin A_1 (PGA_1) with a turnover rate of 15 nmol/min/nmol of P-450 as well as the ω- and (ω-1)-hydroxylation of fatty acids (a turnover rate of 20 nmol/min/ nmol for myristate). PGE_1 and PGE_2 were hydroxylated to much lesser extent (turnover rates of 1.1 and 0.4 nmol/min/nmol, respec- tively). Cytochrome $\underline{b}_5$ was required for the maximal activities in the reconstituted systems. P-450a was inactive toward xenobio-

230

tics. On the other hand, P-450b was an inducible form, and had a monomeric molecular weight of 49,000. Its CO-reduced difference spectral peak was at 451 nm. This form hydroxylated fatty acids preferentially at the (ω-1)-position (a turnover rate of 1.3 nmol/min/nmol for myristate). It metabolized benzphetamine, aminopyrine, 7-ethoxycoumarin and p-nitroanisole with turnover rates of 44.4, 8.3, 5.5 and 7.5 nmol/min/nmol of P-450, respectively. Goat antibody against rabbit hepatic P-450 LM_2 (donated by Prof. R.Sato and Dr. T.Aoyama) was tested with these cytochromes by Ouchterlony double-diffusion technique. The antibody cross-reacted with either P-450a or P-450b. When P-450b was placed on a well adjacent to that of P-450 LM_2 antigen, a complete fussion was observed. By contrast, P-450a formed a spur with the antigen. These cytochromes were subjected to limited proteolysis with Staphylococcus aureus V_8 and papain (Fig. 1). The peptide patterns of hepatic P-450 LM_2 was different from those of P-450a, but similar to those of P-450b. From these results, P-450b appears to have the most resemblance to P-450 LM_2.

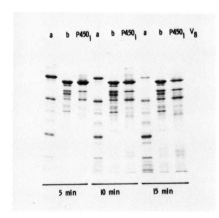 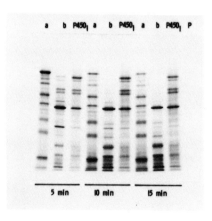

Fig. 1. SDS-PAGE of the peptides generated by proteolytic digestion of P-450a, P-450b and hepatic P-450 LM_2 (P-450$_1$). The samples were incubated with either S. aureus V_8 protease (Left) or papain (Right) for 5, 10, and 15 min.

REFERENCES

1. Ogita, K., Kusunose, E., Ichihara, K., and Kusunose, M. (1982) J. Biochem., 92, 921-928.

2. Ogita, K., Kusunose, E., Yamamoto, S., Ichihara, K., and Kusunose, M. (1983) Biochem. Internatl., 6, 191-198.

© 1983 Elsevier Science Publishers B.V.
Extrahepatic Drug Metabolism and Chemical Carcinogenesis,
J. Rydström, J. Montelius and M. Bengtsson eds.

CYTOCHROME P-450 FROM INTESTINAL MICROSOMES OF RABBITS TREATED WITH 3-METHYLCHOLANTHRENE

KOSUKE ICHIHARA[1], KIYOMI ISHIHARA[1], EMI KUSUNOSE[2], MASATOSHI KAKU[2] AND KIYOKAZU OGITA[2]

[1]Department of Biochemistry, Kawasaki Medical School, Kurashiki 701-01, and [2]Toneyama Institute, Osaka City University Medical School, Toyonaka 560 (Japan)

INTRODUCTION

Since the small intestine is a site which is directly exposed to various carcinogens and other foreign chemicals in the diet, it may be of great importance to characterize the nature of the intestinal cytochrome P-450 (P-450)-dependent monooxygenase systems. Although liver P-450 has been extensively studied, intestinal P-450 was characterized only to a limited extent. Earlier, we reported that at least two different P-450 forms were present in rabbit intestinal mucosa; one preferentially hydroxylating polycyclic hydrocarbons such as benzo(a)pyrene (1), and the other preferentially aliphatic hydrocarbons such as hexadecane (2). In the present study, we have separated two distinct P-450 forms from intestinal mucosa microsomes of rabbits treated with 3-methylcholanthrene (MC).

METHODS

Male rabbits were injected i. p. with 80 mg of MC once daily for 3 days. Two forms of P-450, referred to as P-448a and P-448b, were separated by chromatography on 6-amino-n-hexyl Sepharose 4B, hydroxylapatite, and CM-Sepharose CL-6B columns from the intestinal microsomes of MC-treated rabbits.

RESULTS AND DISCUSSION

Benzo(a)pyrene hydroxylase and 7-ethoxycoumarin O-deethylase activities of intestinal microsomes were increased 7.2- and 4.0-fold by MC treatment, respectively. This treatment caused no change in microsomal P-450 levels, but a shift of absorption maximum of CO-difference spectrum from 450 nm to 449 nm. SDS-PAGE of the intestinal microsomes from MC-treated rabbits revealed the induction of a protein band with a molecular weight of 58,000.

TABLE 1.   SUBSTRATE SPECIFICITY OF P-448a AND P-448b

| Substrate | Activity (nmol/min/nmol of P-450) | |
	P-448a	P-448b
Benzo(a)pyrene	8.54	5.16
7-Ethoxycoumarin	0.92	1.44
7-Ethoxyresorufin	1.27	0.92
Benzphetamine	0	0
Myristate	0	0
Aminopyrine	0	0

Two forms of P-450 were purified from MC-treated rabbits intestinal microsomes as described under METHODS. The specific contents of P-448a and P-448b were 7.4 and 6.3 nmol/mg of protein, respectively. P-448a was apparently homogenous on SDS-PAGE, and its monomeric molecular weight was estimated to be 58,000. SDS-PAGE of P-448b gave a single major protein band with a molecular weight of 55,500. P-448a and P-448b were catalytically active toward some substrates when reconstituted with NADPH-cytochrome c reductase and phosphatidylserine. As shown in TABLE 1, the substrate specificities of these two P-450 were similar. P-448a and P-448b had very high catalytic activities toward benzo(a)pyrene. O-Deethylations of 7-ethoxycoumarin and 7-ethoxyresorufin were also preferred by both the cytochromes. In contrast, these cytochromes had no measurable activities toward benzphetamine, myristate and aminopyrine.

The absorption maxima in the CO-reduced difference spectra of both P-448a and P-448b were observed at 448 nm. The oxidized P-448a had absorbance maxima at 416, 532 and 571 nm, showing that this form is in the low spin state. The reduced form had absorption peaks at 412 and 556 nm. These results indicate that P-448a has properties similar to P-450 Form 6, a major form of hepatic P-450 induced by 2,3,7,8-tetrachlorodibenzo-p-dioxin.

REFERENCES
1. Ichihara, K., Kasaoka, I., Kusunose, E., and Kusunose, M. (1980) J. Biochem. 87, 671.
2. Ichihara, K., Ishihara, K., Kusunose, E., and Kusunose, M. (1981) J. Biochem. 89, 1821.

© 1983 Elsevier Science Publishers B.V.
Extrahepatic Drug Metabolism and Chemical Carcinogenesis,
J. Rydström, J. Montelius and M. Bengtsson eds.

ARYL HYDROCARBON HYDROXLASE (AHH) ACTIVITY IN HUMAN PLACENTA AND ITS RELATION
WITH AIR POLLUTION

FİLİZ HINCAL

Department of Pharmaceutical Toxicology, Faculty of Pharmacy, University of
Hacettepe, Ankara, Turkey

INTRODUCTION

Ankara, the capital city of Turkey is one of the most polluted cities of the
world, due primarily to climatic and topographic conditions and secondarily to
economic and social development problems. In the year of 1982, the mean pollu-
tant values were determined to be 257.48 $\mu g/m^3$ for sulfur dioxide and 126.84
$\mu g/m^3$ for smoke. Pollutants of these high values might have severe adverse
effects on general health and on some enzyme systems as well.

This investigation was done in an effort to see if there was a relationship
between air pollution and aryl hydrocarbon hydroxylase (AHH) activity, the
enzyme system responsible for the metabolism of polycyclic aromatic hydrocarbons
(PAH) which are present in the air of polluted areas as a result of incomplete
combustion.

MATERIALS AND METHODS

Placental AHH activites were measured for a period of 13 months from January
1982 through February 1983, in 152 women who live in Ankara and in 125 control
patients who live out Ankara. Patients were all nonsmokers.

Enzyme activities were determined in the whole homogenates of the placental
tissues essentially by the method of Nebert and Gelboin (1).

RESULTS

As it is shown in Table 1, significantly higher levels ($p < 0.001$) of placental
AHH activities were found in women who live in Ankara.

TABLE 1

VARIATION ANALYSIS OF THE PLACENTAL AHH ACTIVITIES DETERMINED IN TWO GROUPS

Groups	n	(pmol 3-OH-BP/mg protein/30 min)	Significance
ANKARA	152	11.17 ± 5.41	< 0.001
CONTROL	125	6.44 ± 5.48	

Since the variations are quite high, especially in the control group and do

234

not fit in a normal distribution, significance of the difference might be due to these high variations. In order to exclude this possibility and make the analysis more valid, AHH values were transformed by using a square-root $(y = \sqrt{x + 1/2})$ transformation. Even after this treatment there was still a significant difference ($p < 0.05$) between the two groups.

In addition, a strong correlation ($r = 0.89$) was found between the monthly mean values of AHH activities of the group of ANKARA (Fig.1) and monthly mean concentrations of smoke present in the air of the city which in turn contains the PAH's (2).Fig.2 shows this relationship.

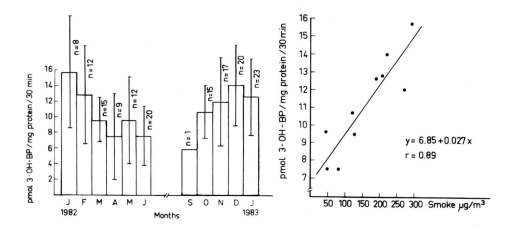

Fig.1.Monthly distribution of AHH activities of the group of ANKARA

Fig.2.The relationship between the monthly mean values of placental AHH and monthly mean smoke concentration

These results suggests that AHH activities in the population of air polluted cities are induced and thus AHH activity can be used as a measure of exposure to environmental carcinogens.

ACKNOWLEDGEMENTS

This study was supported by grant TAG-469 from the Scientific and Technical Research Council of Turkey "TÜBİTAK".

REFERENCES

1. Nebert, D.W., Gelboin, H.V. (1968) J.Biol.Chem., 243,6242.
2. WHO (1979) Enviromental Health Criteria 8, Sulfur Oxides and Suspended Particulate Matter, WHO, Geneva, pp.83.

© 1983 Elsevier Science Publishers B.V.
Extrahepatic Drug Metabolism and Chemical Carcinogenesis,
J. Rydström, J. Montelius and M. Bengtsson eds.

MECHANISMS OF EXTRAHEPATIC BIOACTIVATION OF AROMATIC AMINES: THE ROLE OF HEMO-GLOBIN IN THE N-OXIDATION OF 4-CHLOROANILINE

INES GOLLY AND PETER HLAVICA

Institut für Pharmakologie und Toxikologie der Universität, Nussbaumstrasse 26, D-8000 München 2, Federal Republic of Germany

INTRODUCTION

The metabolic route of N-oxidation of a wide variety of nitrogenous compounds has received increasing attention during the past decade. Two microsomal systems, that is cytochrome P-450 and a flavin-containing monooxygenase (N-oxide forming; EC 1.14.13.8) have been recognized to catalyze oxidative attack on vulnerable nitrogen centres (1). Recently, a monooxygenase-like activity of hemoglobin has been reported (2,3). The present study analyzes the ability of the blood pigment to effect N-oxidation of 4-chloroaniline and discusses the importance of such process under in vivo conditions.

RESULTS AND CONCLUSIONS

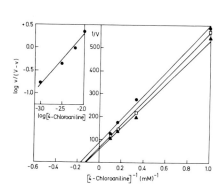

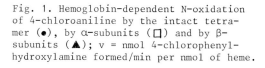

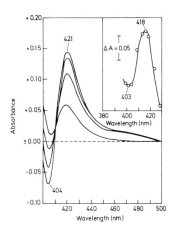

Fig. 1. Hemoglobin-dependent N-oxidation of 4-chloroaniline by the intact tetramer (●), by α-subunits (□) and by β-subunits (▲); v = nmol 4-chlorophenyl-hydroxylamine formed/min per nmol of heme.

Fig. 2. Spectral changes associated with the oxidative metabolism of 4-chloroaniline. The inset of the figure shows the absolute spectrum of the metabolic complex.

Hemoglobin was found to mediate N-oxidation of 4-chloroaniline (4-CA) in a system containing NADPH:cytochrome c(P-450) reductase (EC 1.6.2.4) and reduced

TABLE 1

THE ACTION OF ERYTHROCYTE REDUCTASES IN SUPPORTING HEMOGLOBIN-CATALYZED
N-OXIDATION OF 4-CHLOROANILINE

System	N-Oxygenating activity (nM/min)
A. *"NADPH:methemoglobin reductase"-dependent:*	
Complete	31.8
Minus reductase	17.2
Minus methylene blue	0.0
B. *NADH:cytochrome b_5 reductase-dependent:*	
Complete	37.6
Minus reductase	13.2
Minus cytochrome b_5	9.4

pyridine nucleotide. The reaction is severely blocked by the presence of CO, mannitol or superoxide dismutase (data not shown). The K_m value for the arylamine is 5.9 mM; the turnover number is 0.04 min^{-1} (Fig. 1). The amine interacts with the hemoprotein in a non-cooperative manner (n_H = 1.1; Fig. 1, inset). Lack of cooperativity is moreover evidenced by the ability of highly purified α- and β-chains to promote N-oxidation of 4-CA with K_m and V_{max} values close to those of the intact tetramer (Fig. 1). Metabolism of 4-CA is associated with the formation of a 421 nm absorbing spectral complex (Fig. 2), which might represent a ferryl species or a product adduct. Naturally occurring erythrocyte reductases, such as "NADPH:methemoglobin reductase" or NADH:cytochrome b_5 reductase (EC 1.6.2.2), also sustain N-oxidation of 4-CA in the presence of an appropriate electron carrier (Table 1). Intact rabbit erythrocytes produce 0.57 μM 4-chlorophenylhydroxylamine during a reaction period of 30 min, when incubated with the parent amine in the presence of 6 mM glucose and O_2. Our findings suggest that the red cell deserves serious consideration as being a relevant site of bioactivation of aromatic amines, some of which are potent mutagens and carcinogens.

REFERENCES

1. Hlavica, P. (1982) *CRC Crit. Rev. Biochem.*, *12*, 39.

2. Mieyal, J.J., Ackerman, R.S., Blumer, J.L. and Freeman, L.S. (1976) *J. Biol. Chem.*, *251*, 3436.

3. Blisard, K.S. and Mieyal, J.J. (1981) *Arch. Biochem. Biophys.*, *210*, 762.

© 1983 Elsevier Science Publishers B.V.
Extrahepatic Drug Metabolism and Chemical Carcinogenesis,
J. Rydström, J. Montelius and M. Bengtsson eds.

BIO-ALKYLATION OF BENZO(a)PYRENE IN RAT LUNG AND LIVER

JAMES W. FLESHER, KEVIN H. STANSBURY, ABDELRAZAK M. KARDY AND STEVEN R. MYERS

Department of Pharmacology, College of Medicine and Graduate Center for Toxicology, University of Kentucky, Lexington, KY 40536 (U.S.A.)

Ten years ago, we postulated that polycyclic hydrocarbon carcinogens lacking alkyl substituents, such as benzo(a)pyrene, must be methylated or hydroxy-methylated in the meso-position (or L-region) as a necessary first step in carcinogenesis. In support of this hypothesis, we presented evidence that 6-hydroxymethylbenzo(a)pyrene is a metabolite of benzo(a)pyrene and of 6-methylbenzo(a)pyrene when these substrates are incubated with homogenates or microsomal preparations of liver from Sprague-Dawley rats (1). Recently we reported that S-adenosyl-L-methionine (SAM) is a carbon donor in the conversion of benzo(a)pyrene to 6-hydroxymethylbenzo(a)pyrene by rat liver S-9 (2). However, the formation of 6-methylbenzo(a)pyrene was not detected. The present experiments are part of a series of investigations that deal with the formation and subsequent activation and inactivation of meso-hydroxyalkyl metabolites of carcinogenic hydrocarbons.

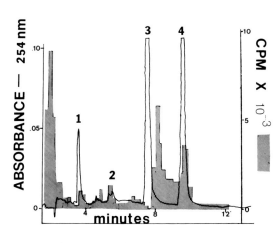

Fig. 1. Identification of tritium labeled metabolites of benzo(a)-pyrene. Reaction conditions: Benzo(a)pyrene (100 nmol), NADPH (800 nmol), MgCl$_2$ (3 µmol) and potassium phosphate buffer (20 µmol, pH 7.4), [methyl-^{3}H]-SAM (3.0 µc, 187 pmoles) and S-105 supernatant fraction equivalent to 2 mg fresh tissue, total volume 1 ml, were incubated in a light-protected Dubnoff shaker at 37°C for 1 hr in air. The reaction was stopped by the addition of 2 ml of cold acetone. The mixture was then extracted 3 times with 2 ml volumes of ethyl acetate. The ethyl acetate extracts were combined, washed with water and evaporated under reduced pressure. The extracted products were re-dissolved in 0.1 ml methanol and analyzed by high pressure liquid chromatography. A Beckman 25 cm x 4.6 mm column packed with ultrasphere-ODS was eluted with 100% methanol, temperature 20°C, flow rate 1.0 ml/min. Ultraviolet absorbance was monitored at 254 nm with an Isco Type 6 UV detector. Eluant fractions were collected at 12 second intervals for counting of tritium in a Packard liquid scintillation counter.

A typical high-performance liquid chromatogram of the products of reaction of benzo(a)pyrene and [methyl-^{3}H]-SAM in the presence of rat lung S-105 supernatant fraction fortified with NADPH and MgCl$_2$ is shown in Figure 1. A radioactive peak (shaded area) is indistinguishable from synthetic 6-hydroxymethylbenzo(a)pyrene added as a marker (peak 1). Peak 2 is probably 6-formylbenzo(a)pyrene, peak 3 is benzo(a)pyrene and peak 4 is indistinguishable from synthetic 6-methylbenzo(a)pyrene. A large radioactive peak eluting just after benzo(a)pyrene (peak 3) is unidentified. A similar pattern of radioactive metabolites was obtained when a S-105 supernatant fraction of rat liver was used as a source of enzyme. In large scale incubations, the identity of 6-methylbenzo(a)pyrene was confirmed by GC/MS. Evidently, the primary reaction which occurs when benzo(a)pyrene and SAM react is methylation rather than hydroxymethylation. The bio-alkylation of benzo(a)pyrene is undoubtedly an electrophilic substitution reaction, which occurs in the meso-position, the 6-position of benzo(a)pyrene being the most reactive center in the molecule.

The data suggest that metabolic activation of unsubstituted carcinogenic hydrocarbons such as benzo(a)pyrene may involve a bio-alkylation substitution reaction mediated by SAM and cytosolic methyltransferases. The methylated hydrocarbon metabolite is then hydroxylated, primarily by microsomal enzymes, to form a meso-hydroxyalkyl metabolite, which according to our hypothesis is a proximate carcinogen (3). The meso-hydroxyalkyl metabolite may undergo further ring oxidation, presumably at the bay-region, or be converted to a reactive ester of the meso-hydroxyalkyl metabolite (4,5). Complete details of this work will be published in due course.

ACKNOWLEDGMENTS

This work was supported by USAID (Peace Fellowship Program), BRSG Grant 2 SO 7RR05374 and the Committee on Research, UKRF.

REFERENCES

1. Flesher, J.W. and Sydnor, K.L. (1973) Int. J. Cancer, 11, 433.

2. Flesher, J.W., Stansbury, K. and Sydnor, K.L. (1982) Cancer Letters, 16, 91-94.

3. Sydnor, K.L., Bergo, C.H. and Flesher, J.W. (1980) Chem.-Biol. Interact., 29, 159-167.

4. Flesher, J.W. and Sydnor, K.L. (1981) J. Supramol. Struct. Cell. Biochem., Suppl. 5, Abstracts Symposia p. 165, #438.

5. J.W. Flesher, Kadry, A.M., Chien, M., Stansbury, K.H., Gairola, C. and Sydnor, K.L. in: Cooke, M. (Ed.), The Seventh International Symposium on Polynuclear Aromatic Hydrocarbons, in press.

© 1983 Elsevier Science Publishers B.V.
Extrahepatic Drug Metabolism and Chemical Carcinogenesis,
J. Rydström, J. Montelius and M. Bengtsson eds.

URINARY METABOLITE PATTERNS AS INDICATORS OF ACTIVATION AND INACTIVATION
REACTIONS IN THE BIOTRANSFORMATION OF m-XYLENE AND ETHYLBENZENE

EIVOR ELOVAARA[1], KERSTIN ENGSTRÖM[2], AND HARRI VAINIO[1]
[1]Institute of Occupational Health, SF-00290 Helsinki 29
[2]Turku Regional Institute of Occupational Health, SF-20500 Turku 50, Finland

Pathways where oxidation occurs at the aromatic nucleus indicate that reactive
intermediates are formed during biotransformation; such pathways are also
known to be involved in the biotransformation of ethylbenzene (EB) and
m-xylene (X) in addition to aliphatic side-chain oxidations. The aim of the
present study was to investigate whether simultaneous exposure to EB and X
alters the relative amounts of urinary metabolites and in this indirect way to
obtain information on the metabolic pathways involved, including the formation
of reactive metabolic species.

Rats were exposed for 5 days (6h/d) to a mixture of X and EB in the air. Four
exposure levels were used: 0+0, 75+25, 300+100, or 600+200 ppm of X+EB. The
urine was collected in two daily portions (6-h and 18-h). The rats showed no
overt toxic response to the treatments.

The composition of average metabolite patterns of the urinary elimination of
the solvents are shown in Fig.1. The measured metabolites of EB were hippuric,
mandelic, phenylglyoxylic, and phenaceturic acids and 1-phenylethanol. The
metabolites of X were methylhippuric acid, methylbenzylalcohol, and dimethylphenols (principally the 2.4-isomer). Phenolic compounds were excreted at detectable levels solely from xylene. Comparisons were made for the daily metabolite patterns, but neither the exposure levels nor the time caused any apparent changes. It should be emphasized that 25 ppm of EB is a low exposure level
that, from an analytical (GC) standpoint, resulted in low amounts of urinary
metabolites. This may partly explain the differences between the metabolic
patterns of EB after exposure to 25 ppm and 100 or 200 ppm (Fig.1).

The excretion of X-metabolites was faster than that of EB-metabolites. Particularly from the second day onwards, X-metabolites were excreted in higher
amounts than expected, both on the basis of the exposure levels alone and in
comparison with the urinary excretion of the first day.

240

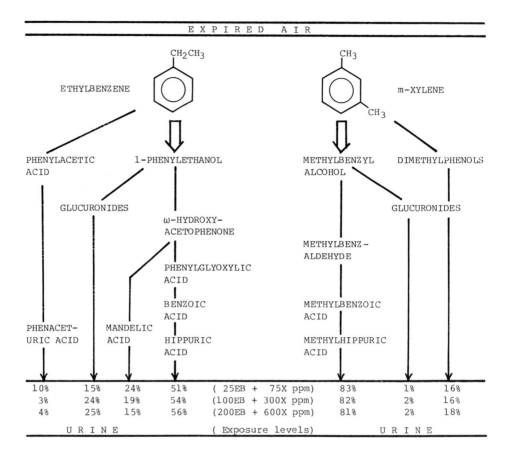

E X P I R E D   A I R

ETHYLBENZENE

m-XYLENE

PHENYLACETIC
ACID

1-PHENYLETHANOL

METHYLBENZYL
ALCOHOL

DIMETHYLPHENOLS

GLUCURONIDES

ω-HYDROXY-
ACETOPHENONE

GLUCURONIDES

METHYLBENZ-
ALDEHYDE

PHENYLGLYOXYLIC
ACID

BENZOIC
ACID

METHYLBENZOIC
ACID

PHENACET-
URIC ACID

MANDELIC
ACID

HIPPURIC
ACID

METHYLHIPPURIC
ACID

10%	15%	24%	51%	(25EB + 75X ppm)	83%	1%	16%
3%	24%	19%	54%	(100EB + 300X ppm)	82%	2%	16%
4%	25%	15%	56%	(200EB + 600X ppm)	81%	2%	18%

U R I N E   (Exposure levels)   U R I N E

Fig.1.   Scheme of the formation of the major metabolites of ethylbenzene, EB,
(M.KIESE & W.LENK; Xenobiotica 4,1974,337) and m-xylene, X, (B.DIEN,
Mutat.Res. 47,1978,75). The percentage amounts of cumulative 24-h
excretion of solvent metabolites (the mean value of 4 days) in the
urine after simultaneous inhalation exposure (6h/day). Exposure levels
for EB and X are denoted in parentheses.

In conclusion, the turnover of EB was slower than that of X after simultaneous
intermittent inhalation exposure. Enhanced microsomal activities of the hepatic drug metabolizing enzymes in vitro and enhanced urinary elimination in
vivo indicated stimulation of the metabolism of the solvents. Metabolic interaction as alterations in the urinary metabolite profiles was not recognized.
As X was detoxified to dimethylphenols, arene oxides may be the potentially
toxic intermediates. This contention agrees with the finding of an up to
12-fold increased urinary excretion of thioethers.

© *1983 Elsevier Science Publishers B.V.*
Extrahepatic Drug Metabolism and Chemical Carcinogenesis,
J. Rydström, J. Montelius and M. Bengtsson eds.

DIMETHYLSULFOXIDE INDUCED ACTIVATION OF RENAL MICROSOMAL ETHOXYCOUMARIN O-DEETHYLATION

ANTTI ZITTING, SINIKKA VAINIOTALO AND EIVOR ELOVAARA
Department of Industrial Hygiene and Toxicology, Institute of Occupational Health, Haartmaninkatu 1, SF-00290 Helsinki 29 (Finland)

INTRODUCTION

Dimethylsulfoxide (DMSO) is a common solvent for many compounds difficult to dissolve for toxicologic studies. Its effects on the hepatic xenobiotic metabolism as well as its hepatotoxicity are minimal but sometimes it probably forms complexes with a xenobiotic and affects in a synergistic fashion (1,2). DMSO can modify the permeability of biological membranes – e.g., blood brain barrier allows the absorption of some compounds after the administration of DMSO (3).

MATERIALS AND METHODS

Male Wistar rats (280-310 g) were injected i.p. with undiluted DMSO (1.5 g/kg) and the kidneys were removed after 4, 12 or 24 h. Renal microsomes were isolated by gel filtration (4) and analyzed for the contents of cytochromes P-450 and b_5 (5) and the activities of 7-ethoxycoumarin O-deethylase (6) and NADPH-cytochrome c reductase (7). Microviscosity of the microsomal membranes was measured with fluorescence polarization of diphenylhexatriene label (8). Polyacrylamide gel electrophoresis was conducted with the standard methodology using a gradient of 5-16 %.

RESULTS AND DISCUSSION

The DMSO-treatments did not affect the renal concentrations of cytochromes P-450 and b_5. The activity of NADPH-cytochrome c reductase remained at the control level during the 48-h follow-up period (Table 1). The activity of 7-ethoxycoumarin O-deethylase, however, increased significantly. The highest activity (twice the control level) was observed 24 h after the DMSO-dosage but 24 h later on this enhancement well-nigh levelled off (Table 1). No effects on the activity were observed in the liver and lung microsomes. The fluorescence polarization measurements of the diphenylhexatriene labelled microsomes did not show any changes after the DMSO-treatment. No effects on the protein composition of the membranes were either detected with polyacrylamide gel electrophoresis. DMSO inhibited competitively ($K_i \approx 20$ mM) the O-deethylation of ethoxycoumarin when incubated with renal microsomes.

TABLE 1. Effects of intraperitoneal injection (1.5 g/kg) of dimethylsulfoxide on rat kidney.

Hours after treatment	Ethoxycoumarin O-deethylase- (pmol/min/mg prot.)	NADPH-cyt. c reductase (nmol/min/mg prot.)
Control	21.8 ± 5.3	22.0 ± 3.8
4	32.0 ± 7.3*	25.5 ± 2.6
24	45.7 ± 9.2***	24.4 ± 2.1
48	23.6 ± 5.0	23.4 ± 1.6
	Cyt. P-450 (nmol/mg prot.)	Cyt. b_5 (nmol/mg prot.)
Control	0.15 ± 0.02	0.092 ± 0.021
4	0.16 ± 0.02	N.D.
24	0.17 ± 0.03	0.099 ± 0.015
48	0.17 ± 0.03	N.D.

Results are the means $\pm$ SD (five rats/group)

*$p < 0.05$, ***$p < 0.001$ (Student's t-test); N.D. = not determined

The induction of enzyme synthesis is an unlikely reason for the observed enhancement of deethylation activity because of its rapid onset and the following decrease. No major effects were either observed in the physical properties of the membrane microenvironment with fluorescence polarization. It can be speculated that DMSO forms complexes with some endogenous compounds which can activate the renal monooxygenase complex.

REFERENCES

1. Mathew, T., Karunanithy, R., Yee, M.H. and Natarajan, P.N. (1980) Lab. Invest., 42, 257.

2. Hietanen, E., Laitinen, M. and Lang, M. (1980) Gen. Pharmac. 11, 169.

3. Broadwell, R.D., Salcman, M. and Kaplan, R.S. (1982) Science 217, 164.

4. Pyykkö, K. (1983) Acta Pharmacol. Toxicol. 52, 39.

5. Omura, T. and Sato, R. (1964) J. Biol. Chem. 239, 2370.

6. Zitting, A. (1981) Anal. Biochem. 115, 177.

7. Phillips, A. and Langdon, R.G. (1962) J. Biol. Chem. 237, 2652.

8. Rouer, E. Dansette, P., Beaune, P. and Leroux, J-P (1980) Biochem. Biophys. Res. Commun. 95, 41.

© 1983 Elsevier Science Publishers B.V.
Extrahepatic Drug Metabolism and Chemical Carcinogenesis,
J. Rydström, J. Montelius and M. Bengtsson eds.

DRUG-METABOLIZING ENZYMES IN *DROSOPHILA MELANOGASTER*, IN RELATION TO GENOTOXICITY TESTING

AALBERT J. BAARS, MARIJKE JANSEN AND DOUWE D. BREIMER

Department of Pharmacology, Subfaculty of Pharmacy, Sylvius Laboratories, University of Leiden, P.O. Box 9503, 2300 RA Leiden, The Netherlands

INTRODUCTION

During biotransformation of xenobiotics, chemicals can be transformed into reactive intermediates (bioactivation). These intermediates are able to interact covalently with cellular macromolecules, leading to toxic effects like carcinogenesis, mutagenesis, tissue necrosis etc. (1). The involvement of reactive intermediates in such processes can be detected via their capacity to induce mutations in suitable animal models. Of these bioassays, the fruitfly *Drosophila melanogaster* is widely used, as it is a genetically well-studied organism, permitting the assessment of a great number of genetic effects (2).

Investigations in our institute as well as in others have indicated the capacity of this species to generate reactive intermediates (3-5). In the present study attention was focussed on epoxide-metabolizing enzymes: glutathione S-transferases and epoxide hydrolases.

MATERIALS AND METHODS

The preparation of subcellular fractions from homogenates of *Drosophila melanogaster*, strain Berlin K, is described in (4). The isozymes of the glutathione S-transferase system as present in the post-microsomal supernatant, were obtained by ion exchange chromatography followed by molecular sieving and hydroxylapatite chromatography. The procedure will be reported in full detail elsewhere (M. Jansen, A.J. Baars and D.D. Breimer, to be published). Enzyme activities were assayed as described in (6).

RESULTS AND DISCUSSION

Epoxides, once generated, can be metabolized further via two enzymatical pathways: conjugation with glutathione catalyzed by the glutathione S-transferase system, and hydrolysis catalyzed by epoxide hydrolases. Cytosolic glutathione S-transferase and microsomal epoxide hydrolase activities were shown to occur in Drosophila in previous studies (3, 5, 6). Recently we could demonstrate the presence of an appreciable epoxide hydrolase activity in the post-microsomal supernatant of Drosophila homogenates (7). However, the Drosophila glutathione S-transferase did not catalyze the conjugation of the two epoxide substrates used: styrene-7,8-oxide and 1,2-epoxy-3(p-nitrophenoxy)-propane. The enzyme activities observed are shown in the table.

In order to investigate the apparent lack of epoxide-conjugating capacity, attempts were made to isolate the isozymes of the Drosophila glutathione S-transferase system. The isozyme pattern as observed in the final hydroxylapatite chromatogram showed three peaks of enzyme activity using 1-chloro-2,4-dinitrobenzene as the electrophilic substrate, while an additional fourth peak was observed with 1,2-dichloro-4-nitrobenzene as the substrate. However, also the isolated isozymes were not active with the mentioned epoxide substrates, although rat liver soluble glutathione S-transferases, isolated by the same procedure, did catalyze the conjugation of these epoxides (results not shown).

TABLE.

EPOXIDE-METABOLIZING ENZYMES IN *DROSOPHILA MELANOGASTER* HOMOGENATES

Enzyme	Substrate	Activity[a]
Glutathione S-transferase (cytosolic)	1-Chloro-2,4-di-nitrobenzene	6100 ± 850 (6)
	Styrene-7,8-oxide	n.d.[b] (4)
	1,2-Epoxy-3(p-nitro-phenoxy)propane	n.d.[b] (3)
Epoxide hydrolase (microsomal)	Styrene-7,8-oxide	30 ± 3 (3)
Epoxide hydrolase (cytosolic)	Styrene-7,8-oxide	38 ± 4 (6)

[a] Activities are expressed as mean ± s.d., in nmoles/min per g body weight.

[b] n.d.: not detectable.

In brackets the number of experiments.

These finding suggest that Drosophila is unable to conjugate at least certain epoxides with glutathione, in contrast to mammalian transferases. This may have consequences in testing compounds that are metabolized via the epoxide-gluta-thione pathway. The results contribute to the quantitative understanding of the disposition in Drosophila of chemicals that are metabolized via the epoxide-diol way and/or the epoxide-glutathione way. This in turn will contribute to a better evaluation of genetic toxicology testing in Drosophila.

REFERENCES

1. Miller, J.A. and Miller, E.C. (1979) in: Emmelot, P. and Kriek, E. (Eds.), Environmental Carcinogenesis - Occurrence, Risk Evaluation and Mechanisms, Elsevier/North-Holland Biomedical Press, Amsterdam, pp. 25-50.

2. Vogel, E. and Sobels, F.H. (1976) in: Hollaender, A. (Ed.), The Function of Drosophila in Genetic Toxicology Testing, Plenum Publishing Co., New York, pp. 93-142.

3. Baars, A.J. (1980) Drug Metab. Revs. 11, 191-221.

4. Baars, A.J., Blijleven, W.G.H., Mohn, G.R., Natarajan, A.T. and Breimer, D.D. (1980) Mutation Res. 72, 257-264.

5. Hällström, I. and Grafström, R. (1981) Chem.-Biol. Interact. 34, 145-159.

6. Baars, A.J., Jansen, M. and Breimer, D.D. (1979) Mutation Res. 62, 279-291.

7. Jansen, M., Baars, A.J. and Breimer, D.D. (1982) in: Proceedings 24th Dutch Federation Meeting, Dutch Foundation - Federation of Medical Scientific Societies, Nijmegen, no. 175.

© 1983 Elsevier Science Publishers B.V.
Extrahepatic Drug Metabolism and Chemical Carcinogenesis,
J. Rydström, J. Montelius and M. Bengtsson eds.

ENHANCEMENT OF EXTRAHEPATIC DRUG METABOLISM BY PHENOXYACID HERBICIDES AND
CLOFIBRATE

MARKKU AHOTUPA[1], EINO HIETANEN[1], EERO MÄNTYLÄ[1] AND HARRI VAINIO[2]
[1]Department of Physiology, University of Turku, Turku (Finland) and
[2]Institute of Occupational Health, Helsinki (Finland)

INTRODUCTION

Phenoxyacid herbicides have a widespread use in agriculture and forestry.
Human exposure to these chemicals takes place either via inhalation or via the
gastrointestinal tract, but also via the skin in occupationally exposed workers.
Clofibrate, a drug structurally related to phenoxyacid herbicides, is clinically used as a hypolipidemic agent. Workers exposed to phenoxyacid herbicides
have an increased incidence of soft tissue sarcomas (1). Clofibrate has been
suspected of liver carcinogenicity (2,3).

In spite of the widespread use of both phenoxyacid herbicides and clofibrate,
there is little experimental data about the biologic effects of these compounds.
In the present study we have investigated the effects of phenoxyacid herbicides
and clofibrate on the activities of extrahepatic drug-metabolizing enzymes. As
representatives of phenoxyacid herbicides, 2,4-dichlorophenoxyacid (2,4-D) and
4-chloro-2-methyl-phenoxyacid (MCPA) were used. For comparison, the effects
of a herbicide not structurally related to phenoxyacids (glyphosate) were also
studied.

MATERIALS AND METHODS

Both of the phenoxyacid herbicides were purchased from Kemira Company (Helsinki, Finland), glyphosate from Monsanto Chemical Corporation (St. Louis, Mo.,
U.S.A.), and clofibrate (Klofiran[R]) from Remeda (Kuopio, Finland). The chemicals were administered intragastrically to 6 - 7 weeks old male Wistar rats.
2,4-D, clofibrate and glyphosate were given at a dose of 1 mmol/kg, MCPA at
a dose of 0.5 mmol/kg. Control animals received an equal volume of saline.
After 2 weeks daily doses the rats were killed 24 h after the last dose. The
kidneys and a 30 cm segment of the proximal small intestine were excised and
a postmitochondrial supernatant was prepared. Kidney supernatant was further
centrifuged to prepare microsomes while the intestinal supernatant was used as
such for the determination of enzyme activities. The following enzyme activities were measured: NADPH cytochrome c reductase; aryl hydrocarbon hydroxylase
(AHH)(radiochemical method); ethoxycoumarin O-deethylase (ECDE); ethoxyresorufin

deethylase; epoxide hydrolase (EH) and glutathione S-transferase with styrene
oxide as the substrate; UDP-glucuronosyltransferase with 4-nitrophenol (4-NP)
or 4-methylumbelliferone (4-MU) as the aglycone.

RESULTS AND DISCUSSION

The effects of herbicides and clofibrate on intestinal and renal drug-
metabolizing enzymes are given in Table 1. The results show that 2,4-D and

TABLE 1

EXTRAHEPATIC DRUG-METABOLIZING ENZYME ACTIVITIES OF RATS EXPOSED TO PHENOXYACID
HERBICIDES, CLOFIBRATE OR GLYPHOSATE

Exposure	AHH[a] Intestine	ECDE[a] Intestine	ECDE[a] Kidney	EH[a] Intestine	EH[a] Kidney	4-NP[a] Intestine	4-MU[a] Intestine	4-MU[a] Kidney
Control	1.3	0.14	0.04	20.8	12.7	32	94	21.8
2,4-D	2.1^+	0.23	0.08^+	19.0	18.8	32	98	15.1
MCPA	2.2^+	0.33	0.08^+	19.5	20.4^+	37	164	15.8
Clofibrate	2.1^+	0.44^+	0.05	20.7	18.3	41	155^+	20.8
Glyphosate	1.4	0.11	0.06	15.6	9.4	28	90	21.5

[a]Mean results from 4 - 7 animals are given. The results are expressed as
nmol/min x g on wet weight basis. Two-tailed t-test: + = 2P < 0.05; ++ =
2P < 0.01.

MCPA enhanced intestinal and renal monooxygenase activities. The latter compound elevated renal epoxide hydrolase activity as well. Intestinal monooxygenases were also enhanced by treatment with clofibrate, which as the only
one of the tested compounds was able to elevate extrahepatic UDP-glucuronosyltransferase activity. In addition to the listed data, no differences were
found in the intestinal ethoxyresorufin deethylase or NADPH cytochrome c reductase activities. Moreover, no changes were found in the intestinal or renal
glutathione S-transferase activities. The renal AHH activity was below the
detection limit of the method.

ACKNOWLEDGEMENTS

This study was supported by grants from The Academy of Finland and NIH RO1
ES-01684.

REFERENCES

1. Hardell,L. and Sandström,A. (1979) Br.J.Cancer 39, 711-714.
2. Reddy,J.K., Azarnoff,D.L. and Hignite,E.E. (1980) Nature 283, 397
3. Svoboda,D.J. and Azarnoff,D.L. (1979) Cancer Res. 39, 3419-3425.

© 1983 Elsevier Science Publishers B.V.
Extrahepatic Drug Metabolism and Chemical Carcinogenesis,
J. Rydström, J. Montelius and M. Bengtsson eds.

CHARACTERIZATION OF EPOXIDE HYDROLASE FROM THE HUMAN ADRENAL GLAND

DIMITRIOS PAPADOPOULOS[*][1], JANERIC SEIDEGÅRD[2], ANTONIS GEORGELLIS[1], AND JAN RYDSTRÖM[1]

[1]Department of Biochemistry, Arrhenius Laboratory, University of Stockholm, S-106 91 Stockholm, Sweden and [2]Wallenberg Laboratory, University of Lund, S-220 07 Lund, Sweden

INTRODUCTION

Several aromatic hydrocarbons can be converted to intermediate arene- or aryl epoxides by the mammalian mixed function oxidase (MFO) system. The potentially reactive and carcinogenic intermediate epoxides can be hydrolyzed by the action of epoxide hydrolase (EH) to dihydrodiols. Some of these dihydrodiols can then be recycled through the MFO system to yield highly toxic diol epoxides. In contrast to e.g. the human liver, the human adrenal has recently been shown to contain a high epoxide hydrolase activity but virtually no MFO activity with polycyclic aromatic hydrocarbons as substrates (1). The present investigation of the properties of epoxide hydrolase was carried out in order to determine the physiological role of this enzyme.

MATERIALS AND METHODS

7[^{3}H]-Styrene-7,8-oxide (10 mCi/mmole) was purchased from the Radiochemical Centre, Amersham, England.[^{3}H]-cis and trans-stilbene oxide (2 Ci/mmole) (2), 17α-epoxy-1,3,5-estratrien-3-ol (estroxide) (3) and 17α-epoxy-androst-4-en-3-one (androstenoxide) (3) were synthesized as described. Metabolism of the epoxide substrate was measured using the extraction procedure (4). Mitochondrial, microsomal and cytosolic fractions from adrenal cortex were prepared according to Ernster et.al. (5).

RESULTS

Subfractionation of adrenal cortex tissue revealed that epoxide hydrolase activity was found mainly in the endoplasmic reticulum. The maximal activity of the microsomal enzyme under optimal conditions (except pH) with styrene-7,8-oxide as substrate was 14,3 nmoles per min and mg protein. Specific activities of microsomal epoxide hydrolase with other epoxide substrates are shown in Table I. The apparent K_m value for styrene-7,8-oxide was estimated to 0.98 mM. The adrenal microsomal epoxide hydrolase activity was also investigated over a wide range of pH. Maximal activity was obtained at pH 9,2 with glycine NaOH buffer. The human adrenal epoxide hydrolase was affected by various modulators such as 1,1,1-trichloropropene-2,3-oxide (TCPO) cyclohexene oxide (CHO), benzil and clotrimazole. Thus, TCPO and CHO were strongly inhibitory whereas benzil and clotrimazole activated the enzyme.

The fact that the high activity of the human adrenal epoxide hydrolase is not associated with a measurable AHH activity suggests that the former enzyme may function primarely with endogeneous substrates. However, even though the characterization of the human adrenal epoxide hydrolase is not complete, the present results indicate that the properties of the human adrenal enzyme are not markedly different from those of, e.g., the human liver enzyme.

TABLE I

ACTIVITIES OF HUMAN ADRENAL EPOXIDE HYDROLASE WITH DIFFERENT SUBSTRATES

Substrate	Concentration of substrate (mM)	Specific activity[a] (nmoles/mg/min)	
c-stilbene oxide	0,025	29,5 $\pm$ 9,3	(4)
t-stilbene oxide	0,025	< 0,006	(4)
Estroxide	0,110	13,1 $\pm$ 3,6	(4)
Androstenoxide	0,280	1,9 $\pm$ 0,2	(4)

(a) mean $\pm$ standard deviation for (n) experiments.

REFERENCES

1. Papadopoulos, D., Seidegård, J. and Rydström, J. (manuscript in preparation)

2. Meijer, J., Birberg, W., Pilotti, Å. and DePierre, J.W. (manuscript in preparation).

3. Sparrow, A.J., Bindel, U. and Oesch, F. (1980) Biochim. Biophys. Acta 227, 692-697.

4. Seidegård, J., DePierre, J.W., Moron, M.S., Johannesen, K.A.M., and Ernster, L. (1977) Cancer Res. 37, 1075-1082.

5. Ernster, L., Siekevitz, P. and Palade, G.E. (1962) J. Cell Biol. 15, 541-562.

© 1983 Elsevier Science Publishers B.V.
Extrahepatic Drug Metabolism and Chemical Carcinogenesis,
J. Rydström, J. Montelius and M. Bengtsson eds.

GENETIC VARIATION AND REGULATION OF THE CYTOCHROME P-450 SYSTEM IN THE FRUIT FLY, DROSOPHILA MELANOGASTER

INGER HÄLLSTRÖM[1] AND AGNETA BLANCK[2]

[1]Dept. of Toxicological Genetics, Wallenberg Laboratory, University of Stockholm, S-106 91 Stockholm, Sweden and [2]Dept. of Medical Nutrition, Huddinge University Hospital, F 69, S-141 86 Huddinge, Sweden

The occurrence of genetic variation in the cytochrome P-450 enzyme system in Drosophila (1,2,3) gives the opportunity to study the regulation of the cytochrome P-450 enzymes in this organism with its outstanding theoretical and practical background in genetical analyses.

Microsomes from insecticide-resistant Drosophila strains have a 3- to 15-fold higher p-nitroanisole demethylation and biphenyl 3-hydroxylation when compared to other strains. A higher protein content in a band with an apparent molecular weight of 54.000 after SDS-polyacrylamide gel electrophoresis of the microsomes is also observed. Crosses with a marker strain (y[3P]; Cy/Pm D/Sb) show the high activity as well as the high protein content to be present only in hybrids carrying at least one second chromosome from the resistant parent (fig 1). The almost completely dominant gene responsible for this trait is probably identical with the gene giving the insecticide resistance and a high vinyl chloride metabolism, located at 64-66 cM on the second chromosome. The enzyme activities in the insecticide-resistant strains are non-inducible. Taken together, this indicates that the resistant strains are carrying a constitutive mutation, probably in a regulator gene.

The resistant Oregon strain also has a higher biphenyl 4-hydroxylase activity and content of a band with m.w. 56.000. The genetic regulation of these characteristics still remains to be analyzed.

Microsomes from the Hikone R strain has a considerably lower capacity for benzo(a)pyrene hydroxylation and 7-ethoxycoumarin deethylation when compared to other strains. In this case the activity is lower in hybrids carrying a third chromosome from Hikone R (fig 2). The intermediate activity of these hybrids indicates a

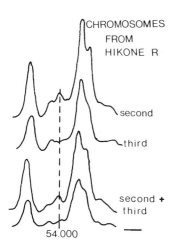

CHROMOSOMES
FROM
HIKONE R

second

third

second + third

54.000

Fig 1. SDS gel electrophoresis of microsomes from hybrids between Hikone R and y[3P]; Cy/Pm D/Sb. Densitometic tracings at 550 nm.

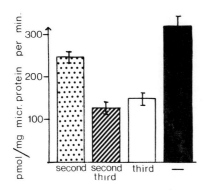

CHROMOSOMES FROM HIKONE R

Fig 2. Benzo(a)pyrene monooxygenase activity in hybrids between Hikone R and y^{3P}; Cy/Pm D/Sb.

semidominant inheritance.

Several enzymatic activities are found not to be concerned by the genes mentioned above; metabolism of ethylmorphine, benzphetamine and aminopyrine, as well as the formation of dihydrodiols from benzo-(a)pyrene, 2-hydroxylation of biphenyl and 7-ethoxyresorufin 0-deethylation. The latter three activities are very low and uninducible in all strains studied, which might indicate a common regulation.

In conclusion, the data demonstrates three structural and/or regulatory genes, being part of the regulation of the multiple-enzyme cytochrome P-450 system in Drosophila.

Table I.

GENETIC LOCALIZATION OF SOME CYTOCHROME P-450-DEPENDENT ACTIVITIES IN DROSOPHILA MELANOGASTER

Localization	Associated activities and features
Second chromosome	p-nitroanisole demethylation biphenyl 3-hydroxylation vinyl chloride metabolism and mutagenicity dimethylnitrosamine toxicity and mutagenicity insecticide resistance protein m.w. 54.000
Third chromosome	benzo(a)pyrene hydroxylation 7-ethoxycoumarin deethylation
Yet unlocalized	biphenyl 4-hydroxylation protein m.w. 56.000

REFERENCES

1. Magnusson, J., Hällström, I. and Ramel, C. (1979) Chem.-Biol. Interact. 24, 287

2. Hällström, I. and Grafström, R. (1981) Chem.-Biol. Interact. 34, 145

3. Hällström, I., Blanck, A. and Atuma, S. (1983) Biochem. Pharmacol., submitted for publication

© 1983 Elsevier Science Publishers B.V.
Extrahepatic Drug Metabolism and Chemical Carcinogenesis,
J. Rydström, J. Montelius and M. Bengtsson eds.

INHIBITION OF RAT LUNG CYTOCHROME P-450 BY CHLORAMPHENICOL*

BIRGITTA NÄSLUND[1,2], INGVAR BETNER[1] AND JAMES HALPERT[1]

[1]Department of Medical Nutrition, Karolinska Institute, Huddinge University
Hospital F69, S-141 86 Huddinge, Sweden and [2]Department of Biochemistry,
Arrhenius Laboratory, University of Stockholm, S-106 91 Stockholm, Sweden

INTRODUCTION

Studies from this and other laboratories suggest that the lung may play an
important role in the metabolism of certain organic solvents of occupational
interest, including xylene and n-hexane (1). Rat lung microsomes have been shown
to have a higher turnover number than liver microsomes for the conversion of
n-hexane to 2-hexanol (1), the precursor of the putative neurotoxic metabolite
2,5-hexanedione. Rat lung microsomes have also been shown to contain significant
constitutive levels of a P-450 isozyme which appears to be very similar to the
major isozyme of rat liver cytochrome P-450 induced by phenobarbital, and which
is inactivated in a suicidal manner by the antibiotic chloramphenicol (2). As
part of our ongoing studies of metabolic interactions between organic solvents
and other xenobiotics, we have undertaken an investigation of the effect of
chloramphenicol on the metabolism of n-hexane in the rat lung.

RESULTS AND DISCUSSION

Inhibition of the formation of 2-hexanol was obtained both upon in vivo administration of chloramphenicol to untreated rats and upon in vitro incubation
of chloramphenicol with lung and liver microsomes from control animals. A dose
of 100 mg/kg chloramphenicol administered i.v. as the succinate ester inhibited
n-hexane metabolism markedly (Table 1). Already after 45 minutes a reduction
in activity from 38 to 14 nmol 2-hexanol $min^{-1}nmol^{-1}$ cytochrome P-450 for the
lung and from 5.6 to 2.6 nmol 2-hexanol $min^{-1}nmol^{-1}$ cytochrome P-450 for the
liver was obtained. This effect was even more marked after treatment of the
animals for 90 minutes. In vitro chloramphenicol caused both reversible and
irreversible inhibition of 2-hexanol formation in control lung microsomes
(Figure 1). The $t_{1/2}$ of the irreversible inhibition was about 3 minutes. The reversible inhibition of the n-hexane metabolism by 50 μM chloramphenicol was 33%.

Studies with radiolabeled compound confirmed the ability of rat lung microsomes to metabolize chloramphenicol to both protein-bound and soluble metabo-

*Supported by grants from the Swedish Medical Research Council and
from the Swedish Work Environment Fund.

lites. Covalent binding to protein reached a maximum of 0.7 nmol/nmol cytochrome P-450 within 30 minutes. Rabbit antibodies to the major phenobarbital-
induced isozyme of rat liver cytochrome P-450 completely inhibited the covalent
binding of chloramphenicol to lung microsomes. The results suggest that chloramphenicol acts as a suicide substrate of an important constitutive isozyme of
rat lung cytochrome P-450 and may prove to be a valuable tool for studying the
role of this isozyme in the metabolism of certain organic solvents.

TABLE 1
METABOLISM OF n-HEXANE IN LUNG AND LIVER MICROSOMES
Adult male Sprague-Dawley rats were treated with 100 mg/kg chloramphenicol (injected i.v. as the succinate ester) for 45 or 90 minutes, respectively. Organs
from 4 animals were pooled and microsomes were prepared (3). The metabolism of
n-hexane was monitored as described previously (1). Microsomes were incubated
at 37° for 10 min in a final volume of 1 ml of 50 mM HEPES buffer, pH 7.4, containing 0.5 mM NADP, 4 mM isocitrate, 15 mM MgCl$_2$, 0.1 mM EDTA, 0.4 unit isocitrate dehydrogenase, and 10 mM n-hexane. The data represent the results of
two incubations per batch of microsomes and are expressed in nmol metabolite
min^{-1} nmol^{-1} cytochrome P-450. CAP = chloramphenicol.

Treatment	lung			liver		
	1-hexanol	2-hexanol	3-hexanol	1-hexanol	2-hexanol	3-hexanol
Control	23.3;26.6	33.8;41.5	9.7;14.1	0.82;0.69	5,9;5.4	0.78;0.77
CAP 45'	21.9;27.3	14.9;12.4	10.4; 9.0	0.48;0.52	2.6;2.6	0.50;0.50
CAP 90'	16.8;17.7	6.6; 7.8	6.2; 7.2	0.58;0.51	2.4;1.9	0.74;0.98

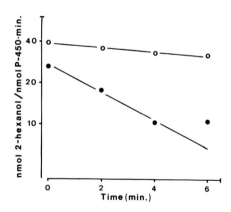

Fig. 1. Inhibition by chloramphenicol
of n-hexane metabolism. Lung microsomes
were preincubated in the same incubation
system as in Table 1 with 0.5 mM NADPH
in the absence (o) or presence (●) of
chloramphenicol (50 µM). At the times
indicated, 10 µmol of n-hexane and
0.5 µmol of NADPH were added, and incubations were allowed to proceed for
another 10 min.

REFERENCES
1.   Toftgård, R. and Nilsen, O.G. (1982) Toxicology, 23, 197.
2.   Halpert, J., Näslund, B. and Betnér, I. (1983) Mol. Pharmacol., 23, 445.
3.   Johannesen, K., DePierre, J.W., Bergstrand, A., Dallner, G. and Ernster,
     L. (1977) Biochim. Biophys. Acta, 496, 115.

© 1983 Elsevier Science Publishers B.V.
Extrahepatic Drug Metabolism and Chemical Carcinogenesis,
J. Rydström, J. Montelius and M. Bengtsson eds.

253

IMMUNOCHEMICAL AND BIOCHEMICAL EVIDENCE OF THE PRESENCE OF CYTOCHROME P-450 MONOOXYGENASE COMPONENTS IN RABBIT HEART AND AORTA

COSETTE J. SERABJIT-SINGH, BARBARA A. DOMIN, JOHN R. BEND AND RICHARD M. PHILPOT
Laboratory of Pharmacology, National Institute of Environmental Health Sciences,
National Institutes of Health, P. O. Box 12233, Research Triangle Park, North
Carolina 27709 (U.S.A.)

INTRODUCTION

A number of investigators have presented enzymatic (1) or immunoc; ιochemical (2) evidence that the vascular endothelium may contain an active cytochrome P-450-dependent monooxygenase system. In this study we have identified specific isozymes of cytochrome P-450, as well as NADPH cytochrome P-450 reductase, in microsomal fractions from rabbit heart and aorta. The experimental approach used establishes the presence of immunoreactive proteins, the molecular weights of the proteins, and the extent to which the antibodies cross-react with proteins other than the primary antigens.

MATERIALS AND METHODS

Microsomal fractions from heart and aorta of male New Zealand White rabbits that were untreated or treated with tetrachlorodibenzo-p-dioxin (TCDD) were electrophoresed on polyacrylamide gels in the presence of sodium dodecyl sulfate. The proteins were then transferred to nitrocellulose sheets (3) and stained by a modification of the immunoperoxidase-bridge method. With this technique, antibodies to the cytochrome P-450 isozymes, forms 2, 5, and 6, and to P-450 reductase reacted specifically with proteins of the same apparent monomeric molecular weights as those of the purified enzymes; 52,000, 58,000, 60,000, and 72,000, respectively. The immunostained bands were quantitated by soft laser (Zenieh) densitometry.

RESULTS

Immunoreactive proteins corresponding to all three isozymes of cytochrome P-450 and P-450 reductase were detected in microsomal fractions from heart and aorta of untreated or TCDD-treated rabbits. The concentrations of isozymes 2 and 5 in microsomal fractions from heart and aorta were about 1% (1-2 pmol/mg protein) of the concentrations in rabbit pulmonary microsomal fractions. Treatment of rabbits with TCDD did not alter the concentrations of isozymes 2 and 5. The concentration of isozyme 6 in heart or aorta fractions was about 20% (1-2 pmol/mg protein) of the concentration in pulmonary fractions. Following treatment with TCDD, the concentration of isozyme 6 increased from 4- to 8-fold in aorta and heart (Figure 1) as compared to a 10- to 20-fold increase in the lung.

254

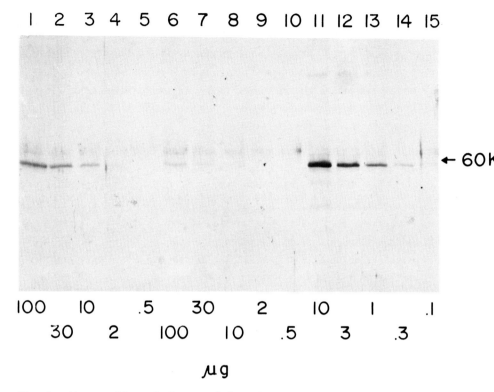

Fig. 1. Western blot of microsomal fractions immunostained for form 6. Samples from hearts of TCDD-treated and untreated rabbits were applied in tracks 1-5 and 6-10, respectively. Pulmonary samples from TCDD-treated rabbits were applied in tracks 11-15.

CONCLUSION

Rabbit heart and aorta appear to contain a monooxygenase system that is composed of NADPH cytochrome P-450 reductase and at least three isozymes of cytochrome P-450.

REFERENCES

1. Bond, J.A., Omiecinski, C.M. and Juchau, M.R. (1979) Biochem. Pharmacol. 28, 305-311.

2. Dees, J.H., Masters, B.S.S., Muller-Eberhard, U. and Johnson, E.F. (1982) Can. Res. 42, 1423-1432.

3. Towbin, H., Staehelin, T. and Gordon, J. (1979) Proc. Natl. Acad. Sci. U.S.A. 76, 4350-4354.

INTESTINAL METABOLISM AND ENTEROHEPATIC CIRCULATION OF CARCINOGENS

© 1983 Elsevier Science Publishers B.V.
Extrahepatic Drug Metabolism and Chemical Carcinogenesis,
J. Rydström, J. Montelius and M. Bengtsson eds.

ENTEROHEPATIC CIRCULATION AND CATABOLISM OF MERCAPTURIC ACID PATHWAY
METABOLITES OF NAPHTHALENE

JEROME BAKKE[1], CRAIG STRUBLE[2], JAN-AKE GUSTAFSSON[3] AND BENGT GUSTAFSSON[4]
[1]Metabolism and Radiation Research Laboratory, Agricultural Research Service,
U.S. Department of Agriculture, Fargo, ND 58105, USA; [2]Animal Science Dept.,
North Dakota State University, Fargo, ND 58105, USA; [3]Depart. Med. Nutrition,
Huddinge Hospital, 141 86 Huddinge, Sweden; [4]Depart. Germfree Research,
Karolinska Institute, S-104 01 Stockholm, Sweden

INTRODUCTION

     Comparison of the metabolic fates of several xenobiotics in germfree rats
and conventional rats have shown that xenobiotic moieties of biliary mercapturic acid pathway (MAP) metabolites can undergo enterohepatic circulation
with concomitant catabolism to methylthio-containing metabolites (methylthiolation) by a process mediated by microfloral C-S lyase activity (1, 2, 3, see
scheme 1). The methylthio-containing metabolites may be oxidized to
methylsulfinyl-, and/or methylsulfonyl-containing metabolites that can be
excreted with either urine or feces. The ability of the intestinal

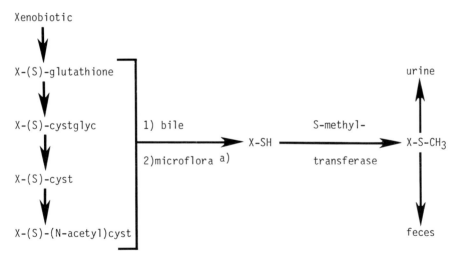

a) The microflora probably convert the biliary MAP metabolites to the
cysteine conjugate before the C-S lyase can function (5).

Scheme 1

microflora to produce thiols from MAP metabolites has recently been verified
in vitro for both aromatic (4) and aliphatic (5) cysteine conjugates. The
physiological site(s) for methylation of these thiols has not been determined
although S-methyl transferase activity has been found in intestinal mucosa
(6). A chemically identical catabolic pathway for MAP metabolites has been
demonstrated in tissues (7), however, the known tissue C-S lyases exhibit
specificity for S-cysteine conjugates in which the prosthetic moieties have
aromaticity at the carbon bonded to the cysteine sulfur (7, 8, 9, 10). These
intestinal and tissue methylthiolation pathways produce new xenobiotics in
kidney, liver and intestine which can require further metabolism before ultimate excretion (3).

Arene oxides of polyaromatic hydrocarbons are conjugated with glutathione
(GSH) to form 1,2-dihydro-1-hydroxy-2-S-glutathionyl conjugates (scheme 2)
[For this discussion, the conjugation of arene oxides with GSH to form
1,2-dihydro-1-hydroxy-2-S-glutathionyl conjugates will constitute entry into
the "premercapturic" acid pathway (preMAP)].

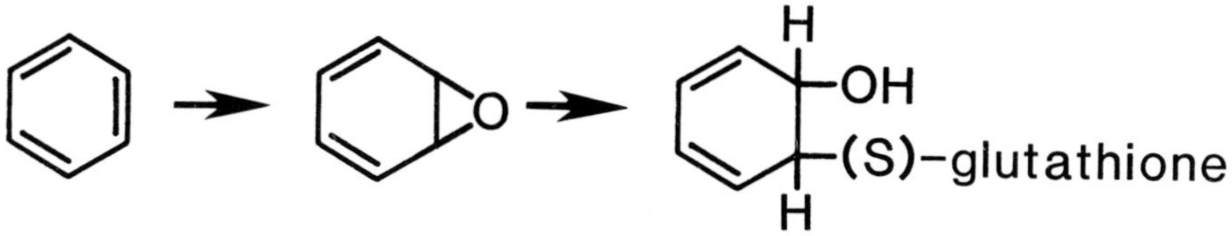

Scheme 2

The specificities of tissue and microfloral C-S lyases for preMAP metabolites
that are formed upon conjugation of arene oxides with GSH have not been determined. C-S lyase mediated catabolism of preMAP metabolites was believed
possible because dihydro-hydroxy-methylthio-metabolites have been isolated
from urine of rats dosed with bromobenzene (11), naphthalene (12) and
phenanthrene (13), and the microfloral C-S lyase system could be involved
because both bromobenzene and naphthalene are metabolized to preMAP metabolites that are excreted in bile (14, 15). The dihydro-methylthio-metabolites
of phenanthrene were proposed to be formed upon dissociation of a sulfonium
ion complex formed between methionine and phenanthrene oxides (13), although
they did not investigate involvement of C-S lyase mediated pathways.

Naphthalene metabolites were selected to serve as a model for studying
preMAP metabolite catabolism because ^{14}C-labeled-1,2-dihydro-1-hydroxy-2-S-

cysteinyl- (I), and -(N-acetyl)cysteinylnaphthalene (II) could be isolated from the bile and urine, respectively, from bile-duct-cannulated rats dosed with ^{14}C-naphthalene in quantities sufficient for dosing rats.

Stillwell et al. (12) identified a series of methylthio-containing metabolites of naphthalene in urine from rats given intraperitoneal doses of naphthalene. The introduction of divalent sulfur into the naphthalene nucleus was proposed to proceed through epoxide formation followed by reaction of the epoxide with sulfur containing nucleophiles (12). Methionine was shown to be a methyl donor for the methylthio groups in these metabolites (16). These authors suggested that the decreased production of methylthio-containing metabolites they observed in antibiotic treated rats dosed with naphthalene was due to lowered yields of preMAP metabolites or a lowered availability of sulfur-containing nucleophiles.

We dosed rats with the cysteine conjugate of naphthalene (I, fig 1) and the mercapturic acid of naphthalene (II, fig 1) to determine if these preMAP metabolites could serve as precursors for the methylthio-containing glucuronide (V) as shown in fig 1.

MATERIALS AND METHODS

Labeled Compounds. The ^{14}C-labeled cysteine conjugate (I-^{14}C) was isolated from bile, and ^{14}C-labeled naphthalene mercapturic acid (II-^{14}C) and ^{14}C-labeled dihydrodiol glucuronide (III-^{14}C) was isolated from urine from rats given single oral doses of ^{14}C-naphthalene (2 mg, 0.5 μCi; Amersham, Arlington Hts., Ill.). Bile-duct-cannulated rats were held in restraining cages (17) after surgery and given laboratory chow and physiological saline ad libitum. Cannulated rats were dosed 12 to 24 hours after surgery.

The I-, II-, and III-^{14}C used for dosing, and the other metabolites listed in tables II and III were isolated using the same methods. The bile and urine collected from 0-24 hours were used for preparation of I-, II-, and III-^{14}C as previously reported (18). For quantitation of metabolites, bile and urine collected from 0-72 hours were used.

I-^{14}C and II-^{14}C were assumed, from previous studies (19), to have the 1,2-dihydro-1-hydroxy structures shown in fig 1. The mass spectra of the trimethylsilyl (TMS) derivatives of I, II (18) and III (18) were compatible with the structures shown in fig 1. No attempts were made to confirm positional or sterochemistry. Radiopurities were determined by paper chromatography (descending: butanol, acetic acid, water 5:1:4, v/v/v), HPLC and GLC to be greater than 95%.

Metabolite Dosing. I-^{14}C, II-^{14}C and III-^{14}C were separately dosed to male Sprague-Dawley rats (250-300 g) as outlined in table I. Oral doses were given in water; intracecal doses, dissolved in physiological saline, were given to anesthetized rats (halothane) through a midline laparotomy. After surgery, the rats given intracecal doses were held in restraining cages (17).

TABLE I

DOSES OF NAPHTHALENE METABOLITES GIVEN TO RATS

compound dosed[a]	dose route	µCi	mg	no. of rats
I-^{14}C	intracecal	0.4	3.3	5
I-^{14}C	oral	0.4	3.3	2
II-^{14}C	intracecal	0.57	5.5	4
II-^{14}C	oral	0.65	6.2	5
III-^{14}C	oral	0.47	5.0	6

[a] See fig 1 for metabolite structures

Four male Sprague-Dawley germfree rats (20, 21) were each given a single oral dose of ^{14}C-naphthalene (2 mg, 1 µCi). The germfree rats were housed within an isolator in stainless steel cages that were designed to separate the urine from the feces. The urine and feces were collected for 72 hours.

Isolation of metabolites. Radiolabeled metabolites were isolated from the urine and bile from the experimental animals by the same procedures used to isolate I-, II- and III-^{14}C (18). Generally, radioactivity was extracted from urine or bile using a Porapak Q column; then chromatographed on LH-20 (H_2O). The radioactive fractions from LH-20 were further purified by HPLC (4.9 mm x 30 cm µ-Bondapak C_{18} column, Waters Assoc., eluted at 2.5 ml/min with a 30 min linear gradient of 100% H_2O to 100% CH_3CN). For the final purification, the samples from HPLC were derivatized with bis-trimethylsilyl trifluoroacetamide containing 1% chlorotrimethylsilane and separated by GLC. Mass spectra were obtained on samples trapped from the gas chromatograph.

For capillary GC-MS analysis, the methods of Horning's group were used (12, 13).

Radioactivity was extracted with methanol from freeze-dried feces from rats given the intracecal doses of I-^{14}C. The soluble ^{14}C (27 to 33% of the dose) was treated in the same manner as the urine samples.

Mass spectrometry was performed using a Varian MAT CH-5 DF mass spectrometer. All samples were introduced with a solid sample probe. Capillary GC/MS was done in a HP 5992A GC-MS with a HP 18740B capillary column unit. The column was fused silica coated with OV-101.

All soluble radioactivity was determined by liquid scintillation spectrometry. Fecal and carcass radioactivity was quantified after solubilization by oxidation in a Model 306 Packard Tri-Carb sample oxidizer.

RESULTS AND DISCUSSION

Recoveries of ^{14}C from conventional and bile-duct-cannulated rats given single oral doses of ^{14}C-naphthalene are given in table II along with quantitation of the ^{14}C-labeled metabolites that were identified. Neither naphthols, naphthol glucuronides nor methylthio-containing metabolite (V) were detected by liquid chromatographic methods in the urine or bile from the bile-duct-cannulated rats dosed with ^{14}C-naphthalene. Naphthols were detected in trace amounts in urine and bile from cannulated rats when capillary GC-MS methods were used, however, methylthio-containing metabolites (aglycone from V and methylthionaphthalene) were only detected in urine from conventional rats using these methods. These results indicated that methylthio-containing metabolites of naphthalene and most of the naphthols excreted by conventional rats were produced from biliary metabolites during enterohepatic circulation. We, therefore, studied the metabolic fate of the biliary metabolites of naphthalene.

Recoveries of ^{14}C from rats dosed with I-, II-, and III-^{14}C are given in table III along with the amounts of these doses recovered as the metabolites listed. The structure was assigned to V from mass spectral data obtained from

TABLE II

RECOVERIES OF ^{14}C IN EXCRETA, TISSUES AND AS METABOLITES FROM CONVENTIONAL AND
BILE-DUCT-CANNULATED RATS 72 HOURS AFTER SINGLE ORAL DOSES OF NAPHTHALENE-^{14}C

	% of ^{14}C dose as metabolites	Recovery of ^{14}C dose
Conventional		
urine		84.3±7.4
mercapturic acid (I)	38.1	
dihydrodiol glucuronide (III)	29.3	
naphthol glucuronide	3.0	
naphthol	1.6	
dihydroxynaphthalene	4.9	
uncharacterized	7	
feces		6.6±1.9
body		2.6±1.0
Bile-Duct-Cannulated		
bile		66.8±13.1
cysteine conjugate (I)	16.9	
mercapturic acid (II)	0.7	
cysteinylglycine conjugate	9.6	
dihydrodiol glucuronide (III)	26.8	
dihydrodiol	6.4	
uncharacterized	6(5)[a]	
urine		32.7±7.5
mercapturic acid (I)	14.4	
dihydrodiol glucuronide (III)	14.5	
dihydroxynaphthalene	1.5	
uncharacterized	3(4)[a]	
feces		‹1
body		‹1

[a]Numbers in parenthesis indicate the number of chromatographic fractions

the per-trimethylsilyl (TMS) derivative and the TMS derivative of the methyl
ester. These spectra have been reported and interpreted (18). After hydrolysis of V with glucuronidase, the TMS derivative of the aglycone gave a mass
spectrum identical with that reported for the TMS derivative of 1-hydroxy-2-
methylthio-1,2-dihydronaphthalene reported by Stillwell et al. (12).

TABLE III

RECOVERIES OF ^{14}C IN EXCRETA, TISSUES AND AS METABOLITES CONTAINING NAPHTHOLS
AND 1,2-DIHYDRO-1-HYDROXY-2-METHYLTHIONAPHTHALENE FROM RATS DOSED WITH [14]C-
LABELED METABOLITES OF NAPHTHALENE

	Metabolite dosed				
	cysteine conjugate (I)		mercapturic acid (II)		dihydrodiol-glucuronide (III)
	oral	intracecal	oral	intracecal	oral
feces	12.3	20.8	n.d.[a]	13.3	6.4
body	2.3	3.5	n.a.	9.6	n.d.
urine	81.6	74.2	73.0	66.2	90.1
naphthols[b]	15.1	21.5	7.3	8.3	trace
1,2-dihydro-1-hydroxy-2-methylthio-naphthalene[b]	1.4	12.4	4.5	34.7	n.d.

[a]n.d. = none detected

[b]percentages are totals of free metabolite and metabolite glucuronides

The isolation of V and naphthol glucuronides from urines from rats dosed
with either I-^{14}C or II-^{14}C showed that preMAP metabolites of naphthalene
could serve as precursors for the aglycone of V and naphthols. The detection
of only traces of naphthols in the urine from rats dosed with III-^{14}C indicate
that the biliary dihydrodiol glucuronide is not a significant precursor for
naphthols.

Naphthols can be produced from preMAP metabolites of naphthalene by
treatment with acid (22), therefore, the naphthols produced from I-^{14}C and
II-^{14}C given orally could have been produced, in part, by contact with stomach
acid. However, when I-^{14}C and II-^{14}C were dosed intracecally, the conversions
to naphthol glucuronides and V were not decreased but actually increased.
These results again indicated involvement of the microflora in production of
both naphthols and V.

The role of the microflora in the formation of naphthols and V was confirmed by dosing germfree rats with naphthalene-[14]C. The methylthio-
containing glucuronide (V) was not detectable by liquid chromatographic

methods and the aglycone of V was not detectable by the capillary GC-MS
method in the urine from the germfree rats. Naphthols were detectable only by
the capillary GC-MS method in the germfree rat urine.

From these studies, the catabolism of naphthalene preMAP metabolites in
vivo in rats is proposed to follow the pathways outlined in fig 1. The preMAP
metabolites are excreted with the bile and are converted to the cysteine conjugate (I) by intestinal enzymes (5). The cysteine conjugate can then proceed

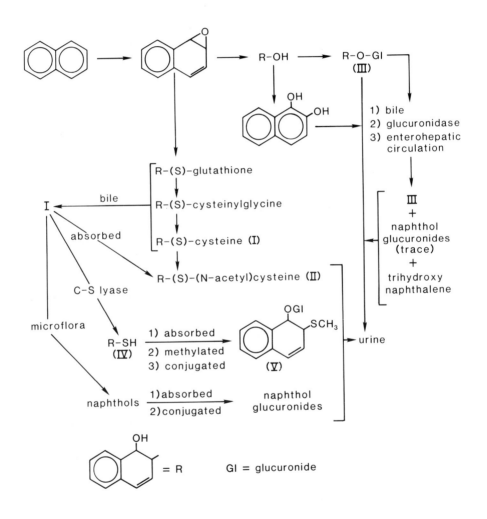

Figure 1. Metabolism of naphthalene in vivo in rats

by at least three routes. It can be absorbed, acetylated and excreted as II. It can be cleaved by microflora C-S lyases to form IV, which is absorbed, methylated, conjugated with glucuronic acid and excreted as V. It can be converted to naphthols by the elimination of either cysteine from I or H_2S from IV. The naphthols are then absorbed, conjugated and excreted. The methylation of IV is thought to take place during or after absorption from the intestinal lumen because IV and naphthols were present in the feces from rats dosed intracecally with I, however, the aglycone of V was not detected in feces. If methylation occurred in the microflora, the aglycone of V would have been expected in the feces unless it was preferentially absorbed from the gut upon formation.

The traces of naphthols that were detected by capillary GC-MS methods in urine and bile could be produced, in part, by degradation of the preMAP metabolites by nonenzymatic means. During the isolation of II-^{14}C, we observed that varying amounts (5 to 30%) of the ^{14}C were lost each time the sample had been stored (-4° to -15°C) and subsequently taken to dryness. HPLC of stored II-^{14}C (without prior evaporation) separated up to four minor radioactive components. These were characterized by capillary GC-MS to be naphthylthiol (tentative), 1- and 2-naphthol and naphthalene. This decomposition of preMAP metabolites may explain the presence of traces of naphthols detected by capillary GC-MS in the bile and urine from bile-duct-cannulated rats and the urine of germfree rats dosed with naphthalene.

The decomposition of preMAP metabolites may also explain the observations of Renwick and Drasar (23) which showed that biliary metabolites of benzo(a)pyrene (presumably containing preMAP metabolites) were converted upon incubation with rat and human feces to dihydrodiols, phenols and quinones, and benzo(a)pyrene, however, incubations in the absence of microorganisms also produced the "hydrolysis" products and benzo(a)pyrene.

The toxicological implications of the existence of the pathways discussed have not been studied, however, any process which regenerates or creates new xenobiotics in the intestinal tract is suspect for chemical carcinogenesis.

REFERENCES

1. Bakke, J.E., Gustafsson, J.A. and Gustafsson, B.E. (1980) Science, 210, 433.

2. Bakke, J.E., Rafter, J.J., Lindeskog, P., Feil, V.J., Gustafsson, J.A. and Gustafsson, B.E. (1981) Biochem. Pharmacol., 30, 1839.

3. Bakke, J.E., Larsen, G.L., Aschbacher, P.W., Rafter, J.J., Gustafsson, J.A. and Gustafsson, B.E. (1981) in: Rosen, J.D., Magee, P.S. and Casida, J.E. (Eds.), Sulfur in Pesticide Metabolism and Function, ACS Symp. Ser. No. 158, American Chemical Society, Washington, D.C., pp. 165-178.

4. Suzuki, S., Tomisawa, H., Ichihara, S., Fukazawa, H. and Tateishi, M. (1982) Biochem. Pharmacol. 31, 2137.

5. Larsen, G.L. and Bakke, J.E. (1983) Xenobiotica, in press.

6. Weisiger, R.A., Pinkus, L.M. and Jakoby, W.B. (1980) Biochem. Pharmacol., 29, 2885.

7. Tateishi, M., Suzuki, S. and Shimizu, H. (1978) J. Biol. Chem., 253, 8854.

8. Collucci, D.F. and Buyske, D.A. (1965) Biochem. Pharmacol., 14, 457.

9. Dohn, D.R. and Anders, M.W. (1982) Analytical Biochem., 120, 386.

10. Stevens, J.L. and Jakoby, W.B. (1982) Federation Proc., 41, 1426.

11. Mizutani, T., Yamamoto, K. and Tajima, K. (1978) Biochem. Biophys. Res. Comm. 82, 805.

12. Stillwell, W.G., Bouwsma, O.J., Thenot, J-P. and Horning, M.G. (1978) Res. Comm. Chem. Pathol. Pharmacol, 20, 509.

13. Lertratanagkoon, K., Horning, M.G., Middleditch, B.S., Tsang, W.-S. and Griffin, G.W. (1982) Drug Metab. Dispos., 10, 614.

14. Sipes, G., Gigon, P.L., and Krishna, G. (1974) Biochem. Pharmacol., 23, 451.

15. Boyland, E., Ramsay, G.S. and Sims, P. (1961) Biochem. J. 78, 376.

16. Stillwell, W.G., Bouwsma, O.J. and Horning, M.G. (1978) Res. Comm. Chem. Pathol. Pharmacol, 22, 329.

17. Bollman, J.E. (1948) J. Lab. Clin. Med., 33, 1368.

18. Bakke, J.E., Feil, V.J. and Struble, C. (1982) Biomed. Mass Spectrom., 9, 246.

19. Jeffery, A.M. and Jerina, D.M. (1975) J. Amer. Chem. Soc., 97, 4427.

20. Gustafsson, B.E. (1948) Acta Pathol. Microbio. Scan. Suppl., 78, 1.

21. Gustafsson, B.E. (1959) Ann. N.Y. Acad. Sci., 78, 17.

22. Jerina, D.M., Daly, J.W., Witkop, B., Zaltman-Nirenberg, P. and Udenfriend, S. (1970) Biochemistry, 9, 147.

23. Renwick, A.G. and Drasar, B.W. (1976) Nature, 263, 234.

© 1983 Elsevier Science Publishers B.V.
Extrahepatic Drug Metabolism and Chemical Carcinogenesis,
J. Rydström, J. Montelius and M. Bengtsson eds.

DISPOSITION AND METABOLISM OF MUTAGENS-CARCINOGENS IN VIVO - INVOLVEMENT OF THE INTESTINAL MICROFLORA

J. RAFTER[1], L. MÖLLER[1], L. NILSSON[1], L. BALL[2], I. BRANDT[3], G. LARSEN[4], M. BLOMSTEDT[1], B. GUSTAFSSON[5] AND J.-Å. GUSTAFSSON[1]

[1]Department of Medical nutrition, Karolinska Institute, Huddinge University Hospital F69, S-141 86 Huddinge, Sweden; [2]Health Effects Research Laboratory, U.S. Environmental Protection Agency, Research Triangle Park, NC, USA; [3]Department of Pharmacology, SLU, Biomedical Centre, Box 573, S-751 23 Uppsala, Sweden; [4]Metabolism and Radiation Research Laboratory, ARS, USDA, State University Station, Fargo, ND 58105, USA; [5]Department of Germfree Research, Karolinska Institute, Box 60400, S-104 01 Stockholm, Sweden.

INTRODUCTION

In the last few years we have been interested in the involvement of the intestinal microflora in the metabolism of xenobiotics. More specifically we have been able to show that metabolism by the microflora is directly involved in the formation of methylthio containing metabolites of a range of xenobiotics. For a review of this work see ref. 1. More recently we have become interested in studying the disposition and metabolism of mutagens-carcinogens in the whole animal, with a particular interest in the role the microflora plays in this process. The main purpose of the latter studies is to attempt to correlate up-take and binding of thse compounds and/or their metabolites in the animal with the target organs of the "in vivo" carcinogenicity tests and, by examining excreted metabolites and mutagenicity, to obtain some information on the levels of circulating "active metabolites" (i.e. capable of DNA binding in vitro) in the animal.

In this article some recent results with representatives from two groups of extremely potent mutagens, i.e. a new series of heterocyclic amines and nitrated polycyclic aromatic hydrocarbons, will be described.

The heterocyclic amines

A new series of heterocyclic amines have been isolated as very potent mutagens from the pyrolysates of various amino acids and proteins by Dr. T. Sugimura´s group at the National Cancer Center Research Institute, Tokyo, Japan. These include 3 amino-1,4-dimethyl-5H-pyrido [4,3-b] indole (Trp-p-1) and 3-amino-1-methyl-5H-pyrido [4,3-b] indole (Trp-p-2) from tryptophan pyrolysates; 2-amino-6-methyldipyrido [1,2-a: 3',2'-d] imidazole (Glu-P-1) and 2-aminodipyrido [1,2-a: 3',2'-d] imidazole (Glu-P-2) from glutamic acid pyrolysates; 2-amino-9H-pyrido [2,3-b]

indole (AαC) and 2 amino-3-methyl-9H-pyrido[2,3-b]indole (MeAαC) from a
pyrolysate of soybean globulin. All of these compounds, which are among the
most mutagenic compounds known today, required metabolic activation to exert
their mutagenicity towards Salmonella typhimurium strains TA 98 and TA 100 (2).
So far all of these compounds which have been tested for carcinogenicity have
proved to be carcinogenic. Trp-P-1, Trp-P-2, Glu-P-1, Glu-P-2, AαC and MeAαC
induced hepatomas in mice, with a higher frequency being observed in female
mice (2). Glu-P-1, Glu-P-2, AαC and MeAαC also induced hemangioendothelial
sarcomas at the interscapular region with the same incidence in both males and
females (2). In addition, recently, it has been observed that administration of
Glu-P-1 to rats resulted in the formation of hepatocarcinomas, squamous cell
carcinomas of the Zymbal glands, brain tumors, skin tumors and tumors in the
small and large intestine (3). The presence of these heterocyclic amines in
various cooked foods has now been confirmed, for example, broiled fish, fried
beef, chicken, chinese mushroom, onion (2). However, while considerable work has
been carried out on studying the metabolism of these compounds "in vitro" so
far no report has appeared in the literature on the disposition and metabolism
of these compounds "in vivo". Therefore we undertook such a study.

Distribution of Trp-P-1 in mice

In order to study the distribution of Trp-P-1 in the whole animal a series of
mice were injected intravenously with Trp-P-1 and were killed and subjected to
whole-body autoradiography at various post-injection times from 10 min to 6 days.
For further experimental details see ref. 4.

Autoradiograms obtained 1-4 h after injection of Trp-P-1 to albino and pigmented
mice showed a pronounced uptake of radioactivity in the lymphatic system (thymus,
lymph nodes, bone marrow and spleen), in the endocrine system (hypophysis, thyroid,
adrenal medulla) and in the liver, kidney medulla and brain. High radioactivity
was present in the excretory pathways, predominantly in the bile/intestinal contents. At longer post-injection times (24 h - 6 days) most of the labelled substance had left the tissues, except for the liver which still retained a high
concentration of radioactivity. The uptake of radioactivity in the liver could
be reduced by pretreatment with 9-hydroxyellipticine suggesting that the observed
accumulation of radioactivity in the liver was partly due to metabolites of Trp-
P-1. After pretreatment with β-naftoflavone (BNF), the administration of Trp-P-1
resulted in a highly selective accumulation of radioactivity in the lung parenchyma, exceeding all other tissues in the body. β-Naftoflavone pretreatment
also increased the uptake of radioactivity in the kidney cortex and small intestinal mucosa. As indicated by a high labelling of the pigmented tissues of the

maternal and fetal eye, the carcinogen and/or its metabolites was accumulated in melanin.

Thus the distribution pattern of Trp-P-1 was characterized by a rapid accumulation of radioactivity in a wide range of tissues including the liver, the endocrine and the lymphatic systems. The high concentration of radioactivity in the bile and intestinal contents during the first hours, after i.v. injection of Trp-P-1, indicates considerable biliary excretion of Trp-P-1 and/or its metabolites.

In contrast to most tissues in the body, where the accumulated radioactivity disappeared at longer post-injection times, the labelled material in the liver remained for the full duration of the study (i.e. up to six days). This indicated a more permanent association of the radioactivity with the hepatic tissue. This is interesting in the light of the observation that Trp-P-1 is a hepatic carcinogen when given orally to mice (2). However, while we observed no difference in uptake of radioactivity in the liver between male and female mice, the latter authors reported that female mice showed higher susceptibilities to Trp-P-1, with regard to hepatocarcinogenicity, than male mice.

Trp-P-1 and Trp-P-2 are metabolized by rat liver microsomes to an N-hydroxylated metabolite, which is mutagenic to S. typhimurium TA 98 (5,6). The metabolite is formed in a reaction catalysed by cytochrome P-448 and binds covalently to DNA in vitro (6). The fact that pretreatment of mice with the selective cytochrome P-448 inhibitor 9-hydroxyellipticine (7,8) resulted in a decreased uptake of radioactivity in the liver conforms with the contention that the pronounced retention of radioactivity in the liver of the control mice was partly due to metabolites of Trp-P-1. Also the decreased excretion of radioactivity to the intestinal contents and the increased retention of radioactivity in extrahepatic tissues (e.g. in the endocrine and lymphatic systems) indicates an overall "slowing down" of the metabolism and excretion of Trp-P-1 in the 9-hydroxyellipticine pretreated mice.

β-Naftoflavone is a selective inducer of cytochrome P-448 in different tissues of mice and rats. The strikingly high accumulation of radioactivity in the lung parenchyma of the BNF pretreated mice indicates formation of a metabolite catalysed by the induced cytochrome P-448. BNF pretreatment also induced an increased binding of radioactivity in the kidney cortex and in some segments of the small intestine, predominantly in the proximal segments. In contrast, the uptake of radioactivity in the liver of the BNF pretreated mice was decreased compared to the control mice. In the liver of the BNF pretreated mice, the radioactivity was preferentially present in the central regions of the lobules, where the highest concentration of cytochrome P-450 has been demonstrated.

Experiments by Yamazoe et al (5) showed that N-hydroxylation of Trp-P-2 by rat liver microsomes increased 200, 80 and 8 times, when rats were treated with PCB, 3-methylcholanthrene and phenobarbital, respectively. Since it has been demonstrated that BNF induces cytochrome P-448 in lung, kidney and liver of rats (9), it seems conceivable that the increased uptake of radioactivity in the lung and kidney cortex in the BNF treated mice was due to an increased formation of N-hydroxylated Trp-P-1. The decreased uptake of radioactivity in the liver of the BNF treated mice is partly explained by the increased binding in the lung, kidney and intestinal mucosa.

In this study Trp-P-1 reached the lung via the circulating blood. The fact that the compounds AαC and MeAαC have been isolated from cigarette smoke condensates (10,11) shows, however, that the heterocyclic amines can be presented to the lung also via the inhaled air. Since it is well established that cytochrome P-448 in lung is induced by a number of factors present in cigarette smoke, mainly by polyaromatic hydrocarbons such as benzo(a)pyrene (12), it seems possible that the metabolism and binding of the heterocyclic amines may be enhanced by inhalation of cigarette smoke.

The rapid and selective accumulation of Trp-P-1 and/or its metabolites in a wide range of tissues of the endocrine and lymphatic systems may indicate a potency of the hepatocarcinogen to produce extrahepatic toxic effects. The fact that the labelled substance left these tissues within a few hours showed, however, that the uptake was not due to a firm binding of metabolites to the tissues.

Metabolism of Trp-P-1 in rats

In this section we report on preliminary results on the metabolism of Trp-P-1 in the rat. A group of five male Sprague-Dawley rats (200-300 g) received a single oral dose of ^{14}C-Trp-P-1 each (3 μCi/4 mg per rat). The administered radioactivity was excreted rapidly with 30% of the dose appearing in the urine and 40% of the dose in the feces within 24 hours. Approximately 70% of the fecal radioactivity was extractable with organic solvents and water. In an additional experiment in which ^{14}C-Trp-P-1 was administered to three bile-fistulated rats, approximately 30% of the dose was recovered in the bile and only 15% in the urine within 24 hours. Further characterization of the radioactive material in the control rat urine, utilizing high pressure liquid chromatography and mass spectrometry, indicated that approximately 30% of the urinary ^{14}C was due to unmetabolized Trp-P-1; approximately 40% of the urinary ^{14}C was due to a number of ring hydroxylated metabolites of Trp-P-1; approximately 8% was due to a ring hydroxylated derivative in which the amino group was acetylated and approximately 2% was due to a metabolite of Trp-P-1 in which the amino group was acetylated. There appeared to be little or no conjugates of Trp-P-1 present in the urine. Interestingly, the pattern of Trp-P-1 and metabolites excreted in the bile and feces was basically similar to that in the urine. Both the urine and fecal extract were mutagenic towards Salmonella typhimurium strains TA 98 and TA 1538. However, both required metabolic activation to exert their mutagenicity.

A similar study was performed using germfree animals. However, preliminary results appear to indicate that there were no major differences in excretion of radioactivity, in the metabolite patterns obtained or in the mutagenicity of the excreta when compared to the conventional animals.

Thus there was considerable metabolism of Trp-P-1 to primary metabolites which appeared to be polar enough to be excreted in the urine and feces without further conjugation. However, at the dose level used, appreciable amounts of unchanged Trp-P-1 were also excreted in the urine and the feces. There appeared to be no direct acting mutagens in either the urine or the fecal extract indicating that the "active" N-hydroxylated metabolite of Trp-P-1 is not excreted as such. In addition, the mutagenic activity present in the urine and fecal extract, which required metabolic activation, appeared to be due mainly to the presence of un-metabolized Trp-P-1. Finally, the preliminary studies with the germfree animals appeared to indicate that the intestinal microflora did not play a major role in the disposition and metabolism of this heterocyclic amine in vivo. However, from the bile fistulation experiments there did seem to be some enterohepatic circula-tion occurring – although this was probably due to Trp-P-1 being reabsorbed, which had been excreted with the bile.

Distribution and metabolism of Glu-P-1 in rats

Some preliminary work carried out in colalboration with Drs. Sato and Sugimura at the National Cancer Center Research Institute, Tokyo, Japan indicate that there is a rough correlation between retention of ^{14}C and cancer target organs after a single oral dose of ^{14}C-Glu-P-1. In addition the radioactivity is excreted rapidly with almost 50% of the dose in the feces and 35% in the urine within 24 hrs. Some-what less appeared in the bile when compared to the above Trp-P-1 experiment. The urine was mutagenic but only after metabolic activation. Thus as in the case of Trp-P-1, none of the "direct acting" mutagenic metabolites of Glu-P-1 were excreted in the urine. The urinary ^{14}C consisted of a small quantity of unmeta-bolized Glu-P-1 and at least two metabolites both of which were mutagenic after metabolic activation. The pattern of metabolites in the bile was similar to that in urine.

Nitrated polycyclic aromatic hydrocarbons

Nitrated polycyclic aromatic hydrocarbons represent another group of extremely potent mutagens which have been detected in combustion emissions. Some research presented elsewhere at this meeting indicates how the intestinal microflora may be involved in the metabolism of this type of compound and in the generation of mutagenic metabolites.

1-Nitropyrene is a representative nitro-aromatic which is among the most abundant in the ambient air. This compound was obtained labelled with ^{14}C and administered by intra-peritoneal injection to germfree and conventional rats of the Agus strain. For further experimental details see ref. 13. The urinary excretion was initially similar between germfree and conventional rats, and the metabolites in both cases consisted principally of 6- and 8-hydroxy-1-nitropyrene (as their glucuronide and sulphate conjugates) and unidentified polar material. Little or no unchanged 1-nitropyrene was seen in the urine at any time after dosing. Beyond 8 hours after dosing, total urinary excretion rose significantly in conventional compared to germfree rats, and 6/8-hydroxy-1-acetamidopyrene (NAAP-OH, mainly as it´s glucuronide conjugate) now accounted for 20 to 30% of the urinary ^{14}C, compared to 2 to 3% in germfree rats and conventional rats at earlier time points.

The mutagenicity of the conventional urines as measured by the Ames assay underwent a concomitant increase in S-9-dependent activity, whereas the urines from the germfree rats continued to exhibit lower levels of mutagenicity which were slightly decreased by addition of S-9. The direct-acting mutagenicity may be associated with the presence of hydroxynitropyrenes in the urine. The S-9-dependent activity was predominantly due to NAAP-OH, which is itself over five-fold more mutagenic than the parent 1-nitropyrene.

The similarity in excretion and metabolite pattern for the first few hours after dosing might indicate that the germfree and conventional rats are not radically different in their hepatic drug-metabolizing or excretion capacities. Results at later time points indicate that about 1/3 of the material excreted into the urine by the conventional rats, at this dose level of 1-nitropyrene, arises from enterohepatic circulation, which is interrupted in the germfree rats. The mutagenic metabolite NAAP-OH is not totally absent from the urines of the germfree rats, and this may reflect the baseline capacity of the liver to reduce nitro-aromatic compounds "in vivo". However, the presence of a functional gut flora and active enterohepatic circulation are demonstrably required to ensure the presence of significant quantities of this compound in the urine.

The occurence of hydroxylated nitropyrenes as early metabolites of 1-nitropyrene suggests that NAAP-OH arises from reductive metabolism of these, primarily by the gut flora. Subsequent acetylation could then occur in the liver or possibly the kidney. NAAP-OH escaping from the enterohepatic circulation cycle would become available for distribution to other organs of the body. A mechanism for genotoxic action for this potent mutagen can then be postulated, by analogy with N-acetylaminofluorene.

2-Nitrofluorene is another potent mutagen which has been identified in ambient air particles. Preliminary metabolism studies using rats have shown that this compound is rapidly (within 24 hr) excreted into the urine after a single oral dose. The urine is mutagenic in the Ames assay with and without metabolic activation. Characterization of the urinary ^{14}C has indicated that many of the metabolites are present as glucuronide and sulphate conjugates. In addition, preliminary experiments with germfree animals have shown that the pattern of urinary metabolites differs significantly between germfree and conventional rats, indicating that the intestinal microflora plays a role in the disposition and metabolism of this nitro-aromatic in the whole animal. The specific nature of this role is at present under investigation in our laboratory.

CONCLUSIONS

Thus it appears that at least with certain of the mutagens-carcinogens studied, the intestinal microflora plays an important role in the disposition and metabolism of these compounds in the whole animal. In view of the now well established fact that components in the diet can affect the biochemical activity of the gut flora it does not seem unreasonable to suggest that one might define a diet which, through its influence on the flora, might result in a decreased formation of mutagenic and potentially carcinogenic metabolites.

ACKNOWLEDGEMENTS

This work was supported by grants from the Swedish Cancer Society and the Swedish Council for Planning and Coordination of Research.

REFERENCES

1. Rafter, J., Bakke, J., Larsen, G., Gustafsson. B. and Gustafsson, J.-Å. (1983) Role of the intestinal microflora in the formation of sulphur-containing conjugates of xenobiotics. Rev. Biochem. Toxicol. Vol V, in press.

2. Sugimura, T. and Sato, S. (1983) Cancer Res. (Suppl.), 43, 2415.

3. Takayama, S. Personal communication.

274

4. Brandt, I., Gustafsson, J.-Å. and Rafter, J. (1983) Distribution of the carcinogenic tryptophan pyrolysis product Trp-P-1 in control, 9-hydroxy-ellipticine and β-naftoflavone pretreated mice. Submitted, Carcinogenesis.

5. Yamazoe, Y., Ishii, K., Kamataki, T., Kato, R. and Sugimura, T. (1980) Chem.-Biol. Interact. 30, 125.

6. Kato, R., Yamazoe, Y., Ishii, K., Mita, S., Kamataki, T. and Sugimura, T. (1982) in: Snyder, R. (Ed.), Biological Reactive Intermediates II, Adv. Exp. Med. Biol. Vol. 136 B. New York Plenum Press, pp. 997-1009.

7. Delaforge, M., Ioannides, C. and Parke, D.V. (1980) Chem.-Biol. Interact. 32, 101.

8. Delaforge, M., Ioannides, C. and Parke, D.V. (1982) Chem.-Biol. Interact. 42, 279.

9. Guengerich, F.P., Wang, P. and Davidson, N.K. (1982) Biochemistry 21, 1698.

10. Yoshida, D. and Matsumoto, T. (1980) Cancer Lett. 10, 141.

11. Matsumoto, T., Yoshida, D. and Tomita, H. (1981) Cancer Lett. 12, 105.

12. Dansette, P.M., Alexandrov, K., Azerad, R. and Frayssinet, Ch. (1979) Europ. J. Cancer 15, 915.

13. Ball, L., Rafter, J., Gustafsson, J.-Å., Gustafsson, B. and Lewtas, J. (1983) Metabolism of 1-nitropyrene in germfree and conventional rats: Role of the gut flora in generation of mutagenic metabolites. This volume.

© 1983 Elsevier Science Publishers B.V.
Extrahepatic Drug Metabolism and Chemical Carcinogenesis,
J. Rydström, J. Montelius and M. Bengtsson eds.

ENTEROHEPATIC CIRCULATION OF THE AROMATIC HYDROCARBONS BENZO(a)PYRENE AND NAPHTHALENE

P.C. HIROM, J.K. CHIPMAN, P. MILLBURN AND M.A. PUE
Department of Biochemistry, St.Mary's Hospital Medical School, London W2 1PG
(U.K.)

INTRODUCTION

Biliary metabolites of xenobiotics are generally polar, unreactive excretory products (1). However, in certain instances mutagenic or pre-mutagenic derivatives may be excreted via this route into the intestine (2). In the case of benzo(a)pyrene (BP) we have shown that metabolites are eliminated extensively in rat and rabbit bile and persist in vivo via the enterohepatic circulation (3-5). Glucuronic acid conjugates of these biliary metabolites are hydrolysed by intestinal microflora to yield a number of potentially reactive aglycones (3-6).

The thio-ether conjugates of BP may also undergo enterohepatic cycling (7) as is the case for such conjugates of propachlor in the rat (8). Many of the conjugated metabolites of naphthalene, including thio-ether derivatives, are excreted in the bile (9), but their enterohepatic circulation has not been investigated. Therefore, we have studied the fate of naphthalene glutathione conjugates (10,11) in the intestine since this may prove instructive with respect to the fate of polycyclic aromatic hydrocarbons such as BP.

METHODS

Chemicals BP Grade I was purchased from Sigma Chemical Co. Ltd. (Poole, Dorset, U.K.). $[7,10-^{14}C]$-BP (sp.act. 27 Ci/mol; 99% radiochemical purity), $[G-^{3}H]$-BP (40 Ci/mmol; 99% pure) and $[1-^{14}C]$-naphthalene (5 µCi/umol; 98% pure) were obtained from Amersham International PLC (Amersham, Bucks., U.K.). Unlabelled and labelled compounds were mixed to give material of the required specific activity. Authentic standards of BP metabolites were obtained from the National Cancer Institute (Carcinogenesis Research Program, Bethesda, Maryland, U.S.A.). Authentic standards S-(1-naphthyl) cysteine and S-(1-naphthyl)- glutathione were gifts from Dr. P. Sims, Institute of Cancer Research, London.

Animals Male New Zealand white rabbits (approx. 2.5 kg) and male Wistar rats (approx. 0.2 kg) were used. Bile- duct-cannulations were performed on animals anaesthetised with sodium pentobarbitone (Sagatal , May & Baker Ltd., Dagenham, Essex, U.K.). Compounds were administered by injection into the ear vein (rabbits) or femoral vein (rats) in 20% aqueous Mulgofen EL-719 (GAF Ltd., Wythenshawe, Manchester, U.K.) – ethanol 1:1 or in 1% bovine serum albumin for high doses of BP in rats (12). Intraduodenal infusions of bile were over a period of 1 h.

Analysis of metabolites Radioactivity was measured by scintillation counting.

Tissue homogenates were solubilised with NCS (Hopkin & Williams, Romford, Essex, U.K.) prior to addition of scintillation fluid.

For BP metabolite identification, bile samples were added to β-glucuronidase with or without saccharo-1,4-lactone, and incubated at pH 5 overnight (37 C) in the dark. The incubates were extracted with ethyl acetate, which was evaporated under a stream of nitrogen, and the samples redissolved in methanol. Identification of BP metabolites was by co-chromatography with authentic standards, using reversed phase HPLC and by spectral analysis (5).

[^{14}C]-naphthalene metabolites were analysed by t.l.c. on aluminium-backed silica gel precoated sheets (Merck, Darmstadt). Butanol/acetic acid/water (4/1/1) was used to develop the chromatograms which were sprayed with ninhydrin or potassium dichromate/silver nitrate, to visualise the glutathione and related conjugates. Naphthalene metabolites were also separated by HPLC using a C18 µbondapak column eluted with a 5-95% methanol in 0.5% acetic acid linear gradient over 15 min. Characterisation of some naphthalene conjugates was achieved by mass-spectrometry.

RESULTS AND DISCUSSION
Biliary excretion and enterohepatic circulation of [^{14}C]-BP Table 1 shows the extent of biliary and urinary excretion of ^{14}C after i.v. dosing of BP to rats and rabbits. In both species the bile is a major excretory route. However, in the rabbit which is less able than the rat to excrete certain anionic metabolites in the bile (13), the urine contains significantly more of the dose. The rabbit is thought to be better model than the rat with respect to the route of excretion of xenobiotics in man (1). The enterohepatic circulation of biliary metabolites shows that some 20% of the intraduodenal dose is re-excreted in the bile of both rats and rabbits, but again urinary excretion is significantly higher in the rabbit.

TABLE 1: EXCRETION AND ENTEROHEPATIC CIRCULATION OF [^{14}C]-BENZO(a)PYRENE
Dose: A, 3 µmol/kg i.v.; B, duodenal [^{14}C]-BP biliary metabolites

Animal	Dose A % Dose Excreted (6h) Bile	Urine	Dose B % Dose ^{14}C re-excreted* Bile	Urine
Rat	59+12 (7)	< 3.0 (7)	19+6.5 (7)	1.3+ 0.7 (7)
Rabbit	30+ 5.6 (5)	12+3.0 (5)	21+7.3 (3)	14 +11 (3)

Data: Mean + S.D. (n)   * rat 30 h, rabbit 23 h

Incubation of bile and urine, from rats administered [^{14}C-BP] i.v., with β-glucuronidase rendered some 40% of the radioactivity extractable into ethyl acetate. HPLC analysis of the ethyl acetate extract shows that BP-4,5-diol is the major aglycone in bile at a dose of 3 µmol/kg of BP (Table 2). When this bile is infused intraduodenally in enterohepatic circulation experiments, the re-excreted bile analysed over 0- 10 h and 20-30 h periods shows essentially the same metabolite pattern as the infused bile. In all these experiments, the proximate carcinogen BP-7,8-diol is either undetectable or at a very low level.

TABLE 2: BILIARY METABOLITES OF [^{14}C]-BENZO(a)PYRENE IN THE RAT

| Metabolite | % Total ^{14}C in: | | |
	Infused 0-2 h Bile (n = 5)*	Re-excreted bile (n = 3) 0-10 h	20-30 h
9,10-diol	< 1.2	< 1.5	< 1.5
4,5-diol	6.5 ±1.3	5.3 ±1.4	7.2 ±1.1
7,8-diol	< 0.5	n.d.	n.d.
3,6-quinone	2.3 +3.1	2.3 ±3.5	2.3 ±2.3
9-hydroxy	2.1 ±0.7	0.9 +0.6	1.7 +1.7
3-hydroxy	2.0 +0.2	1.9 ±1.7	1.1 +0.9

Data: Mean + S.D.
* From rats dosed with [^{14}C]-BP at 3 μmol/kg i.v.

Further experiments were performed in rats fitted with re-entrant cannulae allowing intermittent bile collection. After a single radioactive dose, the label could still be detected in the bile ater 7 days, illustrating the persistence of BP metabolites in the enterohepatic circulation. Analysis of metabolites was possible in bile samples up to 32 h (Table 3) and in this experiment the proximate carcinogen BP-7,8-diol was present as a higher proportion of total ^{14}C than in the acute experiments.

TABLE 3: [^{14}C]-BENZO(a)PYRENE METABOLITES IN INTERMITTENT RAT BILE COLLECTIONS

Dose: 3 μmole/kg i.v. to rats with re-entrant bile duct cannulae

| Metabolite | % of biliary ^{14}C at: | | | |
	1h	6.5h	22h	32h
4,5-diol	5.6	5.0	3.7	2.8
7,8-diol	0.8	3.2	1.2	0.6
3,6-quinone	0.3	1.3	<0.5	1.7
9-hydroxy	1.3	<0.5	<0.5	<0.5
3-hydroxy	1.9	5.7	5.4	1.2

Data are from pooled bile samples from 2 rats collected for 30 min periods at the time points shown.

Influence of dose on species differences in [^{3}H]-BP metabolism Experiments were carried out using [^{3}H]-BP to investigate the influence of dose on the metabolite pattern (Table 4). It can be seen that there is a clear species difference in the main sites of oxidative attack. In the rabbit BP-9,10-diol is the predominant metabolite, particularly at the low dose of 3 μmol/kg, whereas in the rat 4,5-diol formation and the production of quinones (probably originating from phenols (14)) appear to be the main routes of metabolism. This marked species variation may be due to regiospecificity of the mono- oxygenase system. Partially purified cytochromes P-450 from the non-induced livers of rabbits have a very high degree of specificity to form the 9,10-epoxide (15,16). At the high dose in the rabbit, there appears to be a considerable increase in the proportions of the 3- and 9-hydroxy metabolites produced.

TABLE 4: EFFECT OF DOSE ON THE BILIARY METABOLITES OF [^{3}H]-BP
Dose: A, 3 µmol/kg, or B, 40 µmol/kg

	% ^{3}H in bile			
Metabolite	Rat		Rabbit	
	Dose A	Dose B	Dose A	Dose B
Conjugates/- polyhydroxylates	4.3+1.1	2.4+0.8	3.9+1.1	7.1+0.3
BP 9,10-diol	<0.5	<0.5	14.1+1.0	9.9+2.5
BP 4,5-diol	6.4+1.4	3.7+1.1	<0.5	0.8+0.2
BP 7,8-diol	<0.5	<0.5	<0.5	0.7+0.2
BP 1,6-quinone	1.6+0.5	3.7+0.8	1.1+0.1	2.3+0.2
BP 3,6-quinone	5.4+1.8	11.6+0.6	2.7+0.4	1.7+0.2
BP 6,12-quinone	1.4+0.1	3.7+1.1	– not detected –	
9-hydroxy	<0.5	1.0+0.2	<0.5	3.8+0.8
3-hydroxy	<0.5	<0.5	<0.5	4.8+1.6

Mutagenicity of biliary metabolites of BP   Bile from rats and rabbits given [^{3}H]-BP at 40 µmol/kg was tested for mutagenic activity using the bacterial tester strain Salmonella typhimurium TA98 (17). Bile from both species (containing approx. 40 nmol BP metabolites per 100 µl) showed an increase in reverse gene mutation frequency in the presence of β- glucuronidase without S9 fraction. Since an S9 preparation is not needed to produce the mutagenic component, it is unlikely to be derived from BP 7,8-diol or from 3- or 9-OH BP, all of which require further metabolism for mutagenicity (18,19). A reactive intermediate is formed from the glucuronic acid conjugate of 3-OH BP when this is hydrolysed with β - glucuronidase (20). On testing the mutagenicity of benzo(a)pyrene 3-O-glucuronide (17), a significant number of revertants was found using amounts of this conjugate similar to those present in bile samples of animals dosed with BP at 40 µmol/kg. In addition to the mutagenicity, BP metabolites in rabbit bile, when incubated with β -glucuronidase, irreversibly bind to protein and to herring sperm DNA (5).

Distribution of BP metabolites from the intestine   In order to investigate the possible distribution of biliary BP metabolites to intestinal, lung and liver tissues during reabsorption and enterohepatic circulation, bile containing BP metabolites was infused into the duodena of a group of animals and the tissues were removed after 24 h. The distribution of radioactivity in rats is shown in

Table 5. In rabbits a similar distribution was found but with a larger proportion of the dose (23%) in the urine and correspondingly less in the intestine and faeces.

TABLE 5: DISTRIBUTION OF [^{3}H] AFTER DUODENAL ADMINISTRATION OF BILIARY METABOLITES OF [^{3}H]-BENZO(a)PYRENE IN THE RAT

Dose: 2.5 μmol BP metabolites/kg; Sp.Act. 0.625 Ci/mmol

Tissue	% dose of ^{3}H
Lung	0.07 + 0.02
Liver	0.5 + 0.1
Intestinal tissue	1.3 + 0.4
Intestinal contents	17.1 + 5.2
Faeces	59.7 + 6.2
Urine	1.3 + 0.3

Thus, enterohepatic recycling of potentially mutagenic BP metabolites leads to their persistence in vivo; BP metabolites can be detected in the bile of rats possessing an uninterrupted enterohepatic circulation, for at least a week following a single i.v. dose of BP. The fact that radioactivity reaches the urine and lung tissue following the intraduodenal administration of biliary metabolites of [^{3}H]-BP (Table 5), demonstrates that certain metabolites can not only traverse the intestinal wall but can also reach the systemic circulation.

Enterohepatic circulation of glutathione conjugates   The glutathione fraction of BP metabolites has not been studied in detail in vivo. However, we have shown extensive enterohepatic circulation of the glutathione conjugate of naphthalene (10,11).

TABLE 6: EXCRETION OF [^{14}C]-NAPHTHALENE IN THE RAT

Dose: 3 μmol/kg

Time (days)	% Dose excreted	
	Urine	Faeces
0–1	80.4 + 10.1	7.8 + 2.2
1–2	6.1 + 1.7	1.1 + 1.0
2–3	2.5 + 0.7	1.6 + 0.7
3–4	0.8 + 0.3	0.5 + 0.2
4–5	0.5 + 0.2	0.2 + 0.1
Total	90.3 + 7.1	11.1 + 3.8

From Table 6, it can be seen that in normal rats 90% of a dose of [^{14}C]-naphthalene is excreted in the urine. The major urinary metabolite is N-acetyl-S-(1,2-dihydro-1-hydroxy- 2-naphthyl)-cysteine, a "premercapturic acid". However, in bile-duct-cannulated rats, 64% of the dose is excreted in the bile (6

h) with the major metabolite being S-(1,2-dihydro-1- hydroxy-2-naphthyl)-glutathione (76% of biliary ^{14}C in 0-2 h). When [^{14}C]-naphthalene biliary metabolites are infused intraduodenally, absorption and re-excretion occur as shown in Table 7.

TABLE 7: ENTEROHEPATIC CIRCULATION OF [^{14}C]-NAPHTHALENE
BILIARY METABOLITES

Dose: Duodenal infusion of 0.1 µmol [^{14}C]-biliary metabolites

| Route | Time (h) | % Dose excreted [^{14}C]-biliary metabolites | | [^{14}C]-GSH |
		Control	Antibiotic treated	conjugate
Bile	0-1	7.4+ 1.9	3.6+ 1.6	2.5+2.0
	1-2	15.0+ 3.8	15.7+ 2.1	13.3+4.9
	2-3	4.9+ 1.5	6.8+ 1.7	11.4+2.3
	3-4	1.6+ 0.8	2.8+ 2.2	3.5+1.7
	4-5	0.9+ 0.4	1.4+ 1.0	1.8+0.8
	5-6	0.6+ 0.3	0.7+ 0.5	1.1+0.4
	0-24	32.4+ 4.2	32.4+10.0	37.7+2.6
Urine	0-24	27.9+20.3	51.6+ 8.4	44.5+2.5

Values are mean + S.D.

Antibiotic pretreatment (neomycin, tetracycline and bacitracin for 3 days) suppresses the intestinal flora but has no effect on the enterohepatic circulation of the [^{14}C]- naphthalene glutathione conjugate. Also, absorption and re- excretion of ^{14}C in the bile is rapid in the first 3 h and has virtually ceased after 6 h. These observations are in marked contrast to those made with several glucuronides (21), where the enterohepatic circulation is markedly decreased by antibiotic pretreatment and there is a lag period of some 4 h before substantial enterohepatic circulation takes place. Presumably, this lag time is for passage of the glucuronides to the site of maximal bacterial β - glucuronidase hydrolysis (22).

The major urinary metabolite after intraduodenal infusion of the [^{14}C]-naphthalene glutathione conjugate is the corresponding N-acetyl cysteine conjugate confirming that a substantial portion of the urinary "premercapturate" arises from the glutathione conjugate initially excreted in the bile. This process appears not to be dependent on the activity of the microbial flora whichare, however, important in the fission of the C-S bond by bacterial C-S-lyase (23,24).

ACKNOWLEDGEMENTS

This work was supported by a grant from the Cancer Research Campaign. M.A. Pue was in receipt of a research studentship from the Medical Research Council

REFERENCES

1. Millburn,P. (1976) in: Taylor,W. (Ed.), The Hepatobiliary System, Plenum Press, New York, pp.109.

2. Chipman,J.K. (1982) Toxicology, 25, 99.

3. Chipman,J.K., Hirom,P.C., Frost,G.S. and Millburn,P. (1981) Biochem.Pharmacol., 30, 937.

4. Boroujerdi,M., Kung,H.C., Wilson,A.G.E. and Anderson,M.W. (1981) Cancer Res., 41, 951.

5. Chipman,J.K., Bhave,N.A., Hirom,P.C. and Millburn,P. (1982) Xenobiotica, 12, 397.

6. Renwick,A.G. and Drasar,B.S. (1976) Nature, 263, 234.

7. Plummer,J.L., Smith,B.R., Ball,L.M. and Bend,J.R. (1980) Drug Metab.Dispos., 8, 68.

8. Bakke,J.E, Gustaffson,J.A. and Gustaffson,B.E. (1980) Science, 24, 433.

9. Boyland,E., Ramsey,G.S. and Sims,P. (1961) Biochem.J., 78, 376.

10. Pue,M.A., Frost,G.S. and Hirom,P.C. (1982) Biochem.Soc. Trans., 10, 112.

11. Pue,M.A., Frost,G.S. and Hirom,P.C. (1982) Brit.J.Pharm., 77, 421P.

12. Connor,T.H., Forti,G.C., Sitra,P. and Legator,M.S. (1979) Environ.Mutagen., 1, 269.

13. Hirom,P.C., Millburn,P., Smith,R.L. and Williams,R.T. (1972) Biochem.J., 129, 1071.

14. Sims,P. (1967) Biochem.Pharmacol., 16, 613.

15. Wiebel,F.J., Selkirk,J.K., Gelboin,H.V., Haugen,D.A., van der Hoeven,T.A. and Coon,M.J. (1975) Proc.Natl.Acad. Sci.USA, 72, 3917.

16. Deutsch,J., Leutz,J.C., Yang,S.K., Gelboin,H.V., Chiang,Y.L., Vatsis,K.P. and Coon,M.J. (1978) Proc.Natl. Acad.Sci.USA, 75, 3123.

17. Chipman,J.K., Millburn,P. and Brooks,T.M. (1983) Toxicol. Lett., in press.

18. Owens,I.S., Koteen,G.M. and Legraverend,C. (1979) Biochem. Pharmacol., 28, 1615.

19. Wood,A.W., Levin,W., Lu,A.Y.H., Yagi,H., Hernandez,O., Jerina,D.M. and Conney,A.H. (1976) J.Biol.Chem., 251, 4882.

20. Kinoshita,N. and Gelboin,H.V. (1978) Science, 199, 307.

21. Parker,R.J., Hirom,P.C. and Millburn,P. (1980) Xenobiotica, 10, 689.

22. Colburn,W.A., Hirom,P.C., Parker,R.J. and Millburn,P. (1979) Drug Metab.Dispos., 7, 100.

23. Bakke,J.E., Aschbacher,P.W., Feil,V.J. and Gustafsson,B.E. (1981) Xenobiotica, 11, 173.

24. Bakke,J.E. (1982) Biomed.Mass Spectrometry, 9, 74.

© 1983 Elsevier Science Publishers B.V.
Extrahepatic Drug Metabolism and Chemical Carcinogenesis,
J. Rydström, J. Montelius and M. Bengtsson eds.

XENOBIOTICS, THE INTESTINAL FLORA, AND CARCINOGENESIS

RORY P. REMMEL AND PETER GOLDMAN
Departments of Pharmacology and Nutrition, Harvard University, 665 Huntington Avenue, Boston, MA 02115 (U.S.A.)

Xenobiotic compounds that participate in chemical carcinogenesis have been classified as either initiators or promoters. Initiators are compounds that damage DNA either directly or more commonly after transformation to electrophilic metabolites. The electrophilic metabolites have been shown to arise in organs such as the liver but they, or their precursors, may also be formed within the intestinal microflora. Other reactions may eliminate these electrophiles or their precursors; thus, in principle metabolic reactions may either increase or decrease a carcinogen's potency. Metabolism may also affect the action of promoters, compounds that, although not carcinogenic themselves, act to enhance the potency of an initiator, perhaps by stimulating the production of reactive forms of oxygen or other free radicals (1). This presentation will stress the influence of the intestinal microflora on metabolism as it may relate to carcinogenesis. A more comprehensive review of reactions attributed to the intestinal bacteria has been provided by Scheline (2).

Xenobiotic biotransformations that take place in the liver and other tissues have been classified as either phase I or phase II. Phase I reactions introduce new functional groups that usually render a molecule more water soluble. Many phase I reactions are oxidative in character and are catalyzed by the cytochrome P-450 system. Those that have been implicated in carcinogenesis include epoxidation of aromatic hydrocarbons and N-hydroxylation of aminoaromatic compounds. The phase II reaction most strongly implicated in carcinogenesis is conjugation to sulfate.

The reactions catalyzed by the intestinal microflora often oppose the phase I and II reactions of mammalian tissues. The flora is highly anaerobic and therefore tends to

utilize xenobiotic compounds as electron acceptors. The
result is that phase I reactions mediated by the flora are
reductive rather than oxidative. Another contrast is that
bacteria of the flora hydrolyze the conjugates formed in
phase II mammalian reactions. As the flora tends to carry
out either reductive or deconjugative reactions, one may
predict the likelihood that the flora is responsible for a
metabolic reaction in vivo. How then does one assess the
role of the flora in the metabolism of a specific compound?

One method is to incubate a compound or its metabolites with
pure or mixed cultures of fecal or intestinal microorganisms. If
the incubation is carried out under anaerobic conditions, which
are characteristic of the intestinal flora's natural environment,
a preliminary assessment of the flora's capability may be made.
Fecal bacteria, however, are not necessarily representative of
the bacteria that exist normally in the various microenvironments
along the intestinal tract. The bacteria of the feces, which
constitute 10 to 40% of the fecal mass, appear to be similar to
those of the cecum of animals such as the rat, guinea pig and
mouse. In man and rabbits, however, bifidobacteria are a
thousand fold higher in the rectum and the feces than in the
colon. Thus, the feces provide a readily available source of
intestinal bacteria, but only a rough guide to the metabolic
activity of the flora.

The role of the flora may also be assessed by the use of
gnotobiotic animals. If certain metabolites of a compound appear
in the excreta of a conventional rat, but are not found in those
of a germfree rat, then the flora is presumed to be involved.
The presumption becomes more likely if the missing metabolites
appear when bacteria capable of catalyzing the missing reactions
are associated with the germfree rat. However, reactions carried
out by gnotobiotic animals are not necessarily simply the sum of
those carried out by the component mammalian and bacterial enzyme
systems (3, 4).

Experiments with bile acids and steroids, compounds which
have a possible relationship to carcinogenesis, illustrate the
problem of the inconsistencies between in vitro and in vivo
bacterial metabolism. Taurine and glycine conjugates of deoxy-

cholic acid are readily hydrolyzed by strains of some of the many
bacterial genera that comprise the normal flora. Yet relatively
few of these strains confer on the monocontaminated gnotobiotic
rat the capacity to carry out these reactions in vivo (4). Indeed, even if the reaction demonstrated in bacterial culture can
be conferred on the gnotobiotic rat, its extent is less than what
might be anticipated from in vitro reaction rates and the degree
of bacterial colonization. Furthermore, it may be difficult to
isolate in pure culture bacteria that seem so clearly to carry
out a reaction within the host. For example, none of the more
than 100 intestinal bacteria isolated in one study were capable
of catalyzing the 7α-dehydroxylation of bile acids in vitro,
although this reaction affects more than 85% of the bile acids in
the feces (4). Thus, it may not merely be the bacteria per se
but their environment within the host, particularly their association with other organisms, which determines the reactions
carried out by the flora.

Studies in germfree rats established years ago that the flora
was solely responsible for some of the biochemical dehydroxyla-
tions of steroids that occur in vivo (5). Only recently, however, have bacteria been isolated in pure culture that are capable of carrying out these reactions in vitro. Thus, the 21-
dehydroxylation of 11-deoxycorticosterone and the 16α-dehydrox-
ylation of 16α-hydroxyprogesterone, reactions that had previously
been observed only in mixed cultures, have now been demonstrated
in pure cultures of fecal isolates phenotypically resembling
Eubacterium lentum (6). It remains to be determined, however,
whether these bacteria will catalyze these reactions in a
gnotobiotic host.

Supression of the flora by antibiotics has also been used to
implicate intestinal bacteria in the metabolism of a xenobiotic
compound. Neomycin, bacitracin, and tetracycline, first employed
by R. T. Williams, virtually sterilize the feces. However,
several problems are associated with the use of this mixture.
Neomycin and other aminoglycosides cause malabsorption in man and
may interfere with drug absorption. Also, antibiotics may exert
a direct effect on the pharmacokinetics of a compound. Thus,
germ-free rats and ex-germfree rats were found to have similar

volumes of distribution for warfarin (7), but the volume of distribution was decreased when rats in the ex-germfree state were
treated with the antibiotic mixture. Furthermore, clearance was
decreased in antibiotic-treated ex-germfree rats, perhaps as the
result of an inhibition of drug-metabolizing systems by tetracycline. These effects and the possibility of antibiotic-induced
diarrhea, which might influence either the absorption or fecal
elimination of a compound, suggest that the action of antibiotics
may not be limited to the suppression of the flora and its metabolic activity.

Cycasin (methylazoxymethanol-β-D-glucoside), a component of
cycad meal, provides the classic illustration of the flora's
role in chemical carcinogenesis (8). Orally administered cycasin is hepatoxic and produces tumors in the liver, kidney and
intestines of conventional rats. Toxicity seems to require
contact with the flora because cycasin is not toxic after parenteral administration and is not toxic by any route for germfree rats. The importance of metabolism was suggested by finding that cycasin's aglycone, methylazoxymethanol, was toxic to
both conventional and germfree animals. Furthermore, recovery
of cycasin was less than 35% after administration to conventional rats, but was almost complete when administered to germfree
rats. Experiments with gnotobiotic rats provided the final link
between toxicity and bacterial metabolism. Rats associated only
with Streptococcus fecalis, a bacterium with strong glycosidase
activity, developed typical cycasin lesions. Lesions did not
develop, however, when the associated bacteria lacked glucosidase activity and were mild when the associated bacteria had
only limited glucosidase activity (9). Thus, the flora's glucosidase activity was found to be obligatory for the toxicity of
cycasin. This conclusion was extended to glucuronidase activity
as well, by the finding that the cycasin derivative, methyl-
azoxymethanol-β-D-glucosiduronic acid, caused tumors in conventional but not in germfree rats (10).

This study reemphasizes the special in vivo role of bacterial β-glucuronidases. Bacterial enzymes are also obligatory for
the enterohepatic circulation. Glucuronides of both endogenous
and exogenous compounds are excreted in the bile and are hydro-

lyzed in the gut. This process, which permits reabsorption of the parent compound, might be modulated by changes in the flora to alter the exposure of tissues to xenobiotic carcinogens such as benzo(a)pyrene or to endogenous factors such as the bile acids. Similarly, hydrolysis of sulfate conjugates by the flora may affect the pharmacokinetics of an estrogen monosulfate or a proximate chemical carcinogen such as the sulfate of N-hydroxy-2-acetylaminofluorene.

The flora also hydrolyzes the sulfamate bond of cyclamate to yield the weak mutagen, cyclohexylamine. This reaction is of particular interest because the amount of cyclohexylamine formed seems to be quite variable in human subjects (11) and to depend in part on the host's prior exposure to cyclamate. The mechanism of this "induction" of the flora's metabolism in response to exposure to xenobiotic compounds merits further study.

Of the reductive reactions carried out by the flora the most relevant to carcinogenesis are those with compounds containing the nitro and the N-hydroxyl group. 2,4-Dinitrotoluene (2,4-DNT), for example, is an industrial compound that causes hepatic tumors in rats. The flora seems to mediate an effect of this compound on DNA. Thus, an oral dose of 2,4-DNT causes an abnormally high rate of unscheduled DNA synthesis in primary hepatocytes from rats associated with a defined bacterial flora (87% in repair) compared to those from germfree animals (14% in repair) (12). The intestine appears to be the major site of reduction because 2,4-DNT is reduced much more rapidly in rat cecal contents than in liver microsomes and germfree rats excrete almost no amino metabolites. Furthermore, covalent binding of radioactivity in the liver after the administration of ^{14}C-2,4-DNT, is much less in germfree than in conventional rats (13). These experiments with 2,4-DNT provide a good example where the flora is required both for nitro group reduction and for phenomena that may relate to carcinogenesis.

The flora apparently is also responsible for the correlation between nitro group reduction and methemoglobinemia that occurs in response to nitroaromatic compounds such as nitrobenzene. Thus, nitrobenzene causes methemoglobinemia in conventional rats but not in antibiotic-treated or germfree rats (14). The flora, however, is not obligatory for all _in vivo_ nitro group reduction and its consequences. Methemoglobinemia in response to some nitroaromatic compounds is not diminished by antibiotics, perhaps because such compounds can be reduced by erythrocytes (15). Clearly, a case by case analysis must be made to determine the sites at which nitro compounds are reduced, and thus the extent to which the flora may be implicated in their toxicity.

It may be equally difficult to generalize about the role of the flora in the tumorigenicity of the 5-nitrofurans and nitro-imidazoles. The nitroheterocyclic compounds are believed to be activated through a series of reductive reactions such as those shown below.

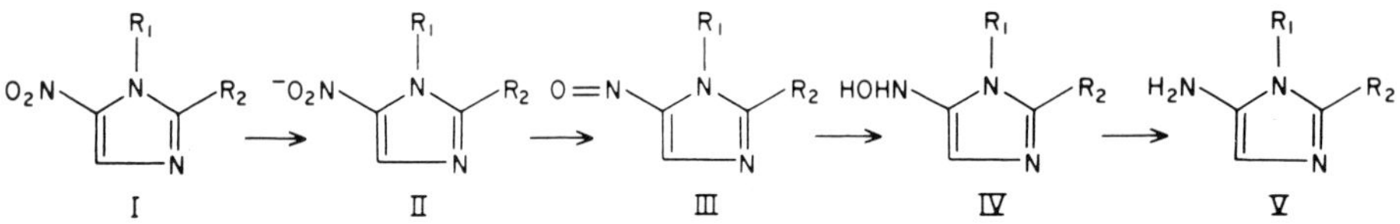

Intermediates comparable to the nitroso (III) and the hydroxyl-amino (IV) derivatives have been proposed in the reduction of nitroaromatic compounds. Similar compounds may mediate the DNA damage caused by nitroheterocyclic compounds. Alternatively, the damage may be mediated by the radical anion (II) acting either directly or through superoxide which forms as the result of an interaction with oxygen (16). To what extent do the flora and mammalian tissues catalyze this critical reaction sequence _in vivo_?

Comparative experiments in germfree and conventional rats have established that the flora carries out the reduction of metroni-dazole (17) and misonidazole (18). When the 5-nitroimidazole, metronidazole is reduced, it fragments to yield the metabolites acetamide and N-(2-hydroxyethyl)oxamic acid. These metabolites are complementary in the sense that they account for all the carbon atoms and all the nitrogen atoms in metronidazole except that in the nitro group. After metronidazole administration both metabolites are excreted by conventional rats, but not by germfree rats (17). Similar experiments establish a role for the flora in the reduction of the 2-nitroimidazole misonidazole. In the metabolism of misonidazole, however, reduction and ring fragmentation are separable. Thus, the urine of a misonidazole-treated rat contains the amino derivative of misonidazole as well as metabolites with the ring fragmented, e.g. urea or 2-hydroxy-3-methoxypropylguanidine (18, 19). These metabolites are merely the stable products that are isolable when a nitroimidazole is reduced; it is not clear whether they arise from a reactive species such as those in the figure above.

Stable products of the reduction of nitrofurazone and misonidazole, but not of metronidazole, can be isolated from the excreta of the germfree rat. This formation of metabolites, which presumably occurs in the tissues of the germfree rat, correlates with the one electron reduction potentials of the parent compounds, that of metronidazole being the most negative and therefore the hardest to reduce (19). Tissue reduction of a 5-nitrofuran may be important because of the suggestion that 5-nitrofurans are tumorigenic in germfree as well as in conventional rats (20). However, further comparisons between toxicity and metabolism of nitroheterocyclic compounds in both germfree and conventional rats must be made before the significance of the flora's metabolism can be assessed.

In the meantime one may speculate about how metabolism by the flora might explain the weak tumorigenicity of the 5-nitroimidazoles. One possibility is that tumorigenicity relates to the formation of acetamide, a metabolite of several of these compounds, and itself a weak tumorigen. Another possibility is that the flora reduces the nitroimidazole to a partially reduced intermediate that has sufficient stability to reach mammalian DNA as well as sufficient reactivity to interact with it. The involvement of free radicals in nitroheterocyclic reduction suggests that these compounds may have promoter activity. Yet their mutagenicity for bacteria as the result of reduction suggests that they act as initiators. In the case of metronidazole its interaction with DNA may be clarified by studies that show bactercidal activity to be related to its reductive metabolism (21). DNA is probably the target for this effect because metronidazole's effectiveness is enhanced in E. coli mutants that are defective in DNA repair (Yeung, McLafferty, Beaulieu and Goldman, unpublished).

N-Hydroxyl metabolites are obligatory intermediates in the activation of the carcinogens 2-acetylaminofluorene (2-AAF) and 4-acetamidobiphenyl (4-AAB). If these N-hydroxyl metabolites were reduced in vivo, as they are in vitro under anaerobic conditions by both the intestinal flora and mammalian tissues (22), the active form of these compounds and therefore their carcinogenicity would be decreased. However, N-hydroxyl compounds also have other fates. They may be conjugated in mammalian tissues either to yield the more carcinogenic sulfate or acetyl derivatives or the less carcinogenic glucuronide. The further metabolism of these conjugates thus provides an additional opportunity for an interaction with the flora. When N-OH-2AAF was administered to germfree rats, it was excreted in the feces conjugated mainly to glucuronic acid, whereas in conventional animals it was found mostly as unconjugated 2-AAF (23). Similar results were found with 4-AAB (24). The significance of these observations is unclear but might be clarified by longterm studies of carcinogenesis in germfree rats.

How the intestinal microflora may influence the potency of carcinogens containing azo bonds or N-oxides is uncertain. Although azo reduction by the flora is obligatory for the metabolism of sulfasalazine (25), the azo bonds of other compounds may be reduced in the liver. There is no evidence that the carcinogenicity of azo dyes, such as a dimethylaminoazobenzene, relate to the activity of the flora. Reduction of a pyrrolizidine alkaloid, indicine-N-oxide, by the flora (26) suggests a role for the flora in the activation of structurally related carcinogenic alkaloids.

The examples discussed in this review, indicate the potential importance of the flora in understanding the mechanism of chemical carcinogenesis. However, one must also recognize the difficulties in studying the flora and in extrapolating findings to man. An effect of diet on the flora, and thus on its metabolic capability, has been proposed to explain the relationship between diet and colon cancer. Diseases and drugs, particularly antibiotics, may also alter the distribution and composition of the flora. Sometimes antibiotics may have a surprisingly long-term effect on the bacterial flora. Marmosets, for example, were found to have a diminished capacity to reduce 4-nitrobenzoic acid many weeks after a course of neomycin, tetracycline, and bacitracin (27). Also, small animals such as the rat, although useful for research, tend to maximize the role of the flora, both because the flora is more extensively distributed throughout their gastrointestinal tracts and because biliary excretion may occur with compounds of lower molecular weight. Consequently, one must be cautious in extrapolating findings in rats and other experimental animals to conclusions concerning the role of the flora in the response of humans to xenobiotic compounds.

ACKNOWLEDGEMENTS

Experimental work by one of us (P.G.) reported in this review was supported in part by U.S. Public Health Service grant CA-15260 from the National Cancer Institute, National Institutes of Health.

REFERENCES

1. Emerit, I. and Cerutti, P. A. (1981) Nature, 293, 144.

2. Scheline, R. R. (1973) Pharmacol. Rev., 25, 451.

3. Peppercorn, M. A. and Goldman, P. (1972) Proc. Nat. Acad. Sci., 69, 1413.

4. Dickinson, A. B., Gustafsson, B. E. and Norman, A. (1971) Acta Path. Microbiol. Scand., Sect. B., 79, 691.

5. Gustafsson, J.-A. and Sjovall, J. (1968) Eur. J. Biochem., 6, 236.

6. Bokkenhauser, V. D. and Winter, J. (1980) Am. J. Clin. Nutr., 33, 2502.

7. Remmel, R. P., Pohl, L. R. and Elmer, G. W. (1981) Drug Metab. Disp., 9, 410.

8. Spatz, M., McDaniel, E. G. and Laqueur, G. L. (1966) Proc. Soc. Exp. Biol. Med., 121, 417.

9. Spatz, M., Smith, D. W. E., McDaniel, E. G. and Laqueur, G. L. (1967) Proc. Soc. Exp. Biol. Med., 124, 691.

10. Laqueur, G. L., Matsumota, H. and Yamamoto, R. S. (1981) J. Natl. Canc. Inst., 67, 1053.

11. Renwick, A. G. and Williams, R. T. (1972) Biochem. J., 129, 869.

12. Mirsalis, J. C., Hamm, T. E. Jr., Sherrill, J. M. and Butterworth, B. E. (1982) Nature, 295, 322.

13. Rickert, D. E., Long, R. M., Krakowka, S. and Dent, J.G.(1981) Toxicol. Appl. Pharmacol., 59, 574.

14. Reddy, B. G., Pohl, L. R. and Krishna, G. (1976) Biochem. Pharmacol., 25, 1119.

15. Facchini, V. and Griffiths, L. A. (1981) Biochem. Pharmacol., 30, 931.

16. Perez-Reyes, E., Kalyanaraman, B. and Mason, R. P. (1980) Mol. Pharmacol., 17, 239.

17. Koch, R. L., Chrystal, E. J. T., Beaulieu, B. B. Jr. and Goldman, P. (1979) Biochem. Pharmacol., 28, 3611.

18. Koch, R. L., Beaulieu, B. B. Jr. and Goldman, P. (1980) Biochem. Pharmacol., 29, 3281.

19. Yeung, T. C., Sudlow, G., Koch, R. L. and Goldman, P. (In press) Biochem. Pharmacol.

20. Wang, C. Y., Croft, W. A. and Bryan, G. T. (1980) The Pharmacologist, 22, 264.

21. Chrystal, E. J. T., Koch, R. L., McLafferty, M. A. and Goldman P. (1980) Antimicrob. Agents Chemother., 18, 566.

22. Williams, J. R. Jr., Grantham, P. H., March, H. H., Weisburger, J. H. and Weisburger, E. K. (1970) Biochem. Pharmacol., 19, 1973.

23. Weisburger, J. H., Grantham, P. H., Horton, R. E. and Weisburger, E. K. (1970) Biochem. Pharmacol., 19, 151.

24. Wheeler, L. A., Soderberg, F. A. and Goldman, P. (1975) Cancer Res., 35, 2962.

25. Peppercorn, M. A. and Goldman, P. (1972) J. Pharmacol. Exp. Ther., 181, 555.

26. Powis, G., Ames, M. M. and Kovach, J. S. (1979) Cancer Res., 39, 3564.

27. Kuzniar, E. J. A. and James, S. P. (1981) Xenobiotica, 11, 675.

© 1983 Elsevier Science Publishers B.V.
Extrahepatic Drug Metabolism and Chemical Carcinogenesis,
J. Rydström, J. Montelius and M. Bengtsson eds.

STUDIES WITH AMARANTH AND OUABAIN IN GERMFREE RATS

DAVID HEWICK AND SYLVIA WILSON*
Department of Pharmacology and Therapeutics, Ninewells Hospital and Medical School,
Dundee. DD1 9SY Scotland.

INTRODUCTION

Germfree (GF) rats may be of value in elucidating the metabolism and disposition of
carcinogens and other xenobiotics where the gut flora are implicated. However, GF
rats exhibit certain differences from conventional (CV) rats making the interpretation of
such studies more difficult (eg. male GF rats; cardiac output is reduced by 30%, hepatic
and intestinal blood flows are reduced by 50% (1)). Since liver blood flow is likely to
affect the biliary excretion of xenobiotics, we initiated studies comparing drug handling
in GF and CV rats using amaranth and ouabain, compounds normally excreted unchanged
solely in the bile (2).

MATERIALS AND METHODS

Littermate pairs of inbred GF and CV BDIX rats (10-12 weeks old) were anaesthetised (urethane 50%, 1.5g/kg, i.m.). Expt.1: the biliary excretion of amaranth (20mg/
ml, 20mg/kg i.v.) in bile duct cannulated rats was determined (2). Expt. 2: ouabain
was infused (7.5mg/ml, 1.9ml/h, i.v.) until cardiac arrest. The heart, liver, stomach and intestines were weighed. Livers from Expt. 2 were used to determine the
hepatocyte nuclear volume proportion (3). Data were compared using Student's paired
t-test ($P<0.05$ significant). Means $\pm$ SE are given.

RESULTS AND DISCUSSION

For GF rats bile flow was reduced by 50 and 16% in males and females respectively, amaranth excretion was initially lower in males but largely unaffected in females
(Fig.1). Expt.2: the lethal dose was 16% lower for GF (16.8 ± 0.6mg/kg) than CV (19.9
±0.5mg/kg) males, and 35% lower for GF (26.9 ± 2.9mg/kg) than CV (41.3 ± 5.9mg/kg)
females. Apart from typical caecal enlargement, and reduced liver weight in the GF rat
(Table 1), relative organ weights were similar to CV. The hepatocyte nuclear volume
proportion was 34% greater for GF (25.6 ± 0.2%) than CV (19.1 ± 0.8%)males, and 24%
greater for GF (24.9 ± 0.5%) than CV (20.1 ± 0.3%) females. Nuclear diameters were

*A recipient of an XNI Award from the Dept. of Education, N.Ireland.

not different. It is puzzling why GF female rats with an unimpaired ability to excrete amaranth in the bile, should be relatively more susceptible to ouabain than GF males. The decreased GF rat liver weight may result from a reduced liver blood flow (1). Hypotrophy is suggested since the increase in GF hepatocyte nuclear volume proportion (without a change in nuclear size) implies a decrease in cytoplasm.

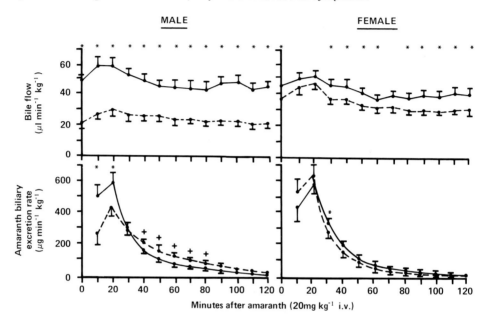

Fig.1. Biliary amaranth excretion in GF •- -• and CV •—• rats (n=7). Means ± SE are given. *CV>GF and +GF>CV (P<0.05).

TABLE 1.BODY AND ORGAN WEIGHT DIFFERENCES IN GF COMPARED TO CV RATS

Organ[a]	Male		Female	
	Expt.1 (n=7)	Expt.2(n=4)	Expt.1(n=7)	Expt.2(n=5)
Liver	24% ↓	27% ↓	28% ↓	18% ↓
Caecum+contents	91% ↑	121% ↑	292% ↑	260% ↑
−contents	nsd	nsd	55% ↑	41% ↑
Body weight	11% ↓	8% ↓	nsd	11% ↓

[a]Calculations on g/kg basis.   nsd - no significant difference.

REFERENCES
1. Gordon H.A. (1968) in : The Germfree Animal in Research. Eds. Coates M.E., Gordon H.A. & Wostmann B.S., Academic Press, London pp 127-150.

2. Klaassen C.D. & Strom S.C. (1978) Drug Metab. & Disposit. 6, 121.

3. Anderson J.M. (1982) in : Histometry. Eds. Bancroft J.D. & Stevens A., Churchill Livingstone, London pp 548-563.

© 1983 Elsevier Science Publishers B.V.
Extrahepatic Drug Metabolism and Chemical Carcinogenesis,
J. Rydström, J. Montelius and M. Bengtsson eds.

METABOLISM OF 1-NITROPYRENE IN GERM-FREE AND CONVENTIONAL RATS: ROLE OF THE GUT FLORA IN GENERATION OF MUTAGENIC METABOLITES.

L.M. BALL[1], J.J. RAFTER[2], J.-A. GUSTAFSSON[2], B.E. GUSTAFSSON[3] and J. LEWTAS[1]
[1] Health Effects Research Laboratory, U.S. Environmental Protection Agency, Research Triangle Park, NC (U.S.A.); [2] Department of Medical Nutrition, Huddinge University Hospital, Huddinge (Sweden) and [3] Department of Germfree Research, Karolinska Institute, Stockholm (Sweden)

INTRODUCTION

Nitropyrenes have been identified in combustion emissions, and may contribute substantially to the mutagenicity of these sources of air pollution. 1-Nitro-[^{14}C]pyrene (NP) underwent extensive metabolism in the rat (1), to urinary mutagens which unlike the parent NP require exogenous metabolic activation (S9). The major urinary mutagenic metabolite of NP was both reduced and acetylated on the nitrogen, and hydroxylated on the aromatic pyrene moiety (NAAP-OH). Since the gut flora are known to reduce nitro compounds in vivo, we compared the metabolism of NP in conventional and germ-free rats of the same strain, to evaluate the role of the intestinal flora in the formation of mutagenic metabolites and the enterohepatic circulation (EHC) undergone by the metabolites of NP.

MATERIALS AND METHODS

Germ-free rats of the AGUS strain, raised and maintained in stainless steel isolators by the methods of Gustafsson, and conventional rats matched for age and sex, were injected ip with 1-nitro[^{14}C]pyrene (2.8μCi/μmol; 1.2 to 1.5 mg per per rat). Urine and faeces were collected and analysed for ^{14}C content by liquid scintillation counting. 8-24h Urines were tested for mutagenicity in the Ames Salmonella plate incorporation assay, and also analysed by HPLC for metabolite content after hydrolysis with β-glucuronidase and sulphatase.

RESULTS

The overall recovery of ^{14}C after 144h was similar (85-100 % of dose) in conventional and in germ-free rats, and excretion patterns were little different between male and female. Total urinary excretion was lower in germfree than in conventional rats (Table 1) indicating that some of the urinary metabolites in conventional rats could arise from recirculation of material originally excreted via the bile. Most of the urinary ^{14}C was recovered from 8 to 24h after dosing (12.7% of dose in conventional, 6-7 % in germ-free rats, ♀ similar to ♂).

TABLE 1

CUMULATIVE EXCRETION OF ^{14}C BY FEMALE RATS DOSED WITH 1-NITRO[^{14}C]PYRENE (%DOSE)

Time after dosing(h)	24		48		144	
Animals (n)	Urine	Faeces	Urine	Faeces	Urine	Faeces
Conventional (3)	14.7±2.8	4.7±4.4	22.0±5.2	34.9±11.5	27.7±3.4	55.5±7.6
Germ-free (3)	8.1±1.2[a]	3.5±4.4	14.2±4.1[a]	23.8±5.0	17.7±4.9[a]	71.8±11.0

[a]Significantly different from conventional, $P \leqslant 0.05$

The percentage of ^{14}C present as NAAP-OH in 8-24h urines from germ-free rats was one-tenth of that in the conventional rats (Table 2). The conventional urines showed low direct-acting mutagenicity in the Ames assay, increased ten-fold by addition of S9. The urines from germ-free rats also contained weak direct-acting mutagens, whose activity was slightly decreased when S9 was added. The specific mutagenicity of the urines correlated with their NAAP-OH content.

TABLE 2

METABOLITES AND MUTAGENICITY IN 8-24H URINE FROM RATS DOSED WITH 1-NITROPYRENE

Female Rats	% of urinary ^{14}C as NAAP-OH	Specific mutagenicity[a] -S9	+S9	Correlation[b] (r^2, n=6)
Conventional (3)	23.4±7.7	8±2	89±26	0.96
Germ-free (3)	2.3±0.5[c]	25±14	16±10[c]	

[a]Revertants/nmole of urinary NP metabolites, assayed in Salmonella TA98
[b]Specific mutagenicity (+S9) versus % of urinary ^{14}C as NAAP-OH
[c]Significantly different from conventional, $p \leqslant 0.05$

DISCUSSION

The gut flora thus contribute to the disposition of NP in vivo by generating specific mutagenic metabolites and by releasing biliary metabolites for EHC.

ACKNOWLEDGEMENTS

LMB was supported by a Resident Research Associateship Award from the National Research Council, Washington, DC (U.S.A.)
"Abstract of a proposed presentation; does not necessarily reflect EPA policy."

REFERENCES

1. Ball, Kohan, Inmon, Claxton & Lewtas: Metabolism of 1-nitro[^{14}C]pyrene in the rat and mutagenicity of urinary metabolites. Submitted, Cancer Res, 1983.

© 1983 Elsevier Science Publishers B.V.
Extrahepatic Drug Metabolism and Chemical Carcinogenesis,
J. Rydström, J. Montelius and M. Bengtsson eds.

KINETIC ASPECTS OF 2-ACETYLAMINOFLUORENE UPTAKE, METABOLISM, EXCRETION AND ENTEROHEPATIC CIRCULATION

LENNART C ERIKSSON[1], JOANN SPIEWAK[2], WAHEED ROOMI[2] AND EMMANUEL FARBER[2]

[1]Department of Pathology, Karolinska Institutet, Huddinge University Hospital, 141 86 Huddinge, Sweden and [2]Department of Pathology, University of Toronto, Toronto, Canada.

INTRODUCTION

In the process of chemical carcinogenesis in the liver, cell populations develop which are resistant to a wide variety of toxic substances, amoung them 2-acetylaminofluorene (1,2). To further understand the mechanisms of this for the process fundamental cell property and its consequences for the progress to malignant neoplasia we have investigated some pharmacokinetic properties of 2-acetylaminofluorene in normal rat, in rats with increased (3-MC) or decreased (Co-heme) metabolism of the drug and in hepatocyte nodules, which represent cell populations resistant to the mitoinhibitory effect of the substance.

MATERIALS AND METHODS

Fischer 344 rats were used. 3-Methylcholanthrene (3-MC), 40 mg/kg/day for 5 days. Cobalt-heme (Co-heme), 100 ug/kg in one subcutaneous dose. The experiments were performed 3 days later when the cyt P-450 levels were 20% of normal. Hepatocyte nodules were produced by the resistant hepatocyte model (3) or by cyclic feeding of 2-acetylaminofluorene for 25 weeks followed by basal diet for 5 weeks. 2-Acetylaminofluorene-9-^{14}C dissolved in rat serum was injected in a branch of the superior mesenteric vein (intra portal injection). Analysis of 2-acetylaminofluorene metabolites was performed using and HPLC method. The de-glucuronidation was done using bacterial -glucuronidase at 37°C for 24 hours. The experiments on enterohepatic circulation were performed using Wistar rats. Bile with excreted drug metabolites was given in the small gut of the experimental animal.

RESULTS

2-Acetylaminofluorene is taken up by the liver very fast. Initially microsomes have a high affinity for the drug, but after 1 h binding is equal to all fractions (Fig.1). Nodular kinetic resembles normal but microsomes retain less and the rate of decrease in drug amount associated to the microsomes is slower than the normal rate.

From Fig. 2 is concluded that drug metabolism is the limiting factor for drug excretion to bile. When liver metabolism and excretion are slow, metabolites are excreted in the urine to a larger extent. (Table 1). The fraction of glucuronic acid conjugated metabolites reflects the activity of the UDP-glucuronyl transferase. The parent compound is not found in bile or urine, but can be extracted from blood and liver.

Experiments on enterohepatic circulation show that only a fraction of the drug is participating in the process. After 25 h 26% of given dose is excreted

to bile and 9% to urine, while 51% is still remaining in the gut. At this
time rates of absorbtion and excretion are very low, around 5% of maximal rate.

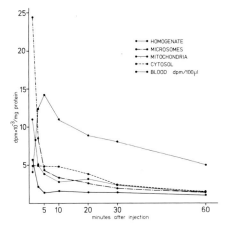

Fig. 1. Intracellular distribution of
radioactivity after intra portal injection of 2-acetylaminofluorene-9-^{14}C.

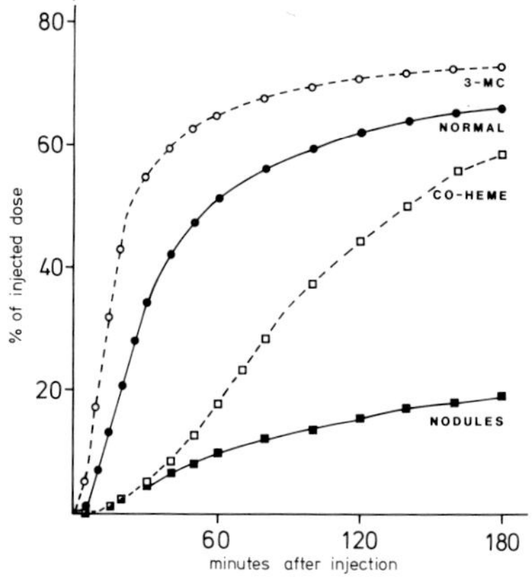

Fig. 2. Appearance of radioactivity in
bile after intra portal administration
of 2-acetylaminofluorene-9-^{14}C.

TABLE 1

Fractionated ether extraction of 2-acetylaminofluorene metabolites excreted in
bile and urine for three hours. % of given dose. 4 exp.

Animals	Ether extractable compound		Extractable after -glucuronidase		Non extractable compound	
	Bile	Urine	Bile	Urine	Bile	Urine
Normal rat	5.8 ± 1.5	0.22	5.9 ± 2.2	3.5	51.8 ± 4.0	15.0
3-MC rat	8.0 ± 2.0	0.13	23.0 ± 3.2	9.8	51.1 ± 2.6	9.0
Co-heme rat	3.0 ± 0.7	0.31	3.6 ± 1.5	3.0	51.3 ± 4.0	8.8
Nodular rat	2.3 ± 0.7	0.8	2.1 ± 0.5	23.6	12.7 ± 2.0	11.8

ACKNOWLEDGEMENTS

This research was supported by grants from the National Cancer Institute of
Canada and the Swedish Medical Research Council.

REFERENCES

1. Farber, e. (1980) Biochim. Biophys. Acta 605, 149.
2. Roberts, E., Ahluwalia, M.B., Lee, G., Chan, C., Sarma, D.S.R. and
   Farber, E. (1983) Cancer Res. 43, 28.
3. Solt, D.B. and Farber, E. (1976) Nature, 263, 701.

© 1983 Elsevier Science Publishers B.V.
Extrahepatic Drug Metabolism and Chemical Carcinogenesis,
J. Rydström, J. Montelius and M. Bengtsson eds.

THE METABOLISM OF BENZO(A)PYRENE IN THE INTESTINE AND THE EFFECT OF
DIETARY FATS

JON D. GOWER AND E. D. WILLS
Department of Biochemistry, Medical College of St. Bartholomew's
Hospital, Charterhouse Square, London, ENGLAND, EC1M 6BQ.

INTRODUCTION

Carcinogens in foodstuffs may be important in human carcinogenesis but polycyclic aromatic hydrocarbons such as benzo(a)pyrene
(BP) are not carcinogenic until they are metabolised to electrophilic epoxides which are mutagenic, carcinogenic and bind to DNA
(1). The rate of this oxidative metabolism in the intestinal
mucosa is therefore likely to be of crucial importance in the
initiation of intestinal cancer and will affect the distribution of
ingested carcinogens and their metabolites to other tissues.

Epidemiological investigations have demonstrated a positive
correlation between dietary fat intake in man and cancer of various
organs including the intestine (2). Furthermore, a high level of
dietary fat and especially polyunsaturated fat increases
tumour incidence in animals treated with a variety of carcinogens
(2) and increases the rate of BP metabolism in the rat liver (3).
This investigation was therefore carried out to study the effects
of various types and quantities of dietary fat on the rate of BP
metabolism in the rat intestinal mucosa.

METHODS

Groups of male Wistar rats, weighing 100-150g were fed for
15-30 days on synthetic diets which contained by weight, 25%
casein, 30% sucrose, 20% wheat starch, 10% dried yeast, 5% Cox's
salt mix, 10% fat and 5000 units of vitamin A and 1000 units of
vitamin D_3/kg. In diets in which the lipid content was other than
10%, the percentage of wheat starch was adjusted accordingly. Some
groups of rats were also fed on Spratts Laboratory Rat Diet No. 1
(Stock diet) which was supplemented with fat (10% by weight).

Rats were killed, the distal half of the intestine (50 cm
nearest the caecum) was removed and washed. The mucosa was scraped
off and suspended in 0.05M Tris-HCl buffer (pH 7.8) (25% w/v)
containing trypsin inhibitor (5mg/g wet weight) and glycerol (20%)

and a post-mitochondrial fraction prepared.

The rate of NADPH-dependent BP hydroxylation was determined fluorimetrically (4), the incubation mixure contained 0.05 M Tris-HCl buffer (pH 7.8), 5mM $MgCl_2$, 320uM NADPH, 6mM BP and 5-10mg protein in a final volume of 2 ml. Alternatively, ^{14}C-BP (20uCi/umol) was used as the substrate and the metabolites of BP produced by the post-mitochondrial fractions were determined by HPLC (5).

The fatty acid composition of the diets and the post-mitochondrial fractions of the intestinal mucosa were determined by GLC.

RESULTS AND DISCUSSION

The rate of hydroxylation of BP in the distal half of the rat intestine was found to be dependent on the quantity and type of fat in the diet. Replacing the stock diet containing 4.5% fat by a fat-free diet caused a fall of 24% in the rate of BP hydroxylation (Table 1). Addition of 10% lard, mackerel oil, cod liver oil, coconut oil or corn oil to the fat free diet significantly increased the rate of BP hydroxylation (Table 1). Increasing the amount of coconut oil or corn oil in the diet from 5% to 20% also significantly ($P < 0.05$) increased the rate of BP hydroxylation (Table 1). The importance of the amount of fat in the diet was also demonstrated by supplementing the stock diet with 10% lard or corn oil which resulted in significant ($P<0.05$) increases in the rate of BP hydroxylation (Table 1).

The proportion of linoleic acid ($C_{18:2}$) in the dietary fat was found to be of particular importance. Feeding a diet containing 10% corn oil (58% $C_{18:2}$) resulted in a BP hydroxylase activity which was significantly greater ($P <0.02$) than when a 10% coconut oil diet (2.0% $C_{18:2}$) was fed (Table 1). The difference in the rate of BP hydroxylation between rats fed corn oil and coconut oil became more pronounced when the amount of these oils in the diet was increased to 20%. Feeding a 10% lard diet (10% $C_{18:2}$) resulted in a rate of hydroxylation which was intermediate between that of the groups fed 10% coconut oil and corn oil diets. Addition of 10% mackerel oil or cod liver oil to the fat-free diet also increased the rate of BP hydroxylation despite the low linoleic acid content of these fats (Table 1). Mackerel oil and cod liver oil contain relatively large proportions of $C_{20:5}$ (8.1% and 17.7% respectively) and $C_{22:6}$ (13.2% and 10.7% respectively) which were not present in

TABLE 1: THE EFFECTS OF VARIATION OF THE LINOLEIC ACID CONTENT OF
THE DIET ON BENZO(A)PYRENE HYDROXYLASE ACTIVITY AND ON THE LINOLEIC
ACID COMPOSITION OF THE INTESTINAL MUCOSA

Diet	Linoleic acid content of diet (g/kg diet)	Linoleic acid content of mucosa (% of total fatty acids)	BP hydroxylase activity (fat-free %) Mean $\pm$ S.E.M
Fat-free	0	9.64	100$\pm$7 (8)
10% lard	1.04	14.19	220$\pm$38 (6)
10% mackerel oil	0.32	5.48	228$\pm$18 (6)
10% cod liver oil	0.77	5.77	258$\pm$23 (8)
5% coconut oil	0.10	ND	131$\pm$23 (6)
10% coconut oil	0.20	10.91	173$\pm$22 (7)
20% coconut oil	0.40	ND	256$\pm$48 (6)
5% corn oil	2.92	16.89	291$\pm$48 (6)
10% corn oil	5.83	21.77	292$\pm$29 (8)
20% corn oil	11.66	21.83	655$\pm$142(6)
Stock (4.5% fat)	0.90	17.14	132$\pm$12 (6)
Stock + 10% lard	1.85	ND	259$\pm$24 (5)
Stock + 10% corn oil	6.64	ND	271$\pm$29 (5)

the other dietary fats. Thus these w-3 polyunsaturated fatty acids
were able to replace the w-6 linoleic acid in supporting a high
rate of BP metabolism.

HPLC analysis of BP metabolites which are determined by the
fluorimetric assay constituted about 20% of the total metabolites
and that about 60% of the metabolites were quinones and 5% were
dihydrodiols. The rate of total metabolite production measured by
HPLC was dependent on the lipid composition of the diet and the
results were similar to those obtained using the fluorimetric
assay. Feeding high concentrations of polyunsaturated fats caused
the mucosa to produce all the metabolites of BP at a faster rate
than after feeding diets containing saturated fats or no fat.

The fatty acid composition of the mucosal endoplasmic reticulum
varied with the type of dietary lipid fed and the percentage of
linoleic acid in the membrane was closely related to the percentage
of this fatty acid in the dietary fat (Table 1). Addition of cod
liver oil or mackerel oil to the fat-free diet caused decreases in
the $C_{18:2}$ content of the mucosal fractions (Table 1) but an

increase in the incorporation of the w-3 polyunsaturated fatty
acids $C_{20:5}$ and $C_{22:6}$. These fatty acids are therefore
incorporated into the membrane at the expense of linoleic acid.

The rate of BP metabolism in the intestinal mucosa was clearly
dependent on the polyunsaturated fatty acid composition of the
endoplasmic reticulum (Fig. 1) The mechanism by which
polyunsaturated fatty acids regulate the rate of oxidative
metabolism of BP is not yet clear. Changes in the fatty acid
composition of the membrane phospholipids may alter the
configuration of active enzymes in the membrane (6). Alternatively
hydroperoxides may be formed _in situ_ from polyunsaturated fatty
acids. Free radicals formed during peroxide formation could then
be responsible for the formation of BP metabolites.

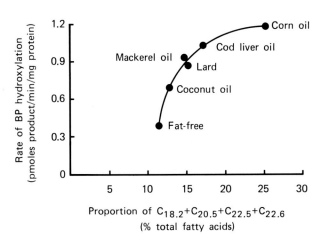

Fig 1. The relationship between the rate of BP hydroxylation and
the proportion of polyunsaturated fatty acids in the mucosal
endoplasmic reticulum.

REFERENCES

1. Gelboin, H.V. (1980) Physiol. Rev. 60, 1107.

2. Carroll, K.K. (1980) J. Environm. Pathol. Toxicol. 3, 253.

3. Lambert, L. and Wills, E.D. (1977) Biochem. Pharmacol. 26,1423.

4. Dehnen, W., Tomingas, R. and Roos, J. (1973) Anal. Biochem.
   53, 373.

5. Stohs, S.J., Grafstrom, R.C., Burke, M.D., Moldeus, P.W. and
   Orrenius, S.G. (1976) Arch. Biochem. Biophys. 177, 105.

6. Wills, E.D. (1980) in: Coon, M.J., Conney, A.H., Estabrook,
   R.W., Gelboin, H.V., Gillette, J.R. and O'Brien, P.J. (Eds)
   Microsomes, Drug Oxidations and Chemical Carcinogenesis,
   Academic Press, New York, pp. 545-548.

© 1983 Elsevier Science Publishers B.V.
Extrahepatic Drug Metabolism and Chemical Carcinogenesis,
J. Rydström, J. Montelius and M. Bengtsson eds.

EFFECT OF DIETHYL MALEATE PRETREATMENT ON GLUTATHIONE LEVELS IN STOMACH, LIVER AND BLOOD OF RATS TREATED WITH GASTRIC DAMAGE INDUCING AGENTS

Paolo Di Simplicio, Antonella Naldini and Maria Teresa Bianco

Institute of Pharmacology, Faculty of Medicine, University of Siena, Italy

INTRODUCTION

Glutathione (GSH) depletion in the glandular portion of rodent stomach has been considered a predisposing factor to the gastric ulcerations caused by ethanol (E)[1]; it has also been reported that rats subjected to stress or treated with diethyl maleate (DEM) present GSH depletion and "also frequently" have gastric erosions[2]. However, more recently, it has been found that DEM at lower doses protects against the E gastric injury while it is ineffective against the aspirin-induced (A) gastric erosions[3].

The effect of DEM pretreatment on the GSH levels in different organs and in blood of rats treated with agents that determine acute gastric erosions has been studied in this report.

MATERIALS AND METHODS

Albino Wistar rats (220-280 g) 14 hr fasted and sacrificed between 8a.m. to 1 p.m. were used.

GSH Determination. GSH was determined with enzymatic method[4] after tissue homogenization following Tietze[5]. Blood was deproteinized with a solution containing 25% trichloroacetic acid and phosphate buffer (0.1 M pH 7.4)(1:3).

RESULTS AND DISCUSSION

No significant difference in GSH concentration exists between the control group and those treated with E, A, or oxyphenbutazone (O)(Table 1). Nevertheless severe gastric erosions were always observed after E and A treatment, while they were less evident in rats treated with O. Rats treated with DEM plus E or A showed a significant decrease in GSH concentration in most tissues, however an increase of the gastric damage was not observed. Rats subjected to stress by physical restraint for 4 hr did not show any GSH depletion except in the liver, while animals treated with DEM and subjected to 4 hr stress showed a decrease in GSH concentration in blood only. No gastric erosions were observed in these groups.

Therefore, in accordance with our data, the GSH depletion of the glandular portion does not result to be an effect of the gastric damage caused by the treatment with E, A, O, and the prior GSH depletion with DEM does not enhance the gastric injury induced by E and A.

TABLE 1

GSH CONCENTRATION IN STOMACH, LIVER (umol/g) AND BLOOD (umol/ml) AFTER TREATMENT WITH GASTRIC DAMAGE INDUCING AGENTS. M $\pm$ SD.

Treatment	Rats	STOMACH		LIVER	BLOOD
		Glandular	Squamous		
Controls	11	1.87 ± 0.21	1.70 ± 0.24	4.56 ± 0.40	0.814 ± 0.093
DEM* 0.35 ml/kg	5	$1.10^{a}\pm0.25$	1.65 ± 0.11	$1.12^{a}\pm0.37$	$0.299^{a}\pm0.110$
DEM* 0.7 ml/kg	5	$0.59^{a}\pm0.30$	$0.58^{a}\pm0.41$	$0.41^{a}\pm0.27$	$0.147^{a}\pm0.083$
E*	5	1.70 ± 0.29	1.94 ± 0.19	4.81 ± 0.72	0.810 ± 0.086
DEM§ 0.35 + E*	3	1.55 ± 0.29	$1.47^{b}\pm0.24$	3.09 ± 1.46	$0.335^{b}\pm0.192$
A**	4	1.73 ± 0.095	1.81 ± 0.08	4.80 ± 0.61	0.742 ± 0.024
DEM§ 0.5 + A**	4	$1.32^{c}\pm0.09$	1.58 ± 0.31	$3.44^{c}\pm1.16$	$0.307^{c}\pm0.046$
Stress	4	2.40 ± 1.05	2.09 ± 0.69	$3.36^{a}\pm0.31$	0.978 ± 0.26
DEM 0.35 + Stress	3	1.96 ± 0.54	1.79 ± 0.26	4.09 ± 0.64	$0.583^{d}\pm0.15$
O**	4	1.76 ± 0.13	1.54 ± 0.23	4.17 ± 0.38	0.813 ± 0.100

E: 2 ml/kg, po; A: 100 mg/kg suspended in 0.5% methyl cellulose containing 0.2 N HCl; O: 100 mg/kg suspended in 0.5% methyl cellulose, po. $P < 0.05$: a vs. control group; b vs. E group; c vs. A group; d vs. stress group. Sacrifice: * 1 hr after treatment; ** 2 hr after treatment. Pretreatment: § 1 hr before E or A treatment. GSSG measured in tissues and blood[5] gave: no GSSG in stomach; 5 and 10% of the GSH content was found in liver and blood, respectively; no significant difference was found between control and treated rats.

REFERENCES

1. Szabo, S., Trier, J.S. and Frankel P.W. (1981) Science, 214, 200.

2. Boyd, S.C., Sasame, H.A. and Boyd M.R. (1979) Science, 205, 1012.

3. Konturek, S.J., Brzozowski, T., Piastuki, I., Radecki, T. and Szabo S. (1982) V Intern. Conference Prostaglandins, Florence, May 18-21, p. 371.

4. Tietze, F. (1969) Anal. Biochem., 27, 502.

5. Klotzsch, H and Bergmeyer H.U. (1965) in Bergmeyer, H.U. (Ed.), Methods of Enzymatic Analysis, Acad. Press, New York, pp. 363-366.

© 1983 Elsevier Science Publishers B.V.
Extrahepatic Drug Metabolism and Chemical Carcinogenesis,
J. Rydström, J. Montelius and M. Bengtsson eds.

EFFECT OF CHOLESTEROL ON PHENOBARBITAL INDUCIBILITY OF BIOTRANSFORMATION
ENZYMES IN THE SMALL INTESTINAL MUCOSA AND LIVER OF THE RAT

EINO HIETANEN[+] AND MARKKU AHOTUPA
Department of Physiology, University of Turku, SF-20520 Turku (Finland)

INTRODUCTION

Dietary factors are of importance in the regulation of hepatic drug metabolism and the inducibility of biotransformation enzymes (1,2). The integral
role of lipids in the membrane structure suggests a close connection between
dietary lipids modifying the membrane composition and the activities of drug-
metabolizing enzymes (3-5). Although the role of dietary fats and their saturation degree in the regulation of hepatic drug metabolism has been rather
extensively studied, fewer studies exist on the role of dietary cholesterol
in the regulation of hepatic biotransformation rates (6). Also the role of
dietary components in the regulation of intestinal biotransformation rates is
little studied (7).

The simultaneous exposure to xenobiotics, while animals are on various lipid
diets, may modify cancer formation in the liver and intestine (8,9). Changes in
the biotransformation enzyme activities in the liver and intestine may alter
the susceptibility to cancer formation.

MATERIALS AND METHODS

Animals and tissues. Weanling male rats were fed either a cholesterol-free
or a high cholesterol (2%) diet for 4 weeks (ICN Nutritional Biochemicals).
After 3 weeks feeding rats were divided into 2 subgroups. One subgroup served
as a control and the other received 0.1 % phenobarbital in drinking water for
1 week. After 4 weeks of feeding rats were killed and liver microsomes and
intestinal postmitochondrial supernatant (20 cm segment distally from pylorus)
were prepared.

Assays. The aryl hydrocarbon hydroxylase (AHH) and ethoxycoumarin O-deethylase (ECDE) activities were determined by fluorometric methods, epoxide hydrolase
(EH) using radiolabelled styrene oxide and the UDPglucuronosyltransferase (UDPGT)
activity was measured 4-methylumbelliferone as an aglycone (for refs.,see 6).
The cholesterol and protein contents of microsomes and postmitochondrial supernatant were determined as described before (10). Student's t-test was applied
for statistical analyses and means are shown.

+Present address: IARC, 150 cours Albert Thomas, 69372 Lyon, France

RESULTS AND DISCUSSION

The hepatic microsomal protein concentration was lower in rats fed 2 % cholesterol diet (30.7 mg/g) than in those fed cholesterol free diet (40.0). Phenobarbital did not cause any significant changes. In the intestinal mucosa no changes were either present. The cholesterol contents and the biotransformation enzyme activities are shown in the table 1.

TABLE 1

CHOLESTEROL CONTENTS AND BIOTRANSFORMATION ENZYME ACTIVITIES IN THE LIVER AND INTESTINE OF RATS FED VARIOUS CHOLESTEROL DIETS

Group	Chol.(umol/g)	AHH	ECDE	EH	UDPGT
Liver					
Chol.free	0.66	0.25	2.5***	48.7***	11.1**
+ PB	0.88	0.14	10.7	162.4	20.0
2% Chol.	0.99**	0.34	5.9***	132.8***/**	19.7***/**
+ PB	0.87	0.25	19.9	319.5	29.2
Intestine					
Chol.free	1.27	0.003	0.17**	22.0	81.6
+ PB	1.30	0.002	0.62	27.0	60.1
2% Chol.	1.70*	0.033***	2.88***	23.1	71.7
+ PB	1.62	0.059	2.92	25.2	67.7

All enzyme activities are expressed as nmoles $\times$ min$^{-1}\times$ g(w.wt)$^{-1}$.
Chol.free is compared to 2 % chol. group. PB to respective control diet.
*: P less than 0.05; **: P less than 0.01 and ***: P less than 0.001.

It is obvious that even the same enzyme responses differently to dietary manipulations (see AHH) and to enzyme inducers (see ECDE) in the intestine as compared to the liver. (Grant: NIH R01 ES 01684 and J. Vainio Foundation).

REFERENCES

1. Basu, T.L. and Dickerson, J.W. (1974) Chem.-Biol. Interact., 8, 193.

2. Hietanen, E. (1977) Acta Pharmac. Tox., 41: Suppl.IV, 30.

3. McLean, A.E.M. (1974) Proc. Nutr. Soc., 33, 197.

4. Marshall, W.J. and McLean, A.E.M. (1971) Biochem. J., 122, 569.

5. Stier, A. (1976) Biochem. Pharmac., 25, 109.

6. Hietanen, E., Ahotupa, M., Heikela, A. and Laitinen, M. (1982) Drug-Nutrient Interact., 1, 313.

7. Hietanen, E. and Laitinen, M. (1978) Biochem. Pharmac., 27, 1095.

8. Reddy, B.S., Watanabe, K. and Weisburger, J.H. (1977) Cancer Res., 37, 4156.

9. Silverstone, H. and Tannenbaum, A. (1951) Cancer Res., 11, 442.

10. Hietanen, E., Ahotupa, M., Heikela, A. et al. (1982) Drug-Nutr. Interact., 1, 279.

© 1983 Elsevier Science Publishers B.V.
Extrahepatic Drug Metabolism and Chemical Carcinogenesis,
J. Rydström, J. Montelius and M. Bengtsson eds.

XENOBIOTIC METABOLISM IN THE SMALL INTESTINAL MUCOSA OF CHILDREN

*EINO HIETANEN[1], TUULA HEINONEN[2], MARJA-LIISA STÅHLBERG[3] AND MARKKU MÄKI[4]

Departments of [1]Physiology and [3]Pediatrics, University of Turku, SF-20520 Turku; [2]Institute of Occupational Health, SF-00290 Helsinki and [4]Department of Pediatrics, University of Tampere, SF-331010 Tampere (Finland).

INTRODUCTION

The intestinal mucosa has quantitatively a minor role in the total metabolic capacity of biotransformation reactions (1). Yet it may have a significant role in the metabolism of xenobiotics entering the body orally in small quantitites (2,3). In the rat small intestine mucosa the aryl hydrocarbon hydroxylase and ethoxycoumarin O-deethylase activities are about 5-20% of that which exists in the liver when calculated on a wet weight basis (4). Although in humans the intestinal mucosa is also the first barrier towards many xenobiotics, very few studies exist on the metabolic capacity of human intestinal mucosa (5).

MATERIALS AND METHODS

Tissues. Children (0.6-16.8 years) were hospitalized at the University Hospitals of Turku and Tampere with suspected glutein enteropathy. After an overnight fast a duodenal biopsy was taken under X-ray control using a capsule technique for the diagnostic purposes. A part of the biopsy specimen was taken for a histological study by a pathologist and a part (0.33-10.52 mg) was used for the enzyme determinations. The sample was frozen (-80°C) whereafter the assays were made within 4 weeks. The patients were divided according to histological diagnosis into 2 groups with or without villus atrophy. Adult male rats were used for the reference tissue in the enzyme determinations.

Enzyme assays. The tissue specimens were homogenized after weighing in 0.15 M KCl. The human samples were used as such and the rat intestinal mucosa was scraped off, homogenized and centrifuged 10000 g x 15 min to prepare a postmitochondrial supernatant. The intestinal alkaline phosphatatase, adenosine triphosphatase and maltase activities were measured as reference enzymes as described before (6). The aryl hydrocarbon hydroxylase (AHH) activity was measured using the radiochemical method as described by DePierre et al. (7).

---

*Present address: International Agency for Research on Cancer, 150 cours Albert-Thomas, 69372 Lyon, Cedex 08, France

The ethoxycoumarin O-deethylase (ECDE) (8), epoxide hydrolase (EH) (9) and UDP-glucuronosyltransferase (10) were measured as described before.

RESULTS AND DISCUSSION

The monoxygenase and epoxide hydrolase activities are shown in Table 1.

TABLE 1

THE INTESTINAL ENZYME ACTIVITIES

Group	AHH	ECDE	EH
Normal (42)	38.2 + 8.3	0.021 + 0.009	$\left\{\begin{array}{l} 38.6 + 157 \\ (n = 23) \end{array}\right.$
Atrophy (10)	33.9 + 14.3	0.042 + 0.029	
Rat intestine	23.1 + 4.5	32.5 + 3.8	353 + 48

All activities are as pmoles $\times$ min^{-1} $\times$ mg (protein)$^{-1}$

The alkaline phosphatase activity was significantly lower in the mucosa of children with villus atrophy (25.6 $\pm$ 6.4 nmol $\times$ min^{-1} $\times$ mg prot^{-1}) than in healthy controls (43.9 $\pm$ 6.4). No differences in the adenosine triphosphatase or malatase activities were found. Only traces of UDP glucuronosyltransferase activity were present in comparison with adult rat intestine (348 $\pm$ 35 pmoles $\times$ min^{-1} $\times$ mg prot^{-1}). The present data suggest that the samll intestinal mucosa of children has a very low capacity for the deethylation and conjugation reactions, possibly increasing the susceptibility to harmful effects of foreign compounds.

REFERENCES

1. Vainio, H. and Hietanen, E. (1980) in: Jenner, P. and Testa, B. (Eds.), Concepts in Drug Metabolism, Marcel Dekker, New York, pp 251-284.

2. Hietanen, E. (1980) Pharmacology, 21, 233.

3. Stohs, S.J., Grafstrom, R.C., Burke, M.D. and Orrenius, S. (1977) Arch. Biochem. Biophys., 179, 71.

4. Ahotupa, M., Hietanen, E., Mantyla, E. and Vainio, H. (1982) J. Appl. Toxicol., 2, 47.

5. Autrup, H. (1982) Drug Metabolism Rev., 13, 603.

6. Hietanen, E. (1973) Academic Diss., University of Turku, Turku, pp 1-76.

7. DePierre, J.D., Moron, M.S., Johannesen, K.A.M. and Ernster, L. (1975) Anal. Biochem., 63, 470.

8. Zitting, A. (1981) Anal. Biochem., 114, 177.

9. Oesch, F., Jerina, D.M. and Daly, J. (1971) Biochem. Biophys. Acta, 227, 685.

10. Arias, I.M. (1962) J. Clin. Invest., 41, 2233.

© 1983 Elsevier Science Publishers B.V.
Extrahepatic Drug Metabolism and Chemical Carcinogenesis,
J. Rydström, J. Montelius and M. Bengtsson eds.

INHIBITION OF THE MUTAGENIC ACTIVITY OF 2-AMINO-3-METHYL-
IMIDAZO(4,5-f)QUINOLINE (IQ) BY RAT INTESTINAL MUCOSA.

GIOVANNA CADERNI, MAURA LODOVICI AND PIERO DOLARA
Institute of Pharmacology and Toxicology, University of
Florence, Viale Morgagni, 65 - 50134 Firenze, Italy.

INTRODUCTION

Potent mutagens are formed during the broiling of meat
or fish, detectable with <u>Salmonella typhimurium</u> strains TA1538
and TA98 with S9 (1). The ones tested so far are also carcinogenic in chronic feeding experiments (1). Since several human
cancers have been associated with the ingestion of low levels
of carcinogenic chemicals in the diet, it interested us to investigate whether components of the intestinal wall could modulate the mutagenic activity of one of these substances, the
2-amino-3-methyl-imidazo(4,5-f)quinoline, known as IQ.

MATERIALS AND METHODS

Intestinal preparations were obtained by scraping the
mucosa from rat small intestines, homogenizing it 1:4 in 0.25M
sucrose. The homogenate was centrifuged at 2,000 g x 20 min,
again at 2,000 g x 20 min. and finally at 22,000 g x 30 min.
After resuspension in 0.1 M Tris-HCl buffer, pH 7.1, the preparation was kept for 2 h at pH 11, centrifuged at 38,000 g x
60 min. and brought back to pH 7.4. Enzymatic activity was
measured spectrophotometrically at 470 nm as described elsewhere
(2). After an incubation of 1 h the samples containing IQ were
tested with strain TA98 with PCB induced rat liver S9 (3).

RESULTS

Preparations of rat intestinal mucosa were capable of inactivating concentrations of IQ up to 5 ng (Figure 1). The
inactivation process was not dependent on the presence of externally added H_2O_2, likely because of the formation of some

310

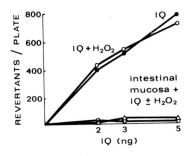

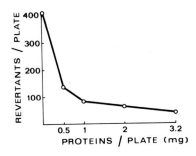

Fig. 1. Mutagenic activity of IQ on strain TA98 + S9 in the presence of 14 mU of intestinal mucosa peroxidase.

Fig. 2. Mutagenic activity of 2 ng of IQ with different concentrations of heat-inactivated rat intestinal mucosa preparations.

hydrogen peroxide by the intestinal preparations rich in peroxidase activity. A decreased mutagenic activity was also observed by incubating IQ with boiled mucosa preparations, the residual activity being related to the amount of proteins present in the plate (Figure 2).

These results indicate that IQ can be deactivated by rat intestinal mucosa, likely by a combination of enzymatic transformation and protein binding. These effects are probably relevant for the toxicology of this group of substances for animals and humans.

ACKNOWLEDGEMENTS

This work was supported by a grant from CNR (Control of Toxic Risk). We thank Dr. Sugimura for his kind gift of pure IQ.

REFERENCES

1. Sugimura, T. (1982) Mutagens, carcinogens and tumor promotors in our daily food. Cancer, 49, 1970.

2. Sgaragli G., Della Corte L., Puliti R., De Sarlo F., Francalanci R., Guarna A., Dolara P. and Komarynsky M. (1980) Oxidation of BHA by horse radish and mammalian peroxidase systems. Biochem. Pharmacol. 29, 763.

3. Ames B.N., McCann J. and Yamasaki E. (1975) Methods for detecting carcinogens and mutagens with the Salmonella-mammalian/microsome mutagenicity test. Mutat. Res, 31,347.

© 1983 Elsevier Science Publishers B.V.
Extrahepatic Drug Metabolism and Chemical Carcinogenesis,
J. Rydström, J. Montelius and M. Bengtsson eds.

THE EFFECT OF HIGH FAT DIET ON THE DISPOSITION OF BENZO[A]PYRENE IN THE GUT

SUSAN BOWES AND ANDREW G. RENWICK

Clinical Pharmacology Group, University of Southampton, Medical & Biological
Sciences Building, Bassett Crescent East, Southampton SO9 3TU, U.K.

INTRODUCTION

Cancer of the colon is one of the commonest tumours in western societies
but not in rural/agricultural communities (1). Environmental differences
which have been implicated include a diet which is high in fat but low in
fibre and also a greater degree of industrialisation. The latter is
accompanied by increased combustion of fossil fuels and environmental
contamination by polycyclic aromatic hydrocarbons like benzo[a]pyrene (BP)
(2). Such compounds are highly lipid soluble and are absorbed in the upper
intestine, and thus have received little attention as potential factors in
colon cancer. However, the bile is the principal route of elimination of BP
in most species (3) and the colonic microflora may be able to hydrolyse
conjugated metabolites and even form the parent hydrocarbon (4). The present
study was designed to investigate the effect of dietary fat on the disposition of BP with particular reference to the colon.

MATERIALS AND METHODS

Animals. Male Duncan-Hartley guinea pigs were given normal, high fat (HF;
17% coconut oil) or high cholesterol (HC; HF + 0.1% cholesterol) diet from
weaning for at least 16 weeks prior to investigation. All data given are the
mean of 6 $\pm$ 2 age-matched animals per treatment group with the standard
deviation indicated (* P<0.05, ** P<0.01, *** P<0.001 by unpaired Student
t-test). In some experiments the animals were pretreated with BP by gavage
(3mg/kg twice weekly for 3 weeks) prior to study.

Enzyme assays. Aryl hydrocarbon hydroxylase (AHH) (5) was determined in
the microsomal pellets obtained from the liver and mucosae of small intestine,
colon and rectum.

Biliary excretion. [^{14}C]BP (25µCi; i.v.) was given to urethane anaesthetised bile-duct cannulated animals. The bile was analysed for total ^{14}C and
for metabolites by tlc and hplc (3) before and after enzymic hydrolysis of
conjugates.

Bacterial incubations. Reference metabolites of BP were incubated with isolated strains of intestinal bacteria under anaerobic conditions for 40h. The incubates were analysed by hplc using fluorescence for detection of metabolic products.

DNA binding. [^{3}H]BP (2-4mCi) was given orally, the animals were sacrificed 3 days later and the DNA of liver and gut mucosae isolated, purified and the ^{3}H content determined.

RESULTS

The bile was the principal route of excretion of [^{14}C]BP in all groups with negligible amounts (<1%) in the urine.

Animals	% dose in bile in 4h
Control	33.2 + 12.5
HF	26.7 + 13.4
HC	36.5 + 14.5

Most of the ^{14}C was present as highly polar conjugates mainly glucuronides, but with a large fraction that did not extract into ethyl acetate even after hydrolysis by sulphatase/glucuronidase or by caecal microflora. BP was not detected in these incubates. HF and HC diets increased the proportion excreted as dihydrodiol conjugates.

Animals	% total excreted in bile (as free + glucuronides)		
	4,5-dihydrodiol	7,8-dihydrodiol	9,10-dihydrodiol
Control	2.4 + 0.9	3.7 + 2.2	2.8 + 0.5
HF	13.5 + 4.1***	4.6 + 0.6	4.9 + 0.9**
HC	11.6 + 3.4***	5.6 + 2.3	6.3 + 1.8**

Incubation of reference BP metabolites with pure strains of intestinal bacteria showed that the glucuronides and to a lesser extent the sulphates of 3- and 9-hydroxy BP were hydrolysed to the primary metabolites. The primary oxidation products (3-, 7- and 9-hydroxy BP and 4,5-, 7,8- and 9,10-dihydrodiols) were stable on incubation with the strains tested (8 x Clostridia, 1 x Bacteroides, 3 x Bifidobacteria). No BP was formed with these strains.

AHH in liver and intestinal mucosa was not altered by HF and HC diets. The levels in mucosae of rectum and colon were below the limit of detection even after pretreatment with BP. BP pretreatment increased the intestinal mucosal AHH in normal but not HF and HC groups, and did not significantly induce the hepatic enzyme.

Animals	AHH activity nmoles 30HBP/mg microsomal protein/h			
	LIVER		SMALL INTESTINE	
	Normal	Pretreated	Normal	Pretreated
Control	0.9 + 0.6	1.3 + 0.7	0.07 + 0.03	0.33 + 0.19*
HF	0.5 + 0.1	0.8 + 0.7	0.03 + 0.04	0.04 + 0.04
HC	0.3 + 0.3	0.8 + 0.8	0.03 + 0.03	0.05 + 0.08

The negligible levels of AHH activity in the hind gut mucosa resulted in only very low levels of ^{3}H incorporation into DNA and much of this could be accounted for by ^{3}H exchange rather than covalent binding. However, HF and HC diets appeared to increase reabsorption (possibly via the increase in the dihydrodiol fraction) since more of the [^{3}H]BP was recovered in the urine and less in the faeces.

Animals	% dose in urine (3days)	% dose in faeces (3 days)
Control	7.8 + 1.8	34.9 + 12.8
HF	12.4 + 3.6*	16.3 + 7.4**
HC	14.4 + 10.8	26.3 + 12.5

CONCLUSION

HF and HC diets increased the biliary elimination of dihydrodiol metabolites, which were stable to microbial metabolism. However, this did not result in increased DNA binding probably due to the absence of measurable AHH activity at this site.

ACKNOWLEDGEMENTS

This work was supported by the Cancer Research Campaign. The authors are grateful to Dr. M. Hill for strains of intestinal bacteria.

REFERENCES

1. Wynder, E. L. (1975) Cancer Res., 35, 3388.

2. Baum, E. J. (1978) in: Gelboin H. V. and Ts'O, P. O. P. (Ed.), Polycyclic Hydrocarbons and Cancer, Volume 1, Academic Press Inc., New York, pp. 45-70.

3. Chipman, J. K., Hirom, P. C., Frost, G. S. and Millburn, P. (1981) Biochem. Pharmacol., 30, 937.

4. Renwick, A. G. and Drasar, B. S. (1976) Nature, 263, 234.

5. Nebert, D. W. and Gelboin, H. V. (1968) J. Biol. Chem., 243, 6242.

© 1983 Elsevier Science Publishers B.V.
Extrahepatic Drug Metabolism and Chemical Carcinogenesis,
J. Rydström, J. Montelius and M. Bengtsson eds.   315

THE CYTOSTATIC HEXAMETHYLMELAMINE, ADMINISTERED ORALLY TO RATS, IS METABOLIZED
IN THE LIVER AND THE GUT WALL

PIERRE KLIPPERT[1], PAUL BORM[1], ABRAM HULSHOFF[2], MARIE-JOSÉ MINGELS[2], GERARD
HOFMAN[1] AND JAN NOORDHOEK[1]
[1]State University of Utrecht, Faculty of Pharmacy, Department of Pharmacology
and Pharmacotherapy and [2]Department of Analytical Pharmacy, Catharijnesingel 60,
3511 GH   Utrecht (The Netherlands)

INTRODUCTION

   Hexamethylmelamine (HMM) has demonstrated its activity against a wide variety
of solid human tumours (1, 2). The drug is usually given in combination with
other chemotherapeutic agents.

   The mechanism of action of HMM is uncertain. It is however not a directly
alkylating agent (3) and probably needs metabolic activation to covalently bind
to tissue macromolecules (4, 5) and thus to express its anti-tumour activity.
Intermediates such as the N-methylolmelamines are significantly more cytotoxic
to tumour cell lines than HMM itself (6, 7).

   In rats and man HMM is metabolized by sequential oxidative N-demethylation (8).
Urinary, biliary and faecal excretion of unchanged HMM are negligible (9).
Mixed function oxygenases, an enzyme system that is present in the liver, the
gastro-intestinal tract and other extrahepatic tissues, may bring about the
demethylation/metabolic activation of HMM and its congeners (4, 10).

   A number of studies indicate that the absorption of HMM is fairly complete
(8, 11). However, the biological availability of HMM administered orally is
very low (11). This is indicative of extensive presystemic elimination in the
liver and/or the gut wall.

   The purpose of this study was to further investigate this presystemic
elimination (first-pass effect) of HMM by analyzing plasma concentration-time
curves after intra-arterial (i.a.), i.v., portal venous (p.v.) and intraduodenal
(i.d.)   administration of HMM (5 and 10 mg/kg) to conscious rats.

MATERIALS AND METHODS

   Chemicals. HMM was obtained from Ofichem (Gieten, The Netherlands, batch no.
790205). The metabolites of HMM used in this investigation were kindly provided
by Dr. D.E.V. Wilman (Institute of Cancer Research, Royal Cancer Hospital,
London, England). Heparin sodium was obtained from Leo Pharmaceutical Products,
Ballerup, Denmark. HMM hydrochloride was prepared as described earlier (12).

GC assay for plasma HMM and metabolites. The extraction procedure of HMM
and its metabolites from plasma and the GC operating conditions have been
reported (13).

Treatment of animals. Male Wistar rats (TNO, Zeist, The Netherlands) weighing
240 ± 10 g were used throughout this study. Rats were anaesthetized with ether
and a PE-50 polyethylene cannula was inserted into the left carotid artery. The
cannula was led under the skin and left the body behind the ears where it was
attached to the skin by suture. This cannula was used for blood sampling.

In the case of i.v. administration another PE-50 cannula was introduced into
the left jugular vein and led in the same way. For p.v. and i.d. administration,
the body was opened through a midline incision in the midabdomen along the
linea alba, PE-50 cannulas were inserted into the ileocolical vein and the
duodenum, respectively and attached by ligatures. The abdomen was then closed
by suture.

In the case of i.a. administration, the rat was fitted with a PE-50 cannula
inserted into the right carotid artery, its tip ending in the aortic arch. This
cannula was used to infuse the drug. A tee was placed in the left carotid
artery. In this way we were able to draw blood from the artery while main-
taining the blood circulation.

30-45 Min after recovering from the ether anaesthesia the rats were placed
in a plexiglass cylinder (15 cm long, 6 cm i.d.) to which they had been
previously conditioned for at least 4 hr. The cylinder was provided with holes
for air ventilation and for the cannulas.

HMM hydrochloride dissolved in saline was administered via an infusion pump
(flow rat 1.90 or 3.80 ml/hr, depending on the dose and the route of administration). Infusion time was 10 min for i.a., i.v. and i.d. administration and
15 min for p.v. administration.

Blood samples (250-500 µl) were removed periodically from the cannula in the
left carotid artery, the cannula was flushed with 150 µl of heparinized saline
(125 IE/ml) and plasma was separated.

RESULTS

Disposition of HMM in the Rat. Plasma concentration-time curves of HMM and
its metabolites are shown in Fig. 1. Plasma levels of HMM can best be described
by a tri-exponential equation. HMM (5 mg/kg) was administered i.a. and i.v.
No significant differences were observed for $t_\frac{1}{2}$ (elimination half-life time)
and AUC (area under the plasma concentration-time curve) see Table 1. These
results indicate that HMM was not appreciably metabolized in the lung.

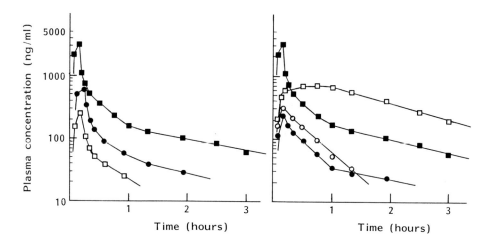

Fig. 1. left: Plasma levels of HMM (5 mg/kg) after i.v. ■–■, p.v. ●–● and i.d. □–□ infusion. right: Plasma levels of HMM (i.v. administration) and metabolites: HMM ■–■, Pentamethylmelamine ●–●, N^2,N^2,N^4,N^6-Tetramethylmelamine o–o and N^2,N^4,N^6-Trimethylmelamine □–□.

TABLE I

SOME PHARMACOKINETIC PARAMETERS FOR HMM

Conscious male Wistar rats received HMM hydrochloride via infusion

Drug	Route	Dose (mg/kg)	AUC_0^∞ (µg min/ml)	$t_{\frac{1}{2}}$ (min)	Clearance (ml/min/kg)
HMM (4)[b]	i.v.	10	122 ± 2^a	87 ± 21^c	82 ± 1^c
HMM (5)	i.a.	5	47 ± 8^c	75 ± 14^c	101 ± 29^c
HMM (6)	i.v.	5	61 ± 12^c	89 ± 12^c	86 ± 22^c
HMM (6)	p.v.	5	16 ± 7^d		
HMM (5)	i.d.	5	5 ± 2^d		

[a] Mean ± S.D.
[b] Figures in parentheses, number of rats
[c] No significant differences ($P > 0.1$) when compared with each other
[d] Significantly different ($P < 0.05$) when compared with each other

Also, HMM follows linear kinetics in the 5-10 mg/kg dose range (Table 1). Thus, no enzyme saturation is observed and total body clearance is dose independent. The biological availability of HMM after an i.d. dose was calculated using the relationship: $F_{id} = AUC_{id}/AUC_{iv}$. $F_{id} = 8 \pm 3\%$. After p.v. administration $27 \pm 12\%$ of the dose was systemically available. The low F_{id} could not be accounted for by incomplete absorption, as judged from metabolite data (results not shown). Moreover, at the end of an i.d. experiment, the intestinal tract was excised, rinsed with 25 ml saline and analyzed for HMM and metabolites. The maximum amount of HMM found corresponded to 0.3-2% of the dose administered. This indicates that HMM absorption from the intestine was essentially complete. Thus, the low F_{id} can only be the result of combined gut wall and liver first-pass metabolism. Intestinal and hepatic extraction ratios (E_G and E_H, respectively) can be calculated: $F_{id} = AUC_{id}/AUC_{iv} = (1-E_H)(1-E_G)$ and $AUC_{pv}/AUC_{iv} = 1-E_H$. Then: $E_H = 73 \pm 12\%$ and $E_G = 71 \pm 15\%$. The above results clearly demonstrate that the low biological availability of orally (or i.d.) administered HMM in rats is the result of simultaneous gut wall and liver metabolism under linear kinetic conditions. The question of how this presystemic elimination can contribute to the mechanism of antineoplastic activity of HMM remains to be investigated.

REFERENCES

1. Johnson, B.L., Fisher, R.I., Bender, R.A., DeVita, V.T., Chabner, B.A. and Young, R.C. (1978). Cancer (Phila.), 42, 2157.
2. Legha, S.S., Slavik, M. and Carter, S.K. (1976). Cancer (Phila.), 38, 27.
3. Rutty, C.J. and Connors, T.A. (1977). Biochem. Pharmacol., 26, 2385.
4. Ames, M.M., Sanders, M.E. and Tiede, W.S. (1981). Life Sci., 29, 1591.
5. Garattini, E., Donelli, M.G., Colombo, T., Paesani, R. and Pantarotto, C. (1981). Biochem. Pharmacol., 30, 1151.
6. Rutty, C.J. and Abel, G. (1980). Chem.-Biol. Interact., 29, 235.
7. D'Incalci, M., Erba, E., Balconi, G., Morasca, L. and Garattini, S. (1980). Br. J. Cancer, 41, 630.
8. Worzalla, J.F., Kaiman, B.D., Johnson, B.M., Ramirez, G. and Bryan, G.T. (1974). Cancer Res., 34, 2669.
9. Colombo, T., Broggini, M., Gescher, A. and D'Incalci, M. (1982). Xenobiotica, 12, 315.
10. Brindley, C., Gescher, A., Langdon, S.P., Broggini, M., Colombo, T. and D'Incalci, M. (1982). Biochem. Pharmacol., 31, 625.
11. Ames, M.M., Powis, G., Kovach, J.S. and Eagan, R.T. (1979). Cancer Res., 39, 5016.
12. Van de Vaart-van Zutphen, H.P.C., Smulders, C.F.A., Renema, J. and Hulshoff, A. (1982). Pharmaceutisch Weekblad Scientific Ed., 4, 25.
13. Hulshoff, A., Neijt, J.P., Smulders, C.F.A., van Loenen, A.C. and Pinedo, H.M. (1980). J. Chromatogr., 181, 363.

© 1983 Elsevier Science Publishers B.V.
Extrahepatic Drug Metabolism and Chemical Carcinogenesis,
J. Rydström, J. Montelius and M. Bengtsson eds.

319

BIOTRANSFORMATION OF HEXAMETHYLMELAMINE IN RAT ISOLATED INTESTINAL EPITHELIAL CELLS AND HEPATOCYTES. ROLE OF MITOCHONDRIAL CYTOCHROME P-450

PAUL BORM[1], PIERRE KLIPPERT[1], MARIE-JOSÉ MINGELS[2], ABRAM HULSHOFF[2], ANK
FRANKHUIJZEN-SIEREVOGEL[1] and JAN NOORDHOEK[1]
[1]Department of Pharmacology and Pharmacotherapy and [2]Department of Analytical
Pharmacy, Faculty of Pharmacy, State University of Utrecht, Catharijnesingel
60, 3511 GH Utrecht, The Netherlands

INTRODUCTION

Hexamethylmelamine (HMM), is a synthetic s-triazine derivative which has
demonstrated activity against a wide variety of solid human tumours (1). The
mechanism of action of HMM is uncertain. Intermediates in metabolic conversion,
such as the N-methylolmelamines which were demonstrated to be produced in vitro
in liver microsomes (2), are significantly more cytotoxic to tumour cell lines
than HMM itself (3, 4).

Recently it was shown in our department that HMM is subject to extensive gut
wall metabolism in vivo (5). It is now reported that mitochondrial and microsomal mixed-function oxidases play an equally significant role in the biotransformation of HMM in rat intestinal mucosal cells. Reported findings may have
important implications for the mechanism of antitumour activity of HMM.

MATERIALS AND METHODS

Animals and cell-preparation. Adult male Wistar rats weighing approximately
250 g (TNO, Zeist, The Netherlands) were used. Animals were killed by decapitation and intestinal mucosal cells were prepared as described previously (6).
Hepatocytes were isolated by sequential Ca^{++}-free and collagenase perfusion
in Hanks' buffer (7). Viability of hepatocytes and intestinal mucosal cells
as judged by trypan blue dye exclusion and leakage of Lactate-dehydrogenase
was always greater than 85 per cent.

Preparation of subcellular fractions. Microsomes and mitochondria were
prepared from cell-suspensions by homogenisation using an Ultra-Turrax (Janke &
Kunkel KG, Staufen im Breisgau, West-Germany) as the homogenizing apparatus.
Exact conditions were described previously (6, 8). Mitochondria were isolated
according to Iemhoff et al. (9) and used within 1 hr after preparation.

Incubations and analysis. Cells obtained from 0.125 g intestine ($7 \cdot 5 \cdot 10^6$
cells) or 0.005 g liver ($2 \cdot 5 \cdot 10^5$ cells) were used in Krebs-glucose-NaHCO$_3$
(3.0 ml total volume). Microsomes and mitochondria obtained from comparable

amounts of tissue were incubated in phosphate-buffer (50 mM, pH 7.4) containing 0.1 mM EDTA. The reaction was started by the addition of 0.5 ml HMM·hydrochloric solution in water. Incubations were stopped by the addition of 375 µl TCA (15%) and subsequently analyzed by HPLC with UV-detection as described previously (8). N-hydroxymethylpentamethylmelamine (HMPMM) was identified by GC-MS after derivatization. Incubations for this purpose were stopped with 2.0 ml ethyl-acetate, 50 µl 0.5 N NaOH was added, vortexed, and 1.0 ml of the organic layer reduced to dryness at 40° C. Mass spectra were obtained as previously described (8).

    Chemicals. NADP, G6-P (disodiumsalt), G6P-DH (grade I), ADP and ATP were purchased from Boehringer Mannheim (Mannheim, West-Germany). HMM was obtained from Ofichem (Gieten, The Netherlands). The N-demethylated metabolites of HMM were kindly provided by Dr. D.E.V. Wilman (Royal Cancer Hospital, London, U.K.). HMPMM was kindly provided by Dr. A. Gescher and Dr. B.P. Langdon (Aston University, Birmingham, U.K.).

RESULTS

    When studying HMM-disposition in isolated cells of rat small intestine and/or liver, a discrepancy was observed between the amount of HMM converted and the amount of pentamethylmelamine (PMM) produced (Fig. 1). Conditions of incubations were selected so that no further demethylation of PMM took place and protein and non-specific binding of HMM or PMM was less than 2 per cent.

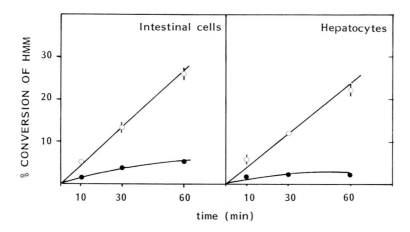

Fig. 1. HMM-conversion (o) and corresponding PMM-formation (●) in intestinal cells and hepatocytes. HMM-concentration was 20 µM and incubations were stopped at different time-intervals. Results are mean ± S.D. of three different cell-batches.

However, it appears that HMM-conversion equals PMM-production in incubations containing subcellular fractions (Table 1). Moreover, summation of HMM-turnover-rates of mitochondria and microsomes conforms to cellular turnover. In hepatocytes and subcellular fractions analogous results to intestinal cells were obtained (data not shown).

TABLE 1

TURNOVER OF HEXAMETHYLMELAMINE IN INTESTINAL CELLS

In vitro-system	HMM[a] conversion	PMM[a] production
Cells[b]	2.37 ± .53	.77 ± .06
Mitochondria[b]	1.29 ± .10	1.15 ± .10
9000 g sup	0.50 ± .09	.46 ± .02
Microsomes[b]	1.00 ± .10	.80 ± .04

[a]Values in nmoles/min.g intestine at 20 μM substrate concentration. Mean ± S.D. of three different cell batches.
[b]Corrected for cell-viability (90%), recoveries and microsomal contamination in mitochondria.

This means, we can explain for cellular turnover of HMM, but somehow PMM or an intermediary metabolite is trapped in the intact cell. Presumably, the mechanism involves the oxidation of HMM to N-hydroxymethyl-PMM and generation of either an imine or iminium intermediate which can be conjugated or bound covalently to macromolecules.

We could establish N-hydroxymethyl-PMM formation in mitochondrial incubations (HPLC, GC-MS) that can be inhibited by SKF-525A and metyrapone (8). At pH 7.4 the methylol dissociates spontaneously to PMM. No methylol could be demonstrated in microsomal incubations.

Activation of HMM is isolated (intestinal) mitochondria helps to clarify its considerable intestinal first-pass, but may also have important implications for the mechanism of the anti-tumour activity of HMM. Present work is concerned in elucidating the nature of the conjugate formed.

ACKNOWLEDGEMENTS

We express our thanks to Dr. M. van der Graft for preparation of isolated liver cells and to Dr. A. Gescher and Dr. P. Langdon for kindly supplying us with standard N-methylolpentamethylmelamine (HMPMM).

322

REFERENCES

1. Legha, S.S., Slavik, M. and Carter, S.K. (1976) Cancer (Phila.), 38, 27.

2. Gescher, A., D'Incalci, M., Fanelli, R. and Farina, P. (1980) Life Sci., 26, 147.

3. D'Incalci, M., Erba, E., Balconi, G., Marosca, L. and Garattini, S. (1980) Brit. J. Cancer, 41, 630.

4. Rutty, C.J. and Abel, G. (1980) Chem.-Biol. Interact., 29, 235.

5. Klippert, P.J.M., Hulshoff, A., Mingels, M.J., Hofman, G.A. and Noordhoek, J. (1983) Cancer Res., accepted for publication.

6. Borm, P.J.A., Frankhuijzen-Sierevogel, J.C. and Noordhoek, J. (1982) Biochem. Pharmac., 31, 3707.

7. Paine, A.J., Williams, L.J. and Legg, R.F. (1979) In: Preisig, R. and Bircher, J. (Eds.), The liver: quantitative aspects of structure and function, Editio Cantor, Aulendorf/Germany, pp. 99.

8. Borm, P.J.A., Mingels, M.J., Hulshoff, A., Frankhuijzen-Sierevogel, J.C. and Noordhoek, J. (1983) submitted for publication.

9. Iemhoff, W.G.J., Van den Berg, J.W.O., De Pijper, A.W. and Hülsmann, W.C. (1970) Biochim. Biophys. Acta, 215, 229.

PITUITARY CONTROL AND ROLE OF CYTOCHROME P-450 IN ENDOCRINE ORGANS

© 1983 Elsevier Science Publishers B.V.
Extrahepatic Drug Metabolism and Chemical Carcinogenesis,
J. Rydström, J. Montelius and M. Bengtsson eds.

METABOLISM OF POLYCYCLIC HYDROCARBONS IN THE MAMMARY GLAND AND THE HORMONE
MIMETIC ACTION OF THE CARCINOGENS

THOMAS L. DAO, CHARLES E. MORREAL AND DILIP K. SINHA
Department of Breast Surgery and Breast Cancer Research Unit, Roswell Park
Memorial Institute, 666 Elm Street, Buffalo, New York 14263 (U.S.A.)

INTRODUCTION

The unique sensitivity or susceptibility of the mammary gland to chemical
carcinogens such as 7,12-dimethylbenz[a]anthracene (DMBA) or 3-methylcholan-
threne (3-MC) has been the subject of investigation for many years (1,2). These
earlier studies led to two important observations: 1) a higher concentration of
the lipid-soluble hydrocarbons in the mammary fat pad and mammary tissues,
resulting in an environment conducive to carcinogenesis; and 2) an interaction
between the carcinogenic hydrocarbon and the ovarian hormones as a requisite
for tumor induction.

The demonstration of the critical role of ovarian hormones in mammary carcinogenesis led to several plausible considerations pertaining to the investigation of the mechanism of carcinogenesis. First, if metabolic activation of
a polycyclic hydrocarbon carcinogen is an essential first step, we suggest that
the formation of proximate carcinogens must necessarily take place in the target tissue, namely, the mammary gland. Second, the sterochemical similarities
which exist between the molecular skeletons of steroids and polycyclic hydrocarbons are probably responsible for a great deal of the similarities in the
biochemical reaction of these two classes of compounds (3), and, thirdly, polycyclic hydrocarbons may be hormone mimetic. In this paper, we discuss in detail these considerations and, in addition, data are presented from our studies
of the estrogenicity of several synthetic compounds (possible metabolites of
polycyclic hydrocarbons) having structural similarities to estrogens.

METABOLISM OF DMBA BY TARGET TISSUE

One pertinent approach toward seeking an answer to the question whether carcinogenic hydrocarbon metabolism is related to tumor induction is to study the
metabolism of hydrocarbons in the target tissue. This author showed earlier
that induction of mammary tumors could occur after in vitro exposure of the
target tissue to DMBA and subsequent transplantation of the mammary gland to
recipient hosts untreated by the carcinogen (4). Later, Dao and Sinha (5)
further demonstrated conclusively the induction of neoplastic change and cancer
in mammary explants in organ culture. These experiments clearly suggest that

if prior metabolism is necessary in carcinogenesis induced in the mammary gland by DMBA, it must occur in the mammary gland since in these above experiments, the carcinogen was not administered systemically.

We have investigated the metabolism of DMBA in both hepatic and mammary tissues of the female rat. Methods for tissue homogenization, incubation, extraction, purification and identification by thin layer chromatography, counter-current distribution and carrier recrystallization were described in detail in our earlier publication (6). The metabolism of DMBA-^{3}H was studied in the liver; in the liver of animals pretreated with 3-MC; in mammary tissues; and in mammary tissues from animals pretreated with 3-MC.

In the liver tissue, we identified radioactive 7-hydroxymethyl-12-methylbenz-[a]anthracene (7-OHM-12-MBA), 12-hydroxymethyl-7-methylbenz[a]anthracene (12-OHM-7-MBA), and 7,12-dihydroxymethylbenz[a]anthracene (7,12-diOHMBA). However, when the rats were pretreated with 3-MC (0.5 mg in DMSO, I.V.) 24 hours prior to tissue incubation, none of the hydroxymethyl compounds were found (Fig. 1,2).

Earlier studies of metabolism of DMBA in the liver have been reported by Boyland and Sims (7). These authors demonstrated the isolation and identification of isomeric monohydroxymethyl derivatives by chromatography and UV absorption. Comparative metabolism of DMBA in the liver and the adrenal of rat has been studied by Jellinck, et al. (8), who found that the isomeric monohydroxymethyl metabolites were present in the liver and adrenal gland of adult rats but absent in the adrenals of immature rats or mice. However, work by Sims (9) showed that the major metabolite of DMBA by the adrenal homogenate was 8,9-dihydro-8,9-dihydroxy-7,12-dimethylbenz[a]anthracene (8,9-diHOH-DMBA), instead of the isomeric monohydroxymethyl derivatives.

The conversion of DMBA by breast tissue is different from both normal and 3-MC treated liver. Mammary tissue homogenate incubated with ^{3}H-DMBA did not form 7,12-dihydroxymethylbenz[a]anthracene. However, prominent peaks were present in CCD patterns of TLC zones corresponding to 7-OHM-12-MBA and 12-OHM-7-MBA (Fig. 3,4). The identities of these compounds were positively verified by carrier recrystallization. Pretreatment of the rat with 3-MC led to an increase in the amount of both polar and water-soluble metabolites. This clearly reflects an increase in aryl hydrocarbon hydroxylase activity. It appears that pretreatment with 3-MC causes different metabolic patterns of DMBA in the liver and the mammary gland. The metabolism of DMBA by the liver was shifted from side chain to ring hydroxylation, but the mammary gland retained its ability to hydroxylate DMBA at the monohydroxy stage. The ability to form the 7-hydroxy derivatives by the mammary gland is markedly decreased as a result of 3-MC pre-

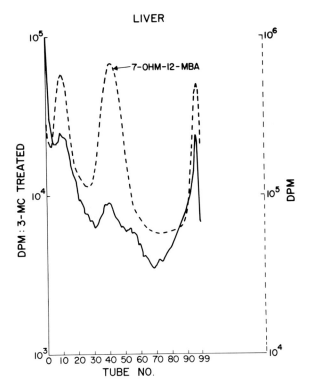

Fig. 1. Counter-current distribution (CCD) in ethanol:H_2O:heptane system of 7-OHM-12-MBA fraction. ---, normal liver; ——, liver from rats pretreated with 3-MC. Reprinted, with permission, from Tamulski (1973).

treatment. This finding suggests that pretreatment with 3-MC stimulates further metabolism to both polar and water-soluble components. Perhaps the most significant contribution of our study is to demonstrate for the first time that enzymes capable of transforming DMBA to hydroxymethyl derivatives were present in the mammary tissue. This observation supports our earlier postulate that conversion to a proximate carcinogen occurs in target tissue.

STUDIES ON HORMONE MIMETIC ACTION OF POLYCYCLIC HYDROCARBONS

The sterochemical similarities which exist between the molecular skeletons of steroids and polycyclic hydrocarbons have been well documented. Attempts to demonstrate the biological similarities of polycyclic hydrocarbons and estrogens have been largely unsuccessful. However, there were two observations that gave convincing evidence to suggest a hormone-mimetic action of polycyclic aromatic hydrocarbons. Dao and Greiner (10) in their studies on the induction of mammary

328

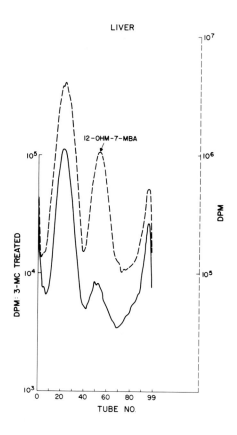

Fig. 2. CCD in ethanol:H$_2$O:heptane system of 12-OHM-7-MBA fraction.
---, normal liver. ———, liver from rats pretreated with 3-MC. Reprinted,
with permission, from Tamulski (1973).

cancer by carcinogenic hydrocarbons in the male rat observed that castrated
males bearing ovarian grafts developed enlargement and hyperplasia of acido-
philes of the pituitary gland. When 3-MC was administered to these rats,
"milk secretion" occurred in the mammary gland, but this phenomenon did not
occur in rats not treated with 3-MC. Later, Moon (11) reported that a single
feeding of 10 mg 3-MC to postpartum Sprague-Dawley rats resulted in an initial
lowering of pituitary prolactin, which was followed by a rebound to the control
level within 24 hr postfeeding. The authors also observed that estrogen-primed
rats treated daily with 10 mg 3-MC for 5 days showed mammary gland of the lac-
tational type, while those treated with the vehicle sesame oil showed varying
degrees of involution. These data suggest that 3-MC caused an increase in the
release of pituitary prolactin. The above observations led to the inevitable

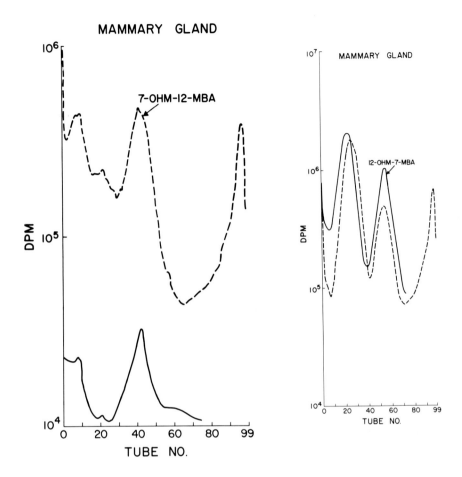

Fig. 3. CCD in ethanol:H$_2$O:heptane system of 7-OHM-12-MBA. ---, normal mammary gland; ———, gland from rats pretreated with 3-MC. Reprinted, with permission, from Tamulski (1973).

Fig. 4. CCD in same system of 12-OHM-7-MBA. ---, normal mammary gland; ———, gland from rats pretreated with 3-MC. Reprinted, with permission, from Tamulski (1973).

conclusion that polycyclic hydrocarbons may play a role in prolactin release or synthesis. Experiments were therefore designed to examine the effects of carcinogenic hydrocarbons such as 3-MC and DMBA and "noncarcinogenic" hydrocarbons such as anthracene, naphthalene, and phenanthrene on plasma and pituitary prolactin levels over a time period of 6, 12, 24, 48 and 72 hr after a single dose (I.M. injection) of any of these agents. In addition, each experimental group was accompanied by a group of rats receiving a single injection of estradiol benzoate for comparison. Each group contained 6 female, 55-60-day-old Sprague-Dawley rats. The blood samples were drawn at the proestrus period and were frozen at -20° until assay. Both serum and pituitary prolactin were assayed by the radioimmunoassay method described by Niswander, et al. (12). Anti-rat prolactin, reference standard prolactin and rat prolactin for iodination were kindly supplied by the National Institutes of Health.

The results of one experiment are shown in Fig. 5. Within 6 hr after a single dose of DMBA, the serum prolactin rose markedly to reach a peak between 6 and 12 hr. The prolactin level returned to the normal range about 48 hr later. In contrast, the pituitary prolactin reached its lowest level at about 12 hours, corresponding to the peak level of serum prolactin, which strongly suggests that prolactin release was markedly enhanced. The effects of DMBA on serum and pituitary prolactin are similar to those of estradiol, except that estradiol increases prolactin synthesis and thus causes a continuous rise of serum levels, even at 72 hr after a single injection.

Studies with noncarcinogenic polycyclic hydrocarbons, phenanthene and naphthalene, showed a lack of effect of these compounds on the release of prolactin. In contrast, 3-MC exerted a profound effect on prolactin release. Altogether, the above experiments and the data reported earlier by Dao (10) and Moon (11) suggest that carcinogenic hydrocarbons exert an effect on the release of prolactin, a phenomenon similarly exhibited by estrogen. It is not understood whether this mechanism by which the action of DMBA and 3-MC on pituitary release of prolactin is similar to that of an estrogen, which inhibits the hypothalamic PIF (pituitary inhibiting factor) and thus causes the release of prolactin by the pituitary. Our findings clearly suggest that carcinogenic polycyclic hydrocarbons are estrogen-mimetic. It is not unreasonable therefore to consider that if a metabolite of a polycyclic hydrocarbon is the active principle in the initiation of mammary cancer, it would probably be structurally related to the estrogenic phenolic steroid.

STUDIES OF BIOCHEMICAL PROPERTIES OF POLYCYCLIC HYDROCARBON DIOLS

In our studies of the metabolism of DMBA by mammary tissues in the rat, we found approximately 35% of the radioactive metabolites to be polar or more polar than 7,12-dihydroxymethylbenz[a]anthracene. This is the zone where diphenols would be expected to be found. The possible presence of appropriate phenol derivatives of the polycyclic hydrocarbons which would be expected to compete with estradiol for the binding sites on the cytoplasmic receptor protein is of great interest.

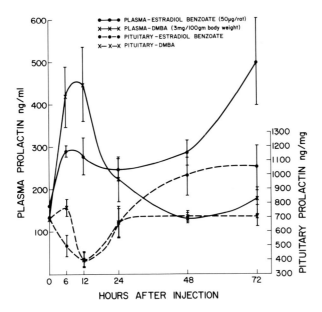

Fig. 5. The effect of DMBA and estradiol benzoate on plasma and pituitary prolactin levels.

Scale models show the great similarity in geometry of the steroid molecules and the carcinogenic polycyclic hydrocarbons; especially conspicuous is the closeness of the distance between the 3 and 17 hydroxy group of estradiol and comparable dihydroxy polycyclic hydrocarbons. The spatial similarities between estradiol, diethylstilbestrol and the appropriate diols are shown in Fig. 6.

The hydroxy phenolic derivatives of DMBA and BA were synthesized in the author's laboratory by Dr. Charles Morreal. These compounds are 7,12-dimethyl-benz[a]anthracene-3,9-diol (13) and 3,9-dihydroxybenz[a]anthracene (14). These two compounds were synthesized because both have the molecular geometry of the steroid nucleus. Our objective is to use these two compounds as a model to investigate their estrogen receptor binding properties, their estrogenic properties, and their possible carcinogenicity.

Estrogen receptor binding properties. These were determined in the uterine cytosol of immature Sprague-Dawley rats by competitive binding experiments with [^{3}H]estradiol and sucrose density centrifugation. The method for the binding assay of the dihydroxy phenolic derivatives of benz[a]anthracene and 7,12-dimethylbenz[a]anthracene was described in two previous papers (15,16). When 3,9-diOHBA was used as competitor, the concentration of the unlabelled compound was from 5.4×10^{-9} to 2.7×10^{-4}M. The concentration of unlabelled 3,9-diOH-

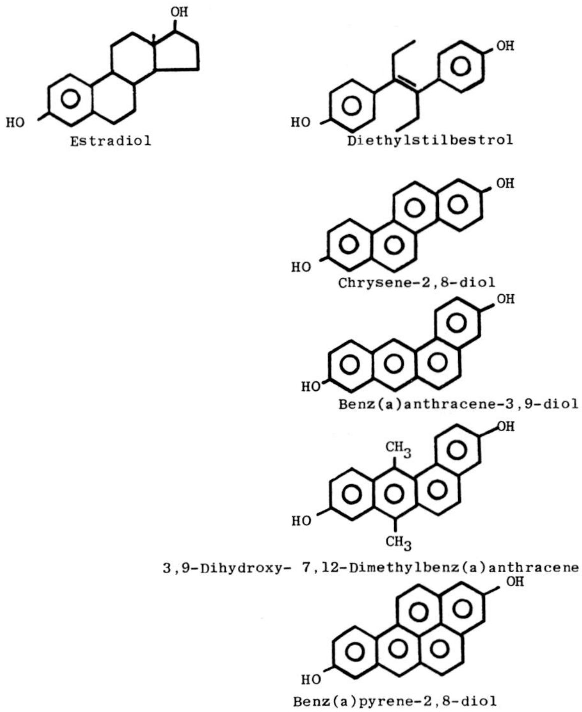

332

OH

HO Estradiol

OH

HO Diethylstilbestrol

OH

HO Chrysene-2,8-diol

OH

HO Benz(a)anthracene-3,9-diol

CH$_3$ OH

HO CH$_3$

3,9-Dihydroxy- 7,12-Dimethylbenz(a)anthracene

OH

HO Benz(a)pyrene-2,8-diol

Fig. 6. Structural formulae of estrogens and synthesized dihydroxy compounds.

DMBA was from 1.7×10^{-9} to 3.3×10^{-5}M. The competition was quantified by the method of Korenman (17). The relative binding affinity (RBA) was calculated from the ratio of the molar concentrations of cold estradiol to 3,9-diOHBA or 3,9-diOHDMBA that inhibits 50% of [^{3}H]estradiol binding. The RAC (relative association constant) was calculated by the formula RAC = (R x RBA)/(R+1- RBA). In this relationship, R is the ratio of free to bound steroid in the presence of only [^{3}H]17β-estradiol.

We analyzed sucrose gradient by using 10-30% sucrose gradients. Cytosol was incubated with [^{3}H]17β-estradiol in the presence or absence of either nafoxidine HCl or 3,9-diOHBA or 3,9-diOHDMBA. After 4 hr at 0°C, labelled cytosols were mixed with charcoal pellets freshly prepared from 0.5 ml of the charcoal suspension. After centrifugation at 800 x g, 150 µl aliquots of cytosol were applied to gradients. Centrifugation was performed in an SW-60 Ti rotor at 50,000 rpm for 16 hr in a Beckman L5-50 preparative centrifuge.

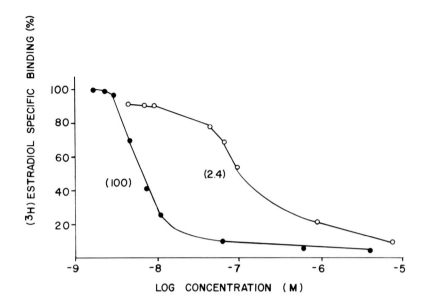

Fig. 7. Competitive binding assay of 3,9-diOHDMBA with rat uterine cytosol. Numbers in parentheses are RAC x 100. Reprinted, with permission, from Morreal (1979).

The results show that RBA for 3,9-diOHBA was 1.12×10^{-2} and that for 3,9-diOHDMBA was 5.2×10^{-2}. The competitive binding assays for these compounds are shown in Fig. 7 and 8. It should be noted that RAC for 3,9-diOHDMBA is 10 times greater than that of 3,9-diOHBA, indicating that 3,9-diOHDMBA binds more tightly to the receptor than 3,9-diOHBA. Inasmuch as 17β-estradiol is known to bind nonreceptor proteins present in the rat uterine cytosol, sucrose density gradient analysis of these two compounds demonstrates the specific binding of these two compounds to 8S protein of the rat uterine cytosol and their inhibition by nafoxidine or 3,9-diOHDMBA (Fig. 9). It shows that 3,9-diOHDMBA inhibited 17β-estradiol binding in the 8S region in the rat uterine cytosol at a concentration of 1×10^{-4}M equal to that of nafoxidine HCl required to inhibit specific binding. At a concentration of 1×10^{-7}M of 3,9-diOHDMBA, approximately 75% of the total 17β-estradiol was inhibited.

Estrogenic activities of polycylic hydrocarbon diols. The estrogenic activity of these diol compounds was assayed by measuring increasing uterine weights in ovariectomized rats. There were five groups of rats (5 rats/group), injected daily with 17β-estradiol in different doses (0.02, 0.2 and 2.0 μg per day) for

334

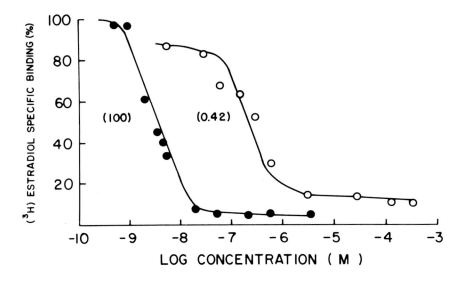

Fig. 8. Competitive binding assay of [^{3}H]estradiol (●—●) and 3,9-diOHBA
(o—o) with rat uterine cytosol. Numbers in parentheses are RAC x 100.
Reprinted, with permission, from Schneider (1976).

7 days and 3,9-diOHBA in doses of 20 and 500 µg daily for 7 days. In another
set of experiments, the dose of 17β-estradiol was the same and the doses of
3,9-diOHDMBA were 40.0 and 400 µg/day. Rats in the control group were given
0.1 ml olive oil for 7 days. The animals were killed 24 hr after the last injection and the uteri were removed, trimmed of fat and weighed.

The results of the bioassay of 3,9-diOHDMBA are summarized in table 1, which
reveals that both these compounds are weakly estrogenic. The results of bioassay indicate that 500 µg of 3,9-diOHBA had the same uterine weight increasing
effect as did 0.14 µg 17β-estradiol and that 500 µg of 3,9-diOHDMBA had the
same uterine weight increasing effect as did 0.112 µg of estradiol.

The above experiments conclusively demonstrated that both these compounds,
3,9-diOHBA and 3,9-diOHDMBA, are effective competitive inhibitors of estradiol
binding to the specific cytoplasmic receptors and they are both weakly estrogenic. These biochemical properties seem to be commensurate with the characteristics of an estrogenic hormone. Whether these compounds are carcinogenic is a
question yet to be answered. Our laboratory will test the carcinogenicity of
3,9-diOHDMBA and if it should prove to be carcinogenic, we will attempt to identify the metabolites in mammary tissue from rats receiving DMBA. We are presently also studying the metabolism of DMBA in the cell culture system.

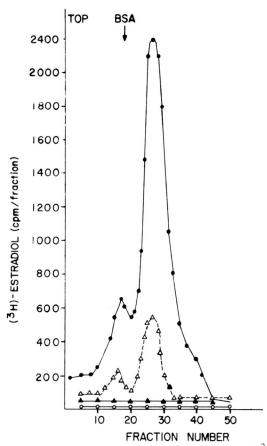

Fig. 9. Sucrose density gradient analysis of binding of [³H]estradiol (2.2 x 10⁻⁹M) to rat uterine cytosol (●—●) in the presence of nafoxidine HCl, 3 x 10⁻⁵M (o—o), and in the presence of 3,9-diOHBA, 1.2 x 10⁻⁵M (△—△). Reprinted, with permission, from Schneider (1976).

TABLE 1

INCREASE IN UTERINE WEIGHTS OF OVARIECTOMIZED RATS

Group No.	Daily dose, μg	Final uterine weight, mg/100 g body wt[a]
1	---	75.21 ± 4.8
2	0.02 17β-estradiol	133.79 ± 10.6
3	0.20 17β-estradiol	187.46 ± 4.1
4	2.00 17β-estradiol	230.09 ± 5.2
5	40.00 3,9-diOHDMBA	101.27 ± 4.7
6	400.00 3,9-diOHDMBA	167.64 ± 7.6

[a]Values are means ± S.E.

Reprinted, with permission, from Morreal (1979).

336

REFERENCES

1. Dao, T.L., Bock, F.G. and Crouch, S. (1959) Soc. Exp. Biol. Med., 102, 635.

2. Dao, T.L. (1962) Cancer Res., 22, 973.

3. Young, N.C., Castro, A.J., Lewis, M. and Wong, T.W. (1961) Science, 134, 386.

4. Dao, T.L. (1970) Proc. Exp. Biol. Med., 133, 416.

5. Dao, T.L. and Sinha, D.K. (1972) J. Natl. Cancer Inst., 49, 591.

6. Tamulski, T.S., Morreal, C.E., and Dao, T.L. (1973) Cancer Res., 33, 3117.

7. Boyland, E. and Sims, P. (1965) Biochem. J., 95, 780.

8. Jellinck, P.H., Coles, S. and Garland, M. (1967) Biochem. Pharmacol., 16, 2449.

9. Sims, P. (1970) Biochem. Pharmacol., 19, 2261.

10. Dao, T.L. and Greiner, M.J. (1961) J. Natl. Cancer Inst., 27, 333.

11. Moon, R.C. (1964) J. Natl. Cancer Inst., 32, 461.

12. Niswender, D., Chen, C.L., Midgeley, A.R., Meites, J. and Ellis, S. (1969) Proc. Soc. Exp. Biol. Med., 130, 393.

13. Morreal, C.E. and Bronstein, R.E. (1978) J. Chem. Eng. Data, 23, 354.

14. Morreal, C.E. and Alks, V. (1975) Org. Chem., 40, 3411.

15. Schneider, S.L., Alks, V., Morreal, C.E., Sinha, D.K., and Dao, T.L. (1976) J. Natl. Cancer Inst., 57, 1351.

16. Morreal, C.E., Schneider, S.L., Sinha, D.K. and Bronstein, R.E. (1979) J. Natl. Cancer Inst., 62, 1585.

17. Korenman, S.G. (1970) Endocrinology, 87, 1119.

© 1983 Elsevier Science Publishers B.V.
Extrahepatic Drug Metabolism and Chemical Carcinogenesis,
J. Rydström, J. Montelius and M. Bengtsson eds.

BENZO(A)PYRENE REPRODUCTIVE TOXICITY AND OVARIAN METABOLISM

DONALD R. MATTISON[1], MARIA S. NIGHTINGALE[1], KEN TAKIZAWA[1], ELLEN K. SILBERGELD[1],

HARUHIKO YAGI[2], AND DONALD M. JERINA[2]

[1]Pregnancy Research Branch, NICHD, and [2]Laboratory of Bioorganic Chemistry,

NIADDK, National Institutes of Health, Bethesda, MD   20205 (U.S.A.)

INTRODUCTION

Reproductive toxicology is gaining attention as our concern for adverse

xenobiotic effects to the reproductive system grows (1-3). Among reports

dealing with female reproductive toxicity, 38% involve menstruation, fertility,

ovarian function or hormone production (Table 1) reflecting hypothalamic,

TABLE 1

REPORTED ADVERSE EFFECTS OF ENVIRONMENTAL CHEMICALS ON FEMALE REPRODUCTION

Adverse Effect	Site of Toxicity[a]	Reported (%)
Miscarriage	E,F,P,O,U,C	23
Pregnancy	E,F,P,O,U,C	21
Menstruation	H,P,O,U	18
Genetalia	S	10
Fertility	H,P,O,U,T	8
Ovary	H,P,O	7
Hormones	H,P,O	5
Uterus	U	4
Cervix	C	3
Vagina	S	1
Libido	CNS,H,P,O	1

[a]Key for site of toxicity: E = embryo, F = fetus, P = placenta, H = hypothalamus, P = pituitary, O = ovary, S = skin, C = cervix, U = uterus, CNS = central nervous system, T = fallopian tube.

pituitary or ovarian toxicity (2). These are interconnected in the human through the follicle complex which controls hypothalamic-pituitary function, menstruation, and to a large extent fertility (32,33). This suggests that human ovarian function may be impaired by xenobiotics, consistent with clinical data demonstrating ovarian toxicity (4-6). Cigarette smoking can also impair fertility, and decrease the age of menopause (7,8). At all ages there are more menopausal women among smokers than non-smokers (Table 2), with a dose effect relationship. Early menopause from xenobiotics may be due to oocyte destruction or increased atresia (9).

TABLE 2

EFFECT OF CIGARETTE SMOKING ON THE AGE OF MENOPAUSE (% MENOPAUSAL)[a]

Age	Never Smoked	Current Smokers	
		1/2 ppd	⩾ 1 ppd
44-45	13	19	14
46-47	23	30	35
48-49	34	44	51
50-51	65	77	82
52-53	77	86	92

[a]Data from Jick et al (8).

These observations suggest the necessity to develop a better understanding of ovarian toxicity. These experiments were designed to explore the effect of benzo(a)pyrene (BP), a known ovotoxin (10-12) on the murine ovary, and compare murine and nonhuman primate ovarian BP metabolism.

MATERIALS AND METHODS

Animals. Inbred DBA/2N (D2) and C57BL/6N (B6) mice, and their (D2xB6)F1 heterozygote (F1) were obtained and maintained as described (13). Cynomolgus

(Cynos) monkeys (Macaca fasicularis) used for ovarian metabolism studies were normal cycling females maintained as described (14).

Chemicals. BP, 3-methylcholanthrene (3MC), NADPH, and NADH were obtained from Sigma. Derivatives used in ip treatment, or HPLC analysis were a gift from the NCI carcinogen repository. BP derivatives used in io injections were synthesized as described (15,16). Generally labeled ^{3}H-BP was obtained from NEN.

Oocyte Destruction Following IP Treatment with BP or Derivatives. D2, B6 and F1 mice were treated with BP (1 to 500 mg/kg) in corn oil or corn oil (ip, 1 ml/20 gms) and 5/dose group sacrificed up to 31 days after treatment.

Oocyte Destruction Following Intraovarian (io) Treatment. Mice were anesthetized with ether, the ovary exteriorized through a small incision and treated with indicated compound in 1 µl of DMSO.

Oocyte Counting. Both ovaries were removed, fixed and processed as described (13). Oocytes were classified as (17): small oocytes or follicles, Types 1 through 3; growing, Types 4 and 5; antral, Types 6 through 8. Dose response curves were calculated as described (18).

Reproductive Capacity. Mice (30/dose and strain) were treated ip with BP (1 to 50 mg/kg) and placed 5/cage. Following placement of the male, cages were inspected daily, pups were counted and removed after littering. Data analysis was performed using the Statistical Analysis System software on the NIH IBM-370.

Ovarian BP Metabolism. Mice were treated with corn oil (1 ml/20 g) or 3MC (100 mg/kg) three days before sacrifice. Ovaries were removed from Cynos and mice randomly during the cycle, cleaned, homogenized with a Polytron and centrifuged at 9,000xg for 20 min. The 9,000xg supernatant (S-9) was used to assay ovarian BP metabolism which was quantitated by reverse phase HPLC on a DuPont Zorbax ODS column (19). Each assay was conducted in duplicate with blanks (S-9 without cofactor).

340

RESULTS AND DISCUSSION

  Differental Follicle Sensitivity and Temporal Evolution of Dose-Response.

Blunted dose response curves for antral and growing follicle destruction were

seen 28 to 31 days following BP treatment (Table 3). B6 treated with 500 or

100 mg/kg, had 82% or 20% of the antral follicles destroyed. F1 had 90% and

60% destruction of antral follicles, and D2 had 60% and 20% destruction follow-

ing treatment with BP. At 28 to 31 days following treatment with 500 or 100

TABLE 3

EFFECT OF BP ON GROWING AND ANTRAL FOLLICLE NUMBER IN B6, F1, AND D2 MICE

ANTRAL FOLLICLES (Percent Remaining)

BP (mg/kg)	B6	F1	D2
500	18	10	40
100	80	40	80

GROWING FOLLICLES (Percent Remaining)

BP (mg/kg)	B6	F1	D2
500	5	25	28
100	22	38	71

---

mg/kg, 95% and 78% of the growing follicles were destroyed in B6, 72% and 29%

were destroyed in D2, and 75% and 62% were destroyed in F1 mice.

  Small follicles were more sensitive to BP ovotoxicity than growing or

antral follicles (Fig. 1). Small oocyte destruction was observed about 50

mg/kg, in B6, D2, and F1 mice, 5 days following BP treatment, and was complete

at 100 mg/kg in B6 mice. Small oocyte destruction was only partially complete

in D2 and F1 mice treated with 500 mg/kg sacrificed on day 5. Small oocyte

destruction began about 10 mg/kg in all three groups of mice 14 days follow-

ing treatment and was complete about 100 mg/kg. The ED50s for small follicle

destruction at 14 days were 45 mg/kg in D2, 64 mg/kg in F1, and 38 mg/kg in B6

SMALL OOCYTE DESTRUCTION BY BENZO(A)PYRENE

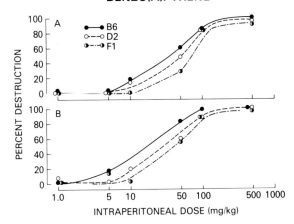

Figure 1. Small follicle destruction in mice sacrificed at: A, 14d; B, D2 and B6-28d; Fl 31d.

mice. Small follicle destruction plateaued after day 14, and on days 28 to 31 ED50s for small follicle destruction were: D2, 37 mg/kg; Fl, 38 mg/kg; and B6, 26 mg/kg.

BP ovotoxicity has been observed previously (10-13, 19-22). The relative insensitivity of growing and antral follicles to destruction by polycyclic hydrocarbons has also been observed (22), however the dose dependence had not been described. Essentially all small follicles were destroyed in D2, B6 and Fl mice treated with 100 mg/kg, while 20% to 60% of the growing and 62% to 78% of the antral follicles were destroyed (Table 3). This difference is striking when it is realized that growing and antral follicles contain rapidly prolifer-ating granulosa cells, with higher metabolic requirements than small follicles. Other investigators have observed similar differential murine follicle sensi-tivity to ionizing radiation, suggesting some common underlying factor such as target molecule (10), or detoxification (23) may account for this difference. The relative insensitivity of growing and antral murine follicles contrasts

with clinical observations and studies using non-human primates which demonstrate toxicity to growing and antral primate follicles (Mattison, unpublished
data; 4,24).

The minimal difference in ED50s for small oocyte destruction at 14 and
28-31 d (Fig. 1) contrasts with early observations (20,21), analysis of the
temporal evolution of the dose response curves reveals the reason for our
initial emphasis on strain differences in murine ovotoxicity. At short times
after PAH treatment there is a considerable difference in ED50s for small
oocyte destruction in B6 vs D2 and F1 mice (21), however, this difference
decreases with time.

Because of 2 to 3 fold greater ovarian aryl hydrocarbon hydroxylase (AHH)
activity after BP treatment in F1 and B6 compared to D2 mice we anticipated
ovotoxicity would parallel ovarian AHH activity. That is not the case. Ovarian
AHH activity and ovotoxicity following ip treatment with PAH do not appear
linked (13,25). This discrepancy between ovarian AHH activity and ovotoxicity
could result from: (i) ovarian toxicity from metabolites formed outside of the
ovary; (ii) more rapid clearance of BP in inducible (B6, F1) than noninducible
(D2) mice; (iii) or the AHH assay may not measure production of ovotoxic metabolites. We have begun to explore these issues by studying ovotoxicity following ip or io treatment.

IP Treatment with BP and Derivatives. Following ip treatment with: BP,
2OH-BP, 3OH-BP, 6OH-BP, 7OH-BP, 9OH-BP, 4,5,-oxide, c-4,5-DHD, t-4,5-DHD,
7,8-oxide, or t-7,8-DHD in doses from 1 to 100 mg/kg the 3OH, and the 9OH
metabolites, contributors to fluorescense in the AHH assay were less ovotoxic
than BP (Fig. 2). All phenols, except 2OH-BP, were less ovotoxic than BP.
The three 4,5-region metabolites and the 7,8 oxide were less toxic, while the
7,8-DHD was more toxic than BP. This suggests that extra-ovarian BP metabolism
may contribute to ovotoxicity.

IO Treatment with BP and Derivatives. A similar pattern of small follicle toxicity was observed following io treatment (Table 4). B6 and D2 mice treated with io BP had 61% and 31% small follicle destruction. The 3-, 7- and 9-phenols were less toxic than BP. The 2-phenol was more toxic than BP in B6 but less toxic in D2 mice. Although little ovotoxicity was observed following ip treatment with the 6-phenol, following io treatment 35% and 49% of the small follicles were destroyed in D2 and B6 mice. As observed following ip treatment the 7,8-oxide is a weak ovotoxin. The (-)-t-7,8-dihydrodiol was as toxic as BP following io treatment.

The most toxic metabolite in this experiment the (+)-DE2 produced 92% and 99% small follicle destruction in D2 and B6 mice. This high degree of ovotoxicity is consistent with observations suggesting that the (+)-DE2 is an ultimate mutagen, carcinogen and tumorigen (26-28). Also of interest is the small strain difference in ovotoxicity for (+)-DE2 compared to the difference for several other derivatives (i.e. 4-5 fold for BP and (-)-t-DHD, and 8 fold for the 2-phenol). This suggests that once (+)-DE2 is formed in the ovary, the target macromolecule(s) and mechanisms of ovarian detoxification are similar in D2 and B6 mice.

These data demonstrate that the ovary can metabolize BP and some BP metabolites to ovotoxic products. Therefore, both ovarian and extraovarian metabolism may contribute to ovotoxicity. The relative contributions made by each may depend on substrate, species, age and ovarian hormonal milieu (36). The potent ovotoxicity of (+)-DE2 suggests that it is an ultimate ovarian toxin formed by ovarian and/or extra-ovarian metabolic processing. Ovotoxicity following io treatment also parallels mutagenicity and carcinogenicity for these polycyclic hydrocarbons (25-27) suggesting that oocyte destruction may represent another useful in vivo assay system for genotoxicity.

Reproduction following BP treatment. D2, B6, and F1 mice treated with BP had dose dependent decreases in reproductive lifespan (Fig. 3). Most F1 mice

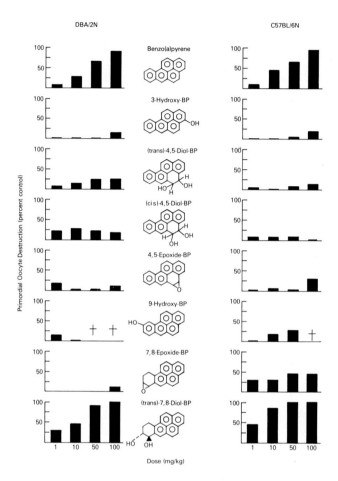

Figure 2. Effect of ip treatment on small follicle destruction.

in the control and BP treated groups achieved 5 litters, and 25/30 of the control and BP treated D2 mice achieved 5 litters. Among B6 mice, 27/30 control and 1 mg/kg treated mice achieved 5 litters, 17/30 of those treated at 10 mg/kg and 16/30 of those treated at 50 mg/kg achieved 5 litters. Similar dose dependent decreases in the number of mice achieving 10 litters was seen among the B6 and D2 mice. F1 mice were more prolific, and except for those treated with BP at 50 mg/kg dose dependent decreases in number of mothers achieving 10 or 15 litters was not evident, however, there were dose dependent decreases in

TABLE 4

SMALL FOLLICLE DESTRUCTION (Percent Destroyed)

Compound (10 µg/ovary)	D2	B6
BP	31	61
2OH	8	87
3OH	4	11
6OH	35	49
7OH	0	1
9OH	0	6
7,8-oxide	0	12
(-)-t-DHD	37	59
+ DE2	92	99

the number of mice achieving 20 and 25 litters. These alterations in fertility were reflected in the total number of pups and litters produced by BP treated mice (Table 5).

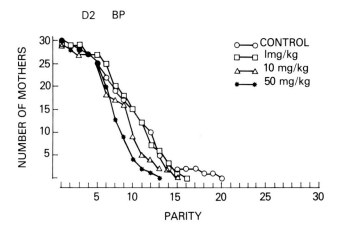

Figure 3. Effect of BP on maximum parity of D2 mice.

TABLE 5

EFFECT OF BP ON FERTILITY IN B6, D2, AND F1 MICE

TOTAL NUMBER OF PUPS	D2	B6	F1
Control	744	1032	3654
BP (50 mg/kg)	662	498	2711

TOTAL NUMBER OF LITTERS	D2	B6	F1
Control	218	248	569
BP (50 mg/kg)	167	128	392

Because BP destroys small, and to a lesser extent growing and antral follicles a decrease in fertility is expected, and consistent with previous observations with BP (29), ionizing radiation (30,31) and alkylating agents (38). In this experiment alterations in fertility were seen with doses of BP below ED50s for small follicle destruction. Even the highest dose of BP tested (50 mg/kg) produced less than 90% oocyte destruction (Fig. 1), suggesting that BP can alter fertility by mechanisms other than follicle destruction, such as increased atresia or alterations of meiosis (34) or steroid metabolism (28).

Ovarian BP Metabolism. As ovarian metabolism contributes to ovarian toxicity we have measured murine and non-human primate ovarian BP metabolism. Basal levels of ovarian BP metabolism were similar in D2, B6, and F1 mice, approximately 1 pmole/mg ovarian S-9/min, (Table 6). Following treatment with 3MC ovarian BP metabolism decreased in D2, while in B6 and F1 mice it increased 2 to 3 fold. The rate of cyno ovarian BP metabolism was considerably higher (i.e. 13 vs 3 pmole/mg/min).

Comparison of the metabolites formed reveals differences between murine and primate ovaries. In mice the "3" and "9" phenol peaks represent about 80%

of the metabolites formed. In cynos these two phenol peaks represent less than 15% of the metabolites formed. In the mouse the 7,8-diol represented about 15% of the metabolites formed, in cynos this metabolite represented 29 to 42% of the metabolites formed. The 9,10-diol also represents a larger proportion of the metabolic profile in cynos than mice. In D2, B6 and F1 mice the 9,10-diol represented 2 to 4% of the metabolite formed, while in cynos the 9,10-diol represented 5 to 7% of the metabolites formed.

These and other data demonstrate that the ovary has enzymes necessary for metabolic processing of xenobiotics to genotoxic products (35-37). To the extent that BP metabolism in the 7,8,9,10 region is important in ovotoxicity (19) this data suggests that cynos and perhaps other primates may be vulnerable to ovarian toxicity dependent on ovarian BP metabolism.

TABLE 6

OVARIAN BP METABOLISM

METABOLITE (% TOTAL)	D2		B6		F1		Cynomolgus
	CO	3MC	CO	3MC	CO	3MC	
9,10-diol	3.3	1.4	4.3	3.5	2.0	2.7	6.5
4,5-diol	4.3	2.7	5.0	1.1	5.0	1.1	17.4
7,8-diol	13.3	13.2	16.3	17.7	12.8	17.6	40.4
1,6-dione	0.5	1.7	0.3	1.2	0	0.1	0
3,6-dione	0.7	0.5	2.9	2.1	6.2	3.6	19.0
6,12-dione	0	0	0	3.1	0	0	0
"9"-phenol	37.3	37.8	34.2	21.4	30.8	23.9	8.0
"3"-phenol	40.7	42.6	37.1	50.0	43.2	51.0	8.7
TOTAL ACTIVITY pmoles/mg/min	1.05	0.43	0.79	2.68	0.75	1.73	13.4

CONCLUSIONS

This data stresses several factors: (i) the ubiquitous xenobiotic BP is indeed a reproductive toxin, destroying small, growing and large follicles; (ii) BP also decreases fertility in mice. This decrease in fertility is due both to oocyte destruction, and other mechanism(s) because it occurs at levels of ovotoxicity lower than would be expected to alter reproductive capacity. Both ovarian and extra-ovarian metabolism may contribute to ovarian toxicity, therefore attempts to correlate ovarian toxicity and ovarian metabolism will be difficult. One way to circumvent this difficulty is to use io injection. This treatment route is useful because it avoids strain or species differences in extraovarian metabolism, distribution, or other factors which may modify ovarian toxicity. This is important because ovarian BP metabolism may be different in murine and primate species. Experiments in progress in our laboratory suggest that the cynomolgus monkey is a suitable model for human ovarian toxicity.

ACKNOWLEDGEMENTS

We would like to thank Ms. L. Baldwin for superb secretarial assistance.

REFERENCES

1. Mattison, D.R. (1983) Reproductive Toxicology, Alan R. Liss, New York, pp. 1-396.

2. Pruett, J.G., Winslow, S.G. (1982) Health Effects of Environmental Chemicals on Human Reproduction. A selected bibliography with abstracts 1963-1981. NLM/TIRC-82/1.

3. Barlow, S.M., Sullivan, F.M. (1982) Reproductive Hazards of Industrial Chemicals. Academic Press, New York, pp. 1-610.

4. Chapman, R.M. (1983) in: Mattison, D.R. (Ed). Reproductive Toxicology, Alan R. Liss, New York, pp. 149-162.

5. Mandl, A.M. (1964) Biol. Rev. 39, 288.

6. Ash, P. (1980) Br. J. Radiol. 53, 271.

7. Mattison, D.R. (1982) Environ. Res. 28, 410.

8. Jick, H., Porter, J., Morrison, A.S. (1977) Lancet 1, 1354.

9. Mattison, D.R., Thorgeirsson, S.S. (1978) Lancet 1, 187.

10. Dobson, R.L., Felton, J.S. (1983) in: Mattison, D.R. (Ed). Reproductive Toxicology, Alan R. Liss, New York, pp. 175-190.

11. Mattison, D.R., Shiromizu, K., Nightingale, M.S. (1983) in: Mattison, D.R. (Ed). Reproductive Toxicology, Alan R. Liss, New York, pp. 191-201.

12. Mackenzie, K.M., Angevine, D.M. (1981) Biol. Reprod. 24, 183.

13. Mattison, D.R., Nightingale, M.S. (1980) Toxicol Appl. Pharmacol. 56, 399.

14. Hodgen, G.D., Tullner, W.W., Vaitukaitis, J.L., Ward, D.N., Ross, G.T. (1974) J. Clin Endocrinol. Metab. 39, 417.

15. Yagi, H., Hernandez, O., Jerina, D.M. (1975) J. Amer. Chem. Soc. 97, 6881.

16. Yagi, H., Holder, G.M., Dansette, P.M., Hernandez, O., Yeh, H.J.C., LeMahieu, R.A., Jerina, D.M. (1976) J. Org. Chem. 41, 977.

17. Pedersen, T., Peters, H. (1968) J. Reprod. Fertil. 17, 555.

18. DeLean, A., Munson, P., Rodbard, D. (1977) Am. J. Physiol. 235, E97.

19. Mattison, D.R., West, D.M., Menard, L.H. (1979) Biochem Pharmac 28, 2101.

20. Mattison, D.R., Thorgeirsson, S.S. (1978) Cancer Res. 38, 1368.

21. Mattison, D.R., Thorgeirsson, S.S. (1979) Cancer Res. 39, 3471.

22. Mattison, D.R. (1980) Toxicol. Appl. Pharmacol. 53, 249.

23. Mattison, D.R., Shiromizu, K., Pendergrass, J.A., Thorgeirsson, S.S. (1983) Pediatric Pharmacology, In Press.

24. Baker, T.G, Neal, P. (1977) in: Zuckerman, S.J., Weir, B.J. (eds) The Ovary Vol III, Second Edition, Academic Press, New York, pp. 1-58.

25. Mattison, D.R., Nightingale, M.S. (1982) Ped. Pharmacol. 2, 11.

26. Gelboin, H.V. (1980) Physiol. Rev. 60, 1107.

27. Pelkonen, O., Nebert, D.W. (1982) Pharmacologic Rev. 34, 189.

28. Conney, A.H. (1982) Cancer Res. 42, 4875.

29. Mattison, D.R., White, N.B., Nightingale, M.S. (1980) Ped. Pharmacol. 1, 143.

30. Peters, H., Levy, E. (1964) J. Reprod. Fertil. 7, 37.

31. Peters, H., Levy, E. (1963) Rad. Res. 18, 421.

32. Mattison, D.R., Nightingale, M.S., Shiromizu, K. (1983) Environ. Health Perspect. 48, 43.

33. Mattison, D.R., Ross, G.T. (1983) in: Vouk, V.B., Sheehan, P.J. (Eds.) Methods for Assessing the Effects of Chemicals on Reproductive Functions. SCOPE pp. 217-246.

34. Basler, A., Rohrborn, G. (1976) Mutat. Res. 38, 327.

35. Heinrichs, W.L., Juchau, M.R. (1980) in: Gram T.E. (Ed.) Extrahepatic Metabolism of Drugs and Other Foreign Compounds, S.P. Medical and Scientific Books, New York pp. 319-332.

36. Bengtsson, M., Rydstrom, J. (1983) Science 219, 1437.

37. Bengtsson, M., Montelius, J., Mankowitz, L., Rydstrom, J. (1983) Biochem. Pharmacol. 32, 129.

38. Generoso, W.M., Stout, S.K., Huft, S.W. (1971) Mutation Res. 13, 171.

© 1983 Elsevier Science Publishers B.V.
Extrahepatic Drug Metabolism and Chemical Carcinogenesis,
J. Rydström, J. Montelius and M. Bengtsson eds.

HORMONAL REGULATION OF CYTOCHROME P-450 DEPENDENT MONOOXYGENASE ACTIVITY AND
BENZOPYRENE METABOLISM IN RAT TESTES.

I. P. LEE[1], K. SUZUKI[2], J. NAGAYAMA[3], H. MUKHTAR[4] AND J. R. BEND[5]

[1]Laboratory of Reproductive and Developmental Toxicology and [5]Laboratory of
Pharmacology, National Institute of Environmental Health Sciences, Research
Triangle Park, North Carolina 27709 (USA), [2]Nippon Veterinary and Zootechnical
College, Tokyo (Japan), [3]Faculty of Medicine, Kyushu University, Fukuoka 812
(Japan) and [4]Dept. of Dermatology, Case Western Reserve University, Cleveland,
Ohio (USA)

INTRODUCTION

All organs and tissues are potential targets for chemical toxicity, with the
testis being one of the more critical since testicular exposure to certain
pollutants might increase the frequency of germ cell mutations and consequently be associated with heritable genetic disease. Polycyclic aromatic hydrocarbons (PAH) have been shown to be toxic to male and female reproductive
organs in various species (1-4). Like many other environmental chemicals, PAH
require metabolic activation by the monooxygenase(s) system before affecting
toxic actions on target organs. In organs other than testes, the toxic effects
of PAH has been attributed to reactive metabolites, epoxides, which may interact with DNA, RNA, and proteins. A steady-state level of epoxide(s) within
the cells of a target organ is obviously a function of the metabolite's rate
of formation and degradation and the sensitivity of the organ to the toxic
metabolite(s). Consequently, the rates of epoxide forming and detoxifying enzyme activities in various tissues or cells may be an important determinant of
tissue specific toxicity. This paper reports the hormonal regulation, the
ontogeny of monooxygenase(s) and epoxide metabolizing enzyme activities and
benzo(a)pyrene metabolism in rat testes.

MATERIALS AND METHODS

Chemicals and hormones. [8-^{14}C]styrene oxide (Spec. act. 0.37 mCi/mmol;
radioactive purity > 98.5%) was obtained from Mallindrodt Chemicals, St. Louis,
MO. [^{3}H]- 4,5-BPO (specific activity, 10 mCi/mmol; radiochemical purity
> 99%) was obtained from Amersham/Searle Corp., Arlington Heights, Ill., and
nonlabeled BPO was purchased from Eastman Organic Chemicals, Rochester, N.Y.
[7,10-^{14}C]BP was purified by HPLC; nonlabeled BP was purified using alumina
column chromatography followed by recrystallization in methanol.

The purity of BP was greater than 99%. Chemically pure BP metabolites, 9,10-diol, 7,8-diol, 4,5-diol, 3-OH, 9-OH, 7-,12-hydroxybenzo(a)pyrene, 1,6-quinone, 3,6-quinone, and 6,12-quinone were obtained from Midwest Research Institute, Kansas City, MO. HPLC quality solvents (acetone, ethyl acetate, and methanol) were purchased from Waters Associates, Milford, Mass. and Preiser Scientific, Durham, N.C. BP was obtained from the Eastman Kodak Organic Chemical Company, Rochester, N.Y. HEPES, glucose 6-phosphate, glucose-6-phosphate dehydrogenase (type XI), and NADP were purchased from Sigma Chemical Company, St. Louis, MO. Other chemicals were of reagent grade and were obtained from standard commercial sources. FSH (NIH-ovine-FSH-S-12) and LH (NIH-ovine LH-S-20) were provided by the Endocrinology Study Section, National Institute of Arthritis, Metabolism, and Digestive Diseases, NIH, Bethesda, MD; the mean relative potencies of FSH and LH were 1.02 to 1.33 units/g and 0.89 to 1.24 units/mg. Testosterone propionate and Vitamin E was obtained commercially.

Animals and experimental design. All animals used in these experiments were CD Sprague-Dawley rats and purchased from Charles River Breeding Laboratories, Inc., Wilmington, MA. To study the ontogeny of cytochrome P-450 dependent monooxygenase(s) activity and epoxide metabolizing enzyme activities, pregnant rats with known plug date and their male offspring were selected and dated. Male rats of desired ages were sacrificed by cervical dislocation to study postnatal development of testicular aryl Hydrocarbon Hydroxylase (AHH), epoxide hydrase (EH), glutathione transferase activities, and cytochrome P-450 content. To study the effects of FSH, LH, and testosterone administration on cytochrome P-450 content and specific AHH, EH, and GSH-T activities of testis and liver, control adult male, sham-operated and hypophysectomized Sprague-Dawley rats (10 weeks old) were used throughout the experiments. Animals were housed 3/cage and allowed free access to a rodent diet (NIH-31S) and drinking water containing 5% dextrose for the first postoperative week. Animals were maintained under stable conditions of illumination (14 hr light, 10 hr dark cycle) and temperature (25^{0}). The experimental groups consisted of control, sham-operated, and hypophysectomized rats. Each group consisted of 60 male rats with the exception of the hypophysectomized animals (240 male rats) which were subdivided into 4 groups. Forty days after surgery, each of the hypophysectomized groups received 3 daily s.c. injections (9 a.m., 1 p.m., and 5 p.m. daily) of either FSH (100 μg), LH (100 μg), or FSH plus LH (100 μg each) in 0.1 ml of 0.15 M NaCl per injection per rat or testosterone (100 μg) in 0.1 ml of corn oil per injection per rat. Groups of control and sham-operated rats were included in each treatment group and they received 0.1 ml s.c.

injections of either 0.15 M NaCl or corn oil (3 times daily).

Preparation of microsomes and cytosolic fractions. Testes were immediately excised, weighted, and homogenized with a Potter-Elvehjem homogenizer fitted with a Teflon pestle in 4 volumes of ice-cold 0.15 M KCl in 0.02 M HEPES (KCl: HEPES), pH 7.4, at 4°. The homogenate was centrifuged for 15 min at 9,000 x g at 4°. The supernatant was removed and centrifuged at 176,000 x g for 45 min to obtain microsomal and supernatant fractions. The microsomal pellet was re-suspended in KCl: HEPES, centrifuged, and washed. The protein concentration for microsomes and supernatant fractions was determined according to the method of Lowry et al. (5).

AHH assay. AHH activity was assayed according to the method described previously (6).

EH and GSH-T assays. The specific activites of EH and GSH-T were determined in 176,000 x g microsomal and supernatant fractions of the testes. Both EH and GSH-T activities were assayed using [4,5-oxide-^{3}H]BP as a substrate (7).

Spectral analysis. Cytochrome P-450 was assayed according to the method of Omura and Sato (8). An extinction coefficient of 91 mM^{-1} cm^{-1} was assayed for the quantitation of P-450. The microsomal protein concentration ranged from 2 to 5 mg/ml in 0.17 M HEPES buffer, pH 7.4. Spectra were recorded with an Aminco DW-2 dual-beam recording spectrophotometer (American Instrument Company, Silver Spring, MD).

Preparation of testis for perfusion studies. Adult rats weighing 250 to 300 g were sacrificed, the testes were immediately removed and placed under a stereomicroscope. The testicular artery was cannulated with a 80-μm-tip glass capillary and perfused it in a perfusion chamber (32 ± 0.5°) with an oxygenated Krebs-Ringer bicarbonate solution containing bovine serum albumin Fraction V (3%) and glucose (0.1%) at the rate of 13 ml/hr/g testis (an average blood flow rate for intact CD rats), using a precision pump. The details of the method has been described previously (6).

The effluent was collected for 60 min from the testicular vein. In order to determine the spontaneous breakdown of [7, 10-^{14}C] BP during perfusion of the isolated testis, the perfusate not passing through the testes was simultaneously collected for 60 min and subjected to HPLC analysis. The background radioactivity profile obtained by HPLC was quantified and subtracted as background.

Isolation of metabolites contained in the perfusion medium. The effluent in each fraction was added to 2 volumes of ethyl acetate:acetone (2:1), v/v) followed by 0.8 mM Vitamin E and 3.5 M NaCl. The addition of Vitamin E during

the extraction procedure minimized spontaneous formation of quinones and did
not interfere with HPLC analysis. The organic and water phases were separated
by centrifugation at 10,000 x g for 10 min; the water phase was subjected to
further extraction. The combined organic extracts were dried over anhydrous
Na_2SO_4. The sample residue was dissolved in 0.1 ml of ethyl acetate for
HPLC analysis.

Isolation of metabolites contained in the testicular tissue. The testicular
tissue was first homogenized with a Polytron homogenizer for 5 min at 0-2^O in
4 volumes of ice-cold 0.15 M KCl in 0.02 M HEPES buffer (pH 7.4). Two volumes
of ethyl acetate:acetone (2:1, v/v) were added and extracted 3 times. The
organic and water phases were separated by centrifugation. The organic and
water phases were separated by centrifugation. The organic extracts were combined, dried over anhydrous Na_2SO_4. The organic layer was further processed
as described above.

HPLC. Chemically pure BP metabolites, 9,10-diol, 4,5-diol, 7,8-diol, 3-OH,
9-OH, 1,6-quinone, 3,6-quinone, 6,12-quinone, and BP dissolved in HPLC grade
methanol were used to establish their HPLC retention times (60 to 100% methanol
gradient). The injection volume of both reference standards and samples was
30 μl. Analysis was performed on a Waters Associates Model ALC/GPC 204 liquid
chromatograph with a 254-nm UV detector. The effluent was collected directly
into scintillation vials. Radioactivity was determined with a Packard Model
2660 liquid scintillation spectrometer.

Statistical methods. Regression analysis and significant differences between
control and treatment groups were determined using MINTAB II statistical computer program and PDP 11-70 and RSX-11M operating system.

RESULTS

Developmental patterns of AHH, EH, GSH-T activities and cytochrome P-450 are
shown in Figure 1. Specific enzyme activities are expressed as total product
formed/min/testis. During the first 20 days after birth, specific testicular
AHH, EH, GSH-T activities and cytochrome P-450 content were very low. However,
specific enzyme activities rose dramatically between days 20 and 40 after
birth. This period corresponds to puberty coincident with increased androgen
synthesis. Beyond 50 days after birth, the specific activities of cytochrome
P-450-dependent monooxygenase(s) and cytochrome P-450 content did not increase
appreciably. On the basis of total organ weight, specific testicular AHH, EH,
GSH-T activity and cytochrome P-450 content were 0.2, 1.5, 5%, and 0.6% of
total hepatic activity, respectively. On the other hand, on the basis of

product formation/min/mg microsomal protein, the relative specific activity of AHH, EH, GSH-T, and cytochrome P-450 content in adult testes were 5, 1, 50%, and 14% of total hepatic activity, respectively (Table 1).

TABLE 1

ARYL HYDROCARBON HYDROXYLASE, EPOXIDE HYDRASE, GLUTATHIONE TRANSFERASE ACTIVITIES AND CYTOCHROME P-450 CONTENT OF MICROSOMES OR 176,000g SUPERNATANT FRACTION FROM ADULT RAT.

Enzyme	Specific activity or content, mean ± SD (n)	
	Testis	Liver
Aryl hydrocarbon hydroxylase pmole 3-hydroxybenzo[a]pyrene formed/min-mg protein (b)	5.17 ± 0.58 (4)	106 ± 8.3 (6)
Epoxide hydrase, nmole product/min-mg protein with benzo[a]pyrene 4,5-oxide substrate (b)	0.98 ± 0.06 (8)	10.85 ± 1.68 (4)
Glutathione transferase, nmole product/min-mg protein with benzo[a]pyrene 4,5 oxide substrate (a)	19.99 ± 1.11 (8)	41.29 ± 2.10 (4)
Cytochrome P-450, nmole/mg protein (b)	0.125 ± 0.018 (4)	0.85 ± 0.03 (6)

(a) 176,000g supernatant.

(b) Microsomes.

Testicular AHH, EH, and GSH-T activities and cytochrome P-450 content of intact control, sham-operated control, and hypophysectomized male rats 40 days after surgery are presented in Table 2. Testicular AHH and EH activities and cytochrome P-450 content were significantly lower in hypophysectomized male rats than in those of intact or sham-operated male rat controls. The specific testicular AHH and EH activities and cytochrome P-450 content in hypophysectomized rat testes were about 6, 40, and 40% respectively, of intact and sham-operated controls. However, testicular glutathione transferase activity (with 4,5-BPO as the substrate) was unchanged in hypophysectomized animals.

The effects of administration of LH and FSH, and testosterone to hypophysectomized rats demonstrated that testicular microsomal AHH activity of male hypophysectomized rats treated continuously with LH or with LH plus FSH for

5, 10, or 15 days after surgery was significantly greater than in hypophysectomized rats treated with 0.15 M NaCl (Table 3).

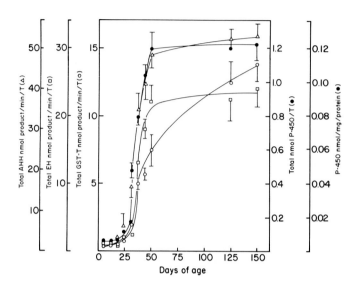

Fig. 1. Ontogeny of testicular AHH, EH, GST-T and cytochrome P-450.

TABLE 2

TESTICULAR AHH, EH, AND GSH-T ACTIVITIES AND CYTOCHROME P-450 CONTENT OF
INTACT CONTROL, SHAM-OPERATED, AND HYPOPHYSECTOMIZED MALE RATS.

Assays were determined simultaneously with preparation from intact control,
sham-operated, and hypophysectomized rats 40 days after hypophysectomy or sham
surgery. Four rats were used for each experiment.

	AHH/(pmol/min/ mg microsomal protein)	EH (nmol/min/mg microsomal pro- tein)	GSH-T (nmol/ min/mg cytosol (protein)	Cytochrome P-450 (nmol/ mg microsomal protein)
Control	5.31 ± 0.12[a]	0.93 ± 0.04	20.00 ± 1.10	0.12 ± 0.01
Sham-operated	5.46 ± 0.17	0.88 ± 0.08	20.30 ± 1.00	0.12 ± 0.004
Hypophysecto- mized[b]	0.84 ± 0.32[c]	0.35 ± 0.05[c]	18.90 ± 0.89	0.05 ± 0.00[c]

[a]Mean ± S.D. for all values.

[b]The mean values of testicular enzyme activities in hypophysectomized rats
were obtained from pooled testes (4 to 6 animals/preparation).

[c]Significantly less than control and sham-operated control values (p<0.01).

When administered to hypophysectomized rats for 15 days, LH and FSH plus LH increased testicular AHH activity about 14 and 7 fold, respectively. However, the diminution of AHH activity with time in the 0.15 M NaCl-treated hypophysectomized controls was the major contributing factor to the magnitude of the changes in AHH activity after 15 days of hormone administration. FSH appears to antagonize the LH-mediated increase of specific AHH activity in testicular microsomes. Testicular AHH activity in hypophysectomized male rats receiving 0.15 M NaCl, FSH alone, or testosterone showed marked decreases in AHH activity between 10 and 15 days of treatment (Table 3).

TABLE 3

EFFECTS OF HORMONES ON TESTICULAR MICROSOMAL AHH ACTIVITY IN HYPOPHYSECTOMIZED MALE RATS

AHH enzyme activity was determined using benzo(a)pyrene as a substrate. For each AHH assay, testes from 4 to 6 hypophysectomized rats were pooled.

Hormones	AHH activity (pmol/min/mg microsomal protein) at following treatment times		
	5 days	10 days	15 days
0.15 M NaCl	0.83 ± 0.26^a	0.93 ± 0.18	0.35 ± 0.16^b
FSH	1.25 ± 0.22	1.05 ± 0.23	0.44 ± 0.08^b
LH	2.31 ± 0.44^c	3.68 ± 0.78^c	4.72 ± 0.93^c
FSH + LH	1.84 ± 0.13^c	2.38 ± 0.20^c	2.36 ± 0.24^c
Testosterone	1.33 ± 0.37	0.75 ± 0.30	0.28 ± 0.07^b

[a]Mean $\pm$ S.D. of 3 experiments for all values.

[b]Significantly less than the 0 time control (prior to hormone treatment); $p < 0.01$ (see Table 2 for 0 time control values).

[c]Significantly greater than the 0.15 M NaCl-treated (hypophysectomized control); $p < 0.01$.

The effects of various hormones on testicular EH activity in hypophysectomized rats were similar to those obtained with AHH activity (Table 4). Testicular EH activity was markedly increased by LH and, to a lesser extent, by LH and FSH in a time-dependent manner after 15 days of treatment. Specific enzyme activities were about 5-fold greater in rats treated with LH and about 4-fold greater in rats given both LH and FSH than in hypophysectomized controls. Testicular EH activity in hypophysectomized rats was not influenced by FSH or testosterone.

As with AHH and EH activity, treatment of male hypophysectomized rats (10 weeks old) with LH and with LH plus FSH caused a significant increase in testicular cytochrome P-450 content; with LH there was almost a 10 fold increase and with LH and FSH the increase was approximately 9 fold (Table 5).

TABLE 4

EFFECTS OF HORMONES ON TESTICULAR MICROSOMAL EH ACTIVITY IN HYPOPHYSECTOMIZED MALE RATS

EH activity was determined using $[^3H]$benzo(a)pyrene 4,5-oxide as substrate. For each EH assay, testes from 4 to 6 animals were pooled.

Hormones	EH activity (nmol diol/min/mg microsomal protein) at following treatment times		
	5 days	10 days	15 days
0.15 M NaCl	0.38 ± 0.08^a	0.35 ± 0.05	0.54 ± 0.09
FSH	0.41 ± 0.11	0.45 ± 0.0	0.78 ± 0.17
LH	0.92 ± 0.13^b	1.77 ± 0.07^b	2.84 ± 0.32^b
FSH + LH	0.82 ± 0.02^b	1.53 ± 0.03^b	2.29 ± 0.15^b
Testosterone	0.56 ± 0.13	0.53 ± 0.17	0.58 ± 0.04

[a]Mean $\pm$ S.D. of 3 experiments for all values.

[b]Significantly greater than the 0.15 M NaCl controls (hypophysectomized); $p<0.01$.

TABLE 5

EFFECTS OF HORMONES ON TESTICULAR CYTOCHROME P-450 CONTENT IN HYPOPHYSECTOMIZED MALE RATS

Testicular cytochrome P-450 was measured in microsomes prepared from the pooled testes of 4 to 6 rats.

Hormones	Testicular cytochrome P-450 content (nmol cytochrome P-450/mg microsomal protein) at following treatment times		
	5 days	10 days	15 days
0.15 M NaCl	0.03 ± 0.0^a	0.02 ± 0.01	0.03 ± 0.0
FSH	0.05 ± 0.01	0.03 ± 0.01	0.03 ± 0.01
LH	0.10 ± 0.01^b	0.21 ± 0.01^b	0.30 ± 0.02^b
FSH + LH	0.10 ± 0.01^b	0.15 ± 0.02^b	0.28 ± 0.02^b
Tesosterone	0.03 ± 0.01	0.02 ± 0.01	0.03 ± 0.01

[a]Mean $\pm$ S.D. of 3 experiments for all values. [b]Significantly different from the 0.15 M NaCl controls (hypophysectomized); $p<0.01$.

In contrast, FSH and testosterone had no effect. For comparison, testicular cytochrome P-450 content in microsomes from hypophysectomized male rats (125 days old; 55 days after surgery) was only about 30% of the values for intact or sham-operted control rats of the same age.

The administration of LH, FSH, FSH plus LH, or testosterone (100 µg 3 times daily) for 5, 10, or 15 days had no significant effect on testicular cytosolic GSH-T activity.

Table 6 demonstrates the distribution of metabolites between the effluent perfusate and testicular tissues of control testes. In the effluent of control testes, the BP metabolites, ranging from the highest to the lowest concentrations, are 9,10-diol, 1,6-quinone, 3,6- and 6,12-quinones, 7,8-diol, 3-OH, 9-OH, and 4,5-diol, respectively. In contrast, BP metabolites in testicular tissues from the highest to the lowest concentration are 9,10-diol, 7,8-diol, 9-OH, 3-OH, quinones, and 4,5-diol. These differences between BP metabolites in the effluent and in the testicular tissue compartment may reflect permeability differences in BP metabolites.

TABLE 6

COMPARISON OF BP METABOLITES IN THE PERFUSATE AND THE TESTICULAR TISSUE

| BP metabolites | Specific activity (pmol/hr/g testis) | |
	Effluent	Testicular tissue
9,10-diol	39.4 $\pm$ 0.7[a] (1.2)[b]	26.9 $\pm$ 4.5 (0.8)[c]
4,5-diol	3.1 $\pm$ 1.0 (0.1)	2.3 $\pm$ 0.7 (0.1)
7,8-diol	9.3 $\pm$ 3.4 (0.3)	12.7 $\pm$ 4.1 (0.6)
9-OH	3.9 $\pm$ 1.5 (0.1)	7.5 $\pm$ 2.5 (0.3)
3-OH	4.7 $\pm$ 2.3 (0.2)	7.1 $\pm$ 1.7 (0.3)
1,6-quinone		
3,6-quinone	8.0 $\pm$ 1.9 (0.3)	3.8 $\pm$ 0.6 (0.1)[c]
6,12-quinone		
Total metabolites	68.3 $\pm$ 10.8 (2.2)	60.3 $\pm$ 14.1 (1.9)
BP	2415.7 $\pm$ 197.1 (79.3)	217.4 $\pm$ 28.8 (7.1)

[a]Mean $\pm$ S.D. from 5 separate experimental values with the exception of 4,5-diol (N = 3).

[b]Numbers in parentheses, percentage of total radioactivity recovered at the end of 60 min of perfusion.

[c]Significantly less than that of effluent metabolites (p<0.05).

DISCUSSION

AHH and epoxide hydrase activity, and cytochrome P-450 are barely detectable in rat testes and liver before puberty, a finding that is in agreement with the ontogeny of xenobiotic metabolizing systems residing in hepatic endoplasmic reticulum (9). Specific epoxide hydrase activity also increases dramatically in testes at the time of puberty. A similar ontogenic pattern of liver epoxide hydrase was reported previously by others (10). Similarly, cytochrome P-450-dependent steroid-metabolizing enzymes such as 17α-hydroxylase and C_{17-20}-lyase have been found to be predominantly associated with Leydig cell microsomes (11).

The results demonstrated that, following hypophysectomy (Hypox), specific testicular microsomal AHH and EH activities and cytochrome P-450 content, but not cytosolic GSH-T activities, were significantly reduced coincident with decreased Leydig cell volume and germ cell degeneration. However, LH hormone treatment for 15 days following Hypox dramatically increased testicular AHH and EH activities and cytochrome P-450 content. In contrast, FSH or testosterone treatment had no effect on testicular AHH and EH activities and cytochrome P-450 levels. Thus, it appears that increases of testicular AHH and EH activities and cytochrome P-450 content are regulated by LH hormone and that the induction of these enzymes in Hypox rats is primarily associated with marked increases in the cellular volume of Leydig cells. On the other hand, specific cytoplasmic GSH-T activity was not affected.

When FSH and LH were administered to Hypox male rats, lower specific testicular AHH and EH activities and decreased cytochrome P-450 contents were observed than in rats treated with LH alone (Tables 3 and 4). This observation apparently is due to an increased number of germ cells by FSH treatment that has low EH, AHH, and cytochrome P-450. FSH has been demonstrated to stimulate Sertoli cells to synthesize androgen-binding protein with the subsequent stimulation of spermatogenic cell differentiation (12). As expected, neither FSH nor testosterone treatment had any significant effect on Leydig cell morphology, testis microsomal AHH and EH activities, or cytochrome P-450 levels.

The molecular basis by which LH induces cytochrome P-450 levels, AHH, and EH enzymes is not clear at the present time. However, interaction between LH receptors of Leydig cells and LH hormone increases intracellular cyclic adenosine 3',5'-monophosphate concentration with subsequent stimulation of testosterone biosynthesis (13), accompanied by increased cytochrome P-450 content, and 17α-hydroxylase and C_{17-20}-lyase activities in the Hypox rat (11). Thus,

LH-associated increases of cytochrome P-450 and EH appear to be related to the LH induction of cytochrome P-450-dependent steroid-biosynthetic enzymes.

In rat testes, in addition to LH induction of monooxygenase activity, other environmental chemicals such as PAH and 2,3,7,8-tetrachlorodibenze-p-dioxin have recently been shown to increase testicular AHH activity from 1.5 to 2 fold in Sprague-Dawley rats (6) and from 85 to 500 fold in C57BL/6 mice (4) respectively. Thus, PAH inducibility of microsomal AHH in various target tissue of hormones is demonstrated to be different.

The results of perfusion studies showed that the major testicular BP metabolites in the organic extractable phase of isolated perfused testis were 9,10- and 7,8-diol, followed by 3-OH and the quinones. Thus, in the CD rat testis, the 9,10 and 7,8 positions are preferentially epoxidated in contrast to the 4,5 position. Epoxidation reaction apparently exceeds that of other metabolic oxidation pathways. In contrast to BP metabolism in the isolated testis, perfusion studies with isolated rat and rabbit lungs demonstrated that the major BP metabolites were phenolic and quinone derivatives of BP (14). Furthermore, the perfusion of isolated lungs from rats pretreated with 3-methylcholanthrene demonstrated that phenolic metabolites increased 7 fold while 7,8-diol production was unchanged (15).

Distribution pattern of BP metabolites between the perfusate effluent and the testicular tissue compartment suggests that quinones and 9,10-diol are lower in the tissues. Therefore, the data suggest that 9,10-diol and quinones move readily from the testicular tissue compartment to the perfusate effluent as compared to the movement of 4,5-diol, 7,8-diol, 3-OH, and 9-OH. If the metabolic pathway leading to the formation of the diol-epoxide is the most important factor of PAH mutagenesis (16), male gonads may be highly susceptible to PAH-induced mutagenesis. Furthermore, if the venous return travels via the unique venous network of pampiniform plexus surrounding the internal spermatic artery and high levels of BP metabolites (especially 7,8-diol-BP) occur, then this may result in reabsorption of BP and BP metabolites into the internal spermatic artery. BP and its metabolites could continue to recycle between the testis and the pampiniform plexus, thus making germ cells even more vulnerable to carcinogenic BP metabolites. Since interstitial cell tumors of the testis have been suggested to be due to the differential presence of steroidogenic enzymes associated with mixed-function oxidase system(s) in Leydig cells of both rodents (17) and humans (18), it is tempting to speculate that environmental factors affecting differential activities of testicular mixed-function oxidases system(s) in testes may play an important role in the chemical carcinogenesis and genetic toxicity of male gonads.

REFERENCES

1. Ford, E. and Huggins, C. (1963) J. Exp. Med., 118, 27-40.

2. Epstein, S.S., Arnold, E., Andrea, J., Bass, W. and Bishop W. (1972) Toxicol. Appl. Pharmacol., 23, 288-325.

3. Generoso, W.M., Cain, K.T., Krishna, M. and Huff, S.W. (1979) Proc. Natl. Acad. Sci. U.S.A., 76, 435-437.

4. Mattison, D.R. and Thorgeirsson, S.S. (1979) Cancer Res., 39, 3471-3475.

5. Lowry, O.H., Rosebrough, N.J., Farr, A.L. and Randall, R.J. (1951) J. Biol. Chem., 193, 265-275.

6. Lee, I.P. and Nagayama, J. (1980) Cancer Res., 40, 3297-3303.

7. Jerina, D.M. and Bend, J.R. (1976) in: Jollow, D., Kocsis, J.J., Snyder, R. and Vainio, H. (Eds.), Reactive Intermediates: Formation, Toxicity and Inactivation, Plenum Publishing Corp., New York, pp. 207-236.

8. Omura, T. and Sato, R. (1964) J. Biol. Chem., 239, 2370-2378.

9. Conney, A.H. (1967) Pharmacol. Rev., 19, 317.

10. Oesch, R. (1976) J. Biol. Chem., 251, 79.

11. Menard, R.H. and Purvis, J.L. (1973) Arch. Biochem. Biophys., 154, 8-18.

12. Means, A.R. and Vaitukaitis, J. (1972) Endocrinology, 90, 39-46.

13. Rommerts, F.F.G., Cooke, B.A. and Van der Molen, H.J. (1974) J. Steroid Biochem., 5, 279-285.

14. Smith, B.R., Philpot, R.M. and Bend, J.R. (1978) Drug Metabol. Dispos., 6, 425-431.

15. Vainio, H., Uotila, P., Hatiala, J. and Pelkonen, O. (1976) Res. Commun. Chem. Pathol. Pharmacol., 13, 259-271.

16. Malaveille, C., Bartsch, H., Grover, P.I. and Sims, P. (1975) Biochem. Biophys. Res. Commun., 66 , 693-700.

17. Inano, H., Machino, A., Tamaoki, B. and Tsubura, Y. (1968) Endocrinology, 83, 659-670.

18. Lipsett, M.B., Sarfaty, G.H., Wilson, H., Bardin, C.W. and Fishman, L.M. (1966) J. Clin. Invest., 45, 1700-1709.

© 1983 Elsevier Science Publishers B.V.
Extrahepatic Drug Metabolism and Chemical Carcinogenesis,
J. Rydström, J. Montelius and M. Bengtsson eds.

REGULATION OF THE METABOLISM OF 7,12-DIMETHYLBENZ(A)ANTHRACENE
IN THE RAT OVARY BY GONADOTROPINS

MARGOT BENGTSSON[1], DONALD R. MATTISON[2] AND JAN RYDSTRÖM[1]
[1]Department of Biochemistry, Arrhenius Laboratory, University of
Stockholm, S-106 91 Stockholm, Sweden and [2]NICHD, NIH, Bethesda,
Maryland 20014, USA

INTRODUCTION

Increasing pollution and spreading of chemicals in the environment is accompanied by several adverse effects on living organisms.
The gonads, being the repository of the germ cells and responsible
for the synthesis of steroid hormones necessary for reproduction,
are very sensitive to mutagenic and carcinogenic agents. Interactions between such compound and the gonads may result in decreased fertility, teratogenicity, mutations and cancer (1).

The toxic and carcinogenic effects of polycyclic aromatic hydrocarbons involve activation of the hydrocarbons to reactive epoxide
intermediates (2-4). The first step in this activation uses the
P-450-dependent monooxygenase, aryl hydrocarbon hydroxylase (AHH)
(5).

Metabolites may bind covalently to DNA or protein and cause cell
destruction and cancer. In the ovary these events are possibly related, i.e. generation of ovary cancer occurs only after oocyte
destruction (1). Reactive intermediates may also be inactivated by
epoxide hydrolase and conjugating enzymes or quinone-reducing DT-
diaphorase.

The activity of AHH has previously been shown to be controlled
by the pituitary hormones in both liver (6), adrenal (7) and testis (8) of hypophysectomized rats. The present investigation concerns the effect of gonadotropins on 7,12-dimethylbenz(a)anthra-
cene-hydroxylase (DMBA-hydroxylase) in the rat ovary of intact
Sprague-Dawley rats. It is shown that DMBA-hydroxylase is regulated by the estrus cycle and pregnant mare's serum gonadotropin
(PMSG), indicating a role in steroid metabolism.

MATERIALS AND METHODS

Female Sprague-Dawley rats weighing 230 g were maintained under a 12 h light, 12 h dark cycle. For the estrus cycle studies, vaginal smears were obtained daily. Only animals showing two consecutive 4-day cycles were used in measurements of estrus-cycle dependent activities. Estrus cycle phases were not checked in rats to be treated with gonadotropins or steroid hormones. Hormones were administered subcutaneously in 0.9% NaCl. Human chorionic gonadotropin (hCG) was administered to rats pretreated with PMSG for 65 hours. Ovaries were removed after decapitation and fractionated immediately as described earlier (9).

DMBA-hydroxylase was assayed with (^{14}C)-DMBA as substrate according to the distribution method (9) or by HPLC separation of metabolites (9). Microsomal epoxide hydrolase (EH) was assayed with (^{3}H)-styrene-7,8-oxide as substrate (10), soluble glutathione-S-transferase (GST) with 1-chloro-2,4-dinitrobenzene (11) and soluble DT-diaphorase (DT) with menadione coupled to reduced cytochrome c (12). Protein was determined according to the Lowry method (13). (^{14}C)-DMBA was purchased from NEN Chemicals (Dreireich, F.R.G.). Purified gonadotropins were provided by NIAMDD (National Institutes of Health, Bethesda, Md). All other chemicals were of analytical grade and purchased from Sigma Chemicals Co (St Louis, Mo).

RESULTS

A single injection of 154 i.u. PMSG to mature female rats gave a maximally 7-fold induction of ovarian DMBA-hydroxylase. The extent of induction increased linearly for at least 48 hours (Fig.1). A maximal activity of about 22 pmoles/min·mg protein was reached after 72 hours (cf. Fig. 3A).

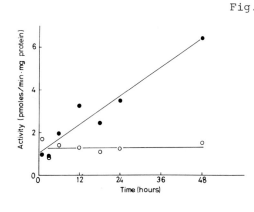

Fig. 1. Time-course of induction of ovarian DMBA-hydroxylase by a single dose of PMSG. At time zero 154 i.u. PMSG was injected s.c.
Open circles indicate control and closed circles PMSG-treated rats.

Repeated treatments every 48 hour with 154 i.u. PMSG resulted in
an increasing activity to a maximal hydroxylase activity after 2
treatments (Fig 2A). Following the third PMSG administration the
activity decreased and reached control level in approximately 72
hours. The weight of the ovary was continously increased by PMSG,
while the weight of the uterus increased 1.5 times and remained
stable after further treatment (Fig 2B). This may reflect that the
increase of the weight of the ovary is due to the gonadotropin
stimulation rather than to enhanced estrogen secretion, since the
weight of the uterus did not change at the same rate.

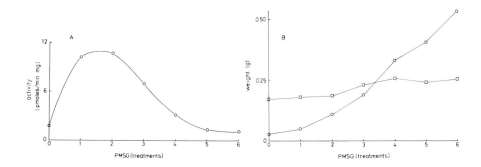

Fig. 2.   Effect of repeated treatments with PMSG every 48 hour
           on DMBA-hydroxylase activity (A)
           on ovarian (o) and uterine (□) weight (B)

Admininstration of hCG to PMSG-pretreated rats resulted in a
rapid decrease in DMBA-hydroxylase activity within 12 hours. hCG
has mainly LH activity, and thus the situation might be compared
to the influence of repeated PMSG injections (Fig 3). A single
treatment with PMSG without following hCG administration, increased the activity 7-fold (Fig 3).

HPLC analysis of the product patterns of PMSG-induced and control microsomes revealed three groups of metabolites, i.e. diols,
quinones and phenols (Fig 4). The PMSG treatment did not result
in new products as was the case with methylcholanthrene-treated
ovaries (14), but rather an overall increase of the same products.
The larger amount of phenols formed by the induced ovarian microsomes led to an incomplete separation between phenols and DMBA.

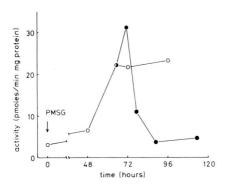

Fig. 3. Effect of hCG on DMBA-
hydroxylase in PMSG-
treated rats. 2 groups
of rats received 154 i.u.
PMSG at time zero; 65
hrs later 200 i.u. hCG
was administered to one
group. Open circles in-
dicate PMSG-treated
rats, closed circles
indicate PMSG plus hCG
treated rats.

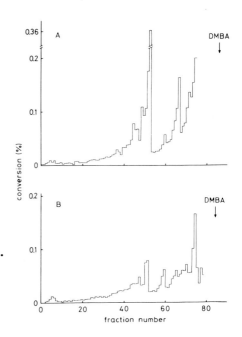

Fig 4. HPLC analysis of DMBA metabolites generated by
PMSG-induced (A) and con-
trol (B) ovarian microsomes.

Different pituitary and steroid hormones were investigated in
order to characterize the induction of ovarian DMBA-hydroxylase.
As may be seen in Table 1, progesterone had no significant effect,
whereas estradiol and its synthetic analogue diethylstilbestrol
(DES) induced ovarian DMBA-hydroxylase 3- and 2-fold, respectively.
Luteinizing hormone (LH) and follicle-stimulating hormone (FSH)
each gave about 3 times induction. In comparison PMSG, which has
both LH and FSH activity (ratio about 1:1), gave 7-fold induction.
Since neither of the pituitary hormones were pure, it is not at
this stage possible to decide whether the LH or FSH effect, or the
combined LH and FSH effects of PMSG, is responsible for the PMSG-
dependent induction of DMBA-hydroxylase.

The combined treatment with estradiol plus PMSG revealed an additive effect, giving more than 10 times induction, suggesting that
there are either two types of ovarian AHH induced by estradiol and
PMSG respectively, or two different mechanisms for the induction
of the same AHH.

TABLE 1

EFFECT OF STEROID AND PITUITARY HORMONES ON OVARIAN
DMBA-HYDROXYLASE

Rats were treated with 100 μg twice daily, for two days with
either estradiol, progesterone, DES, LH or FSH. PMSG was administered only once (154 i.u.). DMBA-hydroxylase was measured after
48 hours.

Treatment	Specific activity (pmoles/min·mg)	Induction (times)
none	1.68 ± 0.29	-
estradiol	4.80 ± 0.31	2.9
progesterone	2.05 ± 0.23	1.2
DES	4.05 ± 0.41	2.4
LH	4.44 ± 0.32	2.6
FSH	4.59 ± 0.80	2.7
PMSG	12.1 ± 0.31	7.2
estradiol + PMSG	17.1 ± 0.30	10.2

These results are consistent with measurements of DMBA-hydroxylase in the different phases of the estrus cycle, where a 4-fold
induction was found in the proestrus/estrus phases (when the gonadotropin levels are maximal), compared to the metestrus/diestrus
phases (Table 2). EH, GST, and DT activities were essentially insensitive to estrus cycle status and PMSG treatment (not shown).

TABLE 2

DMBA-HYDROXYLASE ACTIVITY IN THE DIFFERENT PHASES OF THE
ESTRUS CYCLE

	Phase of the estrus cycle			
	proestrus	estrus	metestrus	diestrus
Activity (pmoles/ min·mg)	4.19 ± 0.39	4.80 ± 0.22	1.80 ± 0.16	1.00 ± 0.08

DISCUSSION

The present data show that treatment of mature female rats with
PMSG causes an induction of ovarian DMBA-hydroxylase, whereas EH,
GST and DT are unchanged. DMBA-hydroxylase is also regulated by
the estrus cycle showing maximal induction in the proestrus/estrus

phase of the cycle, indicating the involvement of FSH and/or LH. Attempts to distinguish between the role of FSH and LH in the induction show that both hormones are active. However, the interpretation of these results are complicated by the impurity of the hormones. Recent experiments with pure FSH and LH indicate that LH may be the main inducing hormone (not shown).

The DMBA-hydroxylase activity induced by a single treatment with PMSG reaches a plateau within 72 hrs. In contrast, the results obtained in experiments with several consecutive PMSG treatments show a transient increase in DMBA-hydroxylase activity. Administration of hCG to rats treated with a maximally inducing dose of PMSG leads to a rapid decrease in activity. Taken together these results are assumed to reflect the FSH and LH activity of PMSG and the LH activity of hCG. Low concentrations of PMSG (a single dose) favours the FSH effect of PMSG leading to an enhanced production of antral follicles. Higher PMSG concentrations favour a high LH activity and increased ovulation; the same effect is caused by hCG. Therefore, it is concluded that DMBA-hydroxylase is located primarely in the large antral follicles, possibly in the granulosa cells. This conclusion is supported by the fact that only antral follicles have LH receptors (15) and is consistent with the previous suggestion that pituitary overstimulation of the ovaries after menopause, where no ovulation occurs, is a possible cause of ovary cancer (16).

ACKNOWLEDGEMENT

Supported by the Swedish Council for Planning and Coordination of Research.

REFERENCES

1. Mattison, D.R. and Thorgeirsson, S.S. (1978) Lancet, 1, 187.
2. Heidelberger, C. (1975) Annu.Rev. Biochem., 24, 79.
3. DePierre, J.W. and Ernster, L. (1978) Biochem.Biophys.Acta, 473, 179.
4. Pitot, H.C. (1979) Annu.Rev.Med., 30, 25.
5. Mattison, D.R. (1978) Cancer Res., 38, 1368.
6. Rumbaugh, R.C. and Colby, H.D. (1980) Endocrinol., 107, 719.

7. Guenthner, T.M., Nebert, D.W. and Menard, R.H. (1979) Mol.Pharmacol., 15, 719.

8. Lee, I.P., Suzuki, K., Mukhtar, H. and Bend, J.R. (1980) Cancer Res., 40, 2486.

9. Montelius, J., Papadopoulos, D., Bengtsson, M. and Rydström, J. (1982) Cancer Res., 42, 1479.

10. Seidegård, J., DePierre, J.W., Moron, M.S., Johannesen, K.A.M. and Ernster, L. (1977) Cancer Res., 37, 1075.

11. Habig, W.H., Pabst, M.J. and Jacoby, W.B. (1974) J.Biol.Chem., 249, 7130.

12. Lind, C. and Höjeberg, B. (1981) Arch. Biochem.Biophys., 207, 217.

13. Lowry, O.H., Rosebrough, N.J., Farr, A.L. and Randall, R.J. (1951) J.Biol.Chem., 193,265.

14. Bengtsson, M., Montelius, J., Mankowitz, L. and Rydström, J. (1983) Biocem.Pharmacol., 32, 129.

15 Ross, G.T., Hillier, S.G., Zeleznik, A.J. and Knazek, R.A. (1979) in: Klopper et.al. (eds.) Research on Steroids, Academic Press, London, 3, 185.

16. Bengtsson, M. and Rydström, J. (1983) Science, 219, 1437.

© 1983 Elsevier Science Publishers B.V.
Extrahepatic Drug Metabolism and Chemical Carcinogenesis,
J. Rydström, J. Montelius and M. Bengtsson eds.

EFFECTS OF ACTH ON METABOLISM AND TOXICITY OF 7,12-DIMETHYLBENZ(a)ANTHRACENE
IN CULTURED RAT ADRENAL CELLS

EINAR HALLBERG AND JAN RYDSTRÖM
Department of Biochemistry, University of Stockholm, Sweden

INTRODUCTION

The adrenal cortex contains a number of different steroid hydroxylases as
well as aryl hydrocarbon hydroxylase (AHH), which are regulated by adrenocorti-
cotrophic hormone (ACTH) (1). In the intact animal the potent carcinogen
7,12-dimethylbenz(a)anthracene (DMBA) selectively generates necrosis of the two
inner zones of the rat adrenal cortex. A prerequisite for the necrosis is ACTH,
since immature and mature hypophysectomized rats are resistant to DMBA treatment (2). The influence of ACTH on the adrenal toxicity of DMBA and it's major
hepatic metabolite 7-hydroxymethyl-12-methylbenz(a)anthracene (7-OHM-12-MBA)
were studied using cultured rat adrenal cells (RAC) as a model system.

MATERIAL AND METHODS

RAC were isolated and cultured as described previously (3) except that L-15
was replaced by MEM, supplemented with 0,1 μM selenium (Na$_2$SeO$_3$), as culture medium in the toxicological experiments.

ACTH, dissolved and stored as described (3) was added directly to the medium. Corticosterone, secreted into the medium, was then estimated fluorimetrically (3).

Conversion of HPLC-purified [^{14}C]-DMBA and analysis of metabolites was
assayed as described previously (4).

RESULTS

In order to study the effect of ACTH on AHH activity, RAC were cultured for
21 hours in the absence of ACTH. The conversion of DMBA in the absence and in
the presence of ACTH was compared (Table 1). Two different concentrations of
DMBA were used, 0,5 μM (equal to Km) and 10 μM (saturating concentration). As
can be seen from table 1 no significant change in AHH activity was observed, although steroidogenesis was dramatically increased. The HPLC-pattern of DMBA metabolites was also unaffected by ACTH (not shown). These results suggest that
the role of ACTH in DMBA-generated adrenolysis is unrelated to short term
steroidogenesis.

In vitro toxicity of DMBA and the major hepatic metabolite 7-OHM-12-MBA,

372

which is not generated by the adrenal, was demonstrated by a decreased ACTH-responsive corticosterone synthesis. After 50 hours exposure of the cells to 20 μM of DMBA or 7-OHM-12-MBA in the presence of ACTH, the corticosterone synthesis declined to 65% and 33%, respectively (fig. 1).

The observed toxic effects are in good agreement with previous data from in vivo experiments (2). Whether adrenal and/or hepatic activation of DMBA and 7-OHM-12-MBA is necessary for adrenal toxicity is presently under investigation.

TABLE 1

EFFECT OF ACTH ON DMBA HYDROXYLASE ACTIVITY IN RAC

Incubations and assays were carried out as described in Materials and Methods. The RAC were incubated in the absence of ACTH for 21 hours before incubation with 0.5 μM and 10 μM DMBA.

Conditions	Concentration of DMBA (μM)	No. of incubations	Specific activity pmol/min · 10^6 cells	P
Control	0.5	4	1.76 ± 0.30	
+ACTH(2 iu/ml)	0.5	4	1.66 ± 0.13	N.S.[a]
Control	10.0	4	5.09 ± 0.53	
+ACTH(2 iu/ml)	10.0	4	4.98 ± 0.34	N.S.[a]

[a] N.S., no statistically significant difference, as compared to control

Fig. 1. Effect of DMBA and 7-OHM-12-MBA on ACTH-induced corticosterone synthesis. Primary cultures of RAC were incubated for 50 hours in the presence of ACTH. Additions were DMSO, 20 μM DMBA and 20 μM 7-OHM-12-MBA dissolved in DMSO (final concentration 2%). The corticosterone produced during the last 4 hours were assayed in duplicate according to methods.

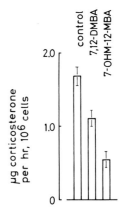

REFERENCES

1. Gunsalus, I.C., Pederson, T.C. and Sligar, S.G. (1979) Anni. Rev. Biochem. 44, 377.

2. Huggins, C.B. (1979) Experimental Leukemia and Mammary Cancer. The University of Chicago Press, Chicago and London.

3. Hallberg, E. and Rydström, J. (1981) Acta Chem. Scand. B 35, 145.

4. Montelius, J., Papadopoulos, D., Bengtsson, M. and Rydström, J. (1982) Cancer Res. 42, 1479.

© 1983 Elsevier Science Publishers B.V.
Extrahepatic Drug Metabolism and Chemical Carcinogenesis,
J. Rydström, J. Montelius and M. Bengtsson eds.

ARE PITUITARY FACTORS ACTING AS MODIFIERS OF LIVER CARCINOGENESIS IN THE RAT ?

AGNETA BLANCK[1], TIIU HANSSON[1], LENNART ERIKSSON[2] AND JAN-ÅKE GUSTAFSSON[1]

[1]Department of Medical Nutrition, Karolinska Institutet, Huddinge University Hospital F 69, S-141 86 Huddinge and [2]Department of Pathology, Huddinge University Hospital F 42, S-141 86 Huddinge, Sweden.

INTRODUCTION

Epidemiological studies show that liver cancer occurs much more frequently in men than in women. Marked sex differences in induction of experimental liver cancer by various carcinogens have also been observed in several strains of rats. Hypophysectomy and lesions in the median eminence area of the hypothalamus in adult rats inhibit the induction of liver tumors by several carcinogens indicating the involvement of the hypothalamo-pituitary system in the regulation of some step(s) in the carcinogenic process.

An experimental model, developed by Solt and Farber (1), offers a new approach to study the early events in liver carcinogenesis. In this model a subcarcinogenic dose of 2-acetylaminofluorene (2-AAF) in combination with partial hepatectomy (PH) is used to create a selective pressure for cells, previously "initiated" by a carcinogen , to grow. The initiated cells resistant to the mitoinhibitory effect of 2-AAF grow to form enzyme altered foci by a week to ten days after cessation of the 2-AAF diet. The majority of the early foci stain positively for γ-glutamyl transpeptidase (γ-GT) activity when studied histochemically and are thus easy to quantitate.

Recent studies show that male Wistar rats develop a larger amount of foci as well as greater foci than females in the Solt-Farber model when diethylnitrosamine (DEN) is used as an initiator. Sex differences in toxicity and carcinogenicity of 2-AAF as well as sex related differences in liver microsomal metabolism of this compound in the rat have been described. The male type of metabolism may be "feminized" by implantation of pituitary grafts under the kidney capsule or by implantation of Alzet osmotic minipumps containing human growth hormone (hGH). The aim of the present study was to investigate whether "feminization" of 2-AAF metabolism in male rat may affect the development of preneoplastic lesions by modifying the selection of DEN-initiated cells by 2-AAF.

RESULTS AND DISCUSSION

DEN (200 mg/kg) was administered i.p. to eight week old male and female Wistar rats. After two weeks the rats were fed a diet containing 0.02% 2-AAF for two weeks and in the middle of this period the animals were subjected to a 70% PH. After a total period of two weeks on 2-AAF diet the rats were fed the stock diet devoid of 2-AAF for further 14 days. At the end of this period they were sacrificed and liver samples were processed for histochemical studies. To study the effect of pituitary factors on the selection of initiated cells one group of male rats were treated as above except that two pituitary glands from female rats were implanted under the kidney capsule one week before the start of the 2-AAF feeding. Another group of male rats received Alzet osmotic minipumps, implanted subcutenously, containing hGH (5 µg/h). In order to quantitate the degree of "feminization" of liver metabolism by these treatments liver samples were taken at the time of PH and assayed for androstenedione metabolism.

EFFECTS OF PITUITARY GRAFTS (PG) OR HUMAN GROWTH HORMONE (hGH) ON THE 2-AAF SELECTION IN THE SOLT-FARBER MODEL

Experiment	Control males (n=7)	Males + hGH (n=10)	Control females (n=10)
PG experiment:			
$\dfrac{\text{Total area of foci}}{\text{Total area}}$ (%)	33.7 ± 11.5[a]	17.6 ± 6.7	11.7 ± 5.9
Number of foci/cm^2	45.2 ± 7.1	51.4 ± 20.3	48.8 ± 19.8
hGH experiment:	Control males (n=8)	Males + hGH (n=8)	Control females (n=7)
$\dfrac{\text{Total area of foci}}{\text{Total area}}$ (%)	34.2 ± 4.9	15.0 ± 8.6	9.7 ± 3.3
Number of foci/cm^2	41.7 ± 5.4	21.2 ± 7.4	26.1 ± 4.1

[a] The data given represent the means $\pm$ standard deviations.

Livers from male rats with pituitary implants or minipumps were "feminized" with regard to androstenedione metabolism (data not shown) during the selection period and exhibited a marked decrease in relative area of γ-GT positive foci when compared to sham-operated male and female rats. The presented data indicate that GH and/or some other pituitary factor(s), modifies the selection of DEN-initiated cells by 2-AAF in the rat, eventually by "feminizing" the hepatic metabolism of 2-AAF.

ACKNOWLEDGMENTS

This work was supported by a grant from the Swedish Medical Research Council (no. 13X-2819).

REFERENCES

1. Solt,D. and Farber,E. (1976) Nature 263, 701.

© 1983 Elsevier Science Publishers B.V.
Extrahepatic Drug Metabolism and Chemical Carcinogenesis,
J. Rydström, J. Montelius and M. Bengtsson eds.

FEMINIZATION OF HEPATIC XENOBIOTIC METABOLISM BY ECTOPIC PITUITARY GRAFTS OR BY
CONTINUOUS INFUSION OF HUMAN GROWTH HORMONE IN MALE RATS

AGNETA BLANCK[1], ANDERS ÅSTRÖM[2], TIIU HANSSON[1], JOSEPH DE PIERRE[2] AND JAN-ÅKE
GUSTAFSSON[1]

[1]Department of Medical Nutrition, Karolinska Institute, Huddinge University
Hospital F69, S-141 86 Huddinge and [2]Department of Biochemistry, Arrhenius
Laboratory, University of Stockholm, S-106 91 Stockholm, Sweden.

INTRODUCTION

Considerable evidence has accumulated that growth hormone (GH) plays a role in
the control of sex differences in the hepatic steroid and xenobiotic metabolism
in the rat (1). The mechanism whereby GH controls the sex differences in hepatic
steroid metabolism has been suggested to be related to the sexually differentiated secretory profile of GH (2). A more "female" like pattern of GH-secretion
in the male rat can be mimicked by implantation of an ectopic pituitary gland
under the kidney capsule or by implantation of an osmotic minipump containing
GH. Both of these treatments result in feminization of hepatic androstenedione
metabolism. The aim of the present study was to investigate whether a more
"female" like pattern of GH secretion in male rat feminizes the hepatic metabolism of three xenobiotic substrates.

RESULTS AND DISCUSSION

Eight week old male Wistar rats received ectopic pituitary grafts under the
kidney capsule or subcutaneous implantation of Alzet osmotic minipumps containing
hGH (5 µg/h). The animals were sacrificed after one week. The liver microsomal
fraction was prepared using a standard procedure. The degree of "feminization"
of liver metabolism were quantitated by measuring the liver microsomal metabolism
of androstenedione. As expected liver microsomes from male rats with pituitary
grafts or minipumps containing hGH were "feminized" with regard to androstenedione metabolism (data not shown). The above treatments feminized the liver microsomal metabolism of benzo(a)pyrene (BP) and 7-ethoxyresorufin (7-EOR) and decreased
the total amount of cytochrome P-450 to female levels in the male rat (Table 1).
The metabolite pattern of 2-acetylaminofluorene (2-AAF) produced by liver microsomes from male rats with pituitary grafts or hGH containing minipumps was
"feminized" as well (Table 2).

TABLE 1

CYTOCHROME P-450 CONTENT, 7-EOR-O-DEETHYLASE AND AHH ACTIVITIES IN LIVER MICRO-
SOMES FROM CONTROL MALE AND FEMALE RATS AND FROM MALE RATS GIVEN hGH OR PITUITARY
GRAFTS (PG).

The values given represent the means $\pm$ standard deviations from four rats in each
group.

Treatment	Cytochrome P-450 nmol/mg protein	Enzyme activity (nmol/min/mg protein) 7-EOR	AHH
Control male	0.38 $\pm$ 0.05	0.154 $\pm$ 0.037	0.122 $\pm$ 0.028
Control female	0.31 $\pm$ 0.04	0.322 $\pm$ 0.091	0.032 $\pm$ 0.014
Male + hGH	0.32 $\pm$ 0.03	0.220 $\pm$ 0.08	0.056 $\pm$ 0.018
Male + PG	0.33 $\pm$ 0.02	0.366 $\pm$ 0.089	0.051 $\pm$ 0.028

TABLE 2

PATTERN OF 2-AAF METABOLITES OBTAINED WITH LIVER MICROSOMES FROM CONTROL MALE AND
FEMALE RATS, AND FROM MALE RATS TREATED WITH hGH OR ECTOPIC PITUITARY GRAFTS (PG).

Treatment	2-AAF metabolites formed (pmol/min/mg protein)					
	7-hydroxy	9-hydroxy	5-hydroxy	3-hydroxy	1-hydroxy	N-hydroxy
Control male	98.9 $\pm$ 6.2	20.1 $\pm$ 3.1	1.48 $\pm$ 0.32	4.01 $\pm$ 0.82	9.12 $\pm$ 2.58	15.4 $\pm$ 3.5
Control female	75.0 $\pm$ 9.1	3.70 $\pm$ 0.59	8.31 $\pm$ 0.59	6.44 $\pm$ 2.89	2.56 $\pm$ 0.52	18.6 $\pm$ 7.8
Male + hGH	81.7 $\pm$ 10.1	6.38 $\pm$ 1.99	6.07 $\pm$ 0.44	6.11 $\pm$ 3.40	3.78 $\pm$ 0.53	23.8 $\pm$ 13.8
Male + PG	73.0 $\pm$ 8.8	5.15 $\pm$ 0.80	4.17 $\pm$ 1.23	4.87 $\pm$ 1.46	3.19 $\pm$ 0.50	17.0 $\pm$ 9.6

In conclusion, our data support the context that the secretion pattern of GH
and/or some other pituitary factor plays a role in the regulation of sex differences in hepatic xenobiotic metabolism.

ACKNOWLEDGEMENTS

This work was supported by a grant from the Swedish Medical Research Council
(No. 13X-2819).

REFERENCES

1. Gustafsson, J.-Å., Mode, A., Norstedt, G., Hökfeldt, T., Sonnenschein, C.,
    Eneroth, P. and Skett, P. (1980) in: Litwack, G. (Ed.), Biochemical Actions
    of Hormones, Vol VII, Academic Press Inc., New York, pp. 47-89.

2. Mode, A., Gustafsson, J.-Å., Jansson, J.O., Edén, S. and Isaksson, O. (1982).
    Endocrinology, 111, 1682.

RECEPTORS AND INDUCTION OF
DRUG-METABOLIZING ENZYMES

© 1983 Elsevier Science Publishers B.V.
Extrahepatic Drug Metabolism and Chemical Carcinogenesis,
J. Rydström, J. Montelius and M. Bengtsson eds.

SEVERAL P-450 GENES REGULATED BY THE *Ah* RECEPTOR

Daniel W. Nebert, Robert H. Tukey, Peter I. Mackenzie,
Masahiko Negishi, and Howard J. Eisen
Laboratory of Developmental Pharmacology, National Institute of Child Health
and Human Development, National Institutes of Health, Bethesda, Maryland 20205
(U.S.A.)

INTRODUCTION

The *Ah* locus (Fig. 1) controls the induction of a small portion of the total
number of forms of P-450[*] (and their corresponding enzyme activities) by
polycyclic aromatic compounds such as TCDD and MC; P_1-450 is one of these
forms. The induction process is mediated by the cytosolic *Ah* receptor
(reviewed in Ref. 2). Numerous relatively planar foreign chemicals bind
avidly (apparent $K_d \sim 1$ nM) to the *Ah* receptor in direct proportion to their
potency as inducers of P_1-450. No endogenous ligand for the *Ah* receptor has
been found. Various assays for quantitating the *Ah* receptor include the use
of [^{3}H-1,6]TCDD (~ 60 Ci/mmol) in combination with dextran-coated charcoal
adsorption, trypsin treatment followed by isoelectric focusing, sucrose
density gradient centrifugation after dextran-charcoal adsorption, a
detergent-washing procedure with purified nuclei, and gel permeation and
anion-exchange chromatography.

The B6 inbred mouse strain was found to express liver microsomal AHH
induction following intraperitoneal MC treatment, whereas the D2 inbred mouse
strain does not express this induction process in liver (2, 3). The genetic
trait was defined as aromatic hydrocarbon responsiveness, with B6 having
Ah^b/Ah^b alleles and D2 having Ah^d/Ah^d alleles. The *Ah* locus recently has been
localized to mouse chromosome 17. AHH (P_1-450) induction is expressed as an
autosomal dominant trait (Fig. 2). When B6 mice are crossed with D2 mice, the

---

[*]Cytochrome P-450 is defined as all forms of CO-binding hemoproteins having
NADPH- and sometimes NADH-dependent monooxygenase activities. "P_1-450" is
defined as that form of polycyclic aromatic-inducible P-450 most closely
associated with polycyclic-aromatic-inducible aryl hydrocarbon hydroxylase
activity. "P_2-450" is defined as that form of isosafrole-induced enzyme which
metabolizes isosafrole best. "P_3-450" is defined as that form of polycyclic-
aromatic-induced enzyme most closely associated with polycyclic-aromatic-
inducible acetanilide 4-hydroxylase activity. Other abbreviations used:
TCDD, 2,3,7,8-tetrachlorodibenzo-*p*-dioxin; MC, 3-methylcholanthrene; AHH, aryl
hydrocarbon (benzo[a]pyrene) hydroxylase (EC 1.14.14.1); B6, the C57BL/6N
inbred mouse strain; and D2, the DBA/2N inbred mouse strain.

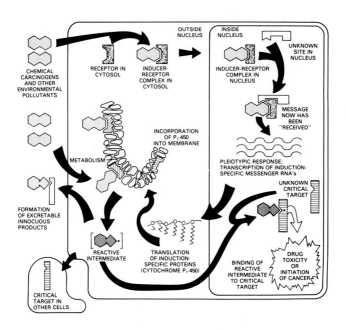

FIG. 1. Diagram of a cell and the hypothetical scheme by which a cytosolic receptor, a product of the regulatory *Ah* gene, binds to inducer (1). The resultant pleiotypic response includes greater amounts of cytochrome P_1-450, P_2-450, and P_3-450, leading to enhanced steady-state levels of reactive intermediates, which are associated with genetic increases in birth defects, drug toxicity, or chemical carcinogenesis. Depending upon the half-life of the reactive intermediate, important covalent binding may occur in the same cell in which metabolism took place, or in nearby cells. Although the "unknown critical target" is illustrated here in the nucleus, there is presently no experimental evidence demonstrating unequivocally the subcellular location of such a target or, for that matter, whether the target is nucleic acid or protein [Reproduced with permission from Dr. W. Junk Publishers].

resultant MC-treated heterozygote has inducible AHH (P_1-450) levels similar to those of the B6 parent. Whereas the cytosolic *Ah* receptor is readily observed in B6 mice, the *Ah* receptor can be detected in the nucleus but not in the cytosol of D2 mice (reviewed in Ref. 2). Of interest, the Ah^b/Ah^d heterozygote exhibits levels of receptor that are midway between those found in the B6 and D2 parents (Fig. 2). P_1-450 is one of many gene products controlled by the *Ah* receptor (2, 3). The definitions of three P-450 proteins regulated by the *Ah* receptor are given in Table 1.

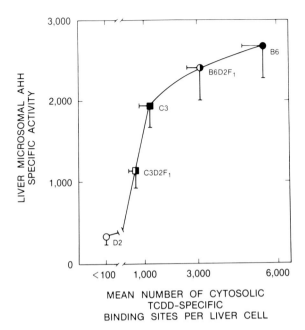

FIG. 2. Maximal hepatic AHH inducibility as a function of number of *Ah* receptor molecules per liver cell among various inbred strains of mice and F_1 hybrids (2). Each value is the mean of five or more individual determinations. C3, the C3H/HeN inbred mouse strain. *Brackets* in both directions denote standard deviations [Reproduced with permission from Academic Press, Inc.].

A relatively specific antibody to P_1-450 ($M_r \sim 55,000$) was developed (4) and used to determine that P_1-450 mRNA was 23 S in size (5). In the remainder of this report we demonstrate primarily the characterization of a P_1-450 cDNA clone and its corresponding genomic P_1-450 clone, λAhP-1.

RESULTS AND DISCUSSION

Colony hybridization

From MC-treated B6 mouse liver 23 S mRNA, double-stranded cDNA was prepared and inserted into the *PstI* site of pBR322. Plasmid DNA from ampicillin-sensitive tetracycline-resistant *E.coli* was fixed on nitrocellulose paper. The probe in this case was labeled cDNA freshly reverse-transcribed from 23 S mRNA from MC-treated B6 or D2 mouse liver. Because there is at least 40 times more P_1-450 mRNA in MC-treated B6 than D2 mice (5), we looked for a colony that was positive in B6 and negative in D2. Two clones, numbers 46 and 68, were found in the first 72 colonies screened (6). Because 46 contained a larger insert than 68, we chose to study clone 46 further.

TABLE 1

Designated name of mouse P-450 protein	One of best substrates in reconstituted enzyme assay	Metabolism that antibody to antigen inhibits most specifically
P_1-450	Benzo[a]pyrene	Benzo[a]pyrene
P_2-450	Isosafrole	Isosafrole
P_3-450	Acetanilide	Acetanilide

Immunologic criteria for cDNA clone

"Positive" and "negative" translation arrest experiments provide classical immunologic proof that the cDNA clone isolated is associated with a particular antibody. The antibody precipitates the protein that has been translated from the mRNA, and this mRNA hybridizes most specifically to the cloned cDNA. There appears to be a problem with hybridization arrest experiments and P-450 membrane-bound proteins. Antibodies to different forms of P-450 are notoriously not monospecific. Even monoclonal antibodies have been reported (7) to recognize two different forms of P-450. We have evidence (R.H. Tukey and D.W. Nebert, manuscript in preparation) that several antibodies--anti-(P_1-450), anti-(P_2-450), and anti-(P_3-450), each of which blocks one catalytic activity and not other activities--all precipitate protein translated from mRNA that hybridizes specifically to P_1-450 cDNA in the translation arrest experiments. Therefore, for reasons at the protein level, translation arrest experiments involving solubilized membrane-bound proteins may lead to difficulties in the interpretation of data. Confusion about which cDNA clone represents P-450b, the major rat phenobarbital-inducible form of P-450, is an example of such problems with hybridization arrest data (reviewed in Ref. 8).

Genetic criteria for cDNA clone

Unfortunately, the only proof available for rabbit and rat cDNA clones is the immunologic criterion, because no genetic polymorphisms have been characterized yet in detail. With the mouse P_1-450 gene, however, we have the additional criterion of *genetic differences* that have been well characterized over the past decade. Hence, when the B6D2F$_1$ heterozygote (Ah^b/Ah^d) is crossed with the D2 parent (Ah^d/Ah^d), among the progeny one finds a 50:50 distribution of Ah^b/Ah^d heterozygotes and Ah^d/Ah^d homozygotes. There is a perfect correlation between the Ah^b allele [*i.e.* induction of AHH activity

(P_1-450)] and the presence of MC-induced P_1-450 (23 S) mRNA that hybridizes to clone 46 (9). This experiment therefore constitutes genetic proof that clone 46 is highly likely to be associated with the P_1-450 cDNA. Additional proof has been obtained via Northern blots involving developmental studies (10, 11), since it is well known (4, 12) that P_1-450 (AHH) induction occurs at least 1 week earlier in gestation than P_2-450 or P_3-450.

No effect on DNA during induction

We have studied DNA from the livers of mice treated with various P-450 inducers (9, 13). There was no evidence for increases in intensity of the blots or changes in the sizes of DNA fragments. We therefore conclude that, during the induction process, neither gene amplification nor some gross form of genomic rearrangement occurs in the area of the P_1-450 gene represented by the clone 46 probe. In other hybridization experiments with B6 sperm, embryo and adult DNA (10), we also were unable to find any evidence for genomic rearrangement during development.

Isolation and characterization of λAhP-1

With clone 46 as the probe, a mouse plasmacytoma MOPC 41 genomic-DNA library was screened by the Benton-Davis plaque-hybridization procedure (14). Mouse tumor DNA had been digested by *EcoRI* and inserted into λ phage Charon 4A, and 50,000 plaques had been fixed to each filter (a generous gift of Dr. Jon Seidman, National Institute of Child Health and Human Development, Bethesda). The entire library consisted of 20 filters, so that we screened a total of about one million plaques. The first positive genomic clone was named λ3NT12 and was found to be 19 kbp in length. By repeating the Benton-Davis plaque hybridization technique, and characterizing three more genomic clones, we have walked up the chromosome with clones λ3NT12, λ3NT13, λ3NT14, and finally λAhP-1. By R-loop analysis, the entire P_1-450 gene was found to reside in λAhP-1, spanning about 4600 bp (Fig. 3). The P_1-450 gene is in the middle of λAhP-1, a clone which has a total length of 15.5 kbp. The P_1-450 genomic gene has at least 5 exons and 4 intervening sequences. Total length of all exons together is about 3000 bp (14).

Clone 46 appears to exist in the 3'-nontranslating region of the P_1-450 gene. With the clone 46 3' probe, it should be emphasized that we are unable to hybridize this probe to any other P-450 gene in mouse genomic DNA (6) or any other mouse P-450 mRNA (13). Clone 46 therefore represents a 3'-unique probe.

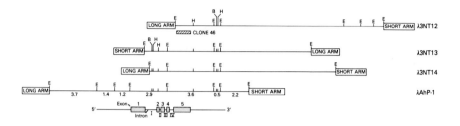

FIG. 3. Restriction maps of four recombinant phage isolated from the mouse genomic-DNA library containing overlapping DNA regions of the P_1-450 chromosomal structural gene (14). The linear DNA maps of individual phage were constructed on the basis of *EcoRI* (E), *HindIII* (H), *BamHI* (B), *PstI*, *SstI*, *XbaI*, and *XhoI* digests alone and in combination. The distances in kbp between the *EcoRI* sites of clone λAhP-1 are indicated, and the relative positions of the overlapping *EcoRI* and *XbaI* sites and clone 46 amongst the four phage are shown. In each of the four recombinant phage, the long and short arms of λ Charon 4A are indicated. By R-loop analysis between λAhP-1 and the P_1-450 (23 S) mRNA from MC-treated B6 liver, the position of the P_1-450 exons and introns was determined and is depicted at *bottom* [Reproduced with permission from Springer-Verlag Inc.].

This laboratory has uncovered several important points of information with the use of the P_1-450 cDNA clone. An association of clone 46 with the P_1-450 protein has been demonstrated by both immunologic and genetic criteria. We know that P_1-450 induction is under transcriptional control, because increased 23 S mRNA and an intranuclear large-molecular-weight mRNA precursor occur concomitantly during the induction process (9). No evidence for gene duplication or gross form of genomic rearrangement has been found, either during induction or during development. P_1-450 mRNA is translated exclusively on membrane-bound polysomes (15). Clone 46 hybridizes with rat and rabbit DNA, and with rat but not rabbit mRNA (10, 16); these data suggest that clone 46 hybridizes to a segment of the rabbit P_1-450 gene that is not transcribed into the messenger. Clone p57, a 1900-bp cDNA clone of P_1-450 that extends 800 bp further 5'-ward than clone 46, has been used successfully to isolate two human genomic genes (17). We found that the P_1-450 gene in adult B6 is *hypo*methylated, compared with the gene in B6 sperm, B6 embryo, or adult D2 mice; this hypomethylation pattern could be related to the increased expressivity of the P_1-450 gene in B6, compared with that in D2 mice (10). Other P-450 inducers, such as benzo[a]anthracene and isosafrole, have been found to induce P_1-450 mRNA, as measured by the clone 46 probe (13). Lastly, we have found an excellent correlation between the intranuclear appearance of the inducer-receptor complex and the induction of P_1-450 mRNA as measured by the clone 46 probe (18).

Sequencing of the entire P_1-450 gene and its flanking regions is underway. We have uncovered an interesting 104-bp sequence (Fig. 4) that includes flanking 10-bp direct repeats. This poly(dG-dT) repeat is consistent with DNA having Z-DNA-forming potential (19, 20). Of additional interest, this stretch of DNA appears to be in the noncoding region of the first exon. Most Pu-Py repeats reported to date occur either upstream from the cap site or in intervening sequences. This preliminary result is under further study.

Other studies in progress

p21, a 1710-bp cDNA clone that hybridizes well to 20 S mRNA (21), is associated with the *Ah* locus and exhibits 5' homology with the P_1-450 gene. This genomic gene has been isolated and clearly differs from the P_1-450 genomic gene (R.H. Tukey and D.W. Nebert, in preparation). Whether p21 represents a cDNA clone for P_2-450 or P_3-450 cannot be answered until we have the necessary protein and nucleotide sequence data completed. The P_2-450 protein has been thoroughly characterized (22).

Benzo[a]pyrene-resistant mutant clones

Benzo[a]pyrene induces high levels of AHH activity in Hepa-1 cells (23). The metabolites of benzo[a]pyrene formed by cytochrome P_1-450 are extremely toxic; exposure of cells to concentrations of benzo[a]pyrene as low as 25 nM is sufficient to produce toxicity and cell death--if the cells possess sufficiently high levels of inducible AHH activity. In the presence of 4 μM benzo[a]pyrene, however, few Hepa-1 cells (~10^{-7} per generation) survive. These benzo[a]pyrene-resistant cells appear to represent somatic mutations in the pathways for AHH induction. Clones derived from such cells have been developed (24) with the intention of examining genetically the multiple steps during the process of AHH induction. By somatic-cell hybridization studies

```
5'  GAAAATAAAA TAGAGAGAGA GTGTGTGTGT GTGTGTGTGT
    GTGTGTGTGT GTGTGTTGTG TGTGTGTGAA TATGATGATT
    AAAATATATT GTGTGAAAAT AAAA  3'
```

FIG. 4. Partial sequence near the 5' end of the P_1-450 gene.

(25), the clones that have been developed are known to represent at least
three distinct complementation groups and therefore reflect mutations in at
least three different genes.

Several clones (Table 2) have normal Ah receptor levels (compared with the
wild-type Hepa-1c1c7 parent), possess normal kinetics for translocation of the
inducer-receptor complex into the nucleus, yet exhibit very low or
nondetectable basal or inducible AHH activity. These clones could represent a
mutation in the P_1-450 structural gene or other genes responsible for the
induced hydroxylase activity. Other clones, c2 and c6, are receptor-
deficient mutants (r⁻), having no more than 10% of wild-type Ah receptor
levels, normal kinetics of nuclear translocation of the inducer-receptor
complex, and no more than 20% of wild-type AHH inducibility by either TCDD or
benzo[a]anthracene. One clone, c4, has normal cytosolic levels of Ah
receptor, is defective in nuclear translocation of the inducer-receptor
complex (nt⁻), and lacks any detectable basal or inducible AHH activity.
These data (23) are an important prelude to our recombinant DNA and
transfection experiments underway that are designed to understand the
regulatory mechanism by which the Ah receptor controls transcription of the
P_1-450 gene during induction by polycyclic aromatic compounds.

TABLE 2

Ah RECEPTOR LEVELS AND MAXIMALLY INDUCIBLE AHH ACTIVITY IN Hepa-1c1c7 PARENT
LINE AND SIX MUTANT CLONES

Cell culture line	Ah receptor (fmol/mg protein)			Maximal AHH activity (units/mg cellular protein)	
	Cytosol, in vitro treatment	Cytosol, exposure in culture	Nuclei, exposure in culture	BzAnth as inducer	TCDD as inducer
Hepa-1c1c7	20	12	6	210	520
c1		7.6	2.0	<0.4	<0.4
c2	2.1	1.7	0.5	42	110
c3		18	3.4	22	16
c4		15	0.3	<0.4	<0.4
c5		6.0	3.4	<0.4	<0.4
c6	1.0	0.5	0.4	4	3

Complementation groups: c1 & c5; c2 & c6; c4. c3 is dominant, and
therefore its complementation group cannot be determined (24, 25). BzAnth,
benzo[a]anthracene.

Concluding remarks

With clone λAhP-1 and the surrounding regions of this mouse chromosome, we hope to understand a great deal about the regulation of P-450 induction, the evolution of the P-450 system, and perhaps the ultimate number of P-450 forms that an individual organism is genetically *capable* of expressing. With this knowledge, we hope to gain insight into the mechanism of chemical carcinogenesis, especially since P_1-450 is directly responsible for the metabolic activation of polycyclic hydrocarbons such as benzo[a]pyrene to the ultimate carcinogenic intermediate, which interacts covalently with DNA. Finally, it may be possible to develop an assay, based on recombinant DNA technology, in order to assess the human *Ah* phenotype (reviewed in Ref. 26); such an assay may predict who is at increased risk for certain types of environmentally-caused cancers.

ACKNOWLEDGMENTS

This work would not have been possible without the combined efforts of Drs. Yuan-Tsong Chen, Michitoshi Nakamura, Toshihiko Ikeda, Mario Altieri, Catherine Legraverend, Tohru Ohyama, Sirpa Kärenlampi, Allan B. Okey, Rita R. Hannah, Dana J. Kessler, Lynn W. Enquist, David C. Swan, and Oliver Hankinson. The expert secretarial assistance of Ms. Ingrid E. Jordan is greatly appreciated.

REFERENCES

1. Nebert, D.W. (1979) Mol. Cell. Biochem., 27, 27.

2. Eisen, H.J., Hannah, R.R., Legraverend, C., Okey, A.B. and Nebert, D.W. (1983) in: Litwack, G. (Ed.), Biochemical Actions of Hormones, Academic Press, New York, pp. 227-258.

3. Nebert, D.W., Negishi, M., Lang, M.A., Hjelmeland, L.M. and Eisen, H.J. (1982) Advanc. Genet., 21, 1.

4. Negishi, M. and Nebert, D.W. (1979) J. Biol. Chem., 254, 11015.

5. Negishi, M. and Nebert, D.W. (1981) J. Biol. Chem., 256, 3085.

6. Negishi, M., Swan, D.C., Enquist, L.W. and Nebert, D.W. (1981) Proc. Natl. Acad. Sci. U.S.A., 78, 800.

7. Thomas, P.E., Reik, L.M., Ryan, D.E. and Levin, W. (1982) Fed. Proc., 41, 297 [Abstract].

8. Nebert, D.W. and Negishi, M. (1982) Biochem. Pharmacol., 31, 2311.

9. Tukey, R.H., Nebert, D.W. and Negishi, M. (1981) J. Biol. Chem., 256, 6969.

10. Chen, Y.-T., Negishi, M. and Nebert, D.W. (1982) DNA, 1, 231.

388

11. Ikeda, T., Altieri, M., Chen, Y.-T., Nakamura, M., Tukey, R.H., Nebert, D.W. and Negishi, M. (1983) Eur. J. Biochem., in press.

12. Guenthner, T.M. and Nebert, D.W. (1978) Eur. J. Biochem., 91, 449.

13. Tukey, R.H., Negishi, M. and Nebert, D.W. (1982) Mol. Pharmacol., 22, 779.

14. Nakamura, M., Negishi, M., Altieri, M., Chen, Y.-T., Ikeda, T., Tukey, R.H. and Nebert, D.W. (1983) Eur. J. Biochem., in press.

15. Chen, Y.-T. and Negishi, M. (1982) Biochem. Biophys. Res. Commun., 104, 641.

16. Chen, Y.-T., Lang, M.A., Jensen, N.M., Negishi, M., Tukey, R.H., Sidransky, E., Guenthner, T.M. and Nebert, D.W. (1982) Eur. J. Biochem., 122, 361.

17. Chen, Y.-T., Tukey, R.H., Swan, D.C., Negishi, M. and Nebert, D.W. (1983) Pediat. Res., in press [Abstract].

18. Tukey, R.H., Hannah, R.R., Negishi, M., Nebert, D.W. and Eisen, H.J. (1982) Cell, 31, 275.

19. Wang, A.H.-J., Quigley, G.J., Kolpak, F.J., Crawford, J.L., van Boom, J.H., van der Marel, G. and Rich, A. (1979) Nature, 282, 680.

20. Nordheim, A., Pardue, M.L., Lafer, E.M., Moller, A., Stollar, B.D. and Rich, A. (1981) Nature, 294, 417.

21. Tukey, R.H., Ohyama, T., Negishi, M. and Nebert, D.W. (1982) Pharmacologist, 24, 207 [Abstract].

22. Ohyama, T., Nebert, D.W. and Negishi, M. (1982) in: Hietanen, E., Laitinen, M. and Hänninen, O. (Eds.), Cytochrome P-450, Biochemistry, Biophysics and Environmental Implications, Elsevier/North-Holland Biomedical Press, Amsterdam, pp. 177-180.

23. Legraverend, C., Hannah, R.R., Eisen, H.J., Owens, I.S., Nebert, D.W. and Hankinson, O. (1982) J. Biol. Chem., 257, 6402.

24. Hankinson, O. (1979) Proc. Natl. Acad. Sci. U.S.A., 76, 373.

25. Hankinson, O. (1981) Somat. Cell. Genet., 7, 373.

26. Nebert, D.W. (1981) Environ. Health Perspect., 39, 11.

© 1983 Elsevier Science Publishers B.V.
Extrahepatic Drug Metabolism and Chemical Carcinogenesis,
J. Rydström, J. Montelius and M. Bengtsson eds.

THE *Ah* RECEPTOR: SPECIES AND TISSUE VARIATION IN BINDING OF
2,3,7,8-TETRACHLORODIBENZO-p-DIOXIN AND CARCINOGENIC AROMATIC HYDROCARBONS

ALLAN B. OKEY, MICHELLE E. MASON AND LYNN M. VELLA
Division of Clinical Pharmacology, Department of Paediatrics, Research
Institute, The Hospital for Sick Children, 555 University Avenue, Toronto,
Ontario CANADA M5G 1X8

INTRODUCTION

The *Ah* receptor, a primary product of the regulatory gene in the *Ah* gene
complex, mediates the induction of aryl hydrocarbon hydroxylase (AHH;
cytochrome P_1-450) and several other pleiotypic responses associated with the
Ah genetic locus (1,2).

Ah receptor in rodent hepatic cytosols has been extensively characterized
using a tritiated form of the potent AHH inducer, 2,3,7,8-tetrachlorodibenzo-
p-dioxin (TCDD, 50 Ci/mmol) as the radioligand (1,2). More recently we have
employed the carcinogenic polycyclic aromatic hydrocarbons (PAHs) [³H]3-
methylcholanthrene (MC, 37 Ci/mmol), [³H]benzo(a)pyrene (BP, 50 Ci/mmol) and
[³H]dibenz(a,h)anthracene (DB(a,h)A, 8.1 Ci/mmol) as radioligands in assays on
extrahepatic and hepatic cytosols from several mammalian species. Binding of
nonradioactive carcinogens to *Ah* receptor is assessed by testing their ability
to compete with the radioligands for specific receptor sites.

With these radioligands we have used sucrose density gradient analyses (3)
to address the following questions:

1) What chemicals bind to the *Ah* receptor?

2) In what tissues does the *Ah* receptor occur?

3) What roles might the *Ah* receptor play in carcinogenesis?

Only a few fragments of experimental evidence concerning these questions can
be presented in this brief review. Please see the cited references for more
complete discussion of specific points.

RESULTS AND DISCUSSION

Direct Detection of Binding of Four Radioligands to *Ah* Receptor in Rodent
Cytosols. Figure 1 illustrates that *Ah* receptor in rat thymic cytosol can be
detected not only by direct binding of [³H]TCDD, but also by direct binding of
the three carcinogenic PAHs: [³H]MC, [³H]BP and [³H]DB(a,h)A. In addition to
binding to *Ah* receptor, the carcinogenic PAHs also bind extensively to a
component (or components) sedimenting at 4-5S.

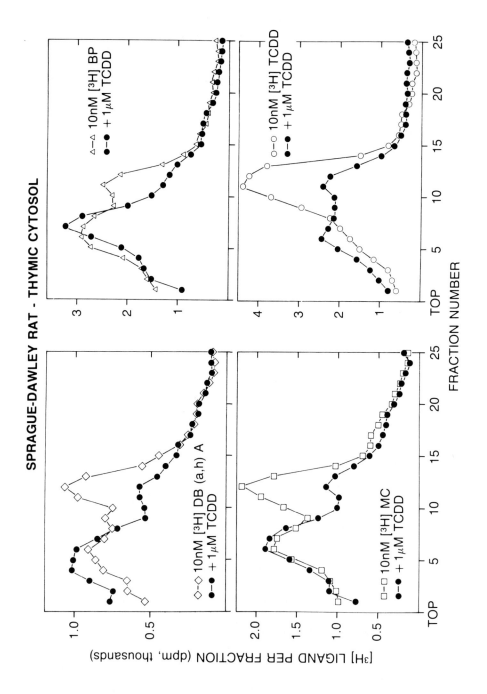

Figure 1. (On Facing Page). Direct Detection of _Ah_ Receptor by Binding of Four Radioligands in Rat Thymic Cytosol.
   Thymic cytosol incubated at 0-40 with the ligands indicated was separated by velocity sedimentation on sucrose density gradients (3). _Ah_ receptor sediments near 9S (Fraction 13 in these assays). Note that binding of each radioligand in the 9S region is competitively eliminated by incubation in the presence of a 100-fold molar excess of nonradioactive TCDD. Binding in the 4-5S region (near Fraction 7 (is not eliminated by TCDD and is not specific for cytochrome P_1-450 inducers.

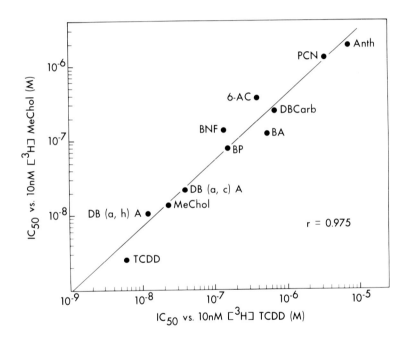

Figure 2. (Above). Competition by Carcinogenic and Non-carcinogenic Chemicals for _Ah_ Receptor Sites in Hepatic Cytosol from C57BL/6J Mice.
   The median inhibitory concentration (IC_{50}) for each chemical was determined by dose-response assays with competitor concentrations for 1 nM to 10 uM against [^{3}H]TCDD and against [^{3}H]MC. DB(a,c)A = dibenz(a,c)anthracene; βNF = βetanaphthoflavone; DBCarb = dibenzocarbazole; 6-AC = 6-aminochrysene; PCN = pregnenolone-16a-carbonitrile; Anth = anthracene; other abbreviations as in test. (Data from Okey & Vella, 1982, ref. 8).

The 4-5S cytosolic component is <u>not</u> specific for chemicals that induce cytochrome P_1-450 and does <u>not</u> segregate with the *Ah* locus in genetic experiments in mice (4,5). Thus the 4-5S binding component does not meet the criteria for a receptor which might regulate induction of AHH. Binding of carcinogenic PAHs to the 4-5S component is of high affinity, however, and may play some role in cellular responses to PAH carcinogens (6,7).

In Sprague-Dawley rats, if *Ah* receptor can be detected in cytosol from a given tissue with [³H]TCDD, receptor also can be detected in that cytosol with [³H]MC, [³H]BP or [³H]DB(a,h)A. The affinity with which [³H]BP binds to *Ah* receptor in rat cytosols (K_d~4 nM) is weaker than with the other radioligands (K_d~1 nM for [³H]TCDD and [³H]MC (5)).

C57BL/6J mice (B6) are genetically "responsive" to induction of AHH by carcinogenic PAHs (1,2). *Ah* receptor in cytosols from several B6 tissues can be detected by direct binding of [³H]TCDD, [³H]MC or [³H]DB(a,h)A. Nonradioactive BP competes with the other radioligands for *Ah* receptor sites in B6 cytosol (Fig. 2), but the affinity of [³H]BP binding in B6 cytosols is too low for *Ah* receptor to be detected by direct binding of [³H]BP in these animals (8). Physicochemical properties and ligand preferences indicate that B6 mouse *Ah* receptor and Sprague-Dawley rat *Ah* receptor are similar, but not identical macromolecules.

DBA/2J mice (D2) are genetically "nonresponsive" to AHH induction by carcinogenic PAHs (1,2); they do, however, demonstrate AHH induction when treated with high doses of TCDD (1,2). In D2 mice, cytosolic *Ah* receptor cannot be detected in any tissue with any available radioligand, including [³H]TCDD (9). See a later section on nuclear uptake of [³H]TCDD·*Ah* receptor complex for further discussion of D2 response mechanisms.

Competition of Nonradioactive Chemicals for *Ah* Receptor Sites. Figure 2 gives an example of how competition experiments versus [³H]TCDD or [³H]MC can be used to estimate the relative affinity with which nonradioactive chemicals interact with *Ah* receptor.

From data in Figure 2 it can be seen that the affinity with which a chemical interacts with *Ah* receptor sites is not a good index of that chemical's carcinogenic potential. For example, β-naphthoflavone is not known to be carcinogenic nor mutagenic, but it has an affinity for *Ah* receptor which is equal to that for the carcinogens BP and BA.

Data in Figure 2 also reveal that the rank-order with which the competitors inhibit [³H]TCDD binding to *Ah* receptor is the same as the rank-order with which they inhibit binding of [³H]MC. This, along with other evidence (5), strongly indicates that [³H]TCDD and [³H]MC are indeed binding to the same receptor and to the same site on that receptor (rather than having a receptor for halogenated aromatic compounds separate from that for polycyclic aromatic hydrocarbon carcinogens). As yet, there is no evidence that any particular tissue contains more than one receptor for "MC-like" inducers of AHH. Variant forms of *Ah* receptor have been detected in certain tissues and cell lines in culture (10,11), but these cells appear still to contain only one form of receptor rather than having multiple species of receptor present in the same cell.

Nuclear Uptake of Inducer·*Ah* Receptor Complexes. Induction of AHH (cytochrome P_1-450) requires that the inducer·*Ah* receptor complex (formed in the cytoplasmic compartment) be translocated into the nucleus. By some unknown mechanism, presence of the inducer·*Ah* receptor complex in the nucleus stimulates production of specific mRNA species that code for cytochrome P_1-450 and associated structural gene products of the *Ah* genetic locus (1).

Nuclear translocation of the inducer·*Ah* receptor complex has been most satisfactorily demonstrated by exposing cells in culture to [³H]TCDD (10,11, 12). Nuclear uptake of the [³H]TCDD·*Ah* receptor complex also can be demonstrated by in vivo injection of [³H]TCDD in mice and rats (12,13,14).

As shown in Figure 3, in vivo injection of [³H]TCDD leads to presence of the [³H]TCDD·*Ah* receptor complex in nuclei from liver, lung and kidney of genetically "responsive" B6 mice and, to a lesser extent, in liver lung and kidney of genetically "non-responsive" D2 mice. Thus nuclear uptake of the inducer·*Ah* receptor complex is not confined to liver, but occurs in nonhepatic tissues as well.

D2 mice appear to have a defective form of cytosolic *Ah* receptor which cannot be detected directly by in vitro incubation with any radioligand. Nuclear uptake in D2 mice injected with high doses of [³H]TCDD in vivo demonstrates that the cytosolic *Ah* receptor is not completely absent in these animals, but is present in a defective form that is competent to translocate to the nucleus only when presented with a high concentration of TCDD.

Nuclear translocation experiments are most easily done with [³H]TCDD since this compound is poorly metabolized in most species. Recently it also has been possible to detect nuclear translocation of the [³H]MC·*Ah* receptor complex in Hepa-1c1 mouse hepatoma cells in culture (11).

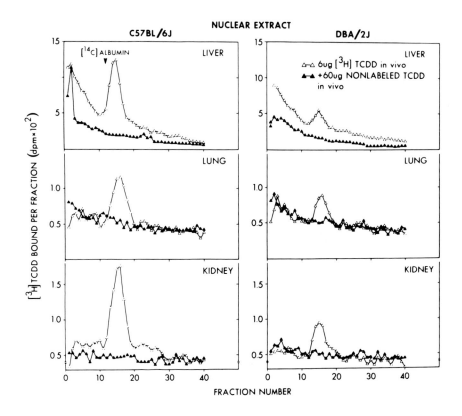

Figure 3. <u>Sucrose Density Gradient Profiles of Binding of [³H]TCDD to Receptor in Nuclear Extracts from Tissues of C57BL/6J and DBA/2J Mice Injected in vivo with the Labeled Dioxin.</u>

[³H]TCDD was injected intraperitoneally (6 μg/mouse = 0.75 μMol per kg body weight). Nuclear extracts were prepared 18 hours later as described in (9). Open triangles represent nuclear binding in mice receiving [³H]TCDD only. To test saturability of nuclear binding sites, pair-matched mice were injected with a 10-fold excess of nonradioactive TCDD 6 hours before injection of [³H]TCDD. (From Mason & Okey, 1981, ref. 9).

Distribution of *Ah* Receptor in Tissues of Various Species.

Table 1 summarizes the various mammalian tissues in which we have detected cytosolic *Ah* receptor. Cytosolic *Ah* receptor was first detected in liver from mice and rats (2, 12); most small laboratory mammals, especially rodents, have abundant hepatic cytosolic *Ah* receptor.

Ah receptor is not confined to the liver, however. Several extrahepatic tissues exhibit high concentrations of cytosolic *Ah* receptor. Many tissues having cytosolic *Ah* receptor are important sites for induction of tumors by chemicals, i.e., lung, gastrointestinal tract, skin, mammary gland and urinary bladder. Carcinogen metabolism, especially of PAHs, has been extensively studied in most of these tissues and experiments now are being done on metabolism (15,16) of carcinogenic PAHs in other receptor-positive tissues such as the ovary (Figure 4).

Most tissues that contain high concentrations of *Ah* receptor also have significant AHH activity and exhibit induction of AHH when donor animals are treated with "MC-like" P_1-450 inducers.

There are several tissues, however, that possess high concentrations of receptor, yet do not have significant levels of AHH or do not exhibit AHH induction when exposed to "MC-like" inducers. Rat thymus has an *Ah* receptor concentration equal to that in liver (Figure 1; refs. 9,13), but the level of AHH activity in thymus is less than 1/1000 that in liver. Adult guinea pig liver and adult rabbit liver have high *Ah* receptor concentrations, but respond only weakly to AHH induction by "MC-like" chemicals (1). Several other examples could be cited which demonstrate that a tissue can have high *Ah* receptor content without having high AHH activity or AHH-induction capacity.

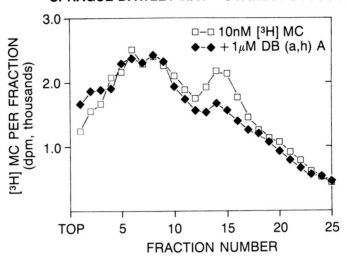

SPRAGUE-DAWLEY RAT - OVARIAN CYTOSOL

Figure 4. Detection of Specific *Ah* Receptor in Rat Ovarian Cytosol with [³H]MC.

INTERPRETATION AND CONCLUSIONS: Possible Roles for the *Ah* Receptor in Carcinogenesis.

It is well-established that the *Ah* receptor plays an important indirect role in chemical carcinogenesis by virtue of its ability to regulate induction of AHH activity by "MC-like" chemicals. Whether carcinogenesis is enhanced or inhibited by AHH induction depends upon the particular chemical involved, the tissue studied and the route of administration (17).

The *Ah* receptor does not appear to be directly involved nor required for initiation of carcinogenesis by chemicals, even though many of the best *Ah* receptor ligands are potent carcinogens. Evidence that the *Ah* receptor is not required for initiation of carcinogenesis is: a) some chemicals such as -naphthoflavone bind to *Ah* receptor with high affinity, but are not carcinogenic nor mutagenic, b) polycyclic aromatic hydrocarbons such as MC, BP, etc. induce tumors in DBA/2J mice even though these animals have a "defective" form of *Ah* receptor that does not functionally bind MC or BP (17), c) C3H/10T1/2 Clone 8 mouse fibroblasts can be malignantly transformed by exposure to MC in

TABLE 1

TISSUES IN WHICH CYTOSOLIC *Ah* RECEPTOR HAS BEEN DETECTED

TISSUE	RAT (Sp-D)	MOUSE (C57BL/6)	G. PIG (Hart)	HAMSTER (GolSyr)	RABBIT (NZW)	MONKEY (Cyno & Rhes)
LIVER	|||	+++	+++	+++	+++	+++
LUNG	+++	++	+	0		+++ F
KIDNEY	+	+	+	0		
STOMACH	++					
SMALL INTESTINE	+	+	0	0		
COLON	++					
THYMUS	+++	+	0	0		+ F
SPLEEN	+	+++	0	0	++	
PANCREAS	+					
SKIN	+					
MAMMARY GLAND	+					
BLADDER	+++	+++				
PROSTATE	0	+				
TESTIS	0	0				
OVARY	+	+				
ADRENAL	0					
SKELETAL MUSCLE	0	0				
HEART	0	0			F = fetal	
BRAIN	0	0			Rhesus	
					tissues	

0 = no detectable specific binding (< 5 fmol/mg cytosol protein)

+ = 5 to 20 fmol/mg cytosol protein

++ = 20 to 40 fmol/mg cytosol protein

+++ = > 40 fmol/mg cytosol protein

Blank spaces in the table indicate that assays have not yet been done on those tissues.

culture, yet MC does not bind *Ah* receptor within these cells in culture nor induce cytochrome P_1-450 (11).

More recently it has been reported that the *Ah* receptor is implicated in promotion of tumorigenesis by agents such as TCDD (18). TCDD binds to the *Ah* receptor in rodent skin and this binding may be the first specific step in tumor promotion by halogenated aromatic hydrocarbons.

Poland and Knutson (2) have described a model in which the *Ah* receptor controls expression of genes that regulate cell division and differentiation. As shown by our survey of mammalian tissues, *Ah* receptor concentrations generally are highest in those tissues that are in close contact with the external environment and have a high proliferative capacity. This distribution tends to support the Poland-Knutson model.

It is clear that *Ah* receptor exists in high concentrations in tissues that do not exhibit significant AHH induction. Thus the *Ah* receptor may be available to regulate cellular functions other than induction of drug-metabolizing enzymes. Although the *Ah* receptor may play an important role in regulation of cell division, cell differentiation and tumor promotion, there is as yet no known endogenous ligand for the *Ah* receptor that might "physiologically" regulate these processes. All high-affinity ligands indentified to this point are xenobiotic chemicals, most of which are highly toxic and/or carcinogenic.

In summary, the *Ah* receptor can be detected by use of several radioligands in many tissues that are susceptible to chemically-induced cancers. The receptor plays an important indirect role in carcinogenesis by regulating induction of AHH (cytochrome P_1-450). Tumor promotion by TCDD and related halogenated compounds also appears to be mediated by the *Ah* receptor.

The relevance of *Ah* receptor mechanisms to human carcinogenesis is unknown. *Ah* receptor has been detected in two primate species -- Cynomolgus and Rhesus monkeys. Human genetic variation in AHH induction is well-established (17) and suggests that *Ah* receptor levels may vary widely among individuals in the human population. Preliminary reports of *Ah* receptor in human tissues have appeared, but thorough characterization of *Ah* receptor in the human population has not yet been accomplished. This is a primary area for further research into the role of the *Ah* receptor in chemical carcinogenesis.

ACKNOWLEDGEMENTS

Supported by grants from the National Cancer Institute of Canada and the Medical Research Council of Canada.

We thank Line P. Babin for typing the manuscript.

REFERENCES

1. Nebert, D.W., Eisen, H.J., Negishi, M., Lang, M., Hjelmeland, L. and Okey, A.B. (1981) Ann. Rev. Pharmacol. Toxicol., 21, 431.

2. Poland, A. and Knutson, J.C. (1982) Ann. Rev. Pharmacol. Toxicol. 22, 517.

3. Tsui, H.W. and Okey, A.B. (1981) Can. J. Physiol. Pharmacol. 59, 927.

4. Hannah, R.R., Nebert, D.W. and Eisen, H.J. (1981) J. Biol. Chem. 256, 4584.

5. Okey, A.B. and Vella, L.M. (1982) Eur. J. Biochem. 127, 39.

6. Holder, G.M., Tierney, B. and Bresnick, E. (1981) Cancer Res. 41, 4408.

7. Zytkovicz, T.H. (1982) Cancer Res. 42, 4387.

8. Okey, A.B., Dube, A.W. and Vella, L.M. (1983) Proc. Amer. Assoc. Cancer Res. 24, 57.

9. Mason, M.E. and Okey, A.B. (1982) Eur. J. Biochem. 123, 209.

10. Legraverend, C., Hannah, R.R., Eisen, H.H., Owens, I.S., Nebert, D.W. and Hankinson, O. (1982) J. Biol. Chem. 257, 6402.

11. Okey, A.B., Mason, M.E., Gehly, E.B., Heidelberger, C., Muncan, J. and Dufresne, M.J. (1983) Eur. J. Biochem. (in press).

12. Okey, A.B., Bondy, G.P., Mason, M.E., Kahl, G.F., Eisen, H.J., Guenthner, T.M. and Nebert, D.W. (1979) J. Biol. Chem. 254, 11636.

13. Lund, J., Kurl, R.N., Poellinger, L. and Gustafsson, J.-A. (1982) Biochim. Biochys. Acta 716, 16.

14. Tukey, R.H., Hannah, R.R., Negishi, M., Nebert, D.W. and Eisen, H.J. (1982) Cell 31, 275.

15. Mattison, D.R. and Nightingale, M.R. (1980) Toxicol. Appl. Pharmacol. 56, 399.

16. Bengtsson, M. and Rydstrom, J. (1983) Science 219, 1437.

17. Nebert, D.W. (1981) Environ. Health Perspect. 39, 11.

18. Poland, A., Palen, D. and Glover, E. (1982) Nature 300, 271.

© 1983 Elsevier Science Publishers B.V.
Extrahepatic Drug Metabolism and Chemical Carcinogenesis,
J. Rydström, J. Montelius and M. Bengtsson eds.

SOLUBLE RECEPTOR PROTEINS IN CONTROL OF GENE EXPRESSION

JAN-ÅKE GUSTAFSSON[1], ÖRJAN WRANGE[1], LORENZ POELLINGER[1], JOHAN LUND[1], FARHANG
PAYVAR[2] AND KEITH YAMAMOTO[2]

[1]Department of Medical Nutrition, Karolinska Institute, Huddinge University
Hospital F69, S-141 86 Sweden and [2]Department of Biochemistry and Biophysics,
University of California, San Fransisco, California 94143, USA.

INTRODUCTION

The mechanism of chemical carcinogenesis for benzo(a)pyrene and other related
polycyclic aromatic hydrocarbons has been well characterized (1,2). Benzo(a)-
pyrene is not carcinogenic in itself but must first undergo activation by metabolism. The enzyme system responsible for the activation of these compounds to
proximal and ultimate carcinogens is a cytochrome P-450-dependent microsomal
monooxygenase system, aryl hydrocarbon hydroxylase (AHH). This enzyme is regulated genetically by the Ah locus (3,4). One of the most potent inducers of AHH is
2,3,7,8-tetrachlorodibenzo-p-dioxin (TCDD). The inductive effect of TCDD on AHH
activity is mediated via an intracellular receptor protein (5,6). This receptor
is stereospecific for TCDD and other hydrocarbons that induce AHH activity. The
receptor binds TCDD with high affinity and low capacity. After binding of TCDD
to the receptor, the complex binds to DNA (7). The receptor can only be found in
those tissues in which TCDD is effective (1,8) and only in the liver cytosol from
those strains of mice that respond to TCDD (5).

Existing physicochemical data on the receptor are very incoherent. In mice
which are sensitive to the induction of AHH activity by polycyclic hydrocarbons
(strain C 57 BL/6 J), a receptor for TCDD sedimenting at approximately 5 S at
high ionic strength has been demonstrated (9). In the same strain of mice, Hannah
et al. (10) reported a sedimentation coefficient of 7.5 S at high ionic strength,
a Stokes radius of 75 Å and a molecular weight of 245,000 for the receptor and a
high degree of nonspecific binding of labeled TCDD. In the Sprague-Dawley rat,
the TCDD receptor in both hepatic and thymic cytosol sediments at 4-5 S at high
ionic strength (11,12). Furthermore, a specific 3-MC-binding protein with a molecular weight of 45,000 and sedimenting at 4.2 S (13) as well as a specific B(a)P
binder sedimenting at 4 S (14) have also been described in the rat. These quite
contradictory and confusing findings from various laboratories do not permit
formulation of a clear concept concerning the mechanism of induction of AHH by
TCDD and polycyclic aromatic hydrocarbons.

In view of these considerations a great need was felt to perform a careful
investigation of the physicochemical characteristics of the TCDD receptor in rats

and mice. It was also considered of value to compare characteristics of the TCDD receptor to those of the glucocorticoid receptor, a well studied steroid receptor protein.

Purification of the glucocorticoid receptor

We have previously purified the [^{3}H]triamcinolone acetonide-labeled glucocorticoid receptor from rat liver cytosol to near homogeneity according to SDS-gel electrophoresis (15). It consisted of one subunit with a molecular weight of 94 K and had one ligand-binding site per molecule. The purification involved sequential chromatography on phosphocellulose, DNA-cellulose twice, and Sephadex G-200. Between the two chromatography steps on DNA-cellulose, the receptor was heat activated. The receptor was affinity eluted from the second DNA-cellulose column with pyridoxal 5'-phosphate. After chromatography on the second DNA-cellulose column, the steroid-receptor complex had a Stokes radius of 6.0 nm and a sedimentation coefficient of 3.4 S in 0.15 M KCl. In the absence of KCl, the sedimentation coefficient was 3.6 S.

Recently, we have found 25 mM MgCl$_2$ in buffer A (1 mM disodium EDTA, 20 mM Tris-HCl, pH 7.8, 10% (w/v) glycerol and 10 mM DTT) to be optimal for elution of the glucocorticoid receptor from the second DNA-cellulose column when considering both purity (63 $\pm$ 19%; n = 6; mean $\pm$ S.D.) and recovery (34 $\pm$ 6%; n = 7) (16). Furthermore, the 25 mM MgCl$_2$-eluted glucocorticoid receptor could be applied directly on a DEAE-Sepharose column and be rapidly eluted with a linear salt gradient resulting in a considerable purification. The recovery in the DEAE-Sepharose step was 66 $\pm$ 7% (n = 5). The purity of DEAE-Sepharose purified glucocorticoid receptor was about 80% according to densitometry scanning of SDS-electrophoresis gels. Except for the 94 K glucocorticoid receptor band there were always two other bands present corresponding to molecular weights of 79 K and 72 K, respectively. The 79 K and 72 K components constituted 9 $\pm$ 3.2% (n = 6) and 12 $\pm$ 1.9% (n = 6), respectively, of the glucocorticoid receptor preparation as measured by densitometry (16).

Proteolytic digestion of the glucocorticoid receptor

Using crude cytosolic preparation, we have previously shown that the rat hepatic glucocorticoid receptor complex has a Stokes radius of 6.1 nm and a sedimentation coefficient of 4.0 S (17). It could be converted to smaller complexes with Stokes radii of 3.6 nm and 1.9 nm by proteolytic digestion with trypsin, α-chymotrypsin (that only gave rise to the 3.6 nm complex, papain, or an extract of the 1,000 x g to 10,000 x g pellet (lysosomal fraction) of liver homogenate. The 6.1 and 3.6 nm complexes had dissociation constants of 6 to 8 x 10^{-9} M and 6 to 9 x 10^{-9} M, respectively, for dexamethasone. The 1.9 nm complex was very labile in the absence of bound ligand and therefore its affinity to dexamethasone could not be determined (18).

Both the 6.1 and 3.6 nm complexes were bound to cell nuclei and DNA-cellulose following heat activation in the presence of ligand. The 6.1 nm complex was eluted from a DNA-cellulose column with a linear KCl gradient at 0.11 to 0.13 M KCl, whereas the 3.6 nm complex was eluted at 0.15 to 0.20 M KCl.

The 1.9 nm complex bound neither to DNA-cellulose nor to cell nuclei. When nuclei or DNA-cellulose containing bound dexamethasone-receptor complex were digested with trypsin and subsequently extracted or eluted at low ionic strength, the recovered dexamethasone-receptor complex had a Stokes radius of approximately 1.9 nm.

It was concluded that the glucocorticoid receptor in liver cytosol may be divided into three parts separable by proteolytic digestion: (a) the steroid-binding site (retained on the 1.9 and 3.6 nm receptor fragments); (b) the DNA-binding site (retained on the 3.6 nm, but absent from the 1.9 nm receptor fragment); and (c) a region with an as yet unknown function and only present on the 6.1 nm receptor (18).

Increasing amounts of trypsin or α-chymotrypsin were also used to study the proteolytic fragmentation pattern of DEAE-Sepharose purified glucocorticoid receptor as judged by SDS-gel electrophoresis. α-Chymotrypsin induced the formation of bands corresponding to molecular weights of 91 K, 50 K, 45 K and 39 K. The 39 K component was relatively resistant towards further degradation by α-chymotrypsin. Protein staining revealed no component of lower molecular weight than 39 K after α-chymotrypsin digestion. The major bands induced by trypsin digestion corresponded to molecular weights of 89 K, 39 K, 27 K and 25 K. With increasing amounts of trypsin only the 27 K and 25 K bands were seen. The 27 K species was relatively resistant towards further proteolysis with trypsin although it could be completely transformed to the 25 K component by high amounts of trypsin (16).

Thus, limited proteolysis of the purified glucocorticoid receptor with trypsin confirmed our previous results with crude cytosol (17,18) that a small and relatively trypsin resistant fragment containing the ligand binding site, the 1.9 nm complex, is formed. The further digestion of the 27 K form (= the 1.9 nm complex) to a 25 K form was not unexpected since a double peak pattern was seen following isoelectric focusing of the glucocorticoid receptor in crude cytosol after treatment with large amounts of trypsin; this further proteolysis did not result in any change in the elution pattern of the 1.9 nm complex from Sephadex G-150 (19).

The 39 K fragment of the glucocorticoid receptor seen both following trypsin and α-chymotrypsin treatment probably corresponds to the previously described 3.6 nm complex which contains the ligand-binding site and which binds to DNA (17,18). No smaller fragment than the 39 K form was detected by silver staining and/or affinity labeling after α-chymotrypsin treatment, in good agreement with our previous findings with crude cytosol.

The 79 K component of the purified glucocorticoid receptor preparation may be a degradation product of the glucocorticoid receptor since i) photoaffinity labeling (20) demonstrated that the hormone bound to both the 94 K and 79 K species (16), ii) antibodies raised against the 94 K species (21) cross-reacted with the 79 K species (16) and iii) α-chymotrypsin treatment seemed to result in degradation of the 94 K glucocorticoid receptor via the 79 K component and further down to the 39 K species (16). It is unclear if the 72 K component of the purified glucocorticoid receptor preparation merely represents a copurifying contaminant or if it constitutes a subunit of the glucocorticoid receptor.

Specific binding of the glucocorticoid receptor to MTV DNA

Biochemical and genetic experiments have demonstrated that steroid receptors associate with DNA (22) and that the hormone strongly increases the affinity of the interaction (23,24); in addition, other chromosomal components have been proposed to participate in the nuclear binding event (for review, see ref. 25). Does receptor binding occur preferentially at specific high-affinity genomic sites? It appears that the bulk of the approximately 10^4 receptors per responsive cell associate non-specifically and with relatively low affinity with nuclei in vivo (26) and in vitro (27), as well as with DNA in vitro (23). However, as elegantly demonstrated with prokaryotic transcriptional regulatory proteins, factors that bind with high affinity to specific DNA sequences also display a reduced but significant affinity for nonspecific sequences (28,29). It was suggested from these observations and from theoretical considerations that the low-affinity nonspecific DNA binding of steroid receptors could preclude detection of a small number of high-affinity genome binding sites that might directly mediate the hormone response (25,30).

Investigation of the process by which glucocorticoids stimulate mammary tumour virus (MTV) gene transcription in cultured cells has revealed that i) sequences are present within the viral DNA itself that are required for hormonal regulation of MTV transcription (31), ii) specific subregions of cloned viral DNA are competent to mediate hormonal regulation upon their reintroduction into cellular genomes by DNA transformation (32), and iii) receptor action appears to stim-

ulate the rate of initiation events from a single preexisting transcriptional
start site within the viral DNA (31). Given this information, together with the
availability of both pure viral sequences on recombinant vectors (32) and purified preparations of glucocorticoid receptors (32), it was of interest to test
the notion that the receptor might selectively recognize and associate with
specific sequences within MTV DNA. In a collaborative study with Dr. Keith
Yamamoto and Dr. Farhang Payvar at the Department of Biochemistry and Biophysics,
University of California, San Fransisco, we examined the selectivity of receptor
binding to DNA by using an assay in which radioactively labeled DNA restriction
fragments that bind to the receptor are selectively retained on a nitrocellulose
filter.

Activated glucocorticoid receptor protein, purified to 40-60% homogeneity from
rat liver extracts, was found to bind selectively in vitro to a cloned fragment
of MTV DNA. The DNA fragment tested contained about half of the sequences present
in intact MTV DNA, and its rate of transcription, like that of the intact viral
element, was strongly stimulated by glucocorticoids when it was introduced into
the genome of a receptor-containing cell. In contrast, the receptor failed to
bind selectively to DNA restriction fragments from E. coli plasmids pBR322 and
RSF2124 or from bacteriophages λ and T4. These studies are consistent with the
notion that steroid receptors may modulate rates of transcription by recog-
nizing specific DNA sequences within or near the regulated genes (33).

In subsequent studies, using both electron microscopic and biochemical
approaches, we have found that purified rat liver glucocorticoid receptor protein
binds specifically to at least four widely separated regions on pure MTV proviral
DNA. One of these specific binding domains, which itself contains at least two
distinct receptor binding sites, resides within a fragment of viral DNA that maps
110-449 bp upstream of the promotor for MTV RNA synthesis. Three other binding
domains lie downstream of the promoter and within the MTV primary transcription
unit (34).

Receptor binding fragments lacking the viral promoter have been fused to a
cloned heterologous promoter and structural gene (the HSV tk gene). Plasmids
containing these DNA sequences have been transfected into XCtk, a line of HAT-
sensitive rat cells. Transformed clones have been isolated that display 30-50-
fold induction of tk transcription by dexamethasone. Thus a receptor binding
fragment from MTV confers hormone responsiveness upon the intact HSV tk promoter
(35). Our results suggest that receptor binding domains defined in vitro are biologically significant in vivo. These properties of receptor binding domains may
have intriguing evolutionary implications: simple transposition of glucocorticoid
receptor binding domains could provide an efficient mechanism for the evolution

of hormone responsive promoters.

Physicochemical characterization of specific and nonspecific polyaromatic hydrocarbon binders in rat and mouse liver cytosol

The aryl hydrocarbon hydroxylase (AHH) inducers 2,3,7,8-tetrachlordibenzo-p-dioxin (TCDD), 3-methylcholanthrene (3-MC) and benzo(a)pyrene (B(a)P) were all shown to bind in a saturable manner to a distinct component in cytosol from both rat and C 57 BL/6 J mouse liver. This component, the so called TCDD receptor, was analyzed by gel permeation chromatography on Sephacryl S-300 and by sucrose density gradient centrifugation and was found to have a Strokes radius of 6.1 nm and a sedimentation coefficient of 4.4 S under high salt conditions. Based on these parameters, which were identical for the rat and mouse receptor, a molecular weight of 111,000 was calculated for the TCDD receptor (36).

The same Stokes radius and sedimentation coefficient were observed regardless of the ligand used for labeling of the receptor protein ($[^3H]$TCDD, $[^3H]$3-MC or $[^3H]$B(a)P). On the other hand, $[^3H]$3-MC and $[^3H]$B(a)P exhibited much more non-specific binding than $[^3H]$TCDD, at least partially due to contaminating serum components, and it cannot be excluded that some previous findings on low-molecular hepatic "receptors" for these polyaromatic hydrocarbons may actually be explained in this way.

The rat hepatic TCDD receptor was also shown to be retained on DEAE-Sepharose (eluted at 0.2-0.3 M NaCl), hydroxylapatite (eluted at 0.15-0.17 M phosphate) and heparin-Sepharose (eluted at 0.3-0.4 M NaCl).

In conclusion, the TCDD receptor showed similar physiochemical and chromatographic characteristics as we have previously found for the glucocorticoid receptor. Thus, the TCDD receptor resembles another well characterized gene regulatory protein not only with respect to its biology but also its biochemistry.

ACKNOWLEDGEMENTS

This work was supported by grants from the Swedish Medical Research Council (No. 13X-2819), the Swedish Cancer Society, the US National Institutes of Health and the American Cancer Society.

REFERENCES

1. Kouri, R.E. and Nebert, D.W. (1977) Cold Spring Harbor Conf. Cell Proliferation 4, 811-835.

2. Poland, A. and Kende, A. (1977) Cold Spring Harbor Conf. Cell Proliferation 4, 847-867.

3. Thomas, P.E., Kouri, R.E. and Hutton, J.J. (1972) Biochem. Genet. 6, 157-168.

4. Nebert, D.W., Goujon, F.M. and Gielen, J.E. (1972) Nature New Biology 236, 107-110.

5. Poland, A., Glover, E. and Kende, A. (1976) J. Biol. Chem. 251, 4936-4946.

6. Carlstedt-Duke, J.M.B., Elfström, G., Snochowski, M., Högberg, B. and Gustafsson, J.-Å. (1978) Toxicol. Lett. 2, 365-373.

7. Carlstedt-Duke, J.M.B., Harnemo, U.-B., Högberg, B. and Gustafsson, J.-Å. (1981) Biochim. Biophys. Acta 672, 131-141.

8. Carlstedt-Duke, J.M.B. (1979) Cancer Research 39, 3172-3176.

9. Okey, A.B., Bondy, G.P., Mason, M.E., Kahl, G.F., Eisen, H.J., Guenthner, T.M. and Nebert, D.W. (1979) J. Biol. Chem. 254, 11636-11648.

10. Hannah, R.R., Nebert, D.W. and Eisen, H.J. (1981) 256, 4584-4590.

11. Poellinger, L., Kurl, R.N., Lund, J., Carlstedt-Duke, J.M.B., Gillner, M., Högberg, B. and Gustafsson, J.-Å. (1982) Biochim. Biophys. Acta 714, 516-523.

12. Lund, J., Kurl, R.N., Poellinger, L. and Gustafsson, J.-Å. (1982) Biochim. Biophys. Acta 716, 16-23.

13. Tierney, B., Weaver, D., Heintz, N.H., Schaeffer, W.I. and Bresnik, E. (1980) Arch. Biochem. Biophys. 200, 513-525.

14. Holder, G.M., Tierney, B. and Bresnik, E. (1981) Cancer Research 41, 4408-4414.

15. Wrange, Ö., Carlstedt-Duke, J.M.B. and Gustafsson, J.-Å. (1979) J. Biol. Chem. 254, 9284-9290.

16. Wrange, Ö., Okret, S., Radojčić, M., Carlstedt-Duke, J.M.B. and Gustafsson, J.-Å. J. Biol. Chem., in press.

17. Carlstedt-Duke, J.M.B., Gustafsson, J.-Å. and Wrange, Ö. (1977) Biochim. Biophys. Acta 497, 507-524.

18. Wrange, Ö. and Gustafsson, J.-Å. (1978) J. Biol. Chem. 253, 856-865.

19. Wrange, Ö. (1979) Biochim. Biophys. Acta 582, 346-357.

20. Nordeen, S.K., Lan, N.C., Showers, M.O. and Baxter, J.D. (1981) J. Biol. Chem. 256, 10503-10508.

21. Okret, S., Carlstedt-Duke, J.M.B., Wrange, Ö., Carlström, K. and Gustafsson, J.-Å. (1981) Biochim. Biophys. Acta 677, 205-219.

22. Yamamoto, K.R. and Alberts, B.M. (1972) Proc. Natl. Acad. Sci. USA 69, 2105-2109.

23. Yamamoto, K.R. and Alberts. B.M. (1974) J. Biol. Chem. 249, 7076-7086.

24. Yamamoto, K.R., Gehring, U., Stampfer, M.R. and Sibley, C.H. (1976) Rec. Progr. Horm. Res. 32, 3-32.

25. Yamamoto, K.R. and Alberts, B.M. (1976) Ann. Rev. Biochem. 45, 721-746.

26. Williams, D. and Gorski, J. (1972) Proc. Natl. Acad. Sci. USA 69, 3464-3468.

27. Chamness, G.C., Jennings, A.W. and McGuire, W.L. (1974) Biochemistry 13, 327-331.

28. Lin, S.-Y. and Riggs, A.D. (1972) J. Mol. Biol. 72, 671-690.

29. Von Hippel, P.H., Revzin, A., Gross, C.A. and Wang, A.C. (1974) Proc. Natl. Acad. Sci. USA 71, 4808-4812.

30. Yamamoto, K.R. and Alberts, B.M. (1975) Cell 4, 301-310.

31. Ucker, D.S., Ross, S.R. and Yamamoto, K.R. (1981) Cell 27, 257.

32. Yamamoto, K.R., Chandler, V.L., Ross, S.R., Ucker, D.S., Ring, J.C. and Feinstein, S.C. (1981) Cold Spring Harbor Symp. Quant. Biol. 45, 687-705.

33. Payvar, F., Wrange, Ö., Carlstedt-Duke, J.M.B., Okret, S., Gustafsson, J.-Å. and Yamamoto, K.R. (1981) Proc. Natl. Acad. Sci. USA 78, 6628-6632.

34. Payvar, F., Firestone, G.L., Ross, S.R., Chandler, V.L., Wrange, Ö., Carlstedt-Duke, J.M.B., Gustafsson, J.-Å. and Yamamoto, K.R. (1982) J. Cell Biochem. 19, 241-247.

35. Yamamoto, K.R., Payvar, F., Firestone, G.L., Maler, B.A., Wrange, Ö., Carlstedt-Duke, J.M.B. and Chandler, V.L. Cold Spring Harbor Symp. Quant. Biol., in press.

36. Poellinger, L., Lund, J., Gillner, M., Hansson, L.-A. and Gustafsson, J.-Å. J. Biol. Chem., in press.

© 1983 Elsevier Science Publishers B.V.
Extrahepatic Drug Metabolism and Chemical Carcinogenesis,
J. Rydström, J. Montelius and M. Bengtsson eds.

IS THE PRIMARY FUNCTION OF THE Ah LOCUS TO REGULATE CYTOCHROME P-450?

JOYCE C. KNUTSON AND ALAN POLAND

McArdle Laboratory for Cancer Research, University of Wisconsin, Madison,
WI 53706 (U.S.A.)

INTRODUCTION

The induction of microsomal monooxygenase activity by the administration
of foreign compounds was first noted about twenty-five years ago (1,2).
The mechanism of this induction is best understood for one group of
xenobiotics, the polycyclic aromatic hydrocarbons and the halogenated
aromatic hydrocarbons. Investigations into this mechanism have been
greatly aided by a) a genetic polymorphism in mice which determines their
inducibility (the Ah locus) and b) 2,3,7,8-tetrachlorodibenzo-p-dioxin
(TCDD), a potent agonist for this response. Further investigations into
the pleiotropic response produced by TCDD indicate that in some tissues,
the response is far more extensive than just the induction of the "drug
metabolizing enzymes", and it is these studies which we wish to review in
this paper.

Pleiotropic Response Produced by Polycyclic Aromatic Hydrocarbons.

The administration of polycyclic aromatic hydrocarbons such as 3-
methylcholanthrene (MC), to laboratory animals induces a battery of
coordinately expressed enzymes in the liver and a variety of other tissues
(for review, see 3). In mouse liver, MC produces a proliferation of the
smooth endoplasmic reticulum, induction of at least two species of
cytochrome P-450 (one of which is often referred to as P_1-450 or P-450c)
with an associated increase in monooxygenase activity, and the induction
of several non-monooxygenase enzyme activities, e.g. UDP-
glucuronosyltransferase, DT-diaphorase, and ornithine decarboxylase. The
enzyme activities expressed in this coordinate response (particularly the
non-monooxygenase activities) vary with the tissue and the animal species.
The induction of aryl hydrocarbon hydroxylase (AHH) activity has
frequently been used as a marker for this pleiotropic response.

Ah Locus

Outbred and many inbred strains of mice (typified by C57BL/6), when challenged with MC, respond with the induction of hepatic cytochrome P_1-450 and AHH activity; however, certain inbred strains (typified by DBA/2) fail to respond (4). In genetic crosses and backcrosses between C57BL/6 and DBA/2, responsiveness to MC (i.e., the induction of AHH activity) is inherited as a simple autosomal dominant trait, and the locus controlling this trait was called the Ah locus (for aromatic hydrocarbon responsiveness) (5). Further understanding of the nature of the Ah locus was provided from studies with TCDD.

TCDD, one of the most potent halogenated aromatic hydrocarbons, serves as a prototype for this class of compounds, which includes dibenzo-p-dioxins, dibenzofurans, azo(xy)benzenes and biphenyls. TCDD (and related halogenated aromatic hydrocarbons) produces a pleiotropic response similar to that elicited by MC; however, TCDD is about 30,000 times as potent as MC (as measured by the induction of AHH activity in mouse and rat liver) (6). The structure-activity relationship for halogenated dibenzo-p-dioxin congeners to induce AHH activity indicates that all agonists have a) at least 3 of the lateral 4 ring positions (i.e., 2,3,7 and 8 positions) occupied by a halogen, b) an order of substitution for potency of Br $>$ Cl $\gg$ F, NO_2 and c) at least one of the ring positions unsubstituted (i.e., the octachloro compound is inactive, but the hepatochloro-congeners are active) (7). The potency of TCDD to induce AHH activity, the capacity to produce a pleiotropic response like that of MC, and the well defined structure-activity relationship among analogues, suggested that TCDD might act by binding to a specific cellular recognition site.

High specific activity ^{3}H-TCDD permitted the identification of a macromolecule in the soluble fraction of mouse and rat liver which had the in vitro binding properties expected of the putative receptor (8). This protein reversibly bound TCDD with a high affinity (K_D = 0.27 nM). For halogenated dibenzo-p-dioxin analogues, the structure-activity relationship for receptor binding corresponded to that for their potency to induce AHH activity. Polycyclic aromatic hydrocarbons which produce the same coordinate enzyme induction as MC also compete for receptor binding. Subsequent studies have a) demonstrated that the ligand-receptor complex translocates to the nucleus (9) b) identified the cytosol receptor in virtually all tissues in which AHH is inducible (10,11), and c) more fully characterized the physicochemical properties of the receptor protein (12).

When TCDD, a far more potent agonist than MC, was administered to mice, hepatic AHH activity was induced in all strains of mice tested, those responsive and nonresponsive to MC (13). The responsive strains, which carry the Ah[b] allele, are sensitive to AHH induction by TCDD and possess a high affinity receptor; the nonresponsive strains (Ah[d] allele) are at least 10 fold less sensitive to induction by TCDD, and have a much lower affinity receptor, which has, as yet, proven difficult to quantify. These observations suggest that the Ah locus is the structural gene for the cytosol receptor which mediates the coordinate enzyme induction produced by polycyclic aromatic hydrocarbons and halogenated aromatic hydrocarbons.

Toxic Responses Produced by Halogenated Aromatic Hydrocarbons

We turn now to our major topic, a much less appreciated component of the pleiotropic response. In some tissues, the Ah locus controls an additional pleiotropic response, one that is distinct from, and apparently unrelated to, the induction of drug metabolizing enzymes.

TCDD and most other halogenated aromatic hydrocarbons are best known as environmental contaminants. These compounds all produce a common pattern of toxic responses which are quite characteristic; however, many of the lesions are highly species-specific (14-16). Following the administration of a lethal dose of TCDD or one of its congeners, virtually all species experience a prolonged wasting syndrome, with loss of adipose tissue, involution of lymphoid organs, and embryotoxicity and/or teratogenicity. In contrast, the more distinctive lesions involve proliferation and/or metaplasia of epithelial tissues such as skin, stomach, intestines and urinary tract, and occur in a limited number of species.

Two independent lines of evidence indicate that the toxic responses produced by TCDD and congeners are mediated by their binding to the induction receptor. First, for a large number of halogenated aromatic hydrocarbons, the rank ordered structure-activity relationship for their receptor affinity or their potency to induce AHH activity corresponds to their toxic potency (measured as the mean lethal dose or dose reported to produce a specific toxic response) (17-19). Secondly, several toxic responses produced by TCDD in mice (thymic involution, teratogenesis, hepatic porphyria) have been shown to segregate with the Ah locus or to follow the strain distribution for the Ah[b] allele (20,21).

While the induction receptor appears essential for the expression of toxicity of the halogenated aromatic hydrocarbons, the presence of the receptor is not sufficient. Many tissues in vivo and cells in vitro respond to TCDD with the induction of AHH activity, and thus possess the receptor, but display no evidence of a toxic response (13,22,23).

HRS/J Mice: Experimental Model for Two Distinct Pleiotropic Responses Controlled by Ah Locus

The characteristic lesion produced by halogenated aromatic hydrocarbons in the skin of humans, rabbits and monkeys is hyperplasia and hyperkeratosis of the epidermis, and metaplasia of the sebaceous gland with the formation of keratinaceous comedones. While TCDD and congeners do not elicit these effects in normal, haired mice, Inagami et al. (24) noted that rice oil contaminated with polychlorinated biphenyls produced similar cutaneous changes in hairless mice. Hairless is a recessive trait in mice controlled by the hr locus on chromosome 14.

HRS/J is an inbred strain of mice segregating for the hr locus; the homozygous hairless (hr/hr) and heterozygous haired (hr/+) mice are genetically "identical" except for one allele at the hr locus. HRS/J (hr/hr) and (hr/+) mice 1) carry the Ah^b allele, i.e they have a high affinity cytosol receptor, and 2) have the same concentration and affinity of cytosol receptor (measured in the liver) (25). Application of TCDD to the skin of HRS/J hr/hr and hr/+ mice induces epidermal AHH activity with a similar time course and dose-response curve in both phenotypes. However, in hr/hr mice TCDD produces a histologic change, epidermal hyperplasia and hyperkeratosis, and sebaceous gland metaplasia, not observed in hr/+ mice (or other haired mice which are wild-type, +/+, at the hr locus).

These histologic changes evoked in the skin of hr/hr mice are mediated through the cytosol receptor, as indicated by two types of studies. First, for a series of halogenated aromatic hydrocarbon congeners, the structure-activity to evoke this response corresponds to that for receptor binding. Secondly, in C57BL/6 and DBA/2 mice which bear the hairless genotype (hr/hr) and their genetic crosses and backcrosses, the histologic changes produced by 3,3',4,4',5,5'-hexabromobiphenyl (a congener of TCDD), segregated with the Ah^b allele (determining the high affinity receptor).

To summarize the most central observation, in the skin of both hr/hr and hr/+ mice, TCDD is recognized as a signal and induces a limited pleiotropic response, e.g., the induction of epidermal AHH activity; however, in the skin of hr/hr mice there is an additional pleiotropic response which results in hyperplasia and metaplasia in the skin, and all of these responses are mediated by the cytosol receptor.

Carcinogenicity and/or Tumor Promotion

HRS/J mice have proved a very useful model in examining the "carcinogenicity" of TCDD. The chronic administration of TCDD (and several other halogenated aromatic hydrocarbons) to rats and mice has resulted in an increased incidence of hepatocellular carcinomas as well as tumors in other tissues (26-28). However, because TCDD has little, if any, mutagenic activity (29,30) and does not bind appreciably to DNA in vivo (31), it has been suggested that this compound is not a complete carcinogen, but rather acts as a tumor promoter enhancing neoplastic expression in already initiated cells. TCDD has been shown to be a potent tumor promoter in a two-stage model of carcinogenesis in rat liver (32), but proven ineffective in the classical model in mouse skin (using CD-1 and Swiss-Webster mice) (33-35). This latter result is not surprising in retrospect, since TCDD does not produce a proliferative response in normal haired (+/+) mouse skin. We examined TCDD as a tumor promoter in HRS/J hr/hr and hr/+ mice (36).

HRS/J (hr/+) haired mice, were initiated with a single dose of the carcinogen 7,12-dimethylbenz(a)anthracene (DMBA) and then, for 25 weeks, given twice weekly topical applications of 1) the classical tumor promoter, 12-0-tetradecanoylphorbol-13-acetate (TPA - 2 μg/mouse); 2) TCDD (50 ng/mouse for 8 weeks and then 20 ㎏g/mouse); or 3) the solvent, acetone. The initiated hr/+ mice treated with TPA developed skin papillomas, those treated with TCDD did not. Mice receiving only DMBA or only repeated application of TPA without prior initiation developed no tumors. In contrast, in HRS/J (hr/hr) hairless mice initiated with DMBA, twice weekly applications of TPA or TCDD produced skin papillomas. Thus, TPA acts as a tumor promoter in the skin of hr/+ and hr/hr mice, TCDD is only effective in hr/hr mice.

Several other halogenated aromatic hydrocarbon congeners or mixtures (2,3,7,8-tetrachlorodibenzofuran, 3,3',4,4',5,5'-hexabromobiphenyl, and Firemaster FF-1 - a commercial mixture of brominated biphenyl isomers) were found to be effective tumor promoters in this two stage model of epidermal carcinogenesis in HRS/J (hr/hr) mice. For the limited number of congeners tested, the structure-activity relationship for tumor promotion corresponded to that for receptor binding.

A General Model of Toxicity

In HRS/J hr/hr and hr/+ mice, the allelic change at the hr locus determines if the skin response to TCDD will consist of induction of AHH activity, or an additional more extensive pleiotropic response involving epidermal hyperplasia and metaplasia. Since hr/+ and hr/hr mice are essentially congenic, differing at only the hr locus or closely linked loci on chromosome 14, hr/+ mice presumably have all the genes necessary for the hyperplastic-metaplastic response, but these genes are not expressed by TCDD.

We propose that this model might be a general one to explain the tissue and species specific toxicity of halogenated aromatic hydrocarbons. In all tissues which contain the receptor, TCDD and congeners produce a limited pleiotropic response (the A response) which consists of the induction of cytochrome P_1-450, microsomal monooxygenase activity, and the expression of other enzymes largely associated with "drug metabolism". However in a few tissues, those which develop morphologic changes (toxicity) in response to TCDD and congeners, the receptor controls an additional battery of genes which control cell proliferation, differentiation and/or involution (the B response). The composition of the additional battery of genes would vary in different tissues.

Unresolved Questions

Finally, we would like to consider some implications of this model and some unresolved questions which might be areas for future research. Historically, the induction of cytochrome P-450 and other drug metabolizing enzymes by a foreign lipophilic chemical has been viewed as an adaptive physiologic response, the "purpose" of which is to increase the rate of metabolism of the foreign chemical and hasten its elimination from the organism. In this view, the focus of regulation is the drug metabolizing enzymes. However, the halogenated aromatic hydrocarbons act on the cytosol receptor to produce two distinct and dissociable responses a) the induction of the drug metabolizing enzymes, and b) in a few tissues a much broader pleiotropic response which involves cell proliferation, differentiation and/or involution. How can we account for these two very different responses being under the control of the same receptor?

One possibility is that the receptor has served two separate roles in the course of evolution. The receptor may have evolved to respond to some physiologic mediator (e.g., a hormone) and controlled cellular proliferation, differentiation and/or involution. Later, this response may have been unnecessary, supplanted by other regulatory mechanisms, and the physiologic ligand ceased to exist. The existing receptor protein may have been reused to respond to foreign chemicals and regulate the drug metabolizing enzymes. Expression of the original proliferation-differentiation response ceased to have selective advantage, and these genes dissociated from receptor control in some tissues. This speculation would explain the induction of the drug metabolizing enzymes in virtually all tissues which possess the receptor but the variable expression of the proliferation/differentiation response in various mammalian tissues tested.

The toxic responses produced by halogenated aromatic hydrocarbons presumably result from the sustained expression of a battery of genes which control cell division and/or differentiation, a pleiotropic response which in higher vertebrates either a) is vestigial, or b) still serves a physiologic role and is expressed more transiently by a postulated mediator. To understand the mechanism of action of these compounds, we must a) identify the gene products which comprise the proliferation/differentiation response (the B response), b) identify the mediators of this response, c) understand the genetic controls which permit or restrict the expression of this pleiotropic response in various tissues, and d) determine if there exists a physiologic ligand for the cytosol receptor in high vertebrates or possibly some lower evolutionary form.

ACKNOWLEDGEMENTS

This work was supported in part by National Institute of Environmental Health Sciences Grant 1 R01 ES 09884 and by National Cancer Institute Core Grant CA-07175. A.P. is a Burroughs Wellcome Scholar in Toxicology.

REFERENCES

1. Conney, A.H., Miller, E.C. and Miller, J.A. (1956) Cancer Res. 16, 450.

2. Remmer, H. (1958) Naturwissenschaften 45, 189.

3. Nebert, D.W., Eiser, H.J., Negishi, M., Lang, M.A., and Hjelmeland, L.M. (1981) Ann. Rev. Pharmacol. Toxicol 21, 431.

4. Nebert, D.W. and Gielen, J.E. (1972) Fed. Proc. 31, 1315.

5. Nebert, D.W., Goujon, F.M., Gielen, J.E. (1972) Nature, New Biology, 236, 107.

6. Poland, A. and Glover, E. (1974) Mol. Pharmacol. 10, 349.

7. Poland, A. and Glover, E. (1973) Mol. Pharmacol. 9, 736.

8. Poland, A., Glover, E., and Kende, A.S. (1976) J. Biol. Chem. 251, 4936.

416

9. Okey, A.B., Bondy, G.P., Mason, M., Nebert, D.W., Forster-Gibson, C.J., Mucan, J. and Dufresene, M.J. (1980) J. Biol. Chem. 255, 11415.

10. Carlstedt-Duke, J.M.B. (1979) Cancer Res. 39, 3172.

11. Mason, M.E. and Okey, A. (1982) Eur. J. Biochem. 123, 209.

12. Carlstedt-Duke, J.M.B., Harnemu, V.-B., Högberg, B. and Gustafsson, J.A. (1981) Biochim. Biophys. Acta 672, 131.

13. Poland, A., Glover, E., Robinson, J.R. and Nebert, D.W. (1974) J. Biol. Chem. 249, 5599.

14. Schwetz, B.A., Norris, J.M., Sparschu, G.L., Rowe, V.K., Gehring, P.J., Emerson, J.L. and Gerbig, C.G. (1973) Environ. Health Persp. 5, 87.

15. Kimbrough, R.D. (1974) CRC Crit. Rev. Toxicol. 2, 445.

16. McConnell, E.E. (1980) in: Kimbrough, R. (Ed.), Halogenated Biphenyls, Terphenyls, Naphthalenes, Dibenzodioxins, and Related Products, Elsevier/North Holland Biomedical Press, Amsterdam, pp. 109-150.

17. McConnell, E.E., Moore, J.A., Haseman, J.K. and Harris, M.W. (1978) Toxicol. Appl. Pharmacol. 44, 335.

18. Poland, A., Greenlee, W.F., and Kende, A.S. (1979) Ann. N.Y. Acad. Sci. 320, 214.

19. Goldstein, J.A. (1980) in: Kimbrough, R. (Ed.), Halogenated Biphenyls, Terphenyls, Naphthalenes, Dibenzodioxins and Related Products, pp. 151-190.

20. Jones, K.G. and Sweeney, G.D. (1980) Toxicol. Appl. Pharmacol. 53, 42.

21. Poland, A. and Glover, E. (1980) Mol. Pharmacol. 17, 86.

22. Bradlaw, D.A. and Casterline, J.L. (1979) J. Assoc. Off. Anal. Chem. 62, 904.

23. Knutson, J.C. and Poland, A. (1980) Toxicol. Appl. Pharm. 54, 377.

24. Inagami, K., Koga, T., Kikuchi, M., Hashmito, M., Takahashi, H., and Wada, K. (1969) Fukuoka Acta Med. 60, 548.

25. Knutson, J.C. and Poland, A. (1982) Cell 30, 225.

26. Kociba, R.J., Keyes, D.G., Beyer, J.E., Carreon, R.M., Wade, C.E., Henber, D.A., Kalnins, R.P., Frauson, L.E., Park, C.N., Barnard, S.D., Hummel, R.A., and Humiston, C.G. (1978) Toxicol. Appl. Pharm. 46, 279.

27. National Toxicol. Program. (1982) Tech. Report Ser 209 (NPT-80-31) NIH Publ. 82-1765.

28. Van Miller, J.P., Lalich, J.J. and Allen, J.R. (1977) Chemosphere 9, 537.

29. Wasson, J.S., Huff, J.E., and Loprieno, N. (1977/1978) Mutat. Res. 47, 141.

30. Geiger, L.E. and Neal, R.A. (1981) Toxicol. Appl. Pharmacol. 159, 125.

31. Poland, A. and Glover, E. (1979) Cancer Res. 39, 3341.

32. Pitot, H.C., Goldsworthy, T., Campbell, H.A., and Poland, A. (1980) Cancer Res. 40, 3616.

33. Giovanni, G., Viaje, A., Berry, D.L., Slaga, T.J. and Juchau, M.R. (1977) Bull. Environ. Contamin. Toxicol. 18, 552.

34. Berry, D.L., DiGiovanni, J., Juchau, M.R., Brachen, W.M., Gleason, G.L. and Slaga, T.J. (1978) Res. Commun. Chem. Pathol. Pharmacol. 20, 101.

35. National Toxicol. Program (1982) Tech. Report Ser 201 (NTP-80-32) NIH Publ. 82-1757.

36. Poland, A., Palen, D. and Glover, E. (1982) Nature 300, 272.

© 1983 Elsevier Science Publishers B.V.
Extrahepatic Drug Metabolism and Chemical Carcinogenesis,
J. Rydström, J. Montelius and M. Bengtsson eds.

MOLECULAR BIOLOGY OF CYTOCHROME P-450

RONALD N. HINES[1], EDWARD BRESNICK[1], CURTIS OMIECINSKI[2] AND JOAN LEVY[1]

[1]Eppley Institute for Research in Cancer and Allied Disease, University of
Nebraska Medical Center, 42nd and Dewey Avenue, Omaha, NE 68105 (U.S.A.)
and [2]Department of Environmental Health Sciences, University of Washington,
Seattle, WA (U.S.A.)

INTRODUCTION

The cytochrome P-450-dependent monooxygenases are widely recognized as
playing a primary role in the detoxification and/or activation of
xenobiotics in hepatic and extrahepatic tissues (1,2). Although the precise
number of individual isozymes for cytochrome P-450 is unknown, at least
eight distinct forms have been characterized (4-6). Pretreatment of animals
with various inducing agents results in increases in the activity and
specific content of particular cytochrome P-450 isozymes (2) and may result
in decreases in the specific content and activity of others (2,3).

Preliminary investigations in our laboratory as well as others have shown
that the increase in cytochrome P-450c, the major 3-methylcholanthrene
inducible isozyme, and cytochrome P-450b, the major phenobarbital inducible
isozyme, is preceded by an increase in specific mRNA levels, suggesting a
role for transcriptional regulation (7,8). Using recombinant DNA technology, our laboratory has cloned cDNA information for the major 3-methyl-
cholanthrene (pEB339) and phenobarbital inducible cytochrome P-450 isozymes
(pPH8) in Sprague Dawley rat liver (9,10). We are continuing our
investigations into the mechanism of regulation for the induction of these
two proteins.

METHODS

Materials. Restriction endonucleases were purchased from either New
England Biolabs (Beverly, MA) or Bethesda Research Laboratories (Gaith-
ersburg, MD). Deoxynucleotide triphosphates were obtained from P-L
Biochemicals (Milwaukee, WI), dideoxynucleotide triphosphates from either
Collaborative Research (Waltham, MA) or P-L Biochemicals. α-^{32}P-dCTP
(either 3,000 Ci/mmol or 800 Ci/mmol) was purchased from Amersham Corp.
(Arlington Heights, IL). Nitrocellulose BA85 membranes were obtained from
Schleicher and Schuell Inc. (Keene, NH). Electrophoresis grade agarose was
purchased from BRL, Inc. Autoradiography was performed using Kodak XAR-5

film in conjunction with a Duport Cranex Quanta II intensifier screen at -70°C.

Methods. Male Sprague Dawley rats (75-100 g) from Charles River Laboratories (St. Constant, Quebec) were pretreated for various times by i.p. injections of either 3-methylcholanthrene in corn oil, 25 mg/kg body weight, or phenobarbital in 0.9% saline, 75 mg/kg body weight. Control animals were untreated. Polysomal poly(A$^+$)RNA was prepared essentially as described earlier (9). Rat liver nuclei were isolated using the methodology of Busch (11). RNA was isolated from the nuclei by suspension in 6 $\underline{M}$ guanidine-HCl, 0.1 $\underline{M}$ 2-mercaptoethanal, 0.025 $\underline{M}$ sodium citrate pH 7.0 and centrifugation through a cushion of 5.7 $\underline{M}$ CsCl, 0.1 $\underline{M}$ EDTA pH 7 as described by Chirgwin et al. (12). RNA dot hybridization and Northern blot hybridization experiments were conducted according to the method of Thomas (13). High molecular weight DNA (>25 kb) for genomic blot hybridizations was isolated as described by Blin and Stafford (14). Southern blot transfers and hybridization to pPH8 or pRSA57 nick-translated probes were conducted as described by Mark et al. (15). DNA sequencing was accomplished using the Messing strains of M13 bacteriophage in conjunction with the Sanger dideoxy chain termination methodology (16).

RESULTS AND DISCUSSION

The cloning and initial characterization of pEB339, a cDNA clone for cytochrome P-450c, has been described in an earlier publication (9). Both Hae III and Sau 3A restriction fragments of pEB339 were sub-cloned into either M13mp7 or M13mp701 and sequenced as described in methods. Unfortunately, no open reading frames were observed that contained any of the known carboxy-terminus amino acid information for cytochrome P-450c. This observation suggested that the mRNA coding for cytochrome P-450c must be considerably larger than the approximately 1.5 kb required for a protein of 55,000 molecular weight. To confirm this, total cytosolic poly(A$^+$)RNA from 3-methylcholanthrene pretreated animals was size fractionated by denaturing formaldehyde/agarose gel electrophoresis and, after Northern transfer to nitrocellulose, hybridized to nick-translated pEB339. A single band was observed at 23s or 3.7 kb. Maximal induction of the 3.7 kb mRNA$_{P-450c}$ was observed 15 h postinjection of 3-methylcholanthrene.

The cloning and initial characterization of pPH8, a cDNA clone for cytochrome P-450b, has been described (10). When total cytosolic poly(A$^+$)-RNA from phenobarbital pre-treated animals was size fractionated as outlined above and hybridized to nick-translated pPH8, a band at 4 kb was observed. This observation is in disagreement with several other reports of a 1.8 kb mRNA for cytochrome P-450b (8,17,18). Several explanations exist for this apparent discrepancy. The 1.8 kb may be a degraded, but fractional mRNA species for cytochrome P-450b or there may be multiple size mRNA species that code for the same protein. It is interesting that in a preliminary experiment, a 2 kb mRNA species may be seen in addition to the 4 kb mRNA by lowering the stringency of hybridization with pPH8. A 14-16 fold maximal induction of the 4 kb $mRNA_{P-450b}$ was observed 16-18 h postinjection phenobarbital (Table I).

TABLE 1

INDUCTION BY PHENOBARBITAL OF P-450b-SPECIFIC mRNA SEQUENCES IN SPRAGUE-DAWLEY RATS

| | | cpms | | |
	Experiment #	Control	Phenobarbital	-Fold Increase
4 kb region of Northern blot	1	336	5376	16
hybridization to PB-8 probe[1]	2	360	4980	14
P-450b immunoprecipitations of	1	150	2339	16
in vitro translations[2]	2	147	2358	16

[1]The 4 kb hybridized region was removed from the hybridization membrane and quantitated for ^{32}P activity by liquid scintillation counting.

[2]Cytochrome P-450b immunoprecipitates of total (poly A^+)RNA translates were subjected to SDS-PAGE and fluorographed. The radioactive bands corresponding to P-450b were excised, solubilized and counted for ^{35}S activity.

When mRNA was isolated from nuclei (see methods), a similar 4 kb RNA species was observed to hybridize to pPH8. Maximal induction of this nuclear RNA was observed 0.5 to 1 h postinjection phenobarbital. By 12 h, nuclear levels of the 4 kb species had returned to near control levels. These data suggest that treatment with phenobarbital results in a rapid increase in transcription of the cytochrome P-450b gene followed by a slower transport out of the nucleus. Sequence studies are currently in progress to better characterize a potential full-length cDNA clone obtained from pPH8 hybrid-selected mRNA.

ACKNOWLEDGEMENTS

Supported in part by NIH Grant ES07974, NCI Grant CA-09286, and Tobacco Research Council Grant 1369.

REFERENCES

1. Lu, A.Y.H. and West, S.B. (1980) Pharmacol. Rev. 31, 277.
2. Conney, A.H. (1967) Pharmacol. Rev. 19, 317.
3. Thomas, P.E., Reik, L.M., Ryan, D.E. and Levin, W. J. Biol. Chem., in press.
4. Guengerich, F.P. (1977) J. Biol. Chem. 252, 3970.
5. Ryan, D.E., Thomas, P.E., Korzeniowski, D. and Levin, W. (1979) J. Biol. Chem. 254, 1365.
6. Haugen, D.A. and Coon, M.J. (1976) J. Biol. Chem. 251, 7929.
7. Bresnick, E., Brosseau, M., Levin, W., Reik, L., Ryan, D.E. and Thomas, P.E. (1981) Proc. Natl. Acad. Sci. USA 78, 4083.
8. Adesnik, M., Bar-Nun, S., Maschio, F., Zunich, M., Lippman, A. and Bard, E. (1981) J. Biol. Chem. 256, 10340.
9. Bresnick, E., Levy, J. and Hines, R.N. (1981) Arch. Biochem. Biophys. 323, 501.
10. Omiecinski, C.J., Bresnick, E., Hines, R.N., Foldes, R.L. and Levy, J.B. (1983) Arch. Biochem. Biophys., submitted.
11. Busch, H. (1967) in: Grossman, L. and Moldaug, K., (Eds.) Methods in Enzymology, Academic Press, NY, pp. 434-439.
12. Chirgwin, J.M., Przybla, A.E., McDonald, R.J. and Rutter, W. (1979) Biochemistry 18, 5294.
13. Thomas, P.S. (1980) Proc. Natl. Acad. Sci. USA 77, 5201.
14. Blin, N. and Stafford, D.W. (1976) Nucleic Acids Res. 3, 2303.
15. Monk, R.S., Meyuhas, O. and Perry, R.P. (1981) Cell 24, 301.
16. Sanger, F., Coulson, A.R., Barrell, B.G., Smith, A.J.H. and Roe, B.A. (1980) J. Mol. Biol. 143, 161.
17. Fujii-Kuriyama, Y., Mizukami, Y., Kawajiri, K., Sogawa, K. and Muramatsu, M. (1982) Proc. Natl. Acad. Sci. USA 79, 2793.
18. Gonzalez, F.J. and Kasper, C.B. (1982) J. Biol. Chem. 257, 5962.

© 1983 Elsevier Science Publishers B.V.
Extrahepatic Drug Metabolism and Chemical Carcinogenesis,
J. Rydström, J. Montelius and M. Bengtsson eds.

BONE MARROW TOXICITY INDUCED BY ORAL BENZO[a]PYRENE: PROTECTION RESIDES AT THE LEVEL OF THE INTESTINE AND LIVER

Catherine Legraverend[1], David E. Harrison[2],
Francis W. Ruscetti[3] and Daniel W. Nebert[1]
[1]Laboratory of Developmental Pharmacology, National Institute of Child Health and Human Development, National Institutes of Health, Bethesda, Maryland 20205, [2]The Jackson Laboratory, Bar Harbor, Maine 04609, [3]Laboratory of Tumor Cell Biology, National Cancer Institute, Bethesda, Maryland 20205 (U.S.A.)

INTRODUCTION

The Ah locus encodes a cytosolic receptor that regulates the induction of a subset of cytochromes P-450 by polycyclic aromatic hydrocarbons. Some inbred mouse strains, such as the B6 strain,[*] have the high-affinity receptor (Ah^b/Ah^b), others like the D2 strain, the poor-affinity receptor (Ah^d/Ah^d). Presence of the high-affinity receptor leads to greater AHH induction by benzo[a]pyrene. If BP is given topically, subcutaneously, or intratracheally, the Ah^b/Ah^b mouse is at greater risk than the Ah^d/Ah^d mouse for tumors or toxicity at the site of application. If BP is given orally, the Ah^d/Ah^d mouse is at greater risk than the Ah^b/Ah^b mouse for bone marrow toxicity or leukemia. This paradox (1) can be explained on the basis of "first-pass elimination" kinetics (2), $i.e.$ the metabolism and excretion of a drug before it has reached a particular target organ. We present here additional support to the first-pass elimination hypothesis.

RESULTS

Effects of BP on marrow cultures

When BP is in the growth medium and therefore in direct contact with marrow cells, Ah^b/Ah^b marrow exhibits greater toxicity than Ah^d/Ah^d marrow (3).

BP metabolism profile

The most critical monooxygenation of BP by P_1-450 is that of the 7,8-bond (4), and this activity can be best detected by hplc analysis of the 7,8-diol

---

[*]Abbreviations used: B6, the inbred C57BL/6N mouse strain; D2, the inbred DBA/2N mouse strain; WB, the WB/ReJ inbred strain; the BALB/c, BALB/cByJ inbred strain; BP, benzo[a]pyrene; AHH, aryl hydrocarbon (benzo[a]pyrene) hydroxylase (EC 1.14.14.1) (cytochrome P_1-450); hplc, high-performance liquid chromatography.

peak. We thus examined BP metabolism profiles from the intestine, liver and marrow of B6 and D2 mice during BP feeding. In the liver, BP induces the 7,8-diol peak in B6 mice but not in D2 mice. In the marrow, BP induces about 2-fold increases in the 3-hydroxy and 9,10-diol peaks in B6 mice and more than 2-fold increases in the 9,10-diol and 7,8-diol peaks in D2 mice (3).

Marrow repopulation

WBB6 F_1 recipients were repopulated with WB or B6 marrow. D2 and BALB/c marrows were interchanged because these strains are both $H\text{-}2^d$ at the major histocompatibility locus. The two sets of mice were chosen mainly because of their Ah phenotype: WB and D2 with the poor-affinity receptor and B6 and BALB/c with the high-affinity receptor. Any intact mouse having the poor-affinity Ah receptor in its intestine and liver died in less than 3 weeks of oral BP treatment--despite what marrow the mouse possessed (3).

The data in this report illustrate a dramatic difference in toxicity, based on a single gene. They are consistent with the fact that toxic BP metabolites formed in the intestine or liver are not transported by the bloodstream to the marrow or spleen where myelotoxicity results. These results are all consistent with our previous hypothesis and pharmacokinetic data (1). If marrow cells are exposed to BP directly, like in culture, Ah^b/Ah^b marrow cells exhibit more $P_1\text{-}450$ induction than Ah^d/Ah^d cells, and therefore more toxic metabolites are formed $in\ situ$. If oral BP is given to the intact animal, the intestine and liver play an important protective role. Enhanced $P_1\text{-}450$ induction in the Ah^b/Ah^b intestine and liver results in detoxication and a smaller dose of BP reaching the marrow. Little or no induction of $P_1\text{-}450$ in the Ah^d/Ah^d intestine and liver results in much less BP metabolism; therefore, a much larger dose of BP reaches the marrow, where BP metabolites are formed and cause toxicity to the myeloid precursors.

REFERENCES

1. Nebert, D.W. (1981) Environ. Health Perspect., 39, 11.

2. Routledge, P.A. and Shand, D.G. (1979) Annu. Rev. Pharmacol. Toxicol., 19, 447.

3. Legraverend, C., Harrison, D.E., Ruscetti, F.W. and Nebert, D.W., manuscript submitted for publication.

4. Legraverend, C., Mansour, B., Nebert, D.W. and Holland, J.M. (1980) Pharmacology, 20, 242.

© 1983 Elsevier Science Publishers B.V.
Extrahepatic Drug Metabolism and Chemical Carcinogenesis,
J. Rydström, J. Montelius and M. Bengtsson eds.

ASSIGNMENT OF THE *Ah* LOCUS TO MOUSE CHROMOSOME 17

Sirpa O. Kärenlampi[1], Catherine Legraverend[1], Peter A. Lalley[2], Christine A. Kozak[3] and Daniel W. Nebert[1]

[1]Laboratory of Developmental Pharmacology, National Institute of Child Health and Human Development, National Institutes of Health, Bethesda, Maryland 20205, [2]Biology Division, Oak Ridge National Laboratory, Oak Ridge, Tennessee 37830 and [3]Laboratory of Viral Diseases, National Institute of Allergy and Infectious Diseases, National Institutes of Health, Bethesda, Maryland 20205 (U.S.A.)

INTRODUCTION

The *Ah* locus controls the induction of numerous drug-metabolizing enzymes induced by polycyclic aromatic compounds such as 2,3,7,8-tetrachlorodibenzo-*p*-dioxin, 3-methylcholanthrene, and benzo[a]anthracene (reviewed in Ref. 1). On the road to understanding the regulation of P_1-450 induction by the *Ah* receptor, it would be advantageous to know the chromosomal localization of both the *Ah* and *P_1-450* genes. In this report, by means of studying 29 somatic cell mouse x hamster hybrid clones, we assign the presence of aryl hydrocarbon hydroxylase inducibility, *i.e.* the *Ah* locus encoding the receptor, to mouse chromosome 17.

RESULTS AND DISCUSSION

Polycyclic-aromatic-inducible aryl hydrocarbon hydroxylase activity is generally regarded as an accurate biochemical marker for determining the presence of the *Ah* receptor. Whereas cell lines having receptor may not express inducible hydroxylase activity (2, 3), the inverse has never been found. We first studied 15 somatic cell hybrids formed by the fusion of BALB/cJ spleen cells with Chinese hamster E36 cells, developed in Oak Ridge by P.A.L. The presence or absence of mouse chromosome 17 correlated with the presence or absence of aryl hydrocarbon hydroxylase inducibility by benzo[a]anthracene in all of these 15 hybrids. Whenever chromosome 17 was present, the hydroxylase activity in the clone was inducible. If the hybrid clone had lost chromosome 17, aryl hydrocarbon hydroxylase activity was not inducible. There were no exceptions. These data (4) strongly suggest that the *Ah* locus encoding the receptor is located on mouse chromosome 17.

426

Several chromosomes were discordant in only three or four of the 15 hybrids studied, however, and thus were still considered suspect. In order to be certain of the chromosomal assignment, we next studied 14 mouse x hamster somatic cell hybrids formed by the fusion of peritoneal cells derived from three different inbred mouse strains with Chinese hamster E36 cells, developed in Bethesda by C.A.K. In 13 out of 14 of these hybrids, aryl hydrocarbon hydroxylase inducibility by benzo[a]anthracene also segregated concordantly with chromosome 17. Our case is substantially strengthened by the fact that one aryl hydrocarbon hydroxylase-inducible hybrid, BE7-2-9-4, retained only mouse chromosome 17. Moreover, all of the chromosomes considered suspect from the Oak Ridge hybrids exhibited discordancy rates of more than 35%. These data (4) thus confirm the assignment of the *Ah* locus to mouse chromosome 17.

It should be noted that, by definition, the *Ah* locus codes for aryl hydrocarbon hydroxylase inducibility by polycyclic hydrocarbons such as benzo[a]anthracene. There are now examples of regulatory genes that control the expression of receptor genes. We thus cannot rigorously rule out the possibility that a regulatory gene on mouse chromosome 17 controls the expression of the *Ah* receptor gene elsewhere in the genome.

REFERENCES

1. Eisen, H.J., Hannah, R.R., Legraverend, C., Okey, A.B. and Nebert, D.W. (1983) in: Litwack, G. (Ed.), Biochemical Actions of Hormones, Academic Press, New York, pp. 227-258.

2. Okey, A.B., Bondy, G.P., Mason, M.E., Nebert, D.W., Forster-Gibson, C., Muncan, J. and Dufresne, M.J. (1980) J. Biol. Chem., 255, 11415.

3. Legraverend, C., Hannah, R.R., Eisen, H.J., Owens, I.S., Nebert, D.W. and Hankinson, O. (1982) J. Biol. Chem., 257, 6402.

4. Legraverend, C., Kårenlampi, S.O., Lalley, P.A., Kozak, C.A. and Nebert, D.W., manuscript submitted for publication.

DRUG METABOLISM, DNA-ADDUCT FORMATION AND DNA REPAIR

© 1983 Elsevier Science Publishers B.V.
Extrahepatic Drug Metabolism and Chemical Carcinogenesis,
J. Rydström, J. Montelius and M. Bengtsson eds.

METABOLISM AND ACTIVATION OF POLYCYCLIC HYDROCARBONS IN MAMMARY AND OTHER
TISSUE

P. L. GROVER[1], D. H. PHILLIPS[1], C. S. COOPER[1], W. H. SWALLOW[1], A. WESTON[1],
P. VIGNY[2], M. O'HARE[3], A. M. NEVILLE[3] and P. SIMS[1]

[1]Chester Beatty Laboratories, Institute of Cancer Research : Royal Cancer
Hospital, Fulham Road, London SW3 6JB (U.K.), [2]Laboratoire Curie, Institut du
Radium, 11, rue Pierre et Marie Curie, 75231 Paris (France) and [3]Ludwig
Institute for Cancer Research, Haddow Laboratories, Institute of Cancer
Research, Sutton, Surrey (U.K.)

INTRODUCTION

The polycyclic aromatic hydrocarbons are of interest as a class of chemical
carcinogens partly because of their ability to induce tumours in many different
tissues in experimental animals, although the target tissues do not usually
include the liver. Almost all tissues including, of course, the liver can
metabolize the hydrocarbons and, in the absence of any direct evidence for the
transport of active metabolites, the presumption is that each target tissue
metabolically activates those hydrocarbons to which it is susceptible. This is
the basis on which the metabolic capabilities of a variety of animal and human
tissues are now being examined. The agents involved in the aetiology of many
human tumours remain unknown and in vitro comparisons between human and animal
tissues may help to identify those human tissues that may be susceptible to
polycyclic hydrocarbon carcinogenesis.

MAMMARY TISSUE

The relatively rapid induction of mammary cancer in rats treated intragastrically or intravenously with 7,12-dimethylbenz(a)anthracene (DMBA) (1)
provides one of the most popular mammary tumour models and the possibility that
polycyclic hydrocarbons might contribute to the initiation of human breast
cancer obviously merits consideration. In our work on hydrocarbon metabolism
and activation by mammary tissue, we have used rat and human mammary epithelial
cells and fibroblasts in culture and rat mammary glands in vivo. The non-
neoplastic human mammary tissue has been obtained from reduction mammoplasties;
both rat and human epithelial cell aggregates and fibroblasts have been
obtained by treating mammary tissue with collagenase and then separating the
epithelial cell aggregates from the fibroblasts by sedimentation (2,3).
Primary cultures have been treated with either benz(a)anthracene (BA), which is
inactive in the rat mammary gland, benzo(a)pyrene (BP), which is weakly carcin-

ogenic in this tissue or DMBA, which is a potent mammary carcinogen. Both epithelial cells, from which mammary tumours are thought to arise (4) and fibroblasts are able to metabolize these three polycyclic hydrocarbons in vitro to a variety of hydroxylated derivatives (3,5,6) including the dihydrodiols that are thought to be involved, through diol-epoxide formation, in metabolic activation, ie, the 3,4- and 8,9-diols of BA, the 7,8-diol of BP and the 3,4-diol of DMBA. Fibroblasts produced relatively more water soluble derivatives than the epithelial cells and there were appreciable inter-individual variations in hydrocarbon metabolism between different human mammary tissue preparations (6,7). All three hydrocarbons became bound to the proteins of mammary cells and both DMBA and BP became covalently bound to DNA: covalent binding of the non-carcinogen BA to mammary cell DNA was not detected however (3).

Some comparisons of hydrocarbon metabolism and activation by human mammary epithelial cells and fibroblasts have been made. These have shown (Table 1) that, in cells from one patient that were treated with DMBA, there were no appreciable differences between epithelial cells and fibroblasts. Cells from patients 2 and 3 were treated with BP and the data show that, in epithelial cells, higher levels of ether-soluble metabolites, including the 7,8-diol, and higher levels of DNA binding occurred than were found in analagous experiments with fibroblasts from the same patients.

TABLE 1

METABOLISM AND ACTIVATION OF HYDROCARBONS BY CULTURED HUMAN MAMMARY TISSUE[a]

Hydro-carbon	Patient No.	Cell type[b]	Ether-soluble metabolites (nmol/mg protein)	Dihydrodiols (pmol/mg protein)	Hydrocarbon-DNA adducts (pmol/mg protein)
				3,4-diol	
DMBA	1	E	0.34	7.3	0.18
		F	0.19	6.8	0.17
				7,8-diol	
BP	2	E	1.7	84	0.27
		F	0.5	27	< 0.05
				7,8-diol	
BP	3	E	2.6	118	0.63
		F	0.6	31	< 0.05

[a]The metabolism and activation of DMBA and BP by epithelial cells and fibroblasts that were prepared from non-neoplastic human mammary tissue was examined. Details of the conditions of maintenance of the mammary cells, their treatment with hydrocarbon (0.8 ug/ml of culture medium), the separation of the metabolites and the analysis of the DNA-hydrocarbon adducts are presented elsewhere (6). [b]E, epithelial cells; F, fibroblasts.

The hydrocarbon-deoxyribonucleoside adducts formed in mammary cells treated with DMBA or BP have been examined using Sephadex LH20 column chromatography, HPLC and photon-counting spectrophotofluorimetry.

DMBA-DNA adducts. The patterns of adducts formed in rat mammary epithelial cells and fibroblasts are similar (3) and possess anthracene-like fluorescence spectra consistent with activation that involves diol-epoxide formation in the 1,2,3,4-ring. The patterns of adducts formed in human mammary cells treated with DMBA differ in some respects from those of rat cells but the differences have not been examined in detail so far.

BP-DNA adducts. Although the BP-DNA adducts formed in human mammary epithelial cells appear to be the same as those formed in mouse skin treated with BP (5), the adducts present in the DNA of rat mammary cells do not appear to arise from BP diol-epoxides of the 'bay-region' type. Sephadex LH20 column elution profiles (Fig. 1) show that the patterns of adducts present in the DNA

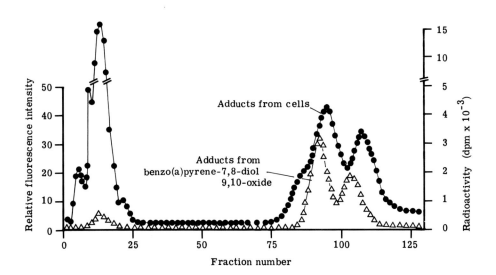

Fig. 1. Sephadex LH20 column chromatography. Hydrolysates of DNA isolated from rat mammary epithelial cells treated with ^{3}H-labelled BP were co-chromatographed with an hydrolysate of DNA that had been reacted with anti-BP-7,8-diol 9,10-oxide.

of cultured rat mammary cells are different from those formed in reactions of the anti-BP-7,8-diol 9,10-oxide with DNA. Further comparisons using HPLC confirm this difference. Fig. 2 shows that when the principal radioactive products present and the marker adducts that eluted with them are examined on a

432

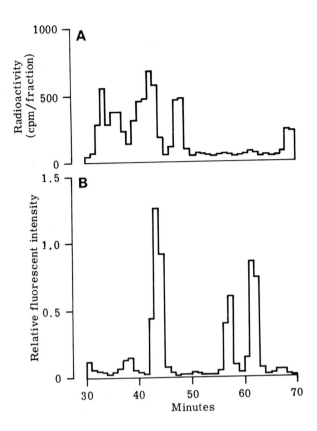

Fig. 2. Hplc of hydrocarbon-deoxyribonucleoside adducts formed in rat mammary epithelial cells treated with BP. The materials present in fractions 78-98 (Fig. 1) were examined by reverse phase hplc on a Zorbax ODS column and the eluate was monitored for the presence of (A) radioactive and (B) fluorescent materials.

reverse phase system, the profiles were again different. Of the four non-radioactive adducts present (Fig. 2B), only one appeared to co-elute with a radioactive product: however, acetylation of the mixture then enabled the radioactive adducts to be separated (Fig. 3) from the marker adduct.

In similar comparisons using a combination of Sephadex LH20 columns and HPLC, the radioactive BP-DNA adducts that are formed by the treatment with ^{3}H-BP of either rat mammary glands in vivo or rat mammary cells in culture have been found to be different from the adducts that arise when (a) syn-BP-7,8-diol 9,10-oxide, anti-BP-9,10-diol 7,8-oxide or BP-4,5-oxide react with DNA, (b) BP-7,8-diol or BP-9,10-diol are activated by metabolism in rat mammary cells or

(c) when 3-hydroxy BP or 9-hydroxy BP are activated by metabolism. In addition, prostaglandin endoperoxide synthetase does not appear to be involved in the generation of the uncharacterized BP-DNA adducts that are formed in rat mammary cells since the presence of either arachidonic acid (100 uM) or indomethacin (100 uM) in the culture medium did not alter the amount of carcinogenDNA binding that occurred.

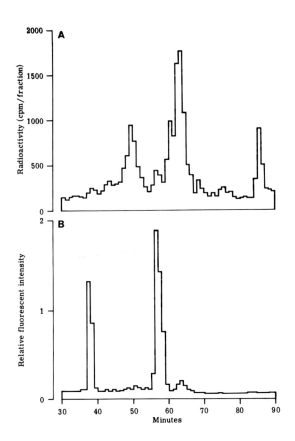

Fig. 3. Hplc of acetylated hydrocarbon-deoxyribonucleoside adducts. The radioactive BP-deoxyribonucleoside adducts and the anti-BP-7,8-diol 9,10-oxide adducts that eluted with them (retention time 41-47 minutes, Fig. 2) were acetylated and re-examined on a Zorbax ODS column: the eluate was monitored for the presence of (A) radioactive and (B) fluorescent materials.

DMBA AND ADRENAL NECROSIS

In addition to inducing mammary tumours in rats, DMBA can also cause a selective destruction of the adrenal cortex (8). The mechanisms by which adrenocortical necrosis is induced by DMBA are not understood, although indirect evidence that DMBA metabolites might be involved exists, since (a) animals can be protected by pretreatment with inducers or inhibitors of hepatic microsomal enzymes (9-11), and (b) 7-hydroxymethyl-12-methylbenz(a)anthracene (7-OHM-12-MBA) is more active than DMBA in inducing adrenal necrosis (12).

Adrenal homogenates can metabolize both these compounds (13) and current candidates for the role of the active adrenocorticolytic agent include the sulphate ester of 7-OHM-12-MBA and a diol-epoxide derived from 7-OHM-12-MBA. In some recent experiments (14), we have examined the metabolism of DMBA and 7-OHM-12-MBA by rat adrenal homogenates and adrenocortical cells in culture. In these systems, a range of metabolites was produced from both substrates and, in brief, the results showed that DMBA was metabolized more extensively than 7-OHM-12-MBA by adrenocortical cells, that more covalent binding to protein occurred in homogenates when 7-OHM-12-MBA was the substrate and that more water-soluble metabolites were formed by cells from DMBA than from 7-OHM-12-MBA. The dihydrodiols detected as metabolites included the 3,4-, 5,6-, 8,9- and 10,11-diols of both substrates and these were present in varying proportions: neither of the 1,2-diols were detected as metabolites, however, using rat adrenal preparations (see below). We have also examined the effect on cell viability, as measured by the trypan blue exclusion test, of incubating rat adrenocortical cells with DMBA or 7-OHM-12-MBA.

As Fig. 4, shows neither of these compounds has a marked cytotoxic effect when they were present at a concentration of 10 ug/ml of medium for up to 72 hr, the time that it takes for adrenal necrosis to develop in vivo in treated rats. In other experiments, the 3,4-diol of 7-OHM-12-MBA (10 ug/ml), the 3-hydroxy derivative of DMBA (10 ug/ml) and the sulphate ester of 7-OHM-12-MBA (1 ug/ml) also failed to reduce the viability of adrenocortical cells. In addition, 2,6-dichloro-4-nitrophenol, which is a potent inhibitor of sulpho-transferases in the rat (15), failed to protect against the adrenocorticolytic effects of 7-OHM-12-MBA in vivo, a result which suggests that the sulphate ester of the 7-hydroxymethyl derivative may not be the active adrenocortico-lytic metabolite of DMBA. Since adrenocortical cells in culture produce a wide range of metabolites from DMBA and 7-OHM-12-MBA, and because neither of these compounds caused appreciable cytotoxicity in such cells (Fig. 4), it appears likely that the mechanism by which adrenal necrosis is induced in rats in vivo by such compounds may be an indirect one.

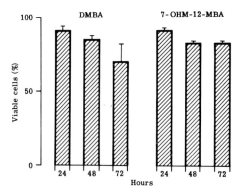

Fig. 4. The effect on cell viability of treating primary cultures of rat adrenocortical cells for up to 72 hr. with DMBA or 7-OHM-12-MBA at a concentration of 10 ug/ml medium.

SKIN

The relative sensitivity of human skin to tumour induction by the polycyclic hydrocarbons has not been established, even though it has been considered for many years to be a target tissue for this class of chemical carcinogens (16). One way in which this sensitivity might be assessed is through comparisons of hydrocarbon activation and metabolism in human skin and in the skin of rodent species that are known to be either susceptible, like the mouse and rabbit, or resistant, like the rat. Some studies of this type are currently in progress using skin samples treated either in vivo or in short-term organ culture with ^{3}H-labelled hydrocarbons. Although no overall conclusions can be drawn as yet, it is apparent that there are qualitative and quantitative differences in the ways in which BP is metabolized and activated by rat and mouse skin in vivo or in short-term organ culture (17). In human skin treated with BP in organ culture, the major hydrocarbon-deoxyribonucleoside adducts formed appear to arise from reactions of the anti-BP-7,8-diol 9,10-oxide with guanosine residues (18).

Epidermal tissues do seem to be capable of forming some hydrocarbon metabolites that have not been detected elsewhere: for example, the 11,12-dihydrodiol of BP has been identified as a metabolite that is produced by rat (19) and human skin (18). Recently another new dihydrodiol metabolite, which has been identified as the 1,2-dihydrodiol of DMBA, has been detected in the media in which rat, mouse or human skin in short-term organ culture has been treated with ^{3}H-DMBA (20): as Fig. 5 shows, this dihydrodiol appears to be a major

436

component of the dihydrodiols that are formed from DMBA by human skin. However, there is no evidence at present to suggest that either the 11,12-diol of BP or the 1,2-diol of DMBA is involved in the metabolic activation of the parent hydrocarbons in epidermal tissues.

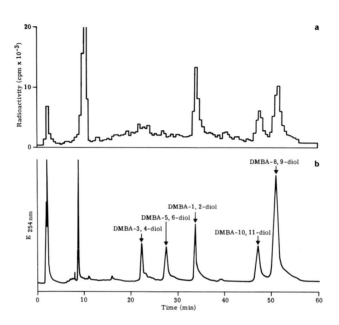

Fig. 5. Hplc of DMBA dihydrodiols. A mixture of the radioactive dihydrodiol metabolites formed when human skin was treated in short-term organ culture with ^{3}H-DMBA was chromatographed in admixture with reference diols of DMBA. The eluate was monitored for (a) radioactive and (b) uv-absorbing materials.

CONCLUSIONS

The basis for the susceptibility or resistance of various mammalian cells and tissues to different classes of chemical carcinogens is not well understood but almost certainly depends upon a combination of factors. For most carcinogens, one factor will concern the balance between the ability of the target cell to activate a carcinogen by metabolism and its ability to inactivate and/or remove the reactive metabolite so formed. For the polycyclic hydrocarbons, adult rat liver provides perhaps the best example of a tissue that is able to metabolize polycyclic hydrocarbons extensively to a range of metabolites, which certainly includes proximate carcinogens, but that is resistant, except in special circumstances, to their carcinogenicity. This resistance may not be based solely upon the ability of hepatic tissue to inactivate the proximate or ultimate carcinogens but may also be due, in part, to comparatively low rates of cell division in normal adult liver.

The relative susceptibility of mammary epithelial cells, in comparison with stromal cells, to hydrocarbons may be partly a reflection of differences in metabolism and activation between the two cell types and, if such differences are genetically determined rather than induced, they could provide a basis for a pre-existing susceptibility to mammary cancer in some individuals. The perplexing results obtained in our studies on the BP-deoxyribonucleoside adducts that are formed in rat mammary tissue treated with BP (see above) indicate that mechanisms of hydrocarbon activation, other than those that simply involve diol-epoxide or phenol-epoxide formation, may also function in mammalian tissues.

The mechanism by which DMBA induces adrenal necrosis in rats is almost certainly different from that by which it induces mammary tumours in the same species. In this case, it now seems possible that the effect of DMBA or 7-OHM-12-MBA on the adrenal cortex is not due to a direct effect of a reactive or toxic metabolite on the adrenocortical cells but is mediated indirectly, perhaps through interference with mechanisms of adrenal control that are exercised by the pituitary. The fact that hydrocarbon metabolism may be both quantitatively and qualitatively different in different tissues is exemplified by the results obtained with rodent and human skin where particular dihydrodiol metabolites have been found that have not been detected in other situations. Together these results all indicate that, for an understanding of polycyclic hydrocarbon carcinogenesis, the traditional biochemical preoccupation with liver may be particularly inappropriate.

ACKNOWLEDGMENTS

This work was supported in part by grants to the Chester Beatty Laboratories, Institute of Cancer Research from the Cancer Research Campaign and the Medical Research Council, and in part by PHS grant no. CA21959 from the National Cancer Institute, DHSS.

438

REFERENCES

1. Huggins, C., Grand, L.C. and Brilliantes, F.P. (1961) Nature, 189, 204.

2. Easty, G.C., Easty, D.M., Monaghan, P., Ormerod, M. and Neville, A.M. (1980) Int. J. Cancer, 26, 577.

3. Cooper, C.S., Pal, K., Hewer, A., Grover, P.L. and Sims, P. (1982) Carcinogenesis, 3, 203.

4. Wellings, S.R. and Jensen, H.M. (1973) J. Natl. Cancer Inst. 50, 1111.

5. MacNicoll, A.D., Easty, G.C., Neville, A.M., Grover, P.L. and Sims, P. (1980) Biochem. Biophys. Res. Commun. 95, 1599.

6. Grover, P.L., MacNicoll, A.D., Sims, P., Easty, G.C. and Neville, A.M. (1980) Int. J. Cancer, 26, 467.

7. Cooper, C.S., Grover, P.L., Hewer, A., O'Hare, M., MacNicoll, A.D., Neville, A.M. and Sims, P. (1982) in: Cooke, M., Dennis, A.J. and Fisher, G.L. (Eds.), Polycyclic Aromatic Hydrocarbons : Physical and Biological Chemistry, Batelle Press, Columbus, pp. 211-219.

8. Huggins, C. and Morii, S. (1961) J. Exp. Med. 114, 741.

9. Huggins, C. and Fukunishi, R. (1964) J. Exp. Med. 119, 923.

10. Wheatley, D.N. (1968) Brit. J. exp. Pathol. 49, 44.

11. Wheatley, D.N., Hamilton, A.G., Currie, A.R., Boyland, E. and Sims, P. (1966) Nature 211, 1311.

12. Boyland, E., Sims, P. and Huggins, C. (1965) Nature, 207, 816.

13. Sims, P. (1970) Biochem. Pharmacol. 19, 2261.

14. Swallow, W.H., Pal, K., Phillips, D.H., Grover, P.L. and Sims, P. (1983) submitted for publication.

15. Mulder, G.J. and Scholtens, E. (1977) Biochem. J. 165, 553.

16. Henry, S.A. (1947) Brit. Med. Bull. 4, 389.

17. Weston, A., Grover, P.L. and Sims, P. (1982) Chem.-Biol. Interactions 42, 233.

18. Weston, A., Grover, P.L. and Sims, P. (1983) Chem.-Biol. Interactions, in press.

19. Weston, A., Grover, P.L. and Sims, P. (1982) Biochem. Biophys. Res. Commun. 105, 935.

20. Weston, A., Grover, P.L. and Sims, P. (1983) submitted for publication.

© 1983 Elsevier Science Publishers B.V.
Extrahepatic Drug Metabolism and Chemical Carcinogenesis,
J. Rydström, J. Montelius and M. Bengtsson eds.

7,12-DIMETHYLBENZ[a]ANTHRACENE-DNA INTERACTIONS IN MOUSE EMBRYO CELL CULTURES AND MOUSE SKIN[1]

ANTHONY DIPPLE, JOSEF T. SAWICKI[2], ROBERT C. MOSCHEL, AND C. ANITA H. BIGGER
Chemical Carcinogenesis Program, LBI-Basic Research Program, NCI-Frederick
Cancer Research Facility, Frederick, MD 21701 (U.S.A.)

INTRODUCTION

7,12-Dimethylbenz[a]anthracene (DMBA) is one of the most potent of the
polycyclic aromatic hydrocarbon carcinogens but its metabolic activation and
mechanism of action have been less thoroughly investigated than those for
other hydrocarbon carcinogens because a convenient synthesis for the putative
active metabolite has not been available. While this has limited the range of
investigations possible, we have continued studies with this carcinogen in the
belief that the interactions of DMBA with cellular DNA may be richer in events
specifically associated with tumor initiation than those interactions for less
potent carcinogens, such as benzo[a]pyrene.

METABOLIC ACTIVATION OF DMBA

As for benzo[a]pyrene (1), initial information on the pathway of metabolic
activation of DMBA came through studies of hydrocarbon-DNA binding. In work
with reactive model compounds related to the methylbenz[a]anthracenes, we had
observed that, unless precautions were taken to protect solutions of 7-bromo-
methyl-12-methylbenz[a]anthracene deoxyribonucleoside adducts from light, pho-
todecomposition products were readily formed (2). However, analogous products
formed with 7-bromomethylbenz[a]anthracene are much more stable, indicating
that this photosensitivity is a function of the hydrocarbon residue (2). Thus,
when the adducts present in DNA isolated from rodent embryo cell cultures
exposed to DMBA were found to be photosensitive, it was possible to obtain
some information on the structure of the hydrocarbon residue present in these
adducts by examining the photosensitivity of various model compounds (3). Of
the compounds examined, only DMBA itself and 9,10-dimethylanthracene (a model
for DMBA saturated in the 1,2,3,4-ring) exhibit photosensitivity similar to
that of DMBA-deoxyribonucleoside adducts, suggesting that the reactive metabolite responsible for DNA binding contains one of these two aromatic systems.

[1]Supported by National Cancer Institute, DHHS, under contract NO1-CO-23909
with Litton Bionetics. [2]Research Training Fellow of the International
Agency for Research on Cancer. J.T.S., permanent address is Dept. Environmental Health Sciences, Medical Academy, Warsaw, Poland.

440

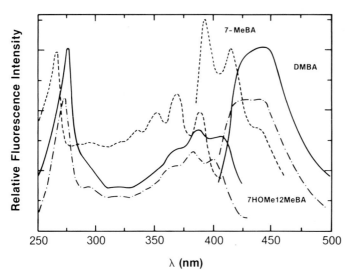

Fig. 1   Fluorescence spectra of hydrocarbon-deoxyribonucleoside adducts in methanol.   7-MeBA, 7-methylbenz[a]anthracene-deoxyribonucleoside adduct excitation (λ_{em}, 415nm) and emission (λ_{ex}, 264nm) spectra.   7-HOMe12MeBA, 7-hydroxymethyl-12-methylbenz[a]anthracene-deoxyribonucleoside adduct excitation (λ_{em}, 430nm) and emission (λ_{ex}, 273nm) spectra.   DMBA, DMBA-deoxyribonucleoside adduct excitation (λ_{em}, 440nm) and emission (λ_{ex}, 274nm) spectra.   Adapted from Moschel et al (14).

To determine whether the DNA bound residue contained the dimethylanthracene, or the intact DMBA, aromatic system, sufficient DMBA-deoxyribonucleoside adducts ($\sim$ 0.1 µg) were recovered from mouse embryo cell cultures for fluorescence measurements (4).   Heretofore, such measurements had been made on hydrocarbon-modified DNA and the presence of the DNA bases had precluded examination of the complete excitation spectra (5-7).   However, by recovering the DMBA-deoxyribonucleoside adducts, we could show that the predominant fluorophore present in these adducts (Fig. 1) was derived from the dimethyl-anthracene fluorophore, suggesting that the reactive metabolite responsible for DNA binding was saturated in the 1,2,3,4-ring and, therefore, was presuma-bly a dihydrodiol epoxide (4).   Subsequently, similar emission spectra were reported by Vigny et al (8) and Ivanovic et al (9) and interpreted in the same way although the latter group pointed out that the active metabolite might be a dihydrodiol epoxide of 7-hydroxymethyl-12-methylbenz[a]anthracene rather than of DMBA itself.   However, the fluorescence spectrum of 7-hydroxymethyl-12-methylbenz[a]anthracene-deoxyribonucleoside adducts recovered from mouse embryo cells is distinguishable from that of DMBA-deoxyribonucleoside adducts (Fig. 1) and, in the same study (10), we found that 7-hydroxymethyl-12-methyl-benz[a]anthracene binds much less efficiently to DNA than does DMBA, and

that the hydrocarbon-deoxyribonucleoside adducts formed from these two hydrocarbons are readily separable by chromatography. Similar findings were reported for mouse skin by MacNicoll et al (11), confirming that, in the mouse at

least, there is no major involvement of this hydroxymethyl metabolite in
DMBA-DNA binding. Further evidence that the active DNA binding metabolite of
DMBA is a 1,2,3,4-ring dihydrodiol epoxide was obtained by showing that DMBA-
DNA binding in mouse embryo cells is inhibited by trichloropropylene oxide,
an inhibitor of epoxide hydrolase, and that adducts eluted as a single peak
from Sephadex LH-20 chromatographic columns can be resolved into two peaks on
the same chromatographic system when sodium borate is added to the eluent
(12). This latter is an indication of the presence of products from both
syn and anti dihydrodiol epoxides. Only the latter contain vicinal cis
hydroxyl groups (Fig. 2) and therefore complex with borate and elute more
rapidly from Sephadex LH-20 in the presence of borate (13). The fact that the
fluorescence spectra of hydrocarbon-deoxyribonucleoside adducts from DMBA and
7-hydroxymethyl-12-methylbenz[a]anthracene (both of which contain a methyl
group in the bay region) are substantially different from those of adducts
with 7-methylbenz[a]anthracene (unsubstituted in the bay region) (Fig. 1)
suggests that the nucleoside is attached near the 12-methyl group in DMBA,
presumably at the 1-position (14). Thus, studies of DNA-bound DMBA indicated
that the metabolic activation pathway for DMBA probably involves the bay region
dihydrodiol epoxide route (Fig. 2) as postulated by Jerina and Daly (15).

Support for this came through studies with the trans-3,4-dihydrodiol of
DMBA obtained both from large scale metabolic reactions (16) and from chemical
syntheses (17,18). Chou and Yang (16) reported that this dihydrodiol bound
much more extensively to DNA in the presence of liver microsomes from phenobarbital treated rats than did DMBA itself, consistent with this dihydrodiol
being on the metabolic activation pathway (Fig. 2). Similarly, the 3,4-dihy-
drodiol exhibits high tumor initiating activity suggesting that the route of
activation for DNA binding is also the route of activation with respect to
tumor initiating activity (19-21). Sims and his colleagues (22) have treated
tetrahydrofuran solutions of the 3,4-dihydrodiol with m-chloroperoxybenzoic
acid, diluted these solutions with ethanol and reacted them directly with DNA
to obtain products which co-chromatograph with DMBA-deoxyribonucleoside adducts
recovered from mouse skin exposed to [^{3}H]DMBA. Nevertheless, the dihydrodiol
epoxides have not yet been isolated so their biological activities remain
unknown and amounts of their reaction products with DNA, sufficient to permit
thorough characterization, are not available.

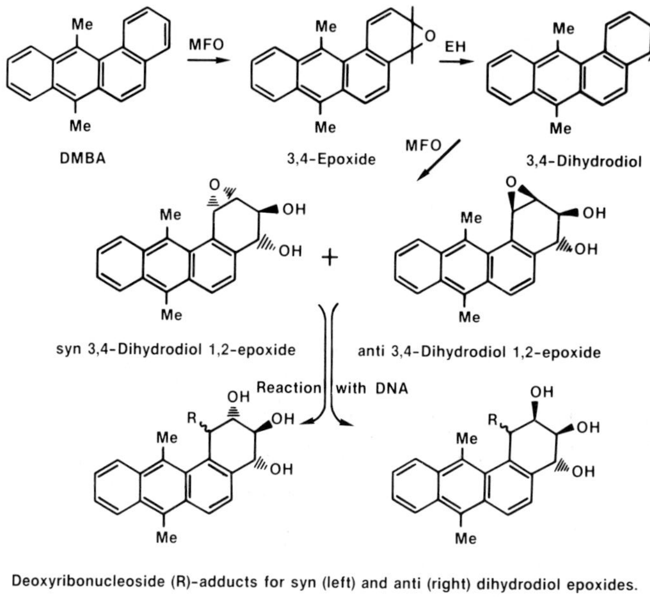

Deoxyribonucleoside (R)-adducts for syn (left) and anti (right) dihydrodiol epoxides.

Fig. 2.   Pathway for metabolic activation of DMBA.   Only relative stereochemistry is implied.   MFO, mixed function oxidase; EH, epoxide hydrolase.

Therefore, we have pursued indirect approaches to obtain more information
about the metabolic activation of DMBA.   Thus, as shown in Figure 2, only
DMBA-deoxyribonucleoside adducts from a bay region anti dihydrodiol epoxide
would contain vicinal cis hydroxyl groups which can complex with borate.
Since m-phenylboronic acid-substituted DEAE-celluloses have been successfully
used as solid phases to separate various RNA fragments, based on binding
to this phase of fragments with free cis hydroxyl groups on the 3'-terminus
(23), we determined whether such celluloses would separate radioactive DMBA-
deoxyribonucleoside adducts into those originating from syn and anti dihydrodiol epoxides (24).   A small column of Servacel DHB separated DMBA-deoxyribonucleoside adducts into two fractions.   One fraction came through the column
in buffer, pH 9, while the second was eluted after adding 10% sorbitol to the
buffer.   These fractions were identified as adducts arising from syn and anti
dihydrodiol epoxides respectively (a) through their behavior on the Servacel
DHB column; (b) because each of the fractions exhibited fluorescence spectra
consistent with those for bay region dihydrodiol epoxide-deoxyribonucleoside
adducts; (c) because further analysis by high pressure liquid chromatography
(hplc) showed that each fraction contained different adducts; and (d) because
the major adducts in each fraction behaved as anticipated for these assignments

when recovered and chromatographed on Sephadex LH-20 either with or without
borate in the eluting solvent (13). In other words, adducts assigned an anti
dihydrodiol epoxide origin (A and D in Fig. 3) eluted more rapidly in the
presence of borate than in its absence while the adduct assigned a syn dihydrodiol epoxide origin (C in Fig. 3) behaved similarly irrespective of the presence or absence of borate. Figure 3 illustrates an hplc profile of DMBA-deoxyribonucleoside adducts from mouse embryo cells where assignments of syn or
anti dihydrodiol epoxide origins are made on the basis of the findings summarized above (24). The most notable aspect of this analysis is that a syn dihydrodiol epoxide makes a substantial contribution to DNA binding for DMBA while
for benzo[a]pyrene in mouse cell systems, little involvement of a syn dihydrodiol epoxide has been found (25-27). In primary mouse embryo cell cultures,
therefore, metabolic activation of DMBA for DNA binding follows the pathway
outlined in Figure 2 leading to both reactive syn and anti bay region dihydrodiol epoxides. In this Figure, only relative stereochemistry is implied and
the two dihydrodiol epoxides illustrated may be enantiomers of the metabolites
actually involved in DNA binding. Nothing is known about the absolute stereochemistry of these DMBA metabolites.

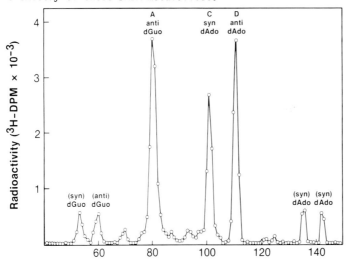

Fraction Number

Fig. 3. Profile of DMBA-deoxyribonucleoside adducts separated by hplc on
Ultrasphere ODS (24). The origin of adducts, i.e. whether they arise from
syn or anti bay region dihydrodiol epoxides and whether the nucleoside
involved is deoxyadenosine (dAdo) or deoxyguanosine (dGuo), is indicated
herein. Where syn or anti is in parenthesis, this indicates that these
adducts elute in this fraction from Servacel DHB (24) but that no confirmatory
data have been collected. The DNA sample illustrated (19.35 μmol DMBA/mol
DNA-P) was obtained from mouse embryo cell cultures exposed to 0.05 μg/ml
of [^{3}H]DMBA.

DMBA-DEOXYRIBONUCLEOSIDE ADDUCTS

To obtain some information on the deoxyribonucleoside moieties involved in adduct formation, mouse embryo cell cultures were grown in the presence of either $[^{14}C]$guanine or $[^{14}C]$adenine prior to exposure to $[^3H]$DMBA. King et al (28) have previously shown that $[^{14}C]$purines were effectively incorporated into the DNA of V-79 Chinese hamster cells and these precursors were similarly effective in mouse embryo cell cultures. $[^{14}C]$Guanine labels deoxyguanosine residues in mouse embryo cell DNA almost exclusively and, in the double-labeling experiment, this precursor was found to be incorporated principally into the DMBA-deoxyribonucleoside adduct labeled A in Figure 3. Thus, DMBA-deoxyribonucleoside adduct A is characterized as an anti bay region dihydrodiol epoxide-deoxyguanosine adduct (29). $[^{14}C]$Adenine labels both deoxyadenosine and deoxyguanosine residues in mouse embryo cell DNA, though the specific radioactivity of the deoxyadenosine residues is some 2.7-3.9 fold higher than that of the deoxyguanosine residues. In these experiments, carbon-14 radioactivity was found to be associated with adducts A, C and D (Fig. 3). However, the ratio of $^3H/^{14}C$ in these peaks was consistent with the earlier conclusion that adduct A was a deoxyguanosine adduct and showed that adducts C and D each contained deoxyadenosine residues. Adducts C and D can be characterized, therefore, as syn bay region and anti bay region dihydrodiol epoxide-deoxyadenosine adducts, respectively (Fig. 3) (29). There is no available evidence on which specific structures can be assigned to these adducts, but our initial finding that the major sites for reaction of aralkylating agents with DNA are the amino groups of the DNA bases (30) has held true for the benzo[a]pyrene dihydrodiol epoxides (31 and references therein). Therefore, the amino groups of the DNA bases would be the most likely site of reaction for the DMBA dihydrodiol epoxides also.

The deoxyadenosine adducts (C and D, Fig. 3) account for a large fraction of the total DMBA-DNA binding in our mouse embryo cell cultures. This also holds true for DNA from mouse skin exposed to $[^3H]$DMBA and, at high DMBA doses in the mouse ($\sim$ 1μmol/mouse), the syn dihydrodiol epoxide-deoxyadenosine adduct (C, Fig. 3) can itself account for about 40% of the total DNA binding (Bigger et al., in preparation). In contrast, analyses of DNA adducts obtained when mouse skin is treated with benzo[a]pyrene indicate that only 2-3% of the total DNA binding is attributable to dihydrodiol epoxide-deoxyadenosine adducts (31). Since DMBA is a considerably more potent initiator of mouse skin tumorigenesis than is benzo[a]pyrene, these findings suggest a possible relationship between tumor initiating activity and reactivity towards deoxyadenosine residues in DNA. Earlier, DiGiovanni et al (32) reported that epidermal homogenate-catalyzed binding of hydrocarbons to polyA correlates better with carcinogenic activity than does binding to polyG. Nevertheless, in their system DMBA binds far more extensively to polyG than to polyA and we have found that the metabolic activation of DMBA in subcellular systems does not mimic the activation occurring in intact cells (33), so that it seems unlikely that the same reactive metabolites are involved in these two systems.

REPAIR RESPONSE TO DMBA-DNA

Few reports on the repair of DMBA damage to DNA are in the literature. Tay and Russo (34) examined the removal of DMBA damage from the DNA of rat mammary epithelial cells in vitro and recorded some 10-35% excision of initial damage in 48 hours depending on the age and parity of the rats from which the cultures were derived. In our mouse embryo cell cultures, we found that DMBA-DNA damage was even less efficiently removed (35). Moreover, cells from the same cell preparations excised DNA damage introduced by 3-methylcholanthrene or 7-bromomethylbenz[a]anthracene much more efficiently than that introduced by DMBA, suggesting that DMBA-DNA adducts may be intrinsically difficult to remove (35). Though the basis for this is not understood, this could contribute to the high tumor initiating activity of DMBA. In earlier studies with 7-bromomethylbenz[a]anthracene, we have observed that in a variety of different cell culture systems the carcinogen-modified deoxyadenosine residues (N^6-(benz-[a]anthracenyl-7-methyl)-2'-deoxyadenosine) are removed more readily than the carcinogen-modified deoxyguanosine residues (N^2-(benz[a]anthracenyl-7-methyl)-2'-deoxyguanosine) (36-39). The excision of individual DMBA-deoxyribonucleoside adducts has not been examined so far and, given the limited overall excision, this may not be very informative anyway. However, it may be of interest that some difficulties have been encountered in the enzymic hydrolysis of DMBA-DNA in vitro and that these indicate that the DMBA-deoxyadenosine adducts can be more difficult to release than the deoxyguanosine adduct. Another feature of DMBA is that it carries a 12-methyl group in the bay region. This structural feature is associated with enhanced tumorigenicity in comparison with the analogue lacking this methyl group, and it is possible that some conformational restraint imposed on DNA adducts by this methyl group may be associated with their limited susceptibility to DNA repair systems (14, 35,40).

DISCUSSION

While our detailed knowledge of the interactions occurring between DMBA and DNA still lags behind that for benzo[a]pyrene-DNA interactions, sufficient progress has been made for some comparison to be worthwhile (Table 1). As a tumor initiator in mouse skin, DMBA is about 30-fold more potent than benzo[a]pyrene. However, the overall DNA binding for DMBA is only about 2-fold higher than for benzo[a]pyrene. It is conceivable, therefore, that the interactions between DMBA and DNA may be richer in tumor initiating events than those for benzo[a]pyrene.

TABLE 1

COMPARISON OF DMBA WITH BENZO[a]PYRENE (BP)

Property	DMBA	BP
Tumor initiation in mouse skin		
Dose for ~ 75% incidence	3 nmol (41)	100 nmol (42)
Tumors /μmol (43)	851	23
Binding to skin DNA		
pmol/mg DNA at a 1 μmol dose (44)	43	23
dAdo adducts in mouse skin	27 - 48%[a]	< 3% (31)
Syn dihydrodiol epoxide adducts	14 - 39%[a]	< 12% (45)

[a] These percentages depend on dose and are from Bigger et al (in preparation).

Although a syn dihydrodiol plays a greater role in DNA binding for DMBA than for benzo[a]pyrene, the most striking difference between these two carcinogens is their different capacities for reaction with deoxyadenosine residues in DNA. Taking into account the higher total binding for DMBA, the modification of adenine residues in DNA by these two carcinogens differs by roughly the same factor (30X) as does their tumor initiating potencies, suggesting that some adenine-rich sequences in DNA may be the key receptors for tumor initiators.

REFERENCES

1. Sims, P., Grover, P.L., Swaisland, A., Pal, K., and Hewer, A. (1974) Nature (London), 252, 326.
2. Rayman, M.P. and Dipple, A. (1973) Biochem., 12, 1202.
3. Baird, W.M. and Dipple, A. (1977) Int. J. Cancer, 20, 427.

4. Moschel, R.C., Baird, W.M. and Dipple, A. (1977) Biochem. Biophys. Res. Commun., 76, 1092.

5. Daudel, P., Crois-Delcey, M., Alonso-Verduras, C., Duquesne, M., Jacquignon, P., Markovits, P. and Vigny, P. (1974) C.R. Acad. Sci. Paris, 278, 2249.

6. Daudel, P., Duquesne, M., Vigny, P., Grover, P.L. and Sims, P. (1975) FEBS Lett., 57, 250.

7. Ivanovic, V., Geacintov, N.E. and Weinstein, I.B. (1976) Biochem. Biophys. Res. Commun. 70, 1172.

8. Vigny, P., Duquesne, M., Coulomb, H., Tierney, B., Grover, P.L. and Sims, P. (1977) FEBS Lett., 82, 278.

9. Ivanovic, V., Geacintov, N.E., Jeffrey, A.M., Fu, P.P., Harvey, R.G. and Weinstein, I.B. (1978) Cancer Lett., 4, 131.

10. Dipple, A., Tomaszewski, J.E., Moschel, R.C., Bigger, C.A.H., Nebzydoski, J.A. and Egan, M. (1979) Cancer Res. 39, 1154.

11. MacNicoll, A.D., Burden, P.M., Ribeiro, O., Hewer, A., Grover, P.L. and Sims, P. (1979) Chem.-Biol. Interact., 26, 121.

12. Dipple, A. and Nebzydoski, J.A. (1978) Chem.-Biol. Interact., 20, 17.

13. King, H.W.S., Osborne, M.R., Beland, F.A., Harvey, R.G. and Brookes, P. (1976) Proc. Natl. Acad. Sci. U.S.A., 73, 2679.

14. Moschel, R.C., Hudgins, W.R. and Dipple, A. (1979) Chem.-Biol. Interact., 27, 69.

15. Jerina, D.M. and Daly, J.W. (1976) in: Parke, D.V. and Smith, R.L. (Ed.), Drug Metabolism, Taylor and Francis, London, pp. 13-32.

16. Chou, M.W. and Yang, S.K. (1978) Proc. Natl. Acad. Sci. U.S.A., 75, 5466.

17. Sukumaran, K.B. and Harvey, R.G. (1979) J. Am. Chem. Soc. 101, 1353.

18. Tierney, B., Hewer, A., MacNicoll, A.D., Gervasi, P.G., Rattle, H., Walsh, C., Grover, P.L. and Sims, P. (1978). Chem.-Biol. Interact., 23, 243.

19. Slaga, T.J., Gleason, G.L., DiGiovanni, J., Sukumaran, K.B. and Harvey, R.G. (1979) Cancer Res. 39, 1934.

20. Chouroulinkov, I., Gentil, A., Tierney, B., Grover, P.L. and Sims, P. (1979) Int. J. Cancer 24, 455.

21. Wislocki, P.G., Gadek, K.M., Chou, M.W., Yang, S.K. and Lu, A.Y.H. (1980) Cancer Res., 40, 3661.

22. Cooper, C.S., Ribeiro, O., Hewer, A., Walsh, C., Grover, P.L. and Sims, P. (1980) Chem.-Biol. Interact., 29, 357.

23. Rosenberg, M., Wiebers, J.L. and Gilham, P.T. (1972) Biochem., 11, 3623.

24. Sawicki, J.T., Moschel, R.C. and Dipple, A. (1983) Cancer Res., 43, in press.

25. Brown, S.H., Jeffrey, A.M. and Weinstein, I.B. (1979) Cancer Res., 39, 1673.

26. Lo, K.-Y. and Kakunaga, T. (1981) Biochem. Biophys. Res. Commun., 99, 820.

27. Shinohara, K. and Cerutti, P.A. (1977) Proc. Natl. Acad. Sci. U.S.A., 74, 979.

448

28. King, H.W.S., Osborne, M.R. and Brookes, P. (1979) Chem.-Biol. Interact., 24, 345.

29. Dipple, A., Pigott, M.A., Moschel, R.C. and Costantino, N. (1983) Cancer Res., 43, in press.

30. Dipple, A., Brookes, P., Mackintosh, D.W. and Rayman, M.P. (1971) Biochem., 10, 4323.

31. Ashurst, S.W. and Cohen, G.M. (1981) Int. J. Cancer, 27, 357.

32. DiGiovanni, J., Romson, J.R., Linville, D., Juchau, M.R. and Slaga, T.J. (1979) Cancer Lett., 7, 39.

33. Bigger, C.A.H., Tomaszewski, J.E., Dipple, A. and Lake, R.S. (1980) Science, 209, 503.

34. Tay, L.K. and Russo, J. (1981) Carcinogenesis, 2, 1327.

35. Dipple, A. and Hayes, M.E. (1979) Biochem. Biophys. Res. Commun., 91, 1225.

36. Lieberman, M.W. and Dipple, A. (1972) Cancer Res., 32, 1855.

37. Dipple, A. and Roberts, J.J. (1977) Biochem., 16, 1499.

38. McCaw, B.A., Dipple, A., Young, S. and Roberts, J.J. (1978) Chem. -Biol. Interact., 22, 139.

39. Dipple, A. and Schultz, E. (1979) Cancer Lett., 7, 103.

40. Moschel, R.C., Bigger, C.A.H., Hudgins, W.R., and Dipple, A. (1980) in: Bjorseth, A. and Dennis, A.J. (Ed.), Polynuclear Aromatic Hydrocarbons: Chemistry and Biological Effects, Battelle Press, Columbus, pp. 663-673.

41. Wislocki, P.G., Gadek, K.M., Chou, M.W., Yang, S.K., and Lu, A.Y.H. (1980) Cancer Res., 40, 3661.

42. Slaga, T.J., Bracken, W.J., Gleason, G., Levin, W., Yagi, H., Jerina, D.M. and Conney, A.H. (1979) Cancer Res., 39, 67.

43. Scribner, N.K., Woodworth, B., Ford, G.P. and Scribner, J.D. (1980) Carcinogenesis, 1, 715.

44. Phillips, D.H., Grover, P.L. and Sims, P. (1979) Int. J. Cancer, 23, 201.

45. Koreeda, M., Moore, P.D., Wislocki, P.G., Levin, W., Conney, A.H., Yagi, H., and Jerina, D.M. (1978) Science, 199, 778.

© 1983 Elsevier Science Publishers B.V.
Extrahepatic Drug Metabolism and Chemical Carcinogenesis,
J. Rydström, J. Montelius and M. Bengtsson eds.

A KINETIC APPROACH TO POLYCYCLIC HYDROCARBON ACTIVATION

COLIN R. JEFCOATE, MARO CHRISTOU, GABRIELA M. KELLER, CHRISTOPHER R. TURNER
AND NEIL M. WILSON

Department of Pharmacology, University of Wisconsin Medical School, Madison,
WI 53706 (U.S.A.)

Xenobiotic-metabolizing enzymes contribute both to the bioactivation of carcinogens and to their detoxication in ways which are dependent on the carcinogen and the particular cell-type undergoing initiation. Polycyclic hydrocarbons initiate carcinogenesis through metabolism to bay-region dihydrodiol oxides (1). This requires a minimum sequence of three reactions consisting of primary mono-oxygenation, oxide-hydration and secondary mono-oxygenation (Fig. 1). An additional step, hydroxylation of the 7- or 12-methyl group of 7,12-dimethylbenzanthracene (DMBA), can precede formation of the 3,4-dihydrodiol 1,2-oxide (2). Carcinogens can be diverted from the activation sequence by (a) alternative mono-oxygenation reactions determined by regio- and stereospecificity of the participating P-450 cytochromes, (b) phenol rearrangement of the primary oxide, or (c) conjugation reactions.

Initiation of carcinogenesis frequently involves exposure to a low level of carcinogen that is fully metabolized. The effectiveness of a carcinogen in modifying DNA in a particular cell then depends upon the fraction passing through the activation pathway as compared to pathways leading to detoxication. Regioselectivity of mono-oxygenation depends on the forms of cytochrome P-450 and their relative amounts, while the remaining partitioning of metabolism is determined by the levels of the transferase enzymes and their cofactors. The fraction of carcinogen that ultimately modifies DNA is the product of the metabolic partition factors for each branching of the activation pathway (3).

At least eight forms of rat liver cytochrome P-450 have been purified (4,5), and the proportion of individual forms of P-450 in a cell is a function of the tissue (6) and the exposure to inducers. The regioselectivity and rate of metabolism of polycyclic hydrocarbons vary greatly between different forms of cytochrome P-450 and indeed can be used to characterize the individual forms. In addition, the proportion of metabolism directed towards the carcinogen activation pathway varies widely among hydrocarbons (1,3). This report compares the regioselectivity which

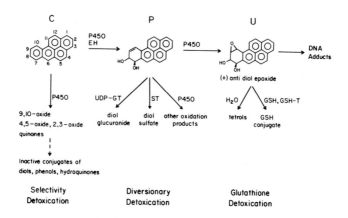

Fig. 1.   Partition of BP metabolism between the carcinogen activation pathway and detoxication pathways.

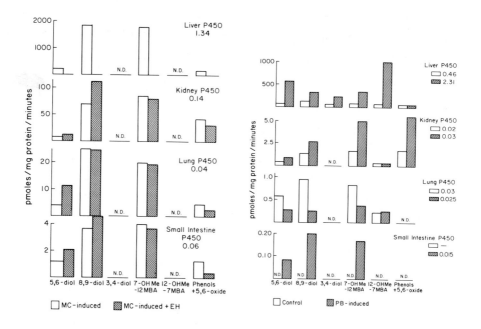

Fig. 2.   Regioselectivity of DMBA metabolism in microsomes from liver and extrahepatic tissues.

different forms of P-450 exhibit in primary and secondary metabolism of benzo(a)pyrene (BP) and DMBA. Both hepatic and extrahepatic rat microsomes and reconstituted vesicles containing purified forms of rat liver cytochrome P-450 were used as enzyme sources. A model for product inhibition of primary and secondary metabolism of BP has been developed and applied to the microsomal system.

The metabolic activity and regioselectivity for BP and DMBA of seven forms of rat liver cytochrome P-450 purified in this laboratory and of three types of microsomes are compared in Tables 1 and 2. While $P-450_c$ is the most active form in metabolizing both BP and DMBA, phenobarbital (PB)-induced $P-450_b$ and $P-450_e$ exhibit rates of DMBA metabolism that are several-fold larger than the corresponding rate of BP metabolism. This agrees with the relatively high rate of DMBA metabolism reported for PB-induced rat liver microsomes (7). BP and DMBA also differ with respect to the effect of inducers on the proportion of the compound passing through the activation pathway. 3-Methylcholanthrene (MC)-induction favors activation of BP, while PB favors detoxication. For DMBA, the reverse was observed; the 3,4-dihydrodiol is formed to a significant extent only in uninduced or PB-induced rat liver microsomes (7). Interestingly, only $P-450_a$ produces DMBA 3,4-dihydrodiol albeit in a a lower proportion than with control or PB-induced microsomes, where this form is only a minor constituent. A second inconsistency occurs for the selectivity between 7- and 12-hydroxylation. 7-Hydroxylation is favored in control and MC microsomes, while 12-hydroxylation is favored in PB microsomes (7). However, $P-450_e$ is the only purified form that produces this reverse selectivity, and again it is a low activity, minor constituent of PB microsomes. It is noteworthy that both hydrocarbons distinguish between $P-450_b$ and $P-450_e$, which possess almost identical antigenic determinants (4). While reconstitution of purified enzymes provides a good account of BP metabolism, major problems remain in understanding the regioselectivity of DMBA metabolism.

In extrahepatic tissues, the levels of cytochrome P-450 were lower than in liver (Fig. 2). The amounts of P-450 reductase and epoxide hydratase in microsomes from rat lung, kidney and small intestine were comparable in uninduced and PB-induced animals and were, respectively, 4- and 10-fold lower than in uninduced liver (see also ref. 8). In the extrahepatic tissues studied, BP and DMBA activities were low in control and PB-induced microsomes, whereas MC induction resulted in substantial increases in

TABLE 1

REGIOSELECTIVITY OF BP METABOLISM BY PURIFIED P-450 CYTOCHROMES

P-450	9,10- diol	4,5- diol	7,8- diol	1,6 Q	3,6 Q	9-OH	3-OH	Activity/ P-450 (min^{-1})
CON-MICS	17	28	14	11	37	18	34	0.7
PB-MICS	6.0	42	3.0	14	28	N.D.[a]	7.5	0.8
a	23	5.5	5.0	8.5	11	3.5	44	1.5
b	2.0	52	1.0	6.0	7.0	3.0	30	1.9
e	1.5	80	N.D.	7.0	5.0	N.D.	6.5	1.2
f	21	45	N.D.	N.D.	N.D.	N.D.	34	0.4
MC-MICS	31	12	17	5.5	15	7.5	13	3.5
c	33	17	15	8.5	12	2.5	13	58
d	23	23	8.0	11	16	4.5	16	0.7

[a] N.D. = not detected.

Microsomal incubations and product analysis by HPLC were carried out as described elsewhere (11). Reconstitutions of enzymes in sonicated vesicles contained 0.1 µM cytochrome P-450, 0.2 µM cytochrome P-450 reductase, 1 µM epoxide hydratase and 20 µg/ml of dilauroylphosphatidyl choline. The substrate concentration was 15 µM.

TABLE 2

REGIOSELECTIVITY OF DMBA METABOLISM BY PURIFIED P-450 CYTOCHROMES

P-450	5,6- diol	8,9- diol	3,4- diol	7HM- MBA	12HM- MBA	HMMBA Metabolite	Phenols	Activity/ P-450 (min^{-1})
CON-MICS	16	16	7.5	32	16	6.0	7.0	0.6
PB-MICS	24	13	7.5	10	23	22	2.0	0.75
a	7.0	8.0	2.0	71	8.5	3.5	N.D.[a]	1.5
b	32	8.5	0.1	33	20	6.0	1.0	9.8
e	18	4.0	0.1	22	46	7.5	N.D.	3.3
f	29	7.0	N.D.	33	31	N.D.	N.D.	0.4
MC-MICS	21	49	0.5	15	N.D.	6.5	8.0	2.3
c	22	28	0.5	30	N.D.	10	7.0	29
d	31	24	N.D.	26	1.5	7.5	10	0.8

[a] N.D. = not detected.

Conditions were as described under Table 1.

metabolism of both substrates; however, only MC kidney showed activity higher than uninduced liver. Regioselectivity in MC-induced extrahepatic microsomes (Table 3; Fig. 2) is typical of P-450$_c$ although formation of dihydrodiols and anti-DE is depressed by deficiency of epoxide hydratase, which is not induced by MC. This is particularly evident in kidney, while in lung a comparable level of epoxide hydratase activity (measured with styrene oxide) effected formation of a substantially higher proportion of dihydrodiols from both BP and DMBA. This suggests a more favorable relationship of P-450$_c$ and epoxide hydratase in the lung. When purified epoxide hydratase was added to MC-induced extrahepatic microsomes, the formation of DMBA 5,6-diol increased. These results support the conclusion that the enzyme is deficient in these microsomes (deficiency: kidney > intestine > lung).

The metabolism of DMBA is nearly fully inhibited in each set of MC-induced microsomes by anti-P-450$_c$ antibodies at 8 mg/nmole P-450 (lung 91%, small intestine 82%, kidney 98% inhibition). Anti-P-450$_c$ also strongly inhibits PB-induced kidney microsomes (88%), while anti-P-450$_b$ produces little inhibition (18%), suggesting that in this tissue PB acts as an inducer at the Ah-receptor. This is consistent with previous results for metabolism of R- and S-Warfarin by kidney microsomes (9). The uninduced lung exhibits regiospecificity for BP and DMBA similar to that of P-450$_b$, while PB induction appears to suppress this cytochrome and leave only P-450$_c$ activity.

Regio- and stereoselectivity at cytochrome P-450 plays an equally important role in the secondary activation of precursor dihydrodiols. MC microsomes and P-450$_c$ converted only 30% of (-)BP 7,8-dihydrodiol to the carcinogenic (+)anti-7,8-dihydrodiol 9,10-oxide (DE) when measured as the 7,10/8,9-tetrol. Since conjugation of dihydrodiols is very slow (10), this selectivity is by far the prime determinant of the partition of metabolism at this step in the pathway. This regioselectivity remains unknown for DMBA 3,4-dihydrodiol although we find that the dominant metabolite formed with MC microsomes is 7HMMBA 3,4-dihydrodiol.

Competition between primary and secondary substrates and the inhibition of both primary and secondary metabolism by other metabolites inevitably must both play important roles in the kinetics of polycyclic hydrocarbon activation. These effects are made apparent by the following features of the kinetics of BP activation by rat liver microsomes (11): (a) BP metabolism declines from linearity after 30-40% metabolism (Fig. 3a);

454

TABLE 3

METABOLISM OF BENZO(A)PYRENE IN LIVER AND EXTRAHEPATIC MICROSOMES[a,b]

	anti-DE[c]	Diols			Quinones		Phenols		Total (nmoles)
		9,10	4,5	7,8	1,6	3,6	9	3	
Liver									
CON, 30'	19[c]	200	350	100	80	200	85	310	1.3
Lung									
CON, 60'	N.D.[d]	3.0	6.0	3.0	3.0	3.0	5.0	10	.03
PB, 60'	N.D.	2.5	3.0	6.5	2.5	6.0	3.0	35	.06
MC, 45'	N.D.	130	190	80	45	105	470	400	1.4
90'	18	170	180	170	70	190	500	700	2.0
Kidney									
CON, 60'	N.D.	2.0	10	10	30	70	100	40	.26
PB, 60'	N.D.	1.5	3.5	6.5	20	50	100	65	.25
MC, 10'	N.D.	50	25	75	65	145	420	580	1.4
45'	12	34	20	100	30	140	240	1040	1.6
Intestine									
PB, 60'	N.D.	N.D.	2.5	5.0	13	7.5	20	13	.06
MC, 45'	N.D.	20	50	35	30	60	125	200	.52
90'	1.7	50	90	95	40	60	180	250	.76

[a] 5 μM BP were incubated with 1 mg/ml microsomal protein.
[b] Activities expressed as pmoles/mg.
[c] Measured as 7,10/8,9-tetrol.
[d] N.D. = not detected.

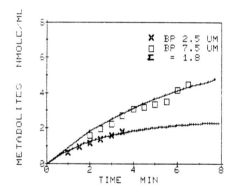
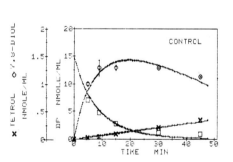

Fig. 3. (a) Nonlinearity of time course for BP metabolism at two concentrations of BP; (b) Time courses for disappearance of BP and formation of 7,8-dihydrodiol and anti-DE (as tetrols). Time course curves were generated to fit the data using experimental values for V, V_D, K_S, K_D and J_D with the best fit values for Σ amd Σ'. Curves were generated on a 48K-Apple II Plus Computer using the method described in the text as a subroutine in the "Scientific Plotter" program, Interactive Microware, Inc.

(b) The onset of the metabolism of 7,8-dihydrodiol to anti-DE is delayed until most of the BP has been metabolized (Fig. 3b). The delay increases as the initial BP concentration is increased; (c) The maximum rate of anti-DE formation reaches only 5% of the rate of metabolism that is reached with the peak concentration of 7,8-dihydrodiol in the absence of BP or metabolites; (d) The addition to microsomes of either UDPGA to activate glucuronyl transferase or of a partially purified sulfotransferase preparation and PAPS results in the removal of inhibitory products. As a consequence, the period of linearity of BP metabolism increases, and the rate of formation of anti-DE and its DNA adduct is enhanced 4-fold. In all experiments, approximately one adduct was formed for every ten anti-DE synthesized (11).

The kinetics of formation of anti-DE from BP are determined by the combined inhibitory effects of (a) all metabolites on primary metabolism, and (b) BP and other metabolites on 7,8-dihydrodiol metabolism. The inhibition of both BP and 7,8-dihydrodiol metabolism by other metabolites has been directly determined. Inhibition is competitive in all cases except with BP 6,12-quinone, which inhibits non-competitively and is not a substrate for $P-450_c$ (12). A marked feature of the inhibition data (Table 4) is the consistently greater sensitivity of 7,8-dihydrodiol metabolism to inhibition. BP phenols were examined for inhibition of BP metabolism by $P-450_c$. It was found that the inhibitory effectiveness of these derivatives correlated closely with their strength of interaction with the heme, as determined by spectral analysis. The combined inhibitory effects of metabolites are measured by two factors, Σ and Σ', which are determined from the fraction of each metabolite formed and from its inhibition constant. The calculated Σ and Σ' values for metabolism of BP and 7,8-dihydrodiol equal 0.5 and 8.0, respectively (Table 4). In each case, the dominant inhibitory effect is due to 1,6- and 3,6-quinone. Both are removed by either glucuronidation or sulfation, which then greatly lowers Σ and Σ'. Product inhibition will also be lowered by any cell constituent that sequesters products, particularly the highly inhibitory quinones. While this may be expected of proteins, DNA exerts a surprising stimulatory effect on BP metabolism, which has been shown to derive from the extremely strong binding of BP quinones to DNA (13).

We have simulated the time course for BP metabolism and anti-DE formation using the Michaelis-Menten equation in differential form with competitive product inhibition. The terms for inhibitor concentration and K_i were replaced by Σ and Σ'; a detailed description of the procedure

TABLE 4

PRODUCT INHIBITION OF BENZO(A)PYRENE AND 7,8-DIOL METABOLISM

Compound	Fraction from BP F	Inhibition of BP Metabolism K_i [μM]	F/K_i [μM^{-1}]	Inhibition of 7,8-Diol Metabolism K'_i [μM]	F/K'_i [μM^{-1}]
9,10-Diol	0.32	30	0.01	8	0.04
4,5-Diol	0.11	5	0.02	0.8	0.14
7,8-Diol	0.14	1.4[a]	0.10	-	-
1,6-Quinone	0.05	0.3	0.17	0.03	5.7
3,6-Quinone	0.10	1	0.10	0.1	1.0
9-Phenol	0.09	1	0.09	0.1	0.90
3-Phenol	0.19	10	0.02	0.7	0.27
BP	-	-	-	1.5	-
			$\Sigma = 0.51$[b]		$\Sigma' = 8.02$[c]

[a] W.E. Fahl, Arch. Biochem. Biophys., 216, 581 (1982).
[b] The Σ value is the sum of all F/K_i fractions.
[c] The Σ' value is the sum of all F/K'_i fractions.

will be presented elsewhere (14). The observed steady state for 7,8-dihydrodiol was lower than predicted from the calculated Σ factors (Table 4). A close fit to the experimental time courses was obtained if Σ was elevated 3.6-fold, while Σ' for 7,8-dihydrodiol metabolism was maintained at the value obtained by direct measurement of inhibition (Fig. 3b). The rate of anti-DE formation was little affected by the elevation of Σ, which indicates that inhibition by BP and the value of Σ' are its major determinants. Since Σ factors depend on the proportions of metabolites, they are a function of the form of cytochrome P-450 and the relative level of epoxide hydratase. The quantitative kinetic model predicting the time-dependent change in primary and secondary metabolites is then applicable to MC-induced extrahepatic microsomes.

Metabolism of DMBA presents a further set of problems from those found for BP. First, the bay-region trans-3,4-dihydrodiol 1,2-oxides can be formed with prior hydroxylation of 7- and 12-positions. As noted above, mono-oxygenation at the methyl group occurs extensively with a selectivity that depends on the form of cytochrome P-450. The extent of formation of hydroxymethyl dihydrodiol oxides depends again to a large degree on the effectiveness of competition between primary metabolism and further mono-oxygenation of 7- and 12HMMBA. The effectiveness of this competition

TABLE 5

INHIBITION OF HEPATIC MICROSOMAL DMBA METABOLISM (15 μM)

Inhibitor (15 μM)	Control $K_i \times 10^{-6}$ M	PB-Induced $K_i \times 10^{-6}$ M	MC-Induced $K_i \times 10^{-6}$ M
7HMMBA	6.2	2.8	1.5
12HMMBA	10.3	2.5	2.0
K_m for DMBA $\times 10^{-6}$ M	15.0	9.5	8.0

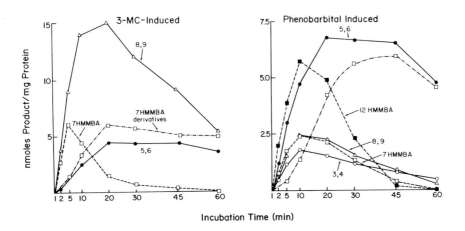

Fig. 4. Time course for DMBA metabolism in MC- and PB-induced rat liver microsomes. Conditions were as described in Table 1. The unlabelled curve in 4b represents 7HMMBA derivatives.

can be seen in two ways. The extent of cross-inhibition indicates that these primary metabolites bind tighter than DMBA to P-450$_c$ in MC-induced microsomes (Table 5). The time course of product formation in liver MC microsomes confirms this preference since 7HMMBA peaks very early in the reaction (Fig. 4), indicating rapid further metabolism in the presence of a large excess of DMBA. DMBA primary metabolism also declines rapidly from linearity, probably due to preferred metabolism of 7HMMBA. 7-Hydroxymethyl dihydrodiols can be formed either by methyl hydroxylation of primary dihydrodiol metabolites or by ring oxygenation of 7HMMBA. Careful analysis of the ratio of 7HMMBA dihydrodiols indicates that in uninduced microsomes, they are predominantly derived from 7HMMBA. Interestingly, MC microsomes produce large amounts of 7HMMBA 10,11-dihydrodiol, even though DMBA or

7HMMBA directly form only very small amounts of 10,11-dihydrodiol. This suggests that secondary oxygenation of 7HMMBA during DMBA metabolism occurs with altered regioselectivity.

Studies presented here indicate that in extrahepatic rat tissues metabolism of polycyclic hydrocarbons derives largely from metabolism by $P-450_c$, and that low levels of epoxide hydrase limit dihydrodiol formation in these tissues. Comparable modification of DNA by DE during metabolism of, respectively, BP and DMBA in the rat tissues suggests that DMBA:DE partitions almost quantitatively towards adduct formation in order to offset the adverse regioselectivity for DMBA:DE formation (3). Studies of the metabolism of both BP and DMBA in the mouse epidermis suggest that regioselectivity is more favorable to DE formation in this target tissue (15). Work presented here also emphasizes that changes in regioselectivity caused by inductive effects of a carcinogen may have an important bearing on carcinogenesis experiments.

REFERENCES

1. Conney, A.H. (1982) Cancer Res., 4, 4875.

2. Joyce, N.J. and Daniel, F.B. (1982) Carcinogenesis, 3, 297.

3. Jefcoate, C.R. (1983) in: Jakoby, W.B. (Ed.), Enzymatic Basis of Detoxication, Vol. 3, Academic Press, New York, pp. 31-76.

4. Ryan, D.E., Thomas, P.E. and Levin, W. (1982) Xenobiotica, 12, 727.

5. Guengerich, F.P., Dannan, G.A. and Kaminsky, L.S. (1982) Xenobiotica, 12, 701.

6. Guengerich, F.P. and Mason, P.S. (1979) Mol. Pharmacol., 15, 156.

7. Chou, M.W., Yang, S.K. and Yang, C.S. (1981) Cancer Res., 41, 1559.

8. Vainio, H. and Hietanen, E. (1980) in: Jenner, P. and Testa, B. (Eds.), Concepts in Drug Metabolism, Part A, Marcel Dekker, New York, pp. 251-284.

9. Kaminsky, L.S., Fasco, M.J. and Guengerich, F.P. (1979) J. Biol. Chem., 254, 9657.

10. Nemoto, N., Takayama, S. and Gelboin, H.V. (1978) Chem. Biol. Interact., 23, 19.

11. Keller, G.M., Turner, C.R. and Jefcoate, C.R. (1982) Mol. Pharmacol., 22, 451.

12. Shen, A.L., Fahl, W.E. and Jefcoate, C.R. (1979) Cancer Res., 39, 4123.

13. Keller, G.M. and Jefcoate, C.R. (1983) Mol. Pharmacol., In press.

14. Keller, G.M. and Jefcoate, C.R. (1983) Manuscript in preparation.

15. DiGiovanni, J., Fischer, S., Slaga, T.J. and Boutwell, R.K. (1980) Carcinogenesis, 1, 41.

© 1983 Elsevier Science Publishers B.V.
Extrahepatic Drug Metabolism and Chemical Carcinogenesis,
J. Rydström, J. Montelius and M. Bengtsson eds.

IN VIVO METABOLISM OF BENZO(A)PYRENE: FORMATION AND DISAPPEARANCE OF BP-
METABOLITE-DNA ADDUCTS IN EXTRAHEPATIC TISSUES VERSUS LIVER

MARSHALL W. ANDERSON AND JOHN R. BEND
Laboratory of Pharmacology, National Institute of Environmental Health Sciences,
National Institutes of Health, P.O. Box 12233, Research Triangle Park, North
Carolina 27709 (U.S.A.)

INTRODUCTION

There is compelling evidence that a large number of mutagens and carcinogens
are able to react with cellular DNA either directly or following metabolic activation to reactive metabolites. If DNA replication proceeds on such a modified
template before altered bases or nucleotides are removed by enzymic repair processes, DNA damage may be genetically fixed. Thus, the extent of carcinogen-
induced promutagenic DNA damage and the capacity of cells to repair such damage
represent critical events in the initiation of carcinogenesis. Polycyclic aromatic hydrocarbons (PAH) such as benzo(a)pyrene (BP) represents a class of
ubiquitous environmental carcinogens. Thus, we have examined the *in vivo* formation and removal of BP metabolite-DNA adducts in target and non-target tissues for BP-mediated neoplasia.

Characterization of *in vivo* BP metabolite-DNA adduct formation. The *in vivo*
formation of BP metabolite-DNA adducts has been examined in various strains and
tissues of mice. As an example, the BP metabolite-DNA binding profiles in lung
and liver of A/HeJ mice 48 hr after an oral dose of BP are shown in Figure 1,
a typical HPLC analysis for BP metabolite-deoxyribonucleoside adducts. Four
peaks were observed in each tissue and in each mouse strain. Peaks II and III
have been previously identified (1) as (-)-7β,8α-dihydroxy-9α,10α-epoxy-7,8,9,-
10-tetrahydrobenzo(a)pyrene (BPDEI)-dGuo, and (+)-BPDEI-dGuo, respectively.
Peak IV was identified as a 7β,8α-dihydroxy-9β,10β-epoxy-7,8,9,10-tetrahydro-
benzo(a)pyrene (BPDEII)-dGuo adduct. Peak I could be either a BP-phenol-oxide-
DNA adduct or a BPDEI-dCyd adduct. In addition to peaks I-IV, uncharacterized
radioactivity eluted in the water fraction (WF) and early in the methanol:wat-
er gradient (1, 2).

In the studies with mice, the *in vivo* binding profiles of BP metabolites to
DNA in all tissues of all strains examined are very similar to those observed
in Figure 1 (see reference 3 for review). The predominant adduct is BPDEI-dGuo
but a BPDEII-dGuo adduct is also observed as well as an adduct corresponding
to peak I (Figure 1). There is also evidence for BPDE-dAdo adducts, although
in relatively small amounts. From the limited data available, it appears that

460

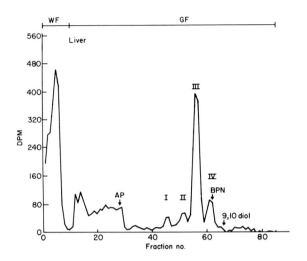

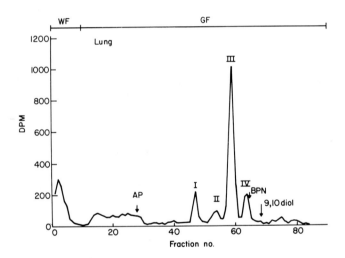

Figure 1. HPLC of BP metabolite:deoxyribonucleoside adducts in lung and liver of A/HeJ mice. Mice were killed 48 hr after a p.o. dose of [^{3}H]-BP (1351 μmol/kg). DNA isolated from these tissues was enzymatically digested and the deoxyribonucleosides were chromatographed on HPLC. WF and GF denote the water and gradient fractions, respectively. Peaks II, III, and IV have been identified as (-)-BPDEI-dGuo, (+)-BPDEI-dGuo, and BPDEII-dGuo, respectively. See text for discussion of peak I.

the *in vivo* adduct binding profiles for other PAH's such as 3-MC and DMBA, are also independent of tissue and mouse strain.

In contrast, the types of BP metabolite-DNA adducts formed are very species-dependent. The predominant adduct formed *in vivo* in lung and liver of the Sprague-Dawley rat is chromatographically identical with peak I (Figure 1) and probably results from the interaction of 9-hydroxy-BP-4,5-oxide with DNA (4). The BPDEI adducts were not detected in rat liver, and only relatively small amounts were observed in lung (3.3% of peak I). Thus, the *in vivo* BP metabolite-DNA adduct profiles obtained in lung and liver of Sprague-Dawley rats are distinctly different from those observed in various mouse strains. This is the only known case in which the BPDE adducts are not the predominant BP metabolite-DNA adducts formed *in vivo*.

In an examination of BP metabolite-DNA adduct profiles in lung and liver of male New Zealand rabbits, BP was administered either orally or i.p. at various doses (5). The DNA adduct profiles were identical with those in mice with one notable difference: in rabbits, the amount of the BPDEII-dGuo adduct was approximately 75% of the BPDEI-dGuo adduct, whereas in mice, there was only 10% as much of the BPDEII adduct as of the BPDEI adduct. This is the only known case *in vivo* in which the BPDEII-deoxyguanosine adduct approaches the BPDEI adduct in amount. The cause of these species differences in adduct profiles is unknown at present but may reflect differences in the hepatic and extrahepatic distribution of various cytochrome P-450 isozymes in the species.

Comparison of extent of *in vivo* BP metabolite-DNA adduct formation between tissues. The specific activities (SA) (pmol per mg DNA) of BPDE-DNA adducts in lung and liver of various mouse strains and New Zealand rabbits are given in Table 1. The amounts of BPDE adducts formed in lung and liver are very similar for each study. Adriaenssens *et al.* (6) examined the BPDE adducts in lung and liver of A/HeJ mice with oral doses of BP ranging from 2 to 1351 µmol/kg and found that the SA of the adducts in lung and liver are similar over the entire BP dose range. Also, the SA of the BPDE adducts in forestomach are very similar to those in lung and liver after oral administration of BP (6-8). The similarity of the amount of BPDE adducts in lung, liver and forestomach is rather surprising, inasmuch as the disposition and rate of metabolism of BP in these tissues are probably very dissimilar.

In a recent study, we examined the extent of adduct formation in various tissues of A/HeJ mice after an oral dose of BP (6 mg per mouse) (5). The levels of these adducts 48 hr after BP treatment were 5.8, 5.8, 5.8, 3.9, 3.2, 3.2, and 3.0 in liver, lung, forestomach, kidney, brain, muscle, and colon,

TABLE 1

FORMATION *IN VIVO* OF BPDE-DNA ADDUCTS IN LUNG AND LIVER OF MICE

Mouse Strain	Tissue	Dose[a] mg/mg	Route	Specific Activity of BPDE-DNA Adducts[b] pmol/mg of DNA	Reference
A/HeJ	Lung	240	P.O.	6.97	9
A/HeJ	Liver	240	P.O.	6.02	9
A/HeJ	Lung	4.8	P.O.	1.68	9
A/HeJ	Liver	4.8	P.O.	0.98	9
ICR/Ha	Lung	240	P.O.	0.42	7
ICR/Ha	Liver	240	P.O.	0.44	7
C57BL/6J	Lung	240	P.O.	5.80	9
C57BL/6J	Liver	240	P.O.	3.50	9
A/J	Lung	0.5	I.V.	0.14, 0.09	18
A/J	Liver	0.5	I.V.	0.10, 0.08	18

[a]Mice assumed to weigh 25 g.
[b]Values represent sums of BPDEI and BPDEII adducts. Adducts determined 48 hr after [^{3}H]-BP dose, except for studies in A/J mice, in which first value is 4 hr after I.V. dose and second is 24 hr after dose. Average of at least two determinations.

respectively. In contrast, there was a marked variation between these tissues in the binding of BP metabolites to protein, the protein binding in liver being 35-times greater than the binding in muscle. These results show that the metabolic capacity of a tissue does not correlate well with the BPDE-DNA adduct levels in the tissue and thus, the transport of BPDE between tissues (cells) may be involved in the *in vivo* formation of BPDE-DNA adducts.

The SAs for the *in vivo* studies reported in Table 1 are calculated on the basis of total DNA in the organ. As the values for the BPDE adducts are not different in lung and liver they do not appear to offer an explanation for the susceptibility of the lung and the resistance of the liver to BP-induced neoplasia in, for example, A/HeJ and A/J mice. However, the amounts of adducts formed in different cell types may vary considerably. This may be an important consideration for organs, such as the lung, that contain a multitude of cell types. Examination of BP adducts in individual cell types might allow differentiation with respect to susceptibility and resistance to PAH-induced neoplasia, although the results discussed in the preceding paragraph obviously complicate this suggestion.

Persistence of BP metabolite-DNA adducts. The mutation and malignant transformation of cells by chemicals may be a consequence of DNA synthesis on parent-strand templates containing unexcised chemically induced lesions. Thus,

the relative persistence of carcinogen-DNA adducts in tissues may be an important consideration in determining organ-specific carcinogenesis.

We examined the persistence of BP metabolite-DNA adducts in lung and liver of
A/HeJ and C57BL/6J mice after a dose of BP (6 mg/mouse) which induces pulmonary
adenomas in A/HeJ mice but not in C57BL/6J mice (9). The disappearance of
BPDEI adduct in A/HeJ mice followed first order kinetics over the time period
examined (28 days), with a half-life of 18 and 9 days in lung and liver, respectively. The decay of this adduct in C57BL/6J mice was biphasic in both
tissues. It should be noted that the *in vivo* disappearance of adducts can be
due to normal DNA turnover without involving any enzymatic excision repair.
Our data on cell turnover suggested that normal DNA turnover can explain the
disappearance of adducts in lung of A/HeJ mice and lung and liver of C57BL/6J
mice, but not in liver of A/HeJ mice. We are currently examining DNA repair
synthesis in liver and lung of mice exposed to BP by measuring unscheduled
DNA synthesis.

Our data on formation and persistence of BP metabolite-DNA adducts and on
cell turnover rates offer no explanation for the strain difference in susceptibility to BP-induced pulmonary adenomas (9). In fact, the data suggest that
the adducts may be more persistent in lungs of the resistant C57BL/6J strain
than in the susceptible A/HeJ strain. Phillips *et al.* (10) and Pelkonen *et al.*
(11) also concluded that the extent of formation and persistence of PAH metabolite-DNA adducts could not explain the strain difference in susceptibility to
PAH-induced neoplasia in skin and subcutaneous tissue. In contrast, Eastman and
Bresnick (2) reported that the persistence of 3-MC metabolite-DNA adducts in
mouse lung correlated with susceptibility of the various mouse strains to 3-MC-
induced pulmonary adenomas. The reasons for the discrepancy between the results of Eastman and Bresnick (2) and the other studies is unclear at present.

Dose-response relationships for binding of BP metabolites to DNA and protein.
Since tumor studies themselves are usually not practical at low doses of a carcinogen, the examination of the dose dependency of pertinent biochemical parameters, i.e., adduct formation, is one way to attempt to extrapolate carcinogenic effects to low doses (12). Adriaenssens *et al.* (6) examined the dose dependency of BP metabolite-DNA adduct levels in lung, liver, and forestomach of A/
HeJ mice following oral doses of BP (2 to 1350 µmol/kg). In lung and liver,
the dose response curves for BPDEI-dGuo adducts were sigmoidal. To compare
protein binding (covalent) and DNA binding of BP metabolites, we plotted the
ratio of BPDEI adduct levels and protein binding levels to BP dose against BP
dose (Figure 2). If a dose response curve is sigmoidal, a plot of the ratio of

the response (adduct levels) to dose against dose gives the type of curves seen in Figure 2 for BPDEI adduct levels in lung and liver. This ratio for BPDEI adduct levels in lung and liver increased rapidly as the dose increased from 2 to 270 μmol/kg, suggesting that the activation of BP to BPDEI increases more rapidly then the inactivation processes in this dose range. The ratios tended to decrease with further increases in dose which is consistent with saturation of the DNA binding in lung and liver. In contrast, there was no indication of saturation of BPDEI-dGuo adduct levels in forestomach.

Pereira *et al.* (13) found a linear relationship between BP dose and the formation of BPDE-DNA adducts in mouse skin following topical applications of BP in doses ranging from 0.01 to 300 μg per mouse. In the study by Adriaenssens *et al.* (6), the dose response curve in forestomach was more linear than the curve for lung and liver. The forestomach was directly exposed to BP in this study just as the skin was in the study by Pereira *et al.* (13). Phillips *et al.* (10) examined the dose-response relationship for DMBA metabolite-DNA adducts in skin after topical application of doses from 0.025 to 1.0 μmol DMBA per mouse. They found that DMBA metabolite-DNA adduct levels in skin varied nonlinearly with dose. However, in each of these studies the dose-response relationship for PAH metabolite-DNA adducts approached linearity at low doses and thus, there does not appear to be a threshold dose below which binding of PAH metabolites to DNA does not occur.

Adriaenssens *et al.* (6) also examined the specific activities (pmol/mg protein) of the binding of BP metabolites to protein of lung, liver, and forestomach as a function of BP dose (Figure 2). In lung the dose-response curve for protein binding is similar to that for BPDEI-dGuo binding whereas in liver the protein binding curve is distinctly different from that for DNA adducts. In liver, the proportion of BP which binds to protein increases rapidly at higher doses. This suggests that the rate of formation of reactive metabolites of BP which bind to protein increases with dose relative to the ability of liver cells to detoxify them. Thus, the dose dependency of the binding of specific metabolites to DNA, i.e., BPDEI, can be very different than the binding of total reactive metabolites to protein.

Effect of AHH inducers and phenolic antioxidants on BP metabolite-DNA adduct formation. The effect of AHH inducers on the *in vivo* binding of BP to DNA has been examined in several tissues of various mouse strains (Table 2). AHH inducers almost completely inhibit *in vivo* BPDE-DNA adduct formation in every tissue of each mouse strain examined. In this respect, the effects of AHH inducers on BPDE adduct formation *in vivo* contrast markedly with their effects

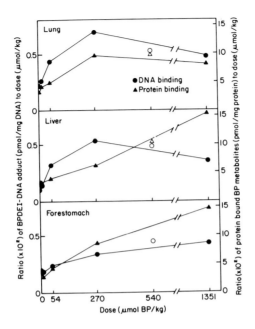

<u>Figure 2</u>. Comparison of dose dependency of binding of BP metabolites to DNA with the binding to protein in lung and liver. On left ordinate is the ratio of BPDEI-dGuo adduct levels to dose (●) and on the right ordinate is the ratio of protein binding levels of BP metabolites to dose (▲).

in vitro, i.e., in microsomes, isolated perfused organs, tissue slices, and hepatocytes. Treatment of animals with AHH inducers stimulates the formation of BPDE adducts *in vitro* (see Wilson *et al*. (14) for references). The reason(s) for the disparity between the *in vivo* and *in vitro* results for BPDE adduct formation is unclear at present.

Induction of AHH has been postulated as a mechanism for the anti-carcinogenic action of a wide variety of compounds (3). In studies by Wilson *et al*. (14) and Cohen *et al*. (15), adduct levels were determined under conditions known to result in inhibition of BP-induced neoplasia by AHH inducers. Their results suggest that AHH inducers, such as β-NF and TCDD, inhibit BP-induced neoplasia by reducing the amounts of BPDE-DNA adducts formed in the target tissue. Whether the prior induction of AHH in the target tissue and/or liver is part of the protective mechanism of AHH inducers against BP-induced neoplasia requires further investigation.

Phenolic antioxidants such as BHA, BHT, and ethoxyquin can also inhibit the induction of tumors in rodents by a variety of carcinogens including BP. Anderson *et al.* (1) and Ioannou *et al.* (7, 8) have shown that dietary BHA inhibits the *in vivo* formation of BPDE-DNA adducts in the lung and forestomach of mice to the same degree that BP-induced neoplasia is inhibited in these tissues by BHA. Recently, Adriaenssens *et al.* (6) showed that dietary BHA inhibits BP metabolite-DNA adduct formation over an oral BP dose range from 2 to 1350 μmol/kg and that the inhibition of adduct was dose dependent in lung and liver but not in forestomach. The results of this study suggest that BHA will inhibit the neoplastic effects of BP at low doses of the carcinogen. Several mechanisms have been proposed to explain the anti-carcinogenic effects of BHA (see references 3, 6, 16 and 17 for discussion). The data from Adriaenssens *et al.* (6), Wattenberg *et al.* (16), and Dock *et al.* (17) are consistent with the hypothesis that dietary BHA shifts the metabolism of BP-7,8-diol to products other than BPDE.

TABLE 2

EFFECT OF AHH INDUCERS ON *IN VIVO* FORMATION OF BPDE-DNA ADDUCTS IN MICE

Strain	Treatment		Tissue	Specific Activity (pmol/mg of DNA) of BPDE-DNA Adducts in Treated Mice % of Control[a]
A/HeJ	β-NF[b]	(Group A)	Lung	15
A/HeJ	β-NF	(Group A)	Liver	0[c]
A/HeJ	β-NF	(Group B)	Lung	8
A/HeJ	β-NF	(Group B)	Liver	0
A/HeJ	TCDD		Lung	5
A/HeJ	TCDD[d]		Liver	0
A/HeJ	Aroclor 1254		Lung	9
A/HeJ	Aroclor 1254		Liver	0
ICR/Ha	β-NF		Lung	16
ICR/Ha	β-NF		Liver	7
ICR/Ha	β-NF		Forestomach	16
Sencar	TCDD		Skin	0
CD-1	TCDD		Skin	0

[a]Data for A/HeJ mice from Wilson *et al.* (14). Data for ICR/Ha mice from Ioannou *et al.* (7). Data for Sencar and CD-1 mice from Cohen *et al.* (15).
[b]β-naphthoflavone.
[c]Zero means adducts were not detected in treated animals.
[d]2,3,7,8-tetrachlorodibenzo-*p*-dioxin.

These studies demonstrate that the relationships between BP metabolism and DNA alkylation *in vivo* are complex. Current investigations are focused on understanding these relationships and the removal of BP metabolite-DNA adducts at the cellular level, especially in lung.

REFERENCES

1. Anderson, M.W., Boroujerdi, M. and Wilson, A.G.E. (1981) Cancer Res., 41, 4309-4315.

2. Eastman, A. and Bresnick, E. (1979) Cancer Res., 39, 2400-2405.

3. National Research Council, Committee on Pyrene and Selected Analogues. Report on "Polycyclic Aromatic Hydrocarbons: Evaluation of Sources and Effects." Chapter 5, Effective Biologic Dose, Washington, D.C., National Academy Press (1983).

4. Boroujerdi, M., Kung, H.C., Wilson, A.G.E. and Anderson, M.W. (1981) Cancer Res., 41, 951-957.

5. Stowers, J.S. and Anderson, M.W. Unpublished data.

6. Adriaenssens, P.I., White, C.M. and Anderson, M.W. Cancer Res., in press.

7. Ioannou, Y.M., Wilson, A.G.E. and Anderson, M.W. (1982) Cancer Res., 42, 1199-1205.

8. Ioannou, Y.M., Wilson, A.G.E. and Anderson, M.W. (1982) Carcinogenesis, 3, 739-745.

9. Kulkarni, M. and Anderson, M.W. Unpublished data.

10. Phillips, D.H., Grover, P.L. and Sims, P. (1978) Int. J. Cancer, 22, 487-494.

11. Pelkonen, O., Boobis, A.R., Yagi, H., Jerina, D.M. and Nebert, D.W. (1978) Mol. Pharmacol., 14, 306-322.

12. Hoel, D.G., Kaplan, N.L., Anderson, M.W. (1983) Science, 219, 1032-1037.

13. Pereira, M.A., Burns, F.A. and Albert, R.E. (1979) Cancer Res., 39, 2556-2559.

14. Wilson, A.G.E., Kung, H.C., Boroujerdi, M. and Anderson, M.W. (1981) Cancer Res., 41, 3453-3460.

15. Cohen, G.M., Bracken, W.M., Iyer, R.P., Berry, D.L., Selkirk, J.K, and Slaga, T.J. (1979). Cancer Res., 39, 4027-4033.

16. Wattenberg, L.W., Jerina, D.M., Lam, L.K.T. and Yagi, H. (1979) J. Natl. Cancer Inst., 62, 1103-1106.

17. Dock, L., Cha, Y.-N., Jernstrom, B. and Moldeus, P. (1982) Chem.-Biol. Interactions, 41, 25-38.

18. Eastman, A., Sweetenham, J. and Bresnick, E. (1978) Chem.-Biol. Interact., 23, 345-353.

© 1983 Elsevier Science Publishers B.V.
Extrahepatic Drug Metabolism and Chemical Carcinogenesis,
J. Rydström, J. Montelius and M. Bengtsson eds.

SPECTROSCOPIC STUDIES OF BENZO(a)PYRENE-7,8-DIHYDRODIOL-9,10-
EPOXIDES COVALENTLY BOUND TO DNA

BENGT JERNSTRÖM[1], PER-OLOF LYCKSELL[2], ASTRID GRÄSLUND[2], ANDERS
EHRENBERG[2] AND BENGT NORDÉN[3]

[1]Department of Forensic Medicine, Karolinska Institutet, Box
60400, S-104 01 Stockholm, [2]Department of Biophysics, University
of Stockholm, Arrhenius Laboratory, S-106 91 Stockholm and
[3]Department of Physical Chemistry, Chalmers University of
Technology, S-412 96 Göteborg (Sweden)

INTRODUCTION

The polycyclic aromatic hydrocarbon benzo(a)pyrene (BP) is carcinogenic after metabolic activation to electrophilic intermediates that subsequently react with cellular constituents. Among
these, DNA is believed to be the most significant target. Of particular relevance regarding BP carcinogenesis is the formation of
syn- and anti-isomers of benzo(a)pyrene-7,8-dihydrodiol-9,10-
epoxide (BPDE). (For a comprehensive review, see ref. 1.)

Figure 1 summarizes some essential steps in the metabolic activation of BP to BPDE. BP is first epoxidized at the 7,8-double
bond by cytochrome P-450 linked monooxygenases and subsequently
hydrolysed by epoxidehydrolase to predominantly (-)-trans BP-7,8-
dihydrodiol. A second epoxidation at the 9,10 position results in
the formation of the BPDE isomers, anti- and syn-BPDE, respectively. The former isomer is preferentially formed and constitutes
about 90% of BPDE formed by rat liver microsomes (1). Both syn-
and anti-BPDE bind to DNA and exhibit biological activity (1)
although the latter, and in particular the (+)-enantiomer, has
been shown to be the most active form (2,3). (+)-Anti-BPDE also
exhibits a higher affinity for DNA than the (-)-analog and binds
more specifically to the exocyclic amino group of deoxyriboguanosine (4,5). Although the ultimate DNA damage required to initiate
the carcinogenic process is not known at present, recent data
however indicate an essential role for deoxyriboguanosine modification (6,7). In order to understand the molecular mechanisms un-

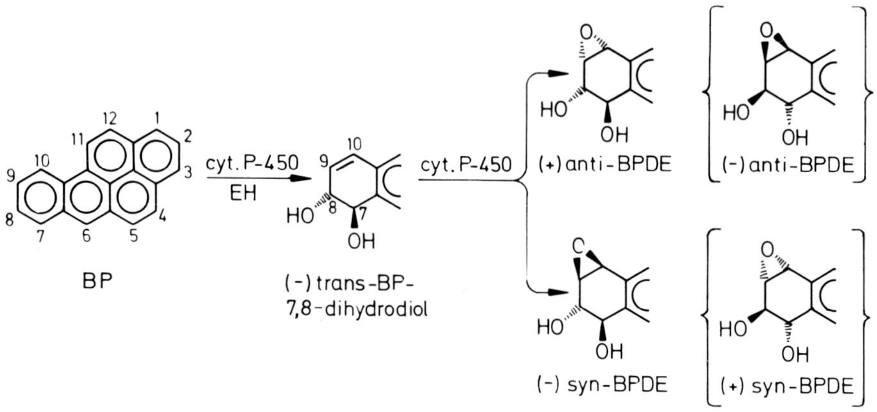

Fig. 1. Microsomal activation of benzo(a)pyrene to benzo(a)-
pyrene-7,8-dihydrodiol-9,10-epoxides. BP, benzo(a)pyrene; EH,
epoxidehydrolase; BPDE, benzo(a)pyrene-7,8-dihydrodiol-9,10-
epoxide.

derlying chemical carcinogenesis one has to identify not only the
ultimate reactive electrophilic intermediates and the appropriate
DNA-targets but also the structures of the resulting complexes
and their possible alterations of normal DNA conformation.

Previous studies on the major bound component from racemic
anti-BPDE have led to suggestions that it is localized outside
the DNA helix with the pyrene-like chromophore in the minor grove
(8), or forms a classical intercalation type complex (9) or results in a wedge-shaped intercalated complex (10). In a previous
study we compared the DNA complexes of racemic anti- and syn-
BPDE in order to reveal possible structural differences to explain
their great difference in tumour initiating activity (11). In this
paper results from our previous work together with recent preliminary findings regarding structural differences of the DNA complexes formed after reaction with the highly carcinogenic (+)- and the
less carcinogenic (-)-enantiomer of anti-BPDE will be discussed.

MATERIALS AND METHODS

Incubations. ^{3}H-labelled or non-labelled racemic syn- or anti-
BPDE or individual enantiomers of anti-BPDE was reacted with calf
thymus DNA for 1 hr at 37°C. One ml of the reaction mixture contained 1 mg DNA, 100-500 nmoles of BPDE in 25 μl dimethylsulfoxide
and 10 μmoles sodium cacodylate adjusted to pH 7.0 with HNO_3.

Extraction of the samples to remove non-covalently bound BPDE
was carried out as previously described (11). Absorption spectra
were recorded on a Cary 219 spectrophotometer and fluorescence
spectra on a Shimadzu RF 510 spectrofluorometer. Linear dichroism
(LD) spectra of flow oriented BPDE-DNA were measured in a Couette
cell on a Jasco 3500 CD spectrometer as described (11).

RESULTS AND DISCUSSION

Table 1 summarizes some experimental properties of DNA-complex-
es derived from racemic anti- and syn-BPDE, respectively. According to the nomenclature of Geacintov *et al.* (12) two spectral
types of complexes can be distinguished; type I with light absorption and fluorescence excitation maxima at 322, 337 and 354 and
type II with maxima at 316, 330 and 345 nm. Spectral analysis revealed that syn-BPDE gave rise to approximately 65% type I and
35% type II. With anti-BPDE the type II complex greatly domina-
ted. A significant difference in chemical stability between syn-
and anti - BPDE - DNA complexes was observed; syn-BPDE-DNA seems to
undergo a continuous degradation as a function of time as judged
by repeated extractions of syn-BPDE-modified DNA with organic
solvent whereas anti-BPDE-DNA is essentially stable on the same
time scale. This may reflect a less specific binding of syn-BPDE
to DNA involving base binding sites that facilitate hydrolysis.
It is also possible that the spatial arrangement of the hydroxyl
groups in syn-BPDE renders the DNA-complex more labile due to
conformational strains.

LD studies revealed that the major DNA bound chromophore from
(±)-syn-BPDE is localized close to perpendicular to the long
axis of DNA probably forming a classical intercalation complex.
It should be mentioned in this context that the physical complex
between (±)-anti-BPDE and DNA has the same spectral properties
as covalently bound syn-BPDE and has been attributed to intercala-

TABLE 1

EXPERIMENTAL PROPERTIES OF THE SPECTRAL TYPES OF DNA COMPLEXES
DERIVED FROM RACEMIC ANTI- AND SYN-BPDE

Observed property	Spectral type of BPDE-DNA complex	
	I	II
Peaks of absorption of fluorescence excitation spectrum	322, 337, 354 nm	316, 330, 345 nm
Major component in	($\pm$)syn-BPDE ($\sim$65%)	($\pm$)anti-BPDE (>90%)
Chemical stability	low	high
Angle between transition moment vector and average DNA axis[a]	>65°	<35°
Fluorescence quenching ratio in presence of various quenchers:		
Ag$^+$ with (Ag$^+$)/(DNA-phosphate) = 0.4	F_0/F[b] = 1	F_0/F = 0.33
O_2, 13 mM	F_0/F = 1.5	F_0/F = 2
O_2, 45 mM	F_0/F = 2.5	F_0/F = 2.5
O_2, 45 mM, denatured DNA	F_0/F = 7[c]	

[a]Orientation axis in linear dichroism measurements
[b]F = fluorescence intensity in presence of quencher
F_0 = fluorescence intensity in absence of quencher
[c]Third spectral type with absorption maxima 316, 332, 351 nm

tion of the pyrene chromophore between base-pairs (12). On the
other hand, the dominating component from covalently bound ($\pm$)-
anti-BPDE has the plane of the chromophore nearly parallel to
the DNA helix axis. This is in agreement with Geacintov et al.
(8) and Hogan et al. (10). It has been suggested that the dominating component from ($\pm$)-anti-BPDE is covalently bound at the outside of DNA and located in one of the grooves (14). For such an
exterior location of the chromophore one would expect external
fluorescence quenching agents such as O_2 and acrylamide to greatly affect the fluorescence intensity. However, results from experiments to probe the microenvironment of the chromophore and its

accessibility to external fluorescence quenching agents are not compatible with exterior binding. For instance, the data from O_2 fluorescence quenching studies summarized in Table 1 (c.f. a more elaborate treatment in ref. 11) indicates that compounds with spectral types I and II in native DNA are equally inaccessible to O_2 compared to the more easily accessible chromophore in denatured DNA.

Moreover, an externally bound chromophore would be sensitive to intramolecular quenching by DNA and upon dilution, an increased relative fluorescence would be expected. No significantly increased fluorescence was observed upon dilution of DNA, or decreased fluorescence upon addition of DNA (10,11). Hogan et al. (10) recently proposed a model where the major chromophore from (±)-anti-BPDE is strongly associated with DNA bases forming intercalation complex with atypical, wedge-type configuration. Our data regarding (±)-anti-BPDE are consistent with such a model.

Figure 2 shows the absorption spectra of DNA after reaction with (+)-anti- and (-)-anti-BPDE. The spectrum of the (+)-enantiomer (λ_{max} 315, 330 and 345 nm) is as expected identical to the spectrum of DNA after reaction with racemic anti-BPDE (11) and similar to that of BP-tetraol in buffer (12) except for a slight shift (∿2 nm) towards longer wavelengths.

The absorption spectrum of the DNA complex of the (-)-enantiomer is significantly different from that of the (+)-enantiomer. It has less resolved peaks and a shoulder at 354 nm, indicating a more heterogeneous distribution of the chromophores. Such heterogeneity is consistent with the finding that the (-)-anti-BPDE binds to DNA with less specificity than the (+)-anti-BPDE (5). The fluorescence spectra of DNA after reaction with the two anti-BPDE enantiomers showed no differences in their intensity maxima (λ_{max} em. 379, 399, 420 nm, λ_{max} ex. 316, 329, 345 nm) although the ratios between individual peaks showed some variation. We also observed that the shoulder in the absorption spectrum of (-)-anti-BPDE at 354 nm was absent in the fluorescence excitation spectrum, indicating that the corresponding adduct has a low or zero fluorescence quantum yield.

Silver ions (Ag^+) bind preferentially to DNA bases and induce conformational changes in DNA (15,16). As shown in Table 1, Ag^+

greatly increased the fluorescence intensity from (±)-anti-
BPDE-modified DNA whereas no effect was observed for syn-BPDE-
DNA. Preliminary studies on the
effect of Ag$^+$ on the fluorescence
intensity on DNA reacted with (+)-
or (-)-anti-BPDE gave the following results: At a ratio of (Ag$^+$)/
(DNA-phosphate) = 0.5, a maximal
7-fold increase in fluorescence
intensity was observed for the
(+)-enantiomer compared to a 3-
fold increase for the (-)-enan-
tiomer. We interpret the effect
of Ag$^+$ to be due to structural
changes in DNA that force the
chromophores from highly quenched
(internal) states to less quenched
(external) ones. This interpretation is supported by our earlier
finding that the increased fluorescence intensity of (±)-anti-
BPDE-DNA in the presence of Ag$^+$
was efficiently quenched by the
external quencher O$_2$ (11).

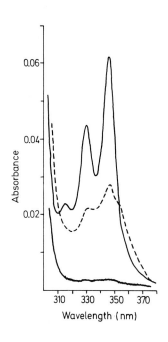

Fig. 2. Light absorption
spectra of (+)-anti-BPDE-
DNA (————) and (-)-anti-
BPDE-DNA (-----).

The complexes between DNA and the two anti-BPDE enantiomers
were further characterized by LD measurements. The results are
summarized in Figure 3. A negative LD signal is obtained for DNA
as expected since the bases and their transition moment vectors
are perpendicular to the long axis of DNA. The LD signal of the
DNA-bound chromophore from (+)-anti-BPDE is positive and consistent with the results from (±)-anti-BPDE modified DNA. In contrast, the LD signal from (-)-anti-BPDE modified DNA is negative
(like that from syn-BPDE-DNA) and the absorption maxima are shifted from 316, 330 and 345 nm (type II complex) for (+)-anti-BPDE
modified DNA to 322, 337 and 354 nm (type I complex). The intensity from (-)-anti-BPDE-DNA is much less although the extent of

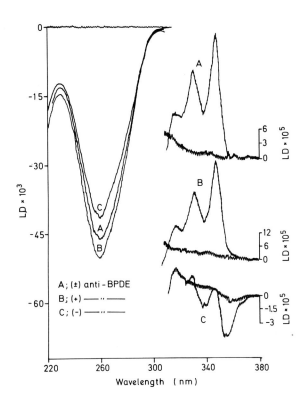

Fig. 3. Linear dichroism spectra of DNA reacted with A; (±)-anti-BPDE (29 nmol BPDE covalently bound per mg DNA) B; (+)-anti-BPDE (49 nmol BPDE covalently bound per mg DNA) C; (-)-anti-BPDE (27 nmol BPDE covalently bound per mg DNA).

binding is similar indicating a more heterogeneous binding distribution.

In conclusion, the present results have shown some characteristic differences between racemic syn- and anti-BPDE-DNA complexes as well as those formed between the (+)- and (-)-enantiomers of anti-BPDE. These differences may be related to their different biological effects. The results on the DNA-binding of the most potent carcinogen (+)-anti-BPDE lead to a picture where the carcinogen is localized parallel òr close to parallel to the helix axis, but with strongly quenched fluorescence probably due to an internal location. This might be explained by the wedge-type binding model proposed by Hogan *et al.* (10). An alternative model is

where the (+)-anti-BPDE chromophore in the type II complex is
strongly associated with the interior of DNA forming an acute
angle with the helix axis. As a consequence, the local DNA conformation must be altered by obstructing the base pairing properties. Since DNA-binding is considered crucial for initiating tumour growth it follows that the unique properties of the Type II
complex may be of fundamental importance in BP-induced carcinogenesis.

ACKNOWLEDGEMENTS

This study was supported by grants from the Swedish Cancer
Society, NIH (No 1RC1 CA 26201), the Swedish Board for Coordina-
tion and Planning of Research, and the Swedish Natural Science
Research Council. The Cancer Research Program of the National
Cancer Institute, Division of Cancer Cause and Prevention
(Bethesda, MD, USA) is gratefully acknowledged for supplying the
benzo(a)pyrene derivatives used in this study.

REFERENCES

1. Gelboin, H.V. (1980) Phys. Rev. 60, 1107.

2. Wood, A.W., Chang, R.L., Levin, W., Yagi, H., Thakker, D.R.,
    Jerina, D.M. and Conney, A.H. (1978) Proc. Natl. Acad. Sci.
    USA, 75, 5358.

3. Slaga, T.J., Bracken, W.J., Gleason, G., Levin. W., Yagi, H.,
    Jerina, D.M. and Conney, A.H. (1979) Cancer Res. 39, 67.

4. Meehan, T. and Straub, K. (1979) Nature, 277, 410.

5. Brookes, P. and Osborne, M.R. (1982) Carcinogenesis, 3, 1223.

6. Ashurst, S.W., Cohen, G.M., Nesnow, S., DiGiovanni, J. and
    Slaga, T.J. (1983) Cancer Res. 43, 1024.

7. Yang, L.L., Maher, V.M. and McGormick, J.J. (1980) Proc. Natl.
    Acad. Sci. USA, 77, 5933.

8. Geacintov, N.E., Gagliano, A., Ivanovic, V. and Weinstein, I.B.
    (1978) Biochemistry, 17, 5256.

9. Drinkwater, N.R., Miller, J.A., Miller, E.C. and Yang, M.C.
    (1978) Cancer Res. 38, 3247.

10. Hogan, M.E., Dattagupta, N. and Whitlock,Jr., J.P. (1981)
    J. Biol. Chem. 256, 4504.

11. Undeman, O., Lycksell, P.O., Gräslund, A., Astlind, T.,
    Ehrenberg, A., Jernström, B., Tjerneld, F. and Nordén, B.
    (1983) Cancer Res. 43, 1851.

12. Ibanez, V., Geacintov, N.E., Gagliano, A.G., Brandimarte, S. and Harvey, R.G. (1980) J. Am. Chem. Soc. 102, 5661.

13. Meehan, T., Gamper, M. and Becker, J.F. (1982) J. Biol. Chem. 257, 10479.

14. Geacintov, N.E., Gagliano, A.G., Ibanez, V. and Harvey, R.G. (1982) Carcinogenesis, 3, 247.

15. Geacintov, N.E., Prusik, T. and Khosrofian, J.M. (1976) J. Am. Chem. Soc. 98, 6444.

16. Dattagupta, M. and Crothers, D.M. (1981) Nucleic Acids Res. 9, 2971.

© 1983 Elsevier Science Publishers B.V.
Extrahepatic Drug Metabolism and Chemical Carcinogenesis,
J. Rydström, J. Montelius and M. Bengtsson eds.

KINETICS OF DNA ADDUCT FORMATION AND REMOVAL IN LIVER AND KIDNEY OF RATS FED 2-ACETYLAMINOFLUORENE

MIRIAM C. POIRIER[1], JOHN M. HUNT[2], B'ANN TRUE[2] and BRIAN A. LAISHES[2]

[1]Laboratory of Cellular Carcinogenesis and Tumor Promotion, National Cancer Institute, NIH, Bethesda, MD 20205 (U.S.A.) and [2]McArdle Laboratory for Cancer Research, University of Wisconsin, Madison, WIS 53706 (U.S.A.)

INTRODUCTION

Studies directed toward determining the structural and functional conse- quences of carcinogen-DNA adduct formation have recently been advanced by the development of immunoassays capable of detecting femtomole quantities of these adducts in DNAs isolated from exposed biological sources (1,2). The immuno- logical approach is uniquely-suited to investigations involving long term chronic chemical exposure since it obviates the necessity for a radioactive carcinogen. In addition, the combination of immunoassay and radiolabeling enables one to address specific aspects of adduct quantitation which might otherwise be virtually impossible.

An antiserum elicited in rabbits against guanosin-(8-yl)-acetylaminofluorene (G-8-AAF) has been shown to be specific for the acetylated and deacetylated guan-(8-yl) (C-8) adducts of 2-acetylaminofluorene (2-AAF) with deoxyguanosine in DNA and does not cross-react with other 2-AAF-DNA adducts, the carcinogen alone, deoxyguanosine or DNA (3,4). The C-8 adducts, N-deoxyguanosin-(8-yl)-AAF (dG-8-AAF) and N-deoxyguanosin-(8-yl)-AF (dG-8-AF), comprise the major portion (90%) of binding products formed upon interaction of 2-AAF, or its activated derivative N-acetoxy-2-acetylaminofluorene (N-Ac-AAF) with DNA in cultured cells (4,5,6) and whole animals (7,8,9). Radioimmunoassay (RIA) has been em- ployed to both quantitate formation and removal of liver and kidney DNA adducts in male Wistar Furth rats fed 0.02% 2-AAF for several weeks, and to determine proportions of acetylated and deacetylated C-8 adducts (10). In addition specific nuclear staining detected by immunonofluorescence has been found to correlate with adduct levels determined in different liver lobes by RIA.

MATERIALS AND METHODS

Animals and Diets. Young adult male Wistar-Furth rats, weighing 130-150g were obtained from Microbiological Associates, Bethesda, MD, and maintained as previously described (9). Animals on a control diet received the purified, semisynthetic basal diet Bio-Mix No. 101 (Bio-Serv, Inc., Frenchtown, NJ). The composition of the diet has been described (9). 2-AAF (m.p. 192-196°, Aldrich Chemical Co., Milwaukee, WI) was added to the control diet (Bio-Mix No. 101) at a concentration of 0.02% (w/w). For the first DNA repair experiment [^{3}H]2-AAF was kindly provided by Dr. F. A. Beland and fed at a specific activity of 131 mCi/mmole. For the second DNA repair experiment [^{3}H]2-AAF purchased from Midwest Research Institute (Kansas City, MO), was fed at a specific activity of 72 mCi/mmole.

Preparation of DNA from Rat Tissues. Tissues were homogenized and samples were were prepared for cesium chloride isopycnic centrifugation as previously described (11). Each tube of the fractionated gradients was read at A_{260}, and the DNA peaks were dialyzed against deionized water.

Radioimmunoassay. Procedures for the synthesis of all adducts for both immunization and RIAs, details of the immunization procedure and characterization of antibody specificity have been previously described (3,4,10). DNAs (250 µg) for RIA were hydrolyzed by 15 µg of P_1 nuclease (Calbiochem, La Jolla, CA) in 0.025 M sodium acetate (pH 5.6) and 0.001 M $ZnSO_4$ for 3 hr. Two types of RIA have been employed in these experiments. First, equal amounts of the same DNA were assayed simultaneously in assays using [^{3}H]G-8-AAF and [^{3}H]G-8-AF as tracers, to approximate the proportion of each C-8 adduct. Secondly, the competition of increasing amounts of modified DNA against [^{3}H]G-8-AAF as tracer was assessed. The proportion of acetylated and deacetylated C-8 adduct in the unknown samples has been determined by RIA with the appropriate standard curves and after evaluation of the data obtained in the above assays. For details see references 10 and 12.

High Pressure Liquid Chromatography. HPLC was performed on hydrolysates of the DNA obtained from livers of rats fed [^{3}H]2-AAF by Ms. Nancy F. Fullerton in laboratory of Dr. F. A. Beland according to previously-published procedures (7).

Immunofluorescence. Frozen sections of liver and kidney were fixed for 20 min. at 4°c in 3:1, methanol: glacial acetic acid, treated with 0.035M NaOH in 70% ETOH for 30 sec. and incubated for 45 min with anti-G-8-AF (13) (diluted 1:20) followed by fluorescein conjugated GOAT-Anti-rabbit IgG (Miles, Elkhardt Ind., diluted 1:80) for 30 min. The procedure used is as described (14).

RESULTS AND DISCUSSION

The Kinetics of Adduct Formation and Removal in Rat Liver and Kidney DNA after 3 and 28 Days of Feeding 0.02% 2-AAF. A combination of DNA adduct detection by RIA and radioactivity has made it possible to monitor the formation and fate of newly-formed (^{3}H), total (RIA) and previously formed (the difference) C-8 adducts at various times during 2-AAF feeding. This approach was initiated as a result of earlier observations from this laboratory that C-8 adducts, although removed efficiently from rat liver and kidney DNA after 3 days of 0.02% 2-AAF feeding, tended to persist and accumulate after 28 days of feeding the carcinogen-containing diet (9).

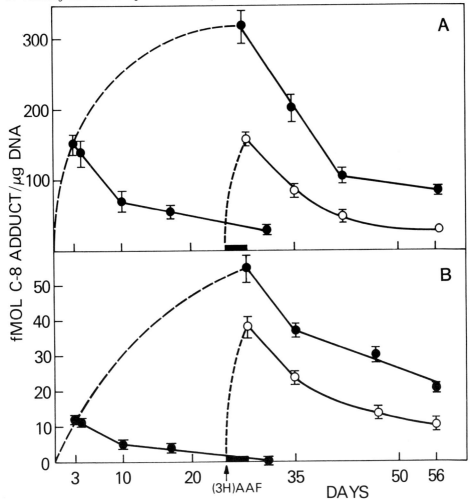

Fig. 1. Guan-(8-yl) adduct formation and removal in DNA of liver (A) and kidney (B) from male Wistar-Furth rats (180 gm) fed either non-radioactive 0.02% 2-AAF for 3 or 25 days (●——●), or [³H]2-AAF (O----O) for 3 days after 25 days of non-radioactive 0.02% 2-AAF diet. Solid lines indicate time of feeding control diet. Closed symbols represent adduct determination by RIA and open symbols represent radioactivity. Note differences in ordinate scale for A and B.

In experiments reported here newly-formed adducts have been determined by RIA after 3 days of feeding non-radioactive 2-AAF to unexposed rats, and by radioactivity after 3 days of feeding $[^3H]$2-AAF to rats previously fed the non-radioactive compound for 25 days. Total C-8 adducts have been determined by RIA in animals fed unlabeled 2-AAF for 25 days and [3H]2-AAF for 3 days. In addition, removal of both newly-formed and total adducts has been monitored during subsequent time intervals (up to 28 days) of feeding control diet. In this (Figure 1,A,B) and one previous experiment (15), qualitatively-similar kinetic profiles were observed for both liver and kidney DNA adducts although the total binding in kidney (which is not a target organ for tumorigenesis) was several-fold lower than in liver.

The kinetics of C-8 adduct formation and removal in liver DNA are shown in Figure 1A. Levels of C-8 adduct formed during three days of feeding non-radioactive 2-AAF to animals not previously exposed (●——●, RIA), or $[^3H]$2-AAF to animals given non-radioactive 2-AAF for 25 days (0----0, radioactivity) were the same (156 fmol/ug DNA and 158 fmol/ug DNA respectively). In addition the rates of removal for these newly-formed adducts were similar when both groups were fed control diet for up to 28 days (Figure 1A, ●——●, 0----0). Although the proportion of dG-8-AF in the newly-formed adduct population has been shown to increase from 80-100% during chronic 2-AAF feeding (9,15) the rates of C-8 adduct formation and removal at both the early (3-day) and later (28-day) times appeared virtually identical. Thus feeding of the 2-AAF diet for up to one month did not alter the capacity of the whole liver to either form or repair new C-8 adducts in DNA.

In animals fed unlabeled 2-AAF for 25 days and $[^3H]$2-AAF for 3 days (a total of 28 days) the level of total C-8 adduct was determined by RIA (Figure 1, 28 days, ●——●). By subtracting the quantity of newly-formed adducts (0----0, radioactivity) from the total adducts (RIA) it is evident that the previously-formed adducts constituted about half of those present at 28 days of feeding 2-AAF. However, in animals subsequently given control diet for 28 days (Figure 1, 56 days), the remaining newly-formed adducts constituted about 25% of the total, suggesting that there was a slow accumulation of persistent previously-formed adducts. In this and other experiments the decrease in adducts with time on control diet (Figure 1A, 28-56 days, solid lines) followed biphasic kinetics, with an early rapid Phase I (the first 7 to 14 days on control diet) and a much slower Phase II (between 14 and 28 days on control diet). The observed persistence of the previously-formed adducts would suggest that Phase II may not have been functioning for these adducts.

In the experiment shown in Figure 1A a decrease in the liver DNA level of
C-8 adducts was monitored during time of feeding control diet. If the repair
rate measured in these rats was artificially slow because there was not a

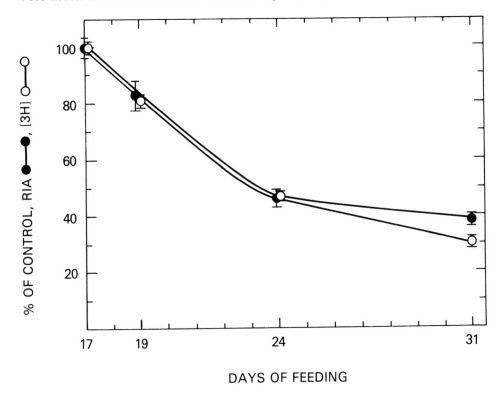

Fig. 2. Removal of C-8 adduct from liver DNA in rats fed either control or
2-AAF diet. Twelve rats were fed unlabeled 0.02% 2-AAF for 14 days and [^{3}H]-
2-AAF for 3 days. At 17 days 3 were sacrificed, the remainder returned to the
unlabeled 2-AAF diet and sacrificed at 2, 7 and 14 days (0——0). Twelve rats
were fed unlabeled 0.02% 2-AAF for 17 days, and 3 were sacrificed. The remainder were given control diet and sacrificed at 2, 7 and 14 days (●——●). Values
are mean $\pm$ S.E. for 3 animals.

continual ingestion of carcinogen, one would expect to observe a different
removal rate after chasing radioactive DNA adducts with a non-radioactive 2-
AAF diet rather than control diet. Figure 2 shows the results of an experiment
in which one group of animals was fed unlabeled 2-AAF for 14 days and [^{3}H]2-AAF
for 3 days, and individuals were sacrificed during a subsequent 14 days of
feeding unlabeled 2-AAF. Dilution of the radioactivity during this time period

indicated removal of radioactive C-8 adducts during 2-AAF feeding, (Figure 2, 0——0). For comparison, another group of animals was simultaneously fed unlabeled 2-AAF for 17 days and individuals sacrificed during a subsequent 14 days of feeding control diet. RIA determination of C-8 adduct removal in the liver DNA of these animals (Figure 2, ●——●) was not significantly different from the radioactive group (Figure 2, 0——0) except at 14 days. Thus the rate of removal of C-8 adducts from rat liver DNA was essentially the same during feeding of either 2-AAF diet or control diet.

TABLE 1

GUAN-(8-yl) ADDUCT FORMATION IN DIFFERENT LIVER LOBES OF MALE WF RATS FED 0.02% 2-AAF FOR 3 DAYS

Liver Lobe	fmol adduct[a] $\overline{\mu g \ DNA}$	%dG-8-AAF
LEFT LATERAL	159.6 + 10.8	18
RIGHT LATERAL	112.6 + 13.2	18
CAUDATE (1)	115.3 + 12.0	--
CAUDATE (2)	123.6 + 29.8	--
MEDIAN	131.0 + 12.7	18
TRIANGULAR	72.0 + 25.7	18

[a] Mean + S.E. for 3 animals

Adduct Localization in Liver Lobes of Rats Fed 0.02% 2-AAF for 3 Days.

Certain aspects of the kinetics of C-8 adduct formation and removal in liver DNA have lead us to postulate compartmentalization of DNA adduct formation in rat liver. For example, at a time when the quantity of total adducts was not increasing with continued dietary administration of 2-AAF, the newly-formed adducts during 3 days of feeding [^{3}H]2-AAF constituted 40-50% of the total. Also, the fact that adduct accumulation continued at the same rate (at least for the first 28 days) suggested that adduct formation might occur in different areas at different times. Evidence that adduct accumulation is not uniform throughout the liver comes from both quantitative assay of adduct levels and immunofluorescence with an anti-G-8-AF antibody.

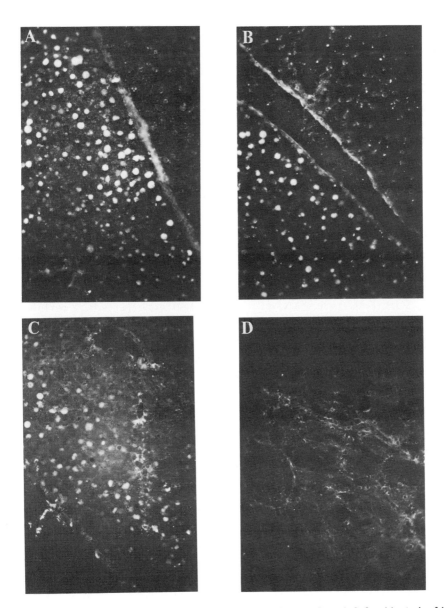

Fig. 3.   Immunofluorescent localization of deacetylated C-8 adduct in liver
nuclei of male Wistar Furth rats fed 0.02% 2-AAF for 3 days.
(A) Adjacent left lateral lobes from animals fed 0.02% 2-AAF (left) or control
    diet (right).
(B) Adjacent median lobes from animals fed 0.02% 2-AAF (left) or control diet
    (right).
(C) Triangular lobe from 2-AAF fed animal.
(D) Kidney from 2-AAF fed animal.

Quantitation of C-8 adduct was carried out by RIA in different liver lobes of 3 male WF rats fed 0.02% 2-AAF for 3 days. The results, shown in Table 1, indicate that at this early time the highest binding levels were in the left lateral lobe, and significantly low levels were observed in the triangular (right posterior sublobe) portion of the median lobe. By RIA, DNA profiles (not shown) confirmed that about 20% of the C-8 adduct in each lobe after 3 days of 2-AAF feeding was acetylated, and therefore that values previously-reported for the liver as a whole reflect the situation in the individual lobes at this time (Table 1).

A similar distribution of adducts was seen by immunofluorescence. In Figure 3A and B the same liver lobes from animals fed 2-AAF and control diet were placed in adjacent positions so both experimental and control tissues could be observed simultaneously. The brightest accumulation of fluorescent nuclei was in the left lateral lobe of 2-AAF fed animals while the triangular lobe (Figure 3, C) contained few fluorescent nuclei. Control livers, and kidney (Figure 3D) from animals fed 2-AAF were negative. Other control experiments were performed in conjunction with those shown here. When the immune (anti-G-8-AF) antiserum was absorbed with dG-8-AF and AF-DNA the nuclear fluorescence disappeared. When the frozen sections were exposed to RNAse (1 mg/ml) for 20 minutes after the NAOH treatment the overall fluorescence was essentially unchanged, suggesting that most of the brightness observed was due to DNA binding.

CONCLUSIONS

Kinetic experiments in which quantitation of 2-AAF guan-(8-yl)DNA adducts has been achieved by both immunoassay and radioactivity have allowed monitoring of newly formed adducts and total adducts, thereby making possible an estimation of previously-formed adducts as the difference between the two. From these studies it is apparent that the rates of formation and removal of C-8 adducts in rat liver DNA were essentially unchanged during the first month of feeding 2-AAF. Removal (either in the presence of 2-AAF or control diet) was biphasic, however, consisting of an early, rapid Phase I (the first 7 to 14 days) and a much slower subsequent Phase II (14-28 days). Since Phase II appeared not to be functioning in animals fed 0.02% 2-AAF for 4 weeks, a slow accumulation of adducts would be predicted, and indeed, a persistent fraction has been observed in this and other experiments (9,15). In the rat kidney virtually identical kinetic profiles of DNA adduct formation and removal suggested that mechanisms similar to those in liver might be functioning to metabolize and detoxify 2-AAF. In kidney, however, adduct levels were always several fold lower than those in liver.

A compartmentalization of liver DNA adduct formation, postulated from various kinetic experiments, has been demonstrated here by both quantitative RIA and immunofluorescence localization. Although still in early stages these studies have demonstrated that all of the liver lobes do not accumulate adducts in a uniform fashion. After three days of 2-AAF feeding adducts levels in DNA of the left lateral lobe were twice as high as those in the right anterior portion (triangular) of the median lobe. Thus, new concepts of carcinogen processing in vivo are being obtained through a combination of quantitative and morphological techniques using antibodies specific for the major DNA binding products of 2-AAF with DNA. These data should strengthen our understanding of molecular mechanisms occurring in both hepatic and extra-hepatic organs during chemical carcinogenesis.

ACKNOWLEDGMENTS

Appreciation for comments and collaborations is extended to Dr. S. H. Yuspa, J. Nakayama, F. Beland and P. Blumberg.

For technical assistance thanks are due to E. Patterson, N. Nguyen, C. Thill, and S. Eng.

REFERENCES

1. Poirier, M.C. (1981) J. Natl. Cancer Inst. (Guest Editorial), 67: 515-519.

2. Muller, R. and Rajewsky, M.F. (1981) J. Cancer Res. CLin. Oncol. (Guest Editorial), 102: 99-113.

3. Poirier, M.C., Yuspa, S.H., Weinstein, I.B. and Blobstein, S. (1977) Nature 270: 186-188.

4. Poirier, M.C., Dubin, M.A. and Yuspa, S.H. (1979) Cancer Res. 39: 1377-1381.

5. Howard, P.C., Casciano, D.A., Beland, F.A. and Shaddock, T.R. Jr. (1981) Carcinogenesis 2: 97-102.

6. Maher, V.M., Hazard, R.M., Beland, F.A., Corner, R., Medrala, A.L., Levinson, J.W., Heflich, R.H. and McCormick, J.J. (1980) Proc. Am. Assoc. Cancer Res. 21: 71.

7. Beland, F.A., Dooley, K.L. and Jackson, C.D. (1982) Cancer Res., 42: 1348-1354.

8. Visser, A. and Westra, J.G. (1981) Carcinogenesis 2: 737-740.

9. Poirier, M.C., True, B.A. and Laishes, B.A. (1982) Cancer Res., 42: 1317-1321.

10. Poirier, M.C., Williams, G.M. and Yuspa, S.H. (1980) Mol. Pharmacol., 18: 234-240.

11. Lieberman, M.W. and Poirier, M.C. (1973) Cancer Res. 33: 2097-2103, 1973.

12. Poirier, M.C. and Connor, R.J. (1982) in: Van Vunakis, H. and Langone J. (Eds.), Immunochemical Techniques, Methods in Enzymology, Volume 84, Academic Press Inc., New York, NY, pp. 607-618.

13. Poirier, M.C., Nakayama, J., Perera, F.P., Weinstein, I.B., and Yuspa, S.H. (1983) In: Milman, H.A., Sell, S. et al. (Eds.), Application of Biological Markers to Carcinogen Testing, Plenum Press, New York, NY, in press.

14. Cornelis, J.J. and Errera, M. (1981) in: Friedberg, E.C. and Hanawalt, P.C. (Eds.), DNA Repair, A Laboratory Manual of Research Procedures, Vol. 1, Marcel Dekker Inc., New York, N.Y., pp. 31-44.

15. Poirier, M.C., True, B.A. and Laishes, B.A, (1982) Second International Conference on Carcinogenic and Mutagenic N-Substituted Aryl Compounds, Environtmental Health Perspectives 49: 93-99.

16. Irving, C.C. and Veazey, R.A. (1971) Proc. Am. Assoc. Cancer Res. 12: 54 (Abstract 213).

© 1983 Elsevier Science Publishers B.V.
Extrahepatic Drug Metabolism and Chemical Carcinogenesis,
J. Rydström, J. Montelius and M. Bengtsson eds.

METABOLISM OF AZO AND HYDRAZINE DERIVATIVES TO REACTIVE INTERMEDIATES

R. A. PROUGH, M. I. BROWN, C. A. AMRHEIN, AND L. J. MARNETT
Department of Biochemistry, The University of Texas Health Science Center at
Dallas, 5323 Harry Hines Blvd., Dallas, TX 75235 (U.S.A.) and Department of
Chemistry, Wayne State University, Detroit, MI 48202 (U.S.A.)

INTRODUCTION

Oral administration of a wide number of hydrazine derivatives to rodents
leads to tumor production (1). In particular, lung appears to be a major site
of tumor formation, even to some extent with organotropic carcinogenic
hydrazines such as 1,2-dimethylhydrazine and procarbazine. The mechanism of
metabolic activation of hydrazine derivatives is not clearly understood, nor
is the organ specific action of the various hydrazines understood. With the
advent of the concept of metabolic activation (3), Druckrey proposed that
1,2-dimethylhydrazine (DMH) is metabolically activated by a series of steps as
seen in equation 1 (3). Methylazoxymethanol has been shown to be chemically
unstable and decomposes to a reactive species similar to diazomethane (4,5).
Grab and Zedeck have also suggested that methylazoxymethanol can serve as a
substrate for alcohol dehydrogenase (6), resulting in increased production of
a reactive intermediate. The 1,2-disubstituted hydrazine, procarbazine
[N-isopropyl-α-(2-methylhydrazino)-p-toluamide, has also been shown to be
metabolized to azo and azoxy derivatives (7-9).

$$\text{DMH} \rightarrow \text{azomethane} \rightarrow \text{azoxymethane} \rightarrow \text{methylazoxymethanol} \quad (1)$$

A number of monosubstituted hydrazines have been shown to be metabolized
by microsomal cytochrome P-450 to form the corresponding hydrocarbon (10,11).
Prough, Wittkop, and Reed suggested that these hydrocarbons were the expected
products of the alkyldiazenes which decompose via a radical intermediate.
Indeed, Augusto et al. (12) have trapped and identified an ethyl free radical
during the NADPH-dependent metabolism of ethylhydrazine. While it is tempting
to speculate that the free radicals formed from diazenes might serve as a
reactive intermediate, it should be pointed out that alkyldiazenes might be
further oxidized to the reactive alkyldiazonium ion.

The focus of the current study was to evaluate the enzyme systems in
rodent lung which might account for the metabolic activation of substituted
hydrazines; namely, cytochrome P-450 (8-11), prostaglandin synthetase (13,14),
and monoamine oxidase (15). Prostaglandin synthetase has been shown to
metabolize certain carcinogens such as benzo(a)pyrene-7,8-dihydrodiol (16) and

various arylamines (17). Hydrazines are known to be potent inhibitors of mitochondrial monoamine oxidase (18) and yet they can be metabolized slowly by this flavoprotein (15,18).

MATERIALS AND METHODS

Methylhydrazine and ethylhydrazine oxalate were purchased from Aldrich Chemical Company (Milwaukee, WI) and procarbazine was a gift from the Hoffman-LaRoche Company, Inc. (Nutley, N.J.). [Ring-^{14}C]-procarbazine was obtained from the Drug Research and Development Program, Division of Cancer Treatment, NCI (Bethesda, MD). Azo-procarbazine was prepared as described previously (8,9). Arachidonic acid was purchased from Nuchek Preps. (Elysian, MN).

Male rats [Crl:CD(SD)BR] (200-250 g) were purchased from Charles Rivers Laboratories, Wilmington, MA and were killed by decapitation. The liver and lungs were perfused with a solution consisting of 0.25 M sucrose and 0.05 M potassium phosphate, pH 7.4, to remove contaminating hemoglobin and red cells (19). The tissue was weighed, minced, and homogenized with 3 volumes of buffered sucrose in a teflon-glass homogenizer. The homogenate was centrifuged at 1000xg for 10 min to sediment cell debri and nuclei and the supernatant fraction was recentrifuged at 17,000xg for 20 min. The mitochondria pellet was resuspended by homogenization and was resedimented at 17,000xg for 20 min. The first post-mitochondrial supernatant was centrifuged at 108,000xg for 60 min to sediment the microsomal fraction. The microsomal and mitochondrial pellets were resuspended by homogenization in a buffer consisting of 0.25 M sucrose, 0.05 M potassium phosphate, pH 7.4. Ram seminal vesicles were prepared as described by Marnett and Wilcox (20). The protein concentrations were determined by the method of Lowry et al. (21).

The oxidative metabolism of methyl- and ethylhydrazine was measured by head space analysis of the respired hydrocarbons (methane or ethane and ethylene) by gas chromatography with a Porapak Q column support at 25° and 35°C, respectively. Mitochondrial or microsomal protein fractions (2 mg/ml) were incubated at 37°C in 5 ml of 0.05 M Tricine, 0.05 M potassium phosphate buffer, pH 7.4, containing 1 mM EDTA in a 25 ml Erlenmeyer flask sealed with a rubber septum. The hydrazines (1 mM) and NADPH (1 mM) were added to initiate the reaction as indicated in the text. The arachidonic acid-dependent consumption of oxygen by ram seminal vesicles (0.5 mg/ml) was measured with a Clark type oxygen electrode as described by Prough and Ziegler (22). The metabolism of procarbazine to its azo derivative was measured as described

previously (8). The metabolism of azo-procarbazine [N-isopropyl-
α-(2-methylazo)-p-toluamide] was determined as shown previously (9).

RESULTS

The time courses of hydrocarbon production from ethylhydrazine by liver
and lung mitochondria are shown in Figure 1. Although the rates of
hydrocarbon production by these tissue fractions were similar, the time course
for ethane and ethylene production in the presence of liver mitochondrial
fractions appeared to be biphasic. Similar results have been shown for liver
and kidney mitochondrial monoamine oxidase (MAO) with monosubstituted
hydrazines (18). The second phase of the reaction in the presence of liver
mitochondria was nearly identical to the rate seen when the liver or lung
mitochondria were boiled for 10 min. Since hydrazines are thought to
irreversibly inactivate MAO, the results of Figure 1 suggested that there may
be differences in the susceptibility of liver and lung MAO to inactivation by
these hydrazines.

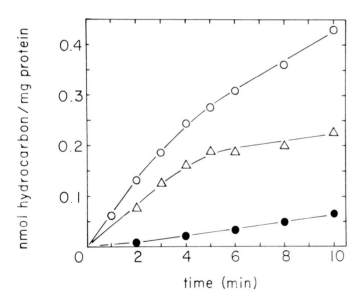

Fig. 1. Time course of hydrocarbon production from ethylhydrazine in the
presence of liver or lung mitochondrial protein fractions. (O), lung
mitochondria; (Δ), liver mitochondria; (●), boiled lung mitochondria.

TABLE 1

THE RATES OF HYDROCARBON PRODUCTION FROM ETHYLHYDRAZINE IN THE PRESENCE OF
TISSUE FRACTIONS FROM RAT LIVER AND LUNG

Tissue Fractions were incubated in either the absence or presence of 1 mM
NADPH as stated in the table.

Tissue Fraction	Metabolic Rate (pmol/min/mg)	Product Ratio (Ethane/Ethylene)
Liver Mitochondria	34^a	4.8
Microsomes	4	2.6
Microsomes + NADPH	101	8.6
Lung Mitochondria	59^a	3.9
Microsomes	29	3.6
Microsomes + NADPH	32	4.6

[a] There was either no effect or a slight inhibition of mitochondrial activity
seen in the presence of 1 mM NADPH.

Table 1 shows the rates of hydrocarbon production from ethylhydrazine by
liver and lung mitochondria and microsomes. Lung mitochondria had a higher
specific activity than did liver mitochondria. Yet, the product ratio
(ethane produced/ethylene produced) obtained with either tissue were not
significantly different. Liver microsomes in the absence of NADPH did not
produce much hydrocarbon, but upon addition of NADPH, the rate of production
increased 25-30 fold as previously seen by Prough et al. (10) and the product
ratio increased to 8.6. However, a significant rate of metabolism of
ethylhydrazine was seen in the presence of lung mitochondria and microsomes
alone; the rate with microsomes only increased 1.1-fold in the presence of
NADPH. This result is not surprising since it was shown that rodent lung

TABLE 2

EFFECT OF VARIOUS TREATMENTS ON HYDROCARBON FORMATION FROM ETHYLHYDRAZINE IN THE PRESENCE OF TISSUE FRACTIONS

The protein fractions (20-30 mg/ml) were incubated at 37°C for 40 min with 1 mM N,N-dimethylpropargylamine (DMPA). An 0.5 ml aliquot of the mixture was added to 10 ml of 0.05 potassium phosphate, pH 7.4, containing 1 mM ethylhydrazine and EDTA; hydrocarbon production was measured subsequently.

Treatment	Metabolic Rate (% of Control)
LUNG MITOCHONDRIA	
None	100[a]
Heat Inactivation	8
DMPA	35
LUNG MICROSOMES	
None	100
Heat Inactivation	11
DMPA	28
LIVER MITOCHONDRIA	
None	100
Heat Inactivation	15
DMPA	37

[a] The control values were 54 pmol/min/mg for lung mitochondria, 24 pmol/min/mg for lung microsomes, and 35 pmol/min/mg for liver mitochondria.

microsomes have a 20-fold lower specific content of cytochrome P-450 than liver microsomes (19). In the presence of NADPH, the mitochondrial activity of liver and lung was slightly suppressed. Similar results were seen with methylhydrazine as a substrate.

Table 2 demonstrates the effects of heat inactivation and an inhibitor of MAO (form B), N,N-dimethylpropargylamine (DMPA). Heat inactivation of lung microsomal protein and liver or lung mitochondrial protein caused a 85-90% loss of activity suggesting that the hydrocarbon production is an enzymic process. After treatment of the microsomal and mitochondrial fractions with 1 mM N,N-dimethylpropargylamine for 40 min, aliquots of the protein fractions were added to the reaction mixtures and hydrocarbon production from ethylhydrazine measured. Pretreatment of the tissue preparations with DMPA caused a 65-70% inhibition of hydrocarbon production. When procarbazine, a 1,2-disubstituted hydrazine, was utilized as a substrate, DMPA inhibited the formation of azo-procarbazine more than 90% (data not shown) indicating that the enzyme responsible for the oxidative metabolism of mono- and 1,2-disubstituted hydrazines was most likely due to monoamine oxidase.

In the presence of the azo derivative of procarbazine, lung and liver mitochondria alone did not catalyze the formation of the azoxy metabolites. In the presence of NADPH and lung microsomes, the formation of the azoxy metabolites from azo-procarbazine was noted, albeit at low rates (data not shown). No metabolism of azo-procarbazine was noted with lung microsomes on addition of 0.3 mM arachidonic acid.

In order to evaluate the role of prostaglandin synthetase in the metabolic activation of mono- and disubstituted hydrazines, we utilized ram seminal vesicles (RSV), a rich source of the enzyme, to study arachidonic acid-dependent metabolism of the hydrazines. As seen in Figure 2, there was a measurable amount of oxidation of ethylhydrazine in the absence of arachidonic acid; this value did not decrease appreciably upon boiling of RSV. Upon addition of 0.3 mM arachidonic acid, there was approximately a 2-fold increase in hydrocarbon production which was somewhat inhibited by the prior addition of 1-10 mM indomethacin. The rates of formation of hydrocarbon by RSV was significantly smaller than those seen with lung microsomes and liver and lung mitochondria. In addition, the product ratio (ethane/ethylene) was approximately 0.2 in contrast to the value of 4 or 8 obtained with mitochondria or liver microsomes, respectively. While the significance of the difference in product ratio is difficult to assess,

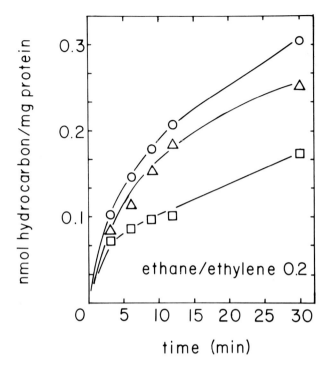

Fig. 2. Time course of hydrocarbon production from ethylhydrazine in the presence of ram seminal vesicles. (□), ram seminal vesicles alone (0.5 mg/ml); (O) ram seminal vesicles in the presence of 0.3 mM arachidonic acid; (△), ram seminal vesicles in the presence of 0.3 mM arachidonic acid and 1 mM indomethacin.

chemical oxidation of ethylhydrazine by potassium ferricyanide (1:2 molar ratio) yielded an ethane/ethylene product ratio of less than 0.5.

Figure 3 shows the effects of 1 mM ethylhydrazine on the oxygen consumption by RSV in the presence of arachidonic acid. Addition of 50 μM arachidonic acid resulted in the consumption of approximately 50 μM oxygen (curve A). The addition of ethylhydrazine either two min prior to or after addition of the unsaturated fatty acid decreased both the rate of O_2 consumption and total amount of O_2 utilized (curve B and C). This result suggests that ethylhydrazine may inhibit prostaglandin synthetase. Further

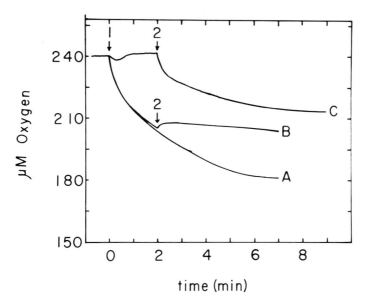

Fig. 3. The effect of 1 mM ethylhydrazine on arachidonic acid-dependent oxygen utilization by ram seminal vesicles. Arachidonic acid (50 μM) was added to ram seminal vesicles (0.5 mg/ml) to initiate oxygen consumption. Curve A. Arachidonic acid was added at 0 min; Curve B. arachidonic acid was added first (0 min) and ethylhydrazine was added second (2 min); Curve C. ethylhydrazine was added first (0 min) and arachidonic acid was added second (2 min). The arrows denote the times of additions.

studies are required to resolve the mechanism of hydrazine inhibition of prostaglandin synthetase.

DISCUSSION

This report has attempted to characterize the relative participation of three oxidative enzymes known to exist in rodent lung and which might be involved in the metabolic activation of hydrazines in lung tissue. The enzymes considered were cytochrome P-450 and prostaglandin synthetase localized in the microsomal fraction and monoamine oxidase localized in the mitochondrial fraction of most tissues. Our results demonstrated that in lung the major enzyme oxidizing ethylhydrazine and procarbazine is apparently monoamine oxidase. Considerable activity was associated with the microsomal fraction; it is not clear whether the presence of MAO in the microsomes is an artifact of the preparation of lung microsomal fractions (19). Only a small amount of NADPH-dependent activity was noted with lung microsomal fractions.

Finally, the differing product ratios of lung microsomal hydrocarbon formation from ethylhydrazine and the low rate of hydrocarbon formation in the presence of arachidonic acid suggested that the oxidation of hydrazines by prostaglandin synthetase is at best a minor metabolic pathway. The results suggest that metabolic studies in those tissues which are susceptible to hydrazine carcinogenesis requires consideration of oxidative enzymes other than cytochrome P-450 and prostaglandin synthetase. This is especially important for compounds with oxidation-reduction potentials like the hydrazines and arylamines.

ACKNOWLEDGEMENTS

This work was supported by American Cancer Society Grants BC-336 (RAP) and BC-244 (LJM), and Robert A. Welch Grant I-616 (RAP). LJM is the recipient of an American Cancer Society Faculty Research Award (FRA 293).

REFERENCES

1. Toth, B. (1975) Cancer Res., 35, 3693.
2. Miller, E.C., and Miller, J.A. (1966) Pharmac. Rev., 18, 805.
3. Druckrey, H. (1970) in: Burdette, W.J. (Ed.), Carcinomas of the Colon and Antecedent Epithelium, C.C. Thomas, Springfield, IL, pp. 267-279.
4. Benn, M.H., and Kazmaier, P. (1972) J. Chem. Soc. Comm., 887.
5. Nagasawa, H.T., Shirota, F.N., and Matsumoto, H. (1972) Nature (London), 236, 234.
6. Grab, D.J., and Zedeck, M.S. (1977) Cancer Res., 37, 4182.
7. Weinkam, R.J., and Shiba, D.A. (1978) Life Sci., 22, 937.
8. Dunn, D.L., Lubet, R.A., and Prough, R.A. (1979) Cancer Res., 39, 4555.
9. Wiebkin, P., and Prough, R.A. (1980) Cancer Res., 40, 3524.
10. Prough, R.A., Wittkop, J.A., and Reed, D.J. (1969) Arch. Biochem. Biophys., 131, 369.
11. Prough, R.A., Wittkop, J.A., and Reed, D.J. (1970) Arch. Biochem. Biophys., 140, 450.
12. Augusto, O., Ortiz de Montellano, P.R., and Quintanilha, A. (1981) Biochem. Biophys. Res. Commun., 101, 1324.
13. Marnett, L.J., Wlodawer, P., and Samuelson, B. (1975) J. Biol. Chem., 250, 8510.

498

14. Sivarajah, K., Anderson, M.W., and Eling, T.E. (1978) Life Sci., 23, 2571.

15. Coomes, M.W., Wiebkin, P., and Prough, R.A. (1980) in: Coon, M.J., Conney, A.H., Estabrook, R.W., Gelboin, H.V., Gillette, J.R., and O'Brien, P.J. (Eds.), Microsomes, Drug Oxidation, and Chemical Carcinogenesis, Academic Press, N.Y., pp. 1133-1136.

16. Reed, G.A. and Marnett, L.J. (1982) J. Biol. Chem., 257, 11368.

17. Josephy, P.D., Mason, R.P., and Eling, T. (1982) Cancer Res., 42, 2567.

18. Patek, D.R., and Hellerman, L. (1974) J. Biol. Chem., 249, 2373.

19. Matsubara, T., Prough, R.A., Burke, M.D., and Estabrook, R.W. (1974) Cancer Res., 34, 2196.

20. Marnett, L.J., and Wilcox, C.L. (1977) Biochim. Biophys. Acta, 487, 222.

21. Lowry, O.H., Rosenbrough, N.J., Farr, A.L., and Randall, R.J. (1951) J. Biol. Chem., 193, 265.

22. Prough, R.A., and Ziegler, D.M. (1977) Arch. Biochem. Biophys., 180, 363.

© 1983 Elsevier Science Publishers B.V.
Extrahepatic Drug Metabolism and Chemical Carcinogenesis,
J. Rydström, J. Montelius and M. Bengtsson eds.

A ROLE FOR ACTIVE OXYGEN-INDUCED DNA DAMAGE IN TUMOR PROMOTION

PETER CERUTTI, JOSEPH FRIEDMAN AND ROBERT ZIMMERMAN
Department of Carcinogenesis, Swiss Institute for Experimental Cancer
Research, CH-1066 Epalinges s/Lausanne, Switzerland

INTRODUCTION

Carcinogenesis is a multistep process. Major steps are initiation and promotion. Initiation involves an irreversible genetic change (e.g. DNA damage, gene-mutation, -amplification or -rearrangement) which does not suffice to produce detectable neoplasms, however. The subsequent repeated treatment with a promotor then completes the transformation process (1-5). It has usually been assumed that promotors modulate gene expression entirely by epigenetic mechanisms. However, recent results indicate that the active ingredient in croton oil, phorbol-myristate-acetate (PMA), induces extensive chromosomal damage in human leukocytes (6,7) and mouse epidermal cells (8) as well as aneuploidy in yeast (9). The formation of chromosomal damage by PMA occurs via indirect action, i.e. the intermediacy of active oxygen species (superoxide radicals O_2^-, hydroxyl-radicals $\cdot OH$, singlet oxygen $^1O_2^*$, hydrogenperoxide H_2O_2), lipid-hydroperoxides and small aldehydes. Indeed, we are suggesting that all DNA damaging agents which operate via indirect action represent candidates for promotional activity and we have classified them into three categories (1) physical agents (2) radiomimetic drugs (3) membrane-active agents. It is conceivable that DNA damage induced by indirect action (e.g. strandbreaks, products of the 5,6-dihydroxy-dihydrothymine-type, apurinic- and apyrimidinic-sites, etc.) represents a trigger for the modulation of the expression of certain genes by promotors (10,11).

In this article we review our work which suggests that active oxygen and lipid-peroxidation play a role in tumor promotion. We will first discuss our model of "membrane-mediated chromosomal damage" (10,11) and then present data which indicates the participation of active oxygen in the induction of ornithine decarboxylase and mouse mammary tumor virus in mouse mammary tumor cells by PMA. A direct indication that active oxygen can exert a promotional effect was obtained with mouse embryo fibroblasts C3H/10T1/2. Cells which had been initiated with a physical or chemical carcinogen could be promoted by repeated treatments with xanthine/xanthine-oxidase which produces a burst of active oxygen species.

(1) The model of "membrane-mediated chromosomal damage"

There are important cellular regulatory molecules which mediate their effect by interacting with specific membrane receptors. Hormones, growth factors and components of the immune system belong to this class of molecules. Certain xenobiotics possess the capability to interact with membranes either by binding to specific receptors or by inducing less defined changes in membrane fluidity and conformation. Such agents can mimic or modulate the action of the physiological effector molecules mentioned above. Phorbol-esters, the complete carcinogens benzo(a)pyrene (BP) and aflatoxin B_1 and particulates such as asbestos and silica fall into this category and may possess tumor promoting capabilities. The model of "membrane-mediated chromosomal damage" proposes that membrane-active xenobiotics induce chromosomal damage because they stimulate the arachidonic acid (AA)-cascade, elicit an oxidative burst and disturb the structural integrity of the membranes. All three mechanisms produce active oxygen, lipid-hydroperoxides and their aldehydic degradation products. These highly reactive secondary products are likely candidates as mediators between the initial events at the membrane and the genome. They may also represent clastogenic factors (CF) which are released by the cell after interaction with the xenobiotic and induce chromosomal- and other macro-molecular damage to neighboring tissues. The model does not imply that chromosomal aberrations are early events on the pathway of tumor promotion. It merely suggests mechanisms by which membrane-active xeno-biotics may induce genetic damage without themselves interacting with DNA. DNA damage induced by these mechanisms may play a role in the modulation of gene expression by promotors (10-12).

The major predictions of the model of "membrane-mediated chromosomal damage" are substantiated for the case of the clastogenic action of PMA on human lymphocytes. The participation of active oxygen was evident because the antioxidants CuZn superoxide dismutase (SOD), 4-methyl-2,6-di-tert-butylphenol, 4-methoxy-2,3-tert-butylphenol and mannitol inhibited the formation of chromosomal aberrations; the involvement of lipid-peroxidation was indicated because the inhibitors of AA metabolism, indomethacin, flufenamic acid, imidazol, nordihydroguaiaretic acid (NDGA), 5,8,11,14-eicosatetraynoic acid (ETYA) were anticlastogenic (6,13). PMA treatment of regular human lymphocyte preparations (which are contaminated with monocytes and some platelets but are usually free of polymorphonuclear leukocytes) induced a low-molecular weight, diffusable CF. The CF could be partially purified by ultrafiltration and is unstable. Its clastogenic activity could be diminished by some of the same agents mentioned above (7). We are speculating that the PMA induced CF consists of free AA plus AA-hydroperoxides and that monocytes and platelets contained in the lymphocyte test system metabolically activate the CF (10).

(2) Antioxidants inhibit the induction of ornithine-decarboxylase by phorbol-myristate-acetate

PMA induces numerous biochemical changes and it is difficult to discern which of them are prerequisites for its promotional effect. For example PMA treatment induces the enzymes plasminogen activator, S-adenosyl-methionine decarboxylase and ornithine decarboxylase (ODC). The latter two enzymes are involved in polyamine biosynthesis which is known to be intimately related to the regulation of DNA synthesis and cell proliferation (1-5). The induction of ODC is probably associated with the activity of PMA as tumor promotor. Specific inhibition of ODC in mouse epidermis by the irreversible antagonist α-difluoromethylornithine which prohibits the accumulation of putrescine in response to PMA treatment has an antipromotional effect (14,15). The induction of ODC by PMA can be inhibited with a variety of steroidal and non-steroidal anti-inflammatory drugs which suppress the stimulation of the AA-metabolism, e.g. inhibitors of phospholipase A_2 (dexamethasone, mepacrine, p-bromophenacylbromide) (16); cyclooxygenase (indomethacin, flufenamic acid, ETYA), lipoxygenase (NDGA, phenidone, BN1015, BW 755C) (17,18). Some of these drugs are anti-carcinogens.

It is not clear whether AA-metabolites are directly involved in the modulation of gene expression by PMA, although prostaglandin E2 has been shown to overcome indomethacin inhibition of the induction of ODC (17). Within the frame of the model of "membrane-mediated chromosomal damage" it is conceivable that the hydroperoxy-AA metabolites 5-,12- and 15-hydro-peroxy-AA (HPETE) and prostaglandin G2 induce DNA damage via indirect action. HPETE's and PG G2 are known to release active oxygen upon their decay to more stable derivatives (19-21). Therefore, we have tested the hypothesis that active oxygen may be involved in the induction of ODC. Mouse mammary tumor cells (Mm5mt/C1) (22) were grown to confluency and treated with PMA in the presence or absence of the antioxidants bovine erythrocyte CuZn superoxide dismutase (SOD), catalase (CAT), a combination of SOD plus CAT and mannitol. As shown in Tabel 1 all these drugs partially suppressed ODC induction with SOD exhibiting the weakest effect. The inhibition by CAT implicates H_2O_2 and by mannitol OH-radicals in ODC induction. In order to test directly whether active oxygen can induce ODC we treated Mm5mt/Cl cells with xanthine/xanthine-oxidase. This enzyme system produces an extracellular burst of O_2^- radicals. A small inductive effect was indeed observed (J. Friedman and P. Cerutti, unpublished). This result may explain ODC induction in mouse skin by ultraviolet B light (24) which is known to produce DNA damage by indirect action (25).

(3) Antioxidants inhibit the induction of mouse mammary tumor virus by phorbol-myristate-acetate

PMA induces mouse mammary tumor virus (MMTV) in the mouse mammary tumor cell line Mm5mt/Cl (26) and Epstein-Barr-Virus in human lymphoblastoid cells (27). Mm5mt/Cl cells originate from a C3H mouse mammary tumor and contain in their genome several exogenous copies of MMTV (22). PMA induced the production of intracellular virus RNA and of virus particles. MMTV is also induced by dexamethasone. The effect of the addition of both PMA and dexamethasone was synergistic (26).

We studied the mechanism of MMTV induction by PMA as a model for the modulation of gene expression by tumor promotors. We used nick-translated MMTV DNA to measure the intracellular levels of MMTV RNA by a spot test. In parallel to our experiments on ODC induction discussed above we measured the effect of antioxidants. SOD and CAT, as well as combinations of the two enzymes, turned out to be good inhibitors; e.g. 25 µg/ml SOD inhibited MMTV induction by 20 ng/ml PMA by approximately 50%. We conclude that active oxygen species, possibly via the formation of DNA damage, are participating in the stimulation of the expression of the MMTV sequences in the Mm5mt/Cl genome. It is conceivable that DNA lesions produced by indirect action such as DNA strand breaks, induce conformational changes in chromatin which open up new domains for transcription (J. Friedman and P. Cerutti, unpublished).

(4) Active oxygen promotes initiated mouse embryo fibroblasts 10T1/2

Two stage carcinogenesis involving initiation and promotion has been first demonstrated in whole animal experiments for skin and later for liver and bladder (1-5). Similar phenomena have been observed in vitro with C3H/

10T1/2 mouse embryo fibroblasts (28). In all these systems the transforming potency of chemical and physical carcinogens could be increased by the subsequent repeated treatment with non-carcinogenic "promoting" substances. The phorbolester PMA has been studied in great detail on mouse skin. As mentioned above it induces a great variety of cellular responses and it is difficult to discern which of them are necessary and responsible for promotion. Experiments on mouse skin and with in vitro culture systems suggest that active oxygen plays a role in promotion. However, most of the evidence is circumstantial and based on the observation that certain anti-oxidants and inhibitors of the arachidonic acid cascade are antipromotional (see refs in 10-12,29).

We have investigated directly whether the extracellular generation of active oxygen could enhance the transformation of carcinogen-initiated 10T1/2 cells and mimic the action of PMA, therefore. We have used non-transforming doses of ^{137}Cs γ-rays and the ultimate benzo(a)pyrene metabolite benzo(a)pyrene-diol-epoxide I (BPDE I) to initiate the cultures and the xanthine/xanthine-oxidase (X/XO) system to generate $0_2^{\bar{}}$ and H_2O_2 extracellularly (23). X/XO treatment was started 48 h after the exposure to the initiator and repeated daily for 3 weeks. X/XO concentrations were chosen which did not inhibit the growth of the cultures and were non-toxic according to daily cell counts and standard clonogenic assays. X/XO treatment following an initiating dose of X-rays resulted in a 3-fold enhancement in the number of transformed foci per dish, 1.25 (foci of type II and III) (30) relative to cultures which received γ-rays alone, 0.45. These results are comparable to those of Kennedy et al. (31) for PMA promotion of X-ray initiated cultures under optimal conditions. Similarly X/XO promoted 10T1/2 cultures which had been initiated with non-transforming doses of BPDE I. In this case the repeated X/XO treatment resulted in foci per dish from 0.3 to 0.6. Again these results are comparable to those obtained in the same culture system with PMA and chemical initiators (28). Addition of 10 U/ml SOD simultaneously with X/XO reduced the promotional effect to one third. Only in one of five experiments did X/XO treatment alone lead to the formation of a small number of foci (0.16 foci per dish). Our results indicate that active oxygen species and in particular $0_2^{\bar{}}$ produced repeatedly under non-toxic conditions possess the capacity to promote initiated 10T1/2 to a degree which is comparable to PMA. They support the notion that at least some of the promotional activities of PMA might be due to the formation of active oxygen. Our results do not allow safe conclusions regarding the mechanism(s) by which active oxygen exerts its promotional activity. In analogy to the mechanism of induction of ODC and MMTV by PMA discussed above modulation of gene expression resulting from DNA damage induced by O_2^-, HO_2^- (perhydroxy-radical), H_2O_2 may play a role. These radicals may also oxidize other cellular components, e.g. membrane phospholipids. Such secondary products may in part act as diffusible clastogenic factors (10). It is known that X/XO treatment of human lymphocytes induces chromosomal damage (32).

Table 1

Inhibition by antioxidants of the induction of ornithine decarboxylase by phorbol-myristate-acetate in mouse mammary tumor cells

	%
PMA	100
PMA + SOD (50 μg/ml)	88
PMA + CAT (50 μg/ml)	64
PMA + SOD (50 μg/ml) + CAT (50 μg/ml)	54
PMA + mannitol (0.1 M)	64

Confluent Mm5mt/Cl cells were treated in fresh, complete medium with 20 ng/ml PMA for 8 h and the ODC activity was determined in the cell lysates (33). PMA induced ODC 30 fold over control levels to 1.52 nmoles CO_2/mg protein, hour.

ACKNOWLEDGEMENTS

This work was supported by grant 3'627.80 from the Swiss National Science Foundation.

REFERENCES

1. Diamond, L., O'Brien, G. and Baird, W. (1980) Adv. Cancer Res. 32, 1-74.

2. Slaga, T., Sivak, A. and Boutwell, R., eds. (1978) "Carcinogenesis", Vol. 2. Raven Press, New York.

3. Hecker, E., Fusenig, N., Kunz, W., Marks, F. and Thielmann, H., eds. (1982) "Carcinogenesis", Vol. 7, Raven Press, New York.

4. Weinstein, I., Mufson, R., Lee, L.-S., Fischer, P., Laskin, J., Horowitz, A. and Ivanovic, V. (1980) in: Pullman, B., Ts'o, P. and Gelboin, H. (eds) Carcinogenesis: Fundamental Mechanisms and Environmental Effects, Reidel Publ., Dodrecht, Netherlands, pp. 543-563.

5. Levin, L. (1981) Adv. Cancer Res. 35, 49-79.

6. Emerit, I. and Cerutti, P. (1981) Nature (London) 293, 144-146.

7. Emerit, I. and Cerutti, P. (1982) Proc. Natl. Acad. Sci. 79, 7509-7513.

8. Fusenig, N. and Dzarlieva, R. (1982) in: Hecker, E., Fusenig, N., Kunz, W., Marks, F. and Thielmann, H. (eds) Cocarcinogenesis and biological effects of tumor promotors, Carcinogenesis, Vol. 7, Raven Press, New York, pp. 201-216.

9. Parry, J.M., Parry, E.M. and Barret, J.C. (1981) Nature 294, 263-265.

10. Cerutti, P., Emerit, I. and Amstad, P. (1983) in: Weinstein, I.B. and Vogel, H. (eds) Genes and Proteins in Oncogenesis, Academic Press, New York, pp. 55-69.

11. Cerutti, P., Amstad, P. and Emerit, I., in: Nygaard, O.F. and Simic, M.G. (eds) Radioprotectors and Anticarcinogens, Academic Press, in press.

12. Ide, M., Kaneko, M. and Cerutti, P., in: McBrien, D. and Slater, T. (eds) Protective Agents in human and experimental cancer, Academic Press, in press.

13. Emerit, I., Levy, A. and Cerutti, P., Mutation Res., in press.

14. Weeks, C., Herrmann, A., Nelson, F. and Slaga, T. (1982) Proc. Natl. Acad. Sci. 79, 6028-6032.

15. Takigawa, M., Verma, A., Simsiman, R. and Boutwell, R. (1982) Biochem. Biophys. Res. Commun. 105, 969-976.

16. Nakadate, T., Yamamoto, S. Ischii, M. and Kato, R. (1982) Cancer Res. 42, 2841-2845.

17. Verma, A., Ashendel, C. and Boutwell, R. (1980) Cancer Res. 40, 308-315.

18. Nakadate, T., Yamamoto, S., Ishii, M. and Kato, R. (1982) Carcinogenesis 3, 1411-1414.
19. Egan, R., Paxton, J. and Kuehl, F.A. (1976) J. Biol. Chem. 251, 7329-7335.
20. Rahimtula, A. and O'Brien, P.J. (1976) Biochem. Biophys. Res. Commun. 70, 893-899.
21. Sujioka, K. and Nakano, M. (1976) Biochim. Biophys. Acta 423, 203-216.
22. Owens, R. and Hackett, A. (1972) J. Natl. Cancer Inst. 49, 1321-1328.
23. Kellogg, E. and Fridovich, I. (1975) J. Biol. Chem. 250, 8812-8817.
24. Verma, A., Lowe, N. and Boutwell, R. (1979) Cancer Res. 39, 1035-1040.
25. Hariharan, P. and Cerutti, P. (1977) Biochemistry 16, 2791-2785.
26. Arya, S.K. (1980) Nature 284, 71-72.
27. Zur Hausen, H., O'Neill, F., Freese, U. and Hecker, E. (1978) Nature 272, 373-375.
28. Mondal, S., Brankow, D. and Heidelberger, C. (1976) Cancer Res. 36, 2254-2260.
29. Benedict, W., Wheatley, W. and Jones, P. (1980) Cancer Res. 40, 2796-2801.
30. Reznikoff, C., Bertram, J., Brankow, D. and Heidelberger, C. (1973) Cancer Res. 33, 3239-3249.
31. Kennedy, A. Murphy, G. and Little, J. (1980) Cancer Res. 40, 1915-1920.
32. Emerit, I., Keck, M., Levy, A., Feingold, J. and Michelson, A. (1982) Mutat. Res. 103, 165-172.
33. Bachrach, U. (1975) Proc. Natl. Acad. Sci. 72, 3087-3091.

© 1983 Elsevier Science Publishers B.V.
Extrahepatic Drug Metabolism and Chemical Carcinogenesis,
J. Rydström, J. Montelius and M. Bengtsson eds.

AROMATIC AMINE INDUCED DNA DAMAGE IN MOUSE HEPATOCYTES

MONA MØLLER, IRENE B. GLOWINSKI AND SNORRI S. THORGEIRSSON
Laboratory of Carcinogen Metabolism, National Cancer Institute, Bethesda, MD
20205 (U.S.A.)

INTRODUCTION

N-Hydroxylation of aromatic amines and amides has been shown to be the rate
limiting step in the in vitro mutagenic activation of these compounds by subcellular fractions from mouse liver (1). In order to examine the relative
roles of metabolic activation vs detoxification pathways in the potential
genotoxicity of carcinogenic aromatic amines and amides, DNA damage was
measured in primary mouse hepatocytes after exposure to 2-acetylaminofluorene
(AAF), 2-aminofluorene (AF) and other AAF derivatives using the alkaline
elution technique (2,3). The importance of N-hydroxylation in the genotoxicity
caused by AF and AAF was studied in intact hepatocytes from aryl hydrocarbon
responsive C57BL/6N (B6) and nonresponsive DBA/2N (D2) mice, after pretreatment
with the cytochrome P_{448} inducer 2,3,7,8-tetrachlorodibenzodioxin (TCDD). In
addition, the metabolites produced from AAF in isolated hepatocytes from both
control and TCDD-treated animals were quantitated using high-pressure liquid
chromatography (HPLC).

RESULTS AND DISCUSSION

Low levels of DNA damage were observed after exposure of hepatocytes to
either AF or AAF (50-200 μM) while both N-hydroxy-2-acetylaminofluorene
(N-OH-AAF) and N-acetoxy-2-acetylaminofluorene (N-OAc-AAF) showed clear dose-
dependent increases in DNA strand breaks (5-100 μM). Treatment of hepatocytes
with paraoxon, an inhibitor of microsomal deacetylase activity, prior to
exposure to either N-OH-AAF or N-OAc-AAF, inhibited the DNA damage caused by
these agents, indicating that these compounds are causing genotoxic effects
after deacetylation.

The deacetylated metabolite, N-OH-AF, caused only low levels of DNA damage.
However, after reducing intracellular glutathione levels by more than 50 percent with diethylmaleate, the damage caused by N-OH-AF was increased in a
dose-dependent manner. This suggests that in untreated hepatocytes, N-OH-AF
is effectively detoxified (reduced) before it can reach the nucleus.

Pretreatment of hepatocytes isolated from B6 and D2 mice with TCDD did not
lead to any significant increase in the amount of damage caused by either AF

or AAF. Furthermore, no difference was observed between the B6 and D2 mice. These results indicate that mouse hepatocytes are capable of either detoxification of the resulting genotoxic metabolites and/or that C-hydroxylation (detoxification) is preferentially induced in B6 mice.

In order to study this in more detail the metabolites produced from AAF in liver cells isolated from B6 mice were quantitated using HPLC. In hepatocytes from control mice, 7-OH-AAF (detoxification) was the major metabolite (174 pmol/min/10^6 cells), and the rate of N-hydroxylation was low (12 pmol/min/10^6 cells) corresponding to approximately 4% of the total AAF metabolism. Pretreatment of the mice with TCDD increased the rate of formation of all metabolites, and even though the rate of N-hydroxylation was increased 20-30 times, C-hydroxylation pathways were still responsible for approximately 90% of the metabolism.

The present results clearly show that mouse hepatocytes have a high capability of detoxifying aromatic amines, mainly through the C-hydroxylation pathways. Since the levels of sulfotransferase and acyltransferase are very low in mouse liver cells, our data suggest that the deacetylase is playing an important role in the genotoxicity of N-OH-AAF. However, even after induction of the N-hydroxylation pathway, the cells are able to detoxify N-OH-AAF, most likely through an increase in glucuronidation (5) and/or an efficient reduction of N-OH-AF by glutathione before it can reach the nucleus.

Intact, isolated liver cells provide a system in which competing metabolic pathways, availability of cofactors, and cellular defense mechanisms are operating. It is therefore an appropriate model for studying the metabolic processes involved in the hepatic genotoxicity and possible carcinogenicity of arylamines in this species.

REFERENCES

1. Felton, J.S., Nebert, D.W. and Thorgeirsson, S.S. (1976) Mol. Pharmacol. 12, 225.

2. Kohn, K.W., Erickson, L.C., Ewig, R.A.G. and Friedman, C.A. (1976) Biochemistry (Wash.), 15, 4629.

3. Erickson, L.C., Osieka, R., Sharkey, N.A. and Kohn, K.W. (1980) Anal. Biochem., 106, 269.

4. Smith, C.L. and Thorgeirsson, S.S. (1981) Anal. Biochem., 113, 62.

5. Owens, I. (1977) J. Biol. Chem., 252, 2827.

© 1983 Elsevier Science Publishers B.V.
Extrahepatic Drug Metabolism and Chemical Carcinogenesis,
J. Rydström, J. Montelius and M. Bengtsson eds.

POSSIBLE SIGNIFICANCE OF A DIRECT INTERACTION BETWEEN NAD(P)H and N-ACETOXY-2-
AMINOFLUORENE ON THE BINDING TO HUMAN LYMPHOCYTE DNA

JANERIC SEIDEGÅRD AND RONALD W. PERO
Wallenberg Laboratory, University of Lund, S-220 07 Lund, Sweden

INTRODUCTION

There is a growing interest in applying knowledge of xenobiotic metabolism,
most of which has been obtained from investigations with experimental animals,
to risk evaluation in human beings. In this regard, circulating lymphocytes
have received much attention since they can be obtained without undue stress
or damage to the individual. The evidence to date indicates that unscheduled
DNA synthesis (UDS) in human lymphocytes is related to risk from genotoxic
damage induced by xenobiotics. There are considerable interindividual variations in UDS in resting lymphocytes and it is important to determine whether
genetic, environmental, and/or methodological factors are involved in these
variations.

We have used N-acetoxy-2-acetylaminofluorene (NA-AAF) to induce UDS in human
lymphocytes in our studies of risk evaluation. It is not known at present
whether the major factor regulating NA-AAF binding to the DNA of lymphocytes
is the result of direct chemical interaction or whether it is mediated via a
metabolic event (1). In our initial experimental design to characterize the
possible role of metabolism, we found unexpectedly that addition of NAD(P)H
alone to NA-AAF in water or buffer results in the chemical transformation of
NA-AAF to mainly 2-acetylaminofluorene (AAF) and two other minor products.

MATERIALS AND METHODS

1-2 mM NADPH or NADH was added to 1-10 μM NA-AAF in aqueous solution and incubation was carried out at room temperature for 45 min before extraction of
the reaction mixture was performed with ethyl acetate. These concentrations
of reactants were chosen to reflect either the cellular situation *in vivo* (i.e.
NAD(P)H), in our test systems (i.e. NA-AAF). Subsequent thin-layer chromatography (TLC) with chloroform:methanol (97:3, v/v) revealed one major product
with an R_f = 0.29 which corresponds to AAF. In one experiment no extraction was
performed although the preincubation was carried out in physiological saline
and then it was added directly to the cell suspension.

Measurement of NA-AAF-induced UDS. About 8-10 x 10^6 lymphocytes were exposed
for 30 min to 10 μM NA-AAF, washed and resuspended in fresh medium containing
10 mM hydroxyurea and tritiated thymidine for an additional 18 hrs incubation.

The lymphocyte DNA was then extracted and purified, and the results were recorded as thymidine incorporated per µg DNA.

<u>Measurement of NA-AAF-binding to DNA</u>. About 8-10 x 10^6 lymphocytes or the corresponding amount of DNA were incubated with 1-5 µM tritiated NA-AAF for 30 min. The lymphocyte DNA or pure DNA was then extracted and quantified, and the results were expressed as NA-AAF bound per µg DNA.

RESULTS AND DISCUSSION

It is now clarified by TLC and HPLC that the major product formed when NA-AAF is incubated with NAD(P)H is AAF. This chemical transformation to AAF is linear with time up to at least 60 min, and at this point in the reaction approximately 50% of the original amount of NA-AAF is degraded. However, when NAD(P)H is excluded from an aqueous incubation with NA-AAF then no AAF was detected, although there was still about 50% of the parent compound (NA-AAF) left.

Interestingly, when this "preincubation medium" was added to lymphocyte suspension only small effects could be detected on UDS or binding of NA-AAF to DNA. However, when NA-AAF was added to a medium containing NADPH (or NADH) and pure DNA, the binding of NA-AAF to DNA was nearly completely inhibited (see table 1), even at concentrations of NADPH that are comparable to the levels that exist in lymphocytes.

TABLE 1

THE INFLUENCE OF NAD(P)H ON BINDING TO DNA IN LYMPHOCYTES OR PURE DNA

Preincubation of NA-AAF (30 min)	% of decrease in:		
	UDS	binding of NA-AAF to DNA in resting lymphocytes	binding of NA-AAF to pure DNA after extraction in ethyl acetate
(1) Water	20	56	53
(2) Water + NADPH	31	60	54
(3) Water + NADH	36	70	53
No preincubation of NA-AAF			
(4) Water (control)	0	0	0
(5) Water + NADPH	0	0	96
(6) Water + NADH	0	0	96

REFERENCE

1. National Cancer Institute Monograph 58 (1980), Carcinogenic and Mutagenic N-substituted aryl compounds, NIH Publication No. 81-2379, National Cancer Institute, Bethesda, pp. 1-258.

© 1983 Elsevier Science Publishers B.V.
Extrahepatic Drug Metabolism and Chemical Carcinogenesis,
J. Rydström, J. Montelius and M. Bengtsson eds.

511

GUANOSINE AND DEOXYGUANOSINE ADDUCTS OF NITROGEN MUSTARDS AND ETHYLENEIMINES
- FORMATION AND DESTRUCTION

KIRSTI SAVELA, SEIJA KALLAMA AND KARI HEMMINKI
Institute of Occupational Health, SF-00290 Helsinki 29, Finland

Nitrogen mustards and ethyleneimines derivatives have been extensively used
in the chemotherapy of malignant disease. Nitrogen mustards are thought to
form a highly reactive ethylenimmonium intermediate, related to ethyleneimine,
before covalent binding to nucleophilic centers. The alkylating activity of
these drugs is studied in relation to the types and stability of guanosine and
deoxyguanosine adducts formed. Four nitrogen mustards are studied: nitrogen
mustard, melphalan, chlorambucil and phosphoramide mustard, a metabolite of
cyclophosphamide, in addition to ethyleneimine, triethylenemelamine (TEM) and
triethylenethiophosphoramide (thio-TEPA).

MATERIALS AND METHODS

Cytostatic drugs were incubated with guanosine or deoxyguanosine in neutral
phosphate buffer. The products were analysed using a C_{18} column in HPLC or
by a fluorescence assay (1). The same techniques were also used to determine
the kinetics of destruction of the products.

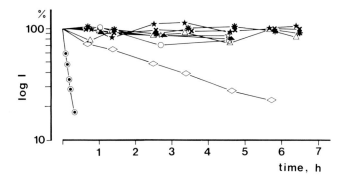

Fig. 1. Decrease in fluorescence (log units) of N-7 alkylguanosines formed by
nitrogen mustard (◇), phosphoramide mustard (○), chlorambucil (✻),
melphalan (✘), ethyleneimine (⊙), TEM (★) and thio-TEPA (△), or of
N-7 alkylguanosine monophosphates formed by phosphoramide mustard (▲) and
ethyleneimine (☆).

512

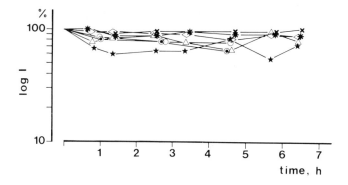

Fig. 2. Decrease of fluorescence (log units) of N-7 alkyldeoxyguanosines
formed by nitrogen mustards and ethyleneimines (symbols as in Fig. 2).

RESULTS AND DISCUSSION

UV- and fluorescence spectra indicated that nitrogen mustard, chlorambucil,
phosphoramide mustard, and ethyleneimine formed an N-7 alkylation product with
guanosine. Fluorescence evidence suggested furthermore that an N-7 alkylguanosine was also afforded by TEM and thio-TEPA.

When the stability of the products was investigated after various periods of
incubation at pH 7.4 it was observed that two kinds of reactions took place:
dechlorination (for nitrogen mustards) and destruction of the imidazole ring
(for nitrogen mustards and ethyleneimines). Dechlorination was assumed to have
taken place when UV-spectra still indicated an intact N-7 alkylguanosine in a
species derived from the initial alkylation product. For ring-opening a typical UV-spectra was taken as an indication. The approximate dechlorination
half-lives for the nitrogen mustards were: 3 min for nitrogen mustard, 2.3 h
for phosphoramide mustard, and 2.7 h for chlorambucil. The half-lives of
imidazole-ring destruction in guanosine, as determined fluorometrically
(Fig. 1), were 6 min for ethyleneimine, 2.5 h for nitrogen mustard, and more
than 6 h for the other compounds studied. Interestingly guanosine monophos-
phate derivatives were much more resistant to ring-opening than the corresponding guanosine derivatives. Imidazole ring of deoxyguanosine was also
markedly more resistant (Fig. 2).

REFERENCE

1. Hemminki, K. (1980) Carcinogenesis, 1, 311.

© 1983 Elsevier Science Publishers B.V.
Extrahepatic Drug Metabolism and Chemical Carcinogenesis,
J. Rydström, J. Montelius and M. Bengtsson eds.

A SENSITIVE REVERSED-PHASE H.P.L.C. METHOD FOR THE DETERMINATION
OF RNA CONTAMINATION IN THE ANALYSIS OF DNA-CARCINOGEN INTERACTIONS.

KEITH R. HUCKLE

Shell Research Ltd., Sittingbourne Research Centre, Sittingbourne,
Kent, ME9 8AG, UK.

INTRODUCTION

   Covalent interactions between chemical carcinogens and DNA are thought to
be an important event in the process of cancer initiation.   In order to
obtain meaningful data on the specificity of binding, the isolation of pure
macromolecular fractions is essential, since electrophilic ultimate chemical
carcinogens interact avidly with nucleophilic sites in the major contaminants
of isolated mammalian DNA preparations, namely cell protein or RNA.   In some
cases, the extent of binding to DNA is somewhat less than that to RNA or to
protein (1).   The presence therefore of even small amounts (<3%) of these
contaminants in the DNA can lead to serious over-estimates in the quantifi-
cation of gross (uncharacterised) covalent binding.   The apparent paucity of
data in the literature concerning the purity of carcinogen-modified DNA
preparations probably reflects the inadequacies of the available methods for
the quantitative determination of such trace contaminants.   Thus, the detection of RNA contamination in DNA samples has in the past, relied upon the use
of colormetric assays; a common procedure, the orcinol method, is insensitive,
non-specific and unreliable, particularly in the presence of a large molar
excess of DNA (2).   The present report describes an alternative assay for the
quantitative estimation of RNA contamination in carcinogen-modified DNA
preparations that is specific, sensitive and reproducible.

MATERIALS AND METHODS

   Enzyme hydrolysis.   Native and carinogen-modified nucleic acid preparations
(in 0.01M Tris/HCl + 0.1M NaCl, pH 7.9, at concentrations up to 1mg/ml) were
treated sequentially at 37° with RNase A (Sigma Type 1A, 8.5×10^{-1} units, 1h),
RNase T_1(Sigma Type V, 6000 units, 1h) and RNase T_2 (Sigma Type V, 1 unit, 2h).
DNase I (Sigma Type DN-EP, 200 units), alkaline phosphatase (Sigma Type III,
5 units) and phosphosdiesterase (Sigma type VII, 2.6×10^{-2} units) were then
added after adjustment of the pH to 9.4 and the addition of $MgCl_2$ (1.5M final
concentration).   The mixture was then reincubated overnight.

Reversed-phase h.p.l.c.   H.p.l.c. of nucleoside standards and nucleic acid
hydrolysates was performed using a μ-Bondapak-C_{18} column (H.P.L.C. Technology,
Macclesfield, UK) and a Co-Pell ODS (Whatman) guard column operating at ambient
temperature and subjected to gradient elution [linear gradient of slope 0 to
25% v/v of an 80% v/v methanol/water solution programmed over 30 min at 1.5 ml/min.
The low strength eluent was 0.1M KH_2PO_4, pH 5.5 (3,4)].   Ribonucleoside
contamination was quantified by peak area integration at 254 nm against a
co-injected internal standard, 8-bromoguanosine.

RESULTS

   Under optimised conditions, complete separation of the major nucleosides
derived from DNA and RNA was achieved in 35 min.   Linear response curves
were obtained for all major nucleosides in the range 0.02 to 100nmol, while
recoveries from the column were 95% in each case.   The detection limit was
ca 20 pmol/nucleoside permitting estimation of ca 0.5% RNA contamination in
samples containing as little as 5 to 10 μg DNA.   Protein did not interfere
with the separation;   crude isolated DNA samples containing 5% to 10%
nucleoprotein contamination were processed with no loss of resolution. Using
thymidine or orotic acid pre-labelled mouse epidermal nucleic acid isolated from
animals treated with benzo(a)pyrene, quantitative enzyme hydrolysis was
observed under the conditions described.

CONCLUSION

   Present procedures for the quantitative determination of small amounts
($\leq$1%) of RNA in the presence of excess DNA are inadequate. The present method
is sensitive, reproducible (relative SD 3% or less) and specific.   Procedural
improvements to commonly used DNA-isolation methods are therefore possible
in order to ensure minimum interference from RNA contamination in carcinogen-
DNA binding studies.

ACKNOWLEDGEMENT

   I would like to thank Dr. R. Davies, Shell Research Ltd., for helpful
discussion of this work.
REFERENCES

1. Koreeda, M; Moore, P.D. Wislocki, P.G. et al (1978) Science, 199, 77.
2. Munro, H.N. and Fleck, A. (1966) Method Biochem. Anal., 14, 113.
3. Hartwick, R.A. and Brown, P.R. (1976) J.Chromatogr., 126, 679.
4. Kuo, C.K; McCune, R.A. and Gehrke, C.W. (1980) Nucleic Acids Res., 8, 4763.

© 1983 Elsevier Science Publishers B.V.
Extrahepatic Drug Metabolism and Chemical Carcinogenesis,
J. Rydström, J. Montelius and M. Bengtsson eds.

DNA REPAIR AS A DETERMINING FACTOR IN THE TRANSPLACENTAL ORGANOTROPIC EFFECT OF N-METHYL-N-NITROSOUREA

ALEXEI J. LIKHACHEV[1], VALERII A. ALEXANDROV[2], VLADIMIR N. ANISIMOV[2], VLADIMIR G. BESPALOV[2], MIKHAIL V. KORSAKOV[2], ANTON I. OVSYANNIKOV[2], IRINA G. POPOVIC, NIKOLAI P. NAPALKOV[2] AND LORENZO TOMATIS[3].
[1]Unit of Mechanisms of Carcinogenesis [1,3]International Agency for Research on Cancer, 150 Cours Albert Thomas, 69372 Lyon Cedex 08, France. [2]N.N. Petrov Research Institute of Oncology, Pesochny 2, 188646 Leningrad, USSR.

It was found in several studies that treatment of pregnant rats with N-methyl-N-nitrosourea (MNU) results in induction of neurogenic and kidney tumours in the offspring (1).

N-nitroso compounds including MNU, are known to alkylate various nucleophilic sites in cellular macromolecules. Of various reaction products, O^6-alkylguanine possesses a miscoding potential and may therefore be the molecular basis of the mutagenic and carcinogenic effects of these agents. In several experimental systems, the principal target organ has appeared to be that in which the persistence of O^6-alkylguanine was highest while non-target organs may be protected from initiation by repair processes which remove this lesion from DNA before replication produces a heritable change in the base sequence (2).

In the present study, we examined whether the repair capacities of various fetal and maternal tissues correspond to the transplacental organotropic carcinogenic effect of MNU.

MATERIALS AND METHODS

Groups of white outbred rats obtained from a Rappolovo Animal Farm of the USSR Academy of Medical Sciences, Leningrad, USSR, were given buffered solution of N-[^{14}C]MNU, synthesized from [^{14}C]methylamine hydrochloride (v/o Isotop, Leningrad, USSR; spec. activity 14.5 mCi/mmol) in a dose of 20 mg/kg bw intravenously. This treatment was followed by administration by the same needle of [^{3}H] thymidine (v/o Isotop, Leningrad, USSR; spec. activity 22 Ci/mmol) on day 21 of pregnancy. Animals were killed 2, 24, 48 or 168 h later, and DNA from livers, kidneys and brains of both dams and offspring was isolated, chromatographed, and concentrations of methylated purines were determined as previously described (3).

Other groups of animals were given MNU (20 mg/kg) intravenously on day 21 of pregnancy. Untreated control was available. Animals were kept while moribund, tissues showing macroscopic lesions were fixed in 10% formalin and paraffin sections were stained with hematoxylin/eosin.

RESULTS

Administration of MNU to rats was followed by the induction of tumours in their offspring, which appeared predominantly within the second year of post-natal onthogenesis. Malignant tumours of central and peripheral nervous system (malignant neurinomas and gliomas of various types) developed in 33% of descendants, whereas kidney tumours (adenosarcomas) were found in 15% of animals. No such tumours developed in control animals.

Initial extent of DNA methylation, under these conditions, was similar in various maternal and foetal tissues, indicating an even distribution of MNU and a lack of placental barrier for it. The loss of 7-methylguanine in DNA occurred at a higher rate in fetuses, than in corresponding maternal tissues, evidently because of the higher rate of DNA turnover and hence its dilution, as indicated by incorporation of radioactive thymidine which was considerably more extensive in DNA of foetal than of corresponding maternal tissues. A rapid loss of 3-methyladenine occurred in all tissues. A considerable difference was observed in the repair of 0^6-methylguanine (0^6-meG) in DNA of different organs. Its faster repair occurred in liver, especially of the dams. In maternal and foetal kidney DNA, this 'promutagenic' adduct was more stable, and it repaired in foetus to a lesser extent. The weakest repair of 0^6-meG occurred in brain DNA and a considerably higher proportion of this adduct remained in the foetus.

The data give further support to the concept (4) that carcinogenesis is initiated by alkylating agents as a consequence of a complex interaction between the alkylation, repair and replication of DNA.

REFERENCES

1. IARC Monographs on the Evaluation of the Carcinogenic Risk of Chemicals to Humans, Vol. 17, Lyon, France: International Agency for Research on Cancer, 1978.

2. Montesano, R. J. of Supramol. Struct. and Cell. Biochem., 17, 259-273, 1981.

3. Montesano, R., Brésil, H. and Margison, G.P. Cancer Res., 39, 1798-1802, 1979.

4. Likhachev, A.J., Ivanov, M.N., Brésil, H., Planche-Martel, G., Montesano, R. and Margison, G.P. Cancer Res., 43, 829-833, 1983.

© 1983 Elsevier Science Publishers B.V.
Extrahepatic Drug Metabolism and Chemical Carcinogenesis,
J. Rydström, J. Montelius and M. Bengtsson eds.

SINGLE-STRAND BREAKS IN DNA OF VARIOUS ORGANS OF MICE INDUCED BY ADMINISTRATION OF STYRENE

S.A.S. WALLES AND I. ORSÉN
Unit of Occupational Toxicology, Research Department, National Board of
Occupational Safety and Health, S-171 84 Solna, Sweden.

Styrene is known to be mutagenic in several organisms and thus cause
DNA-damage. The capability of styrene to induce single-strand breaks (SSB) in
DNA was studied in various organs of mice.

Styrene (175-1050 mg/kg) dissolved in Tween 80 was given i.p. to male
mice (NMRI-type, 25-30 g). The mice were sacrificed 1-24 h after administration. The following organs were removed: liver, lung, kidney, spleen, testis
and brain. Cell nuclei were prepared by a method of Parodi (1). The level of
SSB of DNA was determined by the DNA-unwinding technique (2). The amount of
DNA was measured by means of fluorometry by addition of 4',6-diamidino-2-phenyl
indole 2HCl (DAPI) to the DNA-solution (3). The fraction of double-stranded
DNA (F_{DS}) was calculated as the ratio of the amount of double-stranded DNA
(DS) and the total amount of DNA (DS+SS) (SS= single-stranded DNA) (4). All
these methods were applied for studying SSB induced in vivo (5).

Fig. 1 shows the dose-response curve for damage of kidney-DNA by styrene.
The level of SSB differed in the various organs (Table I). The highest level
was obtained in liver-DNA at 1h but in kidney-DNA not until 4h post-treatment.
In brain-DNA there was an enhanced level of SSB between 4 and 24h after administration.

The capability of metabolizing styrene to styrene-7,8-oxide is different
in various organs (6). The amount of styrene-7,8-oxide 1h after i.p. administration of styrene to mice was about 10 times higher in kidney than in brain
and lung (9).

It seems as if the level of SSB is related to the concentration of
styrene-7,8-oxide in the tissues. Moreover the change in the level of SSB as
a function of time is also influenced by excision repair of damaged DNA bases
(5).

518

TABLE 1

THE LEVEL OF SSB $\pm$ SE (N) IN DNA OF VARIOUS ORGANS DIFFERENT TIMES AFTER I.P. INJECTION OF STYRENE (865 mg/kg IN 100 μl TWEEN 80). THE CONTROL RECEIVED 100 μl TWEEN 80.

| Organ | $-\log F_{DS}$ | | | |
| | time (h) | | | |
	1	4	24	Control
Liver	0.13 $\pm$ 0.01 (7)	0.08 $\pm$ 0.01 (11)	0.07 $\pm$ 0.02 (4)	0.06 $\pm$ 0.01 (22)
Lung	0.04 $\pm$ 0.01 (8)	0.06 $\pm$ 0.01 (10)	0.07 $\pm$ 0.01 (9)	0.05 $\pm$ 0.01 (24)
Spleen	0.02 $\pm$ 0.01 (4)	0.03 $\pm$ 0.01 (5)	0.03 $\pm$ 0.01 (3)	0.04 $\pm$ 0.01 (8)
Kidney	0.08 $\pm$ 0.01 (11)	0.13 $\pm$ 0.01 (12)	0.10 $\pm$ 0.01 (7)	0.06 $\pm$ 0.01 (44)
Testis	0.04 $\pm$ 0.01 (10)	0.05 $\pm$ 0.01 (4)	0.05 $\pm$ 0.01 (3)	0.03 $\pm$ 0.01 (10)
Brain	0.05 $\pm$ 0.01 (5)	0.09 $\pm$ 0.01 (7)	0.10 $\pm$ 0.01 (10)	0.06 $\pm$ 0.01 (26)

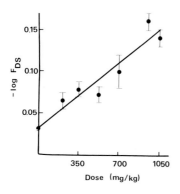

Fig 1. Fraction of double-stranded DNA as a function of the dose 4h after administration of styrene

REFERENCES

1. Parodi, S., Mulivor, R.A., Martin, J.T., Nicolini, C., Sarma, D.S.R., and Farber, E. (1975). Biochim. et Biophys. Acta, 407, 174.

2. Ahnström, G. and Erixon, K. (1981) in: Friedberg, E.C. and Hanawalt, P.C. (Eds.), DNA Repair. Marcel Dekker, New York and Basel, pp. 403-418.

3. Kapuściński, J. and Skoczulas, B. (1977) Anal. Biochem. 83, 252.

4. Erixon, K. and Ahnström, G. (1979) Mutation Res. 59, 257.

5. Walles, S. and Erixon, K. (1983) To be published.

6. Pantarotto, C., Salmona, M., Szczawinska, K., and Bidoli, F. (1980) in Albaiges, J. (Ed) Analytical Techniques in Environmental Chemistry, Pergamon Press, Oxford, pp. 245-280.

7. Nordqvist, M., Löf, A., Ljungquist, E., and Lundgren, E. (1982) Acta Soc. Med. Suec. Hyg., 91, 125.

© 1983 Elsevier Science Publishers B.V.
Extrahepatic Drug Metabolism and Chemical Carcinogenesis,
J. Rydström, J. Montelius and M. Bengtsson eds.

INVESTIGATION OF ABSORPTION, METABOLISM AND DNA BINDING OF PARTICLE ADSORBED
PAH IN THE ISOLATED PERFUSED AND VENTILATED RAT LUNG.

SAM TÖRNQUIST[1], LARS WIKLUND[2] AND RUNE TOFTGÅRD[1]

[1]Department of Medical Nutrition, Karolinska Institutet, Huddinge University
Hospital, F69, S-141 48 Huddinge, Sweden, [2]IVL, Swedish Environmental Research
Institute, Box 21060, S-100 31 Stockholm, Sweden.

INTRODUCTION

Experiments in animal models have shown that after administration of PAH
adsorbed to particulate matter, such as ferric oxide, a significant increase in
lung tumors is obtained, compared to when the PAH is administered as such. The
synergistic effect of combined asbest and cigarette smoke exposure may possibly
reflect a similar phenomenon. In this study perfusion experiments were carried
out with the aim to study differences in the release of unmodified benzo(a)pyrene
(BP) and polar metabolites (PM) to the perfusate buffer and covalent binding to
DNA, following intratracheal administration (i.tr.) of BP in two different forms
of suspension; microcrystalline (MCr) or adsorbed to urban air particles (UAP).

MATERIALS AND METHODS

Perfusions were carried out with lungs from 200 g male Sprague-Dawley rats. BP
was administered at a dose level of 100 µg or 1.3 µg. In one series of experiments, BP was administered directly to the recirculating perfusate buffer (i.b.).
Samples were drawn from the buffer reservoir and venous outflow from the lung,
at fixed time intervals and anlyzed for BP and polar metabolites according to
Van Cantfort et al (1). The fraction of administered dose, remaining in the lung
to be absorbed at time t, (FLu_t), was calculated as a numerical point-area decon-
volution from i.tr. and i.b. concentration time data. DNA was purified from the
lung tissue by hydroxyapatite chromatography and the covalently bound metabolites
were quantified by liquid scintillation counting. BP metabolites present in the
perfusate buffer were separated by HPLC and data was evaluated statistically by
the Mann-Whitney test.

RESULTS AND DISCUSSION

After intratracheal administration of 100 µg BP, different steady state levels
of BP concentration were reached in the perfusate buffer. The lower steady state
level obtained with the UAP preparation was not due to an increased metabolism
rate. In fact the PM concentration at t = 150 min was significantly lower with
the UAP; 80 ± 20 pmol/ml, compared with the MCr; 149 ± 21 pmol/ml. To assess BP

release from the lung at a lower dose, 1.3 µg, BP was administered i.tr. and i.b.
(Fig. 1).   Table 1.

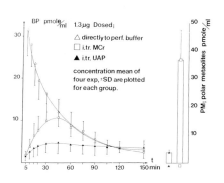

ETHYLACETATE EXTRACTABLE BP METABO-
LITES FROM PERFUSATE BUFFER,100 ug.

	MCr	UAP
9,10 diol	23 + 5.0	39 + 0.9
4,5 -diol	12 + 2.3	7 + 1.2
7,8 -diol	10 + 2.2	14 + 1.1
quinones	10 + 6.0	9 + 0.9
9-OH-phenol	9 + 2.1	8 + 0.5
3-OH-phenol	20 + 4.0	16 + 2.2

% of total ethylacetate extractable
metabolites + S.D. n=4.

FLu$_t$ was calculated and the rate constants for BP disappearence from the lung
were determined to be k_{r1} = 0.051 $\pm$ 0.030 min^{-1} and k_{r2} = 0.007 $\pm$ 0.002 min^{-1},
n = 4, for MCr and UAP respectively. This difference is statistically significant,
p < 0.025. At this dose level the difference in PM concentrations is even more
pronounced (Fig. 1). The levels of BP metabolites covalently bound to DNA were
not markedly different between the two groups; MCr 0.08 pmol/mg DNA and UAP,
0.05 pmol/mg DNA. As shown in Table 1, the metabolic pattern differed to some
extent between the two groups. Small but statistically significant increases in
the formation of BP-9,10-diol and BP-7,8-diol were observed.

In conclusion adsorption of BP into urban air particles would seem to result
in a prolonged local exposure to BP in the lung. Whether or not changes in metabolite pattern or in covalent binding to DNA is significantly affected by particle adsorption of PAH requires further study.

ACKNOWLEDGEMENTS

This investigation was supported by the Swedish Environmental Protection Board;
Project: Air Pollution in Urban Areas. We thank Lillianne Boij for excellent
technical assistance.

REFERENCES

1. Van Cantfort, J. De Graeve and J.E. Gielen (1977) Biochem. Biophys. Res.
    Comm. 79, 505-512.

© 1983 Elsevier Science Publishers B.V.
Extrahepatic Drug Metabolism and Chemical Carcinogenesis,
J. Rydström, J. Montelius and M. Bengtsson eds.

GENETIC CONTROL OF N-ACETOXY-2-ACETYLAMINOFLUORENE (NA-AAF) INDUCED UN-
SCHEDULED DNA SYNTHESIS AND NA-AAF BINDING TO DNA DETERMINED IN MONONUCLEAR
LEUKOCYTES OF TWINS

RONALD W. PERO, CARL BRYNGELSSON, TOMAS BRYNGELSSON AND ÅKE NORDÉN
Wallenberg Laboratory, Biochemical and Genetic Ecotoxicology, University of
Lund, Box 7031, S-220 07 Lund, Sweden

Human genetic variation in response to medical and environmental agents
is now recognized and has been defined as pharmacogenetics and ecogenetics
respectively (1). The best example of an ecogenetic factor is the heritable
capacity of human lymphocytes to induce metabolism of polycyclic hydrocarbons
by aryl hydrocarbon hydroxylase activity.

The carcinogen, 2-acetylaminofluorene (AAF), is also metabolized via ring-
and N-hydroxylations by microsomal mixed function oxygeneases. A metabolic
derivative of AAF, N-acetoxy-2-acetylaminofluorene (NA-AAF), is considered
by most researchers to be either the proximate or ultimate carcinogenic form
of AAF because of its strong electrophilic character and DNA covalent binding
properties. We have assessed the interindividual variation in the response of
cultured mononuclear blood cells to a standardized dose of NA-AAF by estimating the induced levels of unscheduled DNA synthesis (UDS) and the amount of
NA-AAF binding to DNA. Individual variation was considerable and segregated
to age, blood pressure, sex, and genotoxic exposures (2-6).

Here we report on a twin study designed to determine if any of the individual
variation in the NA-AAF method can be explained by genetic factors. We have
examined mononuclear leukocyte samples from both monozygotic (16 pairs) and
dyzygotic (16 pairs) twins for their levels of NA-AAF induced UDS and NA-AAF
binding to DNA. The twins were selected from the Swedish Twin Registry to be
males between 25-35 yr of age, to be concordant for smoking habits and type of
occupation. The intraclass correlation coefficients for NA-AAF induced UDS
were $r_{MZ}=0.86$ and $r_{DZ}=0.46$ and for NA-AAF binding to DNA they were $r_{MZ}=0.85$
and $r_{DZ}=0.22$ (Fig. 1-2). Statistically significant (p< 0.05) heritability
estimates $[\hat{h}_2=2(r_{MZ}-r_{DZ})]$ were calculated as 0.80 and 1.26 respectively. These
data clearly demonstrate that the levels of NA-AAF induced UDS and NA-AAF
binding to DNA are strongly under genetic control.

522

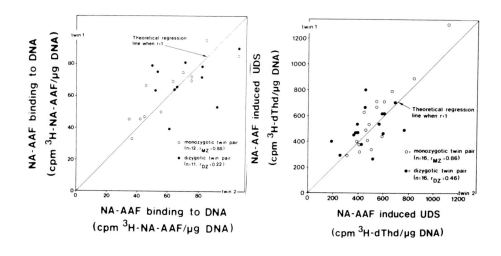

Fig. 1   Fig. 2

REFERENCES

1. Human genetic variation in response to medical and environmental agents:
   Pharmacogenetics and Ecogenetics. (1978) (Vogel, F., Buselmaier, W., Reich-
   ert, W., Kellermann, G. and Berg, P., eds) Human Genetics, Suppl. 1, 1-192.

2. Pero, R.W., Bryngelsson, C., Mitelman, F., Thulin, T. and Nordén, Å. (1976)
   High blood pressure related to carcinogen-induced unscheduled DNA synthesis,
   DNA carcinogen binding, and chromosomal aberrations in human lymphocytes.
   Proc. Natl. Acad. Sci (USA), 73, 2496-2500.

3. Pero, R.W., Bryngelsson, C., Mitelman, F., Kornfält, R., Thulin, T. and Nordén, Å. (1978) Interindividual variation in the responses of cultured human
   lymphocytes to exposure from DNA damaging chemical agents. Mutation Res. 53,
   327-341.

4. Pero, R.W. and Nordén, Å. (1981) Mutagen sensitivity in peripheral lymphocytes as a risk indicator. Environ. Res. 24, 409-424.

5. Pero, R.W., Bryngelsson, T., Högstedt, B. and Åkesson, B. (1982) Occupational and in vitro exposure to styrene assessed by unscheduled DNA synthesis
   in resting human lymphocytes. Carcinogenesis 3:6, 681-685.

6. Pero, R.W., Bryngelsson, T., Widegren, B., Högstedt, B. and Welinder, H.
   (1982) A reduced capacity for unscheduled DNA synthesis in lymphocytes from
   individuals exposed to propylene oxide and ethylene oxide. Mutation Res. 104
   193-200.

© 1983 Elsevier Science Publishers B.V.
Extrahepatic Drug Metabolism and Chemical Carcinogenesis,
J. Rydström, J. Montelius and M. Bengtsson eds.

AGE AND DIET DEPENDENT BINDING OF ^{14}C-DIMETHYLNITROSAMINE METABOLITES TO MOUSE LIVER CHROMATIN

MARIA KLAUDE AND ALEXANDRA VON DER DECKEN
The Wenner-Gren Institute, Norrtullsgtan 16, S-113 45 Stockholm, Sweden.

INTRODUCTION

The object of the investigation is to study the protective influence of dietary proteins on the methylation of nuclear macromolecules by the pro-carcinogen dimethylnitrosamine (DMN). A prerequisite for such studies is to use methods sensitive enough to measure the methylation caused by low concentrations of DMN. Low concentrations of DMN are more likely to be influenced by nutritional conditions. Furthermore, DMN taken up from the environment or formed in the body from precursors is present at concentrations below 5 mg/kg body weight.

MATERIALS AND METHODS

Male mice were fed ad libitum a diet containing 10 % protein. The protein sources were methionine deficient ground peas or ground peas supplemented with DL-methionine (1.7 g/kg diet). The amino acid increases the nutritional quality of the protein. After 6 days mice were injected i.p. with ^{14}C-DMN (2.5 μCi, 5 mg/kg body weight). After 45 min. liver nuclei were isolated, the DNA precipitated and hydrolysed. The apurinic acid, methylated purines and purines were separated by Sephadex G-10 column chromatography (1).

RESULTS AND DISCUSSION

Young growing mice. Young growing mice at 30 days of age were used. Animals fed ground peas showed a lower methylation of the nuclear nucleoprotein complex than mice fed ground peas supplemented with methionine (Table 1). No significant differences were obtained between the dietary groups in the methylation of isolated DNA or purine bases. The results show that growing animals on a diet containing proteins of high nutritional quality have a high DMN-metabolizing capacity. Methylation of nuclear proteins rather than that of DNA changed drastically with the quality of the dietary proteins.

Adult mice. Adult mice at 60 days of age showed no differences between the dietary groups in methylation of the nuclear nucleoproteins, isolated DNA or purine bases (Table 1). In adult mice the differences between the two sources of protein had little effect on the level of methylation of chromatin.

524

TABLE 1

AGE AND DIET DEPENDENT METHYLATION BY DMN OF NUCLEAR DNA AND PROTEIN

Age Days	Protein Source	pmol -CH$_3$ per mg Nucleo-protein	DNA	Ratio DNA/Nucleo-protein	Methylation μmol/mol of Parent Base 3-mA	7-mG	0^6-mG
30	Ground peas	3 480^a	1 870^a	0.54^a	114^a	1 430^a	115^a
	Ground peas plus meth	7 010^b	2 070^a	0.30^b	131^a	1 630^a	122^a
60	Ground peas	5 180^c	1 780^a	0.34^c	98^a	1 430^a	177^b
	Ground peas plus meth	5 120^c	1 920^a	0.38^c	93^a	1 900^a	204^b

[a,b,c] The significance between results were calculated using the two way analysis of variance. Data sharing a common superscript letter within one column are not significantly different; otherwise P<0.05.

Age dependent methylation. In young growing mice the metabolism of DMN in liver varied with the quality of the dietary proteins. In adult mice the capacity of DMN metabolism was little affected by the protein diet. The reason is that in adult animals the proteins are utilized for maintenance metabolism rather than for growth (2). The extent of methylation of purified DNA seemed independent of both diet and age of the animals. Methylation of DNA relative to that of nucleoproteins showed differences which in the young mice were associated with the dietary conditions used (Table 1, column 3). The ratio of methylation of DNA to nucleoprotein was highest in young animals fed ground peas. The level of methylation of 0^6-guanine was not diet but strictly age dependent. It was higher in the adult as compared with the young animals.

The results emphasize the complexity of interaction between diet, age of the animal and metabolism of the procarcinogen DMN. The data obtained will be utilized to establish dietary conditions which at the same time will give a high metabolism of DMN and a reduced level of DNA methylation.

ACKNOWLEDGEMENT
    Support: The Swedish Cancer Society, Project No. 1820-B83-01X.

REFERENCES
1 Montesano, R., Brésil, H. and Margison, G.P. (1979) Cancer Res., 39, 1798.
2 Simon, O., Hernandez, M. and Bergner, H. (1981) Arch. Tierernähr., 31, 751.

IN VIVO AND *IN VITRO* MODEL SYSTEMS
OF CHEMICAL CARCINOGENESIS

© 1983 Elsevier Science Publishers B.V.
Extrahepatic Drug Metabolism and Chemical Carcinogenesis,
J. Rydström, J. Montelius and M. Bengtsson eds.

METABOLISM OF N-NITROSAMINES AND EFFECTS OF FORMALDEHYDE ON DNA
REPAIR IN CULTURED HUMAN TISSUES AND CELLS

ROLAND C. GRAFSTRÖM[1,2] AND CURTIS C. HARRIS[1]

[1]Laboratory of Human Carcinogenesis, National Cancer Institute,
National Institutes of Health, Bethesda, Maryland 20205, (U.S.A.)
and [2]Department of Forensic Medicine, Karolinska Institutet,
S-104 01 Stockholm (Sweden).

INTRODUCTION

Since many chemical carcinogens require metabolic activation
before they can exert their mutagenic and carcinogenic effects,
it is important to determine if human target tissues can metabolize these procarcinogens into their ultimate carcinogenic forms.
Investigations of chemical carcinogenesis in human tissues have
been facilitated by the progress made in the culture of human
epithelial tissues and cells during the last decade (1). Methods
have been developed to culture normal tissues and cells from the
major sites of human cancer. Chemically defined media have been
devised both for explant culture of human bronchus, colon, esophagus, and pancreatic duct and for culture of isolated human
bronchial epithelial cells (2) and skin keratinocytes (3). These
in vitro model systems now provide an important bridge between
epidemiology and studies using experimental animals in the investigation of carcinogenesis.

Important aspects of studying carcinogenesis in cultured human
tissues and cells include the elucidation of the possible role
of metabolism, DNA damage and its repair in relationship to the
relative organ specificity shown by many chemical carcinogens.
For example, N-nitrosamines are potent and organotropic carcinogens in experimental animals. N-Nitrosamines are both found in
the environment and formed by in vivo nitrosation of secondary
amines. Following metabolic activation, N-nitrosamines will give
rise to alkylcarbonium ions, nitrogen and aldehydes (Figs 1 and
2).

Metabolism of N-nitrosodimethylamine (DMNA) gives rise to at
least two products that can react with nucleophilic sites in
cellular macromolecules; methylcarbonium ions by alkylation and

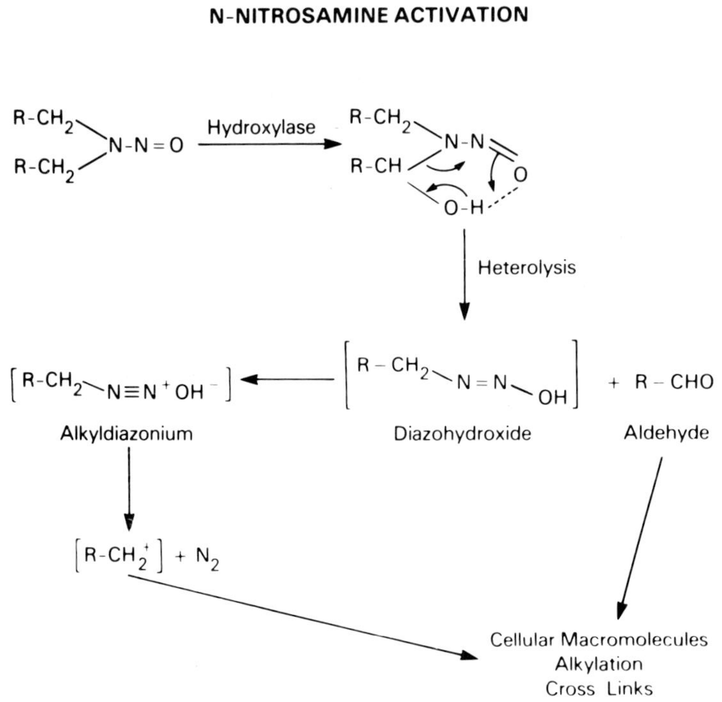

N-NITROSAMINE ACTIVATION

Fig. 1. Metabolic activation of N-nitrosamines.

formaldehyde via formation of unstable methylol derivatives with amine groups (R-HN-CH$_2$OH). These hydroxymethylated derivatives can by a slow spontaneous secondary reaction yield stable methylene bridges between macromolecules. The amounts of methylcarbonium ion and aldehyde bound to macromolecules are dependent on many physicochemical factors (4,5). Formaldehyde may also be rapidly oxidized in the cell to formate and ultimately to CO$_2$ by the involvement of different enzymatic pathways (Fig. 2). Both formaldehyde and formate may eventually enter the one-carbon pool as N^5,N^{10}-tetrahydrofolate derivatives and subsequently become incorporated into a variety of cellular products (cf 6 for references).

Since formation of the alkylcarbonium ion is regarded as essential for initiation of N-nitrosamine carcinogenesis, a possible contribution of aldehydes has received less attention and study. However, formaldehyde, formed by metabolic activation of DMNA, and by demethylation of a variety of other xenobiotics (7) has been shown to be mutagenic in several species (4) including cultured human cells (8) as well as a respiratory carcinogen in rodents (9). Therefore, formaldehyde can be considered as a potential carcinogen in humans (6).

We have investigated metabolism of N-nitrosamines and DNA damage caused by their metabolites in cultured human tissues and cells, and have assessed the potential of formaldehyde to damage DNA, as well as to inhibit the repair of DNA damage caused by either chemical or physical carcinogens.

MATERIALS AND METHODS

Normal appearing human tissues were obtained at the time of either surgery or immediate autopsy, and kept at 4° in L-15 medium until cultured as explants (1). These explants were cultured for 1-7 days to reverse any cellular ischemia and to minimize residual effects of therapeutic treatment, if any, of the donor. Subsequently explants were exposed to radioactive labeled N-nitrosamines at a non-toxic dose, as determined by morphological criteria. After incubation for 24 hrs, the mucosa was collected from the supporting tissues, and DNA was isolated for quantitation of metabolic activation rates as measured by the amount of radioactivity associated with cellular DNA, and by qualitative analysis of carcinogen-DNA adducts (10). The levels of methylated DNA purines after exposure to alkylating agents were analyzed by hydrolyzing DNA in 0.1 N HCl at 70° for 60 minutes followed by subsequent separation of the released purines by high pressure liquid chromatography (HPLC) using a Partisil SCX column and 0.05 M ammonium formate (pH 4.0, 1 ml/min) (11). Optical markers for guanine, adenine, O^6-methylguanine and N7-methylguanine were included.

The alkaline alution technique (12) was used to assess DNA damage by formaldehyde. To measure DNA single-strand breaks the cells were collected onto polycarbonate filters (2 μM pore size; Nucleophore) and lysed with 5 ml of 2 percent sodium dodecyl sulfate (SDS), 0.1 M glycine, and 0.02 M EDTA (pH 9.6). Subsequently, 2 ml of the same solution containing Proteinase K

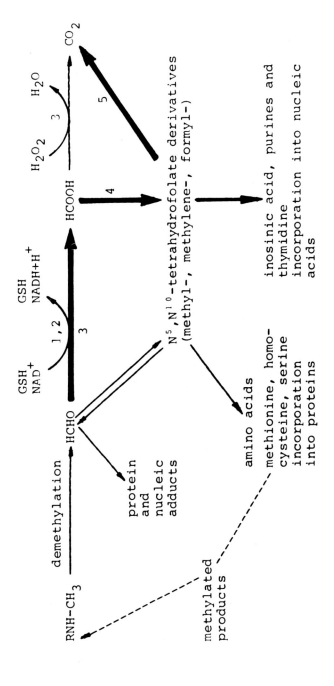

Fig. 2.   Major pathways of formaldehyde metabolism

1, formaldehyde dehydrogenase;   2, S-formylglutathione hydrolase;   3, catal
4, 10-formyltetrahydrofolate dehydrogenases;   5, 10-formyltetrahydrofolate
dehydrogenase

(0.5 mg/ml) was filtered at 0.03 ml/min and followed by 40 ml of a solution containing EDTA (0.02 M; acid form), 0.1 percent SDS, and tetrapropyl ammonium hydroxide at pH 12.2. Eluted fractions were collected and assayed for radioactivity. The combination of the polycarbonate filters, Proteinase K digestion, and SDS in the eluting solution completely removed the DNA protein cross-linking effect of formaldehyde concentrations up to 1 mM. An internal standard ((^{3}H) thymidine-labeled L 1210 cells that received 300 rad at 4°C) was included in each assay. Estimates of the frequency of single-strand breaks and level of DNA protein crosslinks were quantitated by methods described by Fornace (13).

Unscheduled DNA synthesis from exposure to formaldehyde and either (+)-(7β,8α)-dihydroxy(9α,10α)-epoxy-7,8,9,10-tetrahydro-benzo(a)pyrene (BPDE) or UV radiation was measured in confluent bronchial fibroblasts by incorporation of ^{3}H-TdR into DNA in the presence of hydroxyurea by methods previously described (14).

Cytotoxicity of the various agents was determined by plating either 500 bronchial fibroblasts or 5000 epithelial cells/60 mm^2 tissue culture dish and the colony forming efficiency (CFE) determined from colonies containing at least 16 cells after 8 days posttreatment culture of duplicate dishes.

RESULTS

DNA damage and metabolism of N-nitrosamines

Both acyclic and cyclic N-nitrosamines can be activated to metabolites that are associated with DNA in cultured human epi-thelial tissues and cells (Table 1; 15,16). Human bronchus can activate all of the N-nitrosamines tested to date. Radioactivity associated with DNA was observed in human colon incubated with N-nitrosopyrrolidine but no detectable radioactivity was found with N-nitrosopiperidine. Neither of these cyclic N-nitrosamines was activated to metabolites associated with DNA in cultured human esophagus although radioactivity associated with proteins was observed. In contrast, cultured rat esophagus can readily activate cyclic N-nitrosamines to metabolites associated with DNA including the potent organotrophic carcinogen in the rat, i.e., N-nitrosomethylbenzylamine (16). A preference for metabolic α-oxidation at the methyl group was indicated by 10-fold higher

TABLE 1

N-NITROSOAMINES ACTIVATED TO FORM METABOLITES ASSOCIATED WITH DNA BY CULTURED ADULT HUMAN TISSUES AND CELLS

N-Nitrosamine	Bronchus	Colon	Esophagus	Pancreatic duct	Bladder
N-Nitroso-dimethylamine	+[a]	+	+	+	+
N-Nitroso-diethylamine	+	+	+		
N-Nitroso-pyrrolidine	+	+	-		+
N-Nitroso-piperazine	+	-	-		
Dinitroso-piperazine	+	+			
N-Nitroso-methylbenzyl-amine			-		

[a] (+) positive;   (-) nondetectable;   blank space indicates not studied

levels of benzaldehyde than formaldehyde and CO_2. The activation of N-nitrosopyrrolidine was higher in human bronchus and colon than in other human tissues, but a even higher level of DNA binding was seen in the corresponding rat tissues. Both N7- and O^6-methylguanine adducts were detected after incubation of human tissues with ^{14}C-DMNA. However, a significant amount of radioactivity was associated with guanine and adenine due to the metabolic incorporation of C-1 fragments. Considerable amount of radioactivity in DNA was also due to the alkylation of the phosphate groups. When cultured human bronchial epithelial cells were exposed to DMNA most of the radioactivity in DNA was associated with phosphate and methylation at the N7-position of guanine (17).

DNA damage by formaldehyde

Human bronchial epithelial cells and fibroblasts exposed to formaldehyde developed both DNA-protein crosslinks and single strand breaks (SSB) in DNA (14). The number of DNA-protein cross-links induced by 100 μM formaldehyde in epithelial cells and fibroblasts was similar (0.65 and 0.83 unit, respectively), and the frequency of these crosslinks was proportional to the concentration of formaldehyde. The rate at which these crosslinks were removed was also similar in the two cell types; the half-removal time was approximately 2 hours (data not shown): this is consistent with results obtained in mouse L 1210 cells (18). Formaldehyde-induced DNA single-strand breaks were also detected after removal of the crosslinks with proteinase K. The frequency of DNA single-strand breaks induced by 500 μM formaldehyde was 4.2 per 10^{10} daltons in epithelial and 3.5 per 10^{10} daltons in fibroblastic cells and was dose-dependent. The removal rate of the single-strand breaks was also similar in the two cell types (data not shown).

By incubating cells in the presence of the DNA polymerase inhibitor combination of arabinofuranosyl cytosine (AraC) (0.01 mM) and hydroxyurea (2 mM), SSB formed during excision repair can be efficiently accumulated (13). Cells were initially incubated with formaldehyde for 1 hr and then allowed to "repair incubate" without formaldehyde for 3 hrs in the presence of polymerase inhibitors. The frequency of the SSB caused by formaldehyde (attributed to excision repair) was estimated by substracting the background level induced by the polymerase inhibitor combination alone. Exposure to formaldehyde alone with this protocol did not result in any significant numbers of SSB in either bronchial epithelial cells or fibroblasts. In the presence of the AraC/hydroxyurea, SSB accumulated at similar levels (10-12 SSB per 10^{10} daltons) in both epithelial cells and fibroblasts (17). Normal skin fibroblasts and bronchial cells respond similarly to formaldehyde, whereas in two types of xeroderma pigmentosum cells few SSB accumulate (13).

Effects of formaldehyde on DNA repair

The possibility that formaldehyde may inhibit rejoining of SSB induced by exposure to γ-rays was investigated in human bronchial epithelial cells and fibroblasts (Fig. 3; 14). For these experiments, formaldehyde was used at a concentration of 100 μM which

534

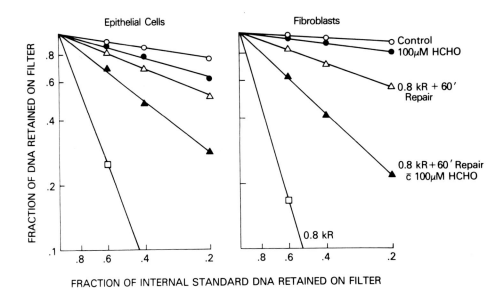

Fig. 3. Effect of formaldehyde on the repair of γ-ray induced DNA single strand breaks in human bronchial epithelial cells and fibroblasts.

causes only a small number of SSB. Exposure of cells to 0.8 krad resulted in high numbers of SSB and a rapid elution of DNA. If the cells were allowed to repair by incubating for 1 hr, the number of SSB decreased substantially. The presence of 100 µM formaldehyde significantly inhibited rejoining of the SSB in both epithelial cells and fibroblasts. Neither methanol, formate, acetaldehyde, benzaldehyde nor acetone had any influence on the rejoining of γ-ray-induced SSB (17).

The influence of formaldehyde on UDS induced by either UV radiation or BPDE was investigated in confluent bronchial fibroblasts (Fig. 4; 14). Exposure of cells to formaldehyde alone did not significantly stimulate UDS. Exposure to UV or BPDE stimulated UDS 6- and 3-fold, respectively. Concentrations of 600 µM formaldehyde or more were required to inhibit UDS caused by either agent. No detectable inhibition of UDS was obtained at 100 µM formaldehyde which was the concentration required to significantly inhibit rejoining of γ-ray-induced SSB. These results suggest that formaldehyde inhibits the ligation step of excision repair.

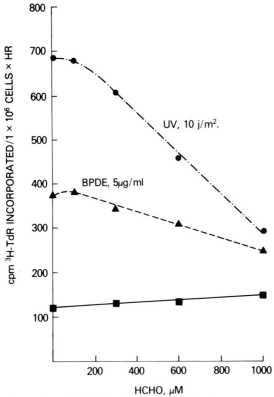

Fig. 4. Effect of formaldehyde on unscheduled DNA synthesis induced by ultraviolet radiation and BPDE in confluent human bronchial fibroblasts. ■, cells exposed to formaldehyde alone; ▲, cells exposed to BPDE; ●, cells exposed to ultraviolet radiation.

The biological consequences of exposure to formaldehyde alone and formaldehyde inhibition of DNA repair processes were further investigated. When human bronchial epithelial cells or fibroblasts were exposed to formaldehyde up to 300 μM for 1 hr only slight toxicity was observed (Fig. 5). Inhibition of colony forming efficiency (CFE) was only slightly greater at 300 μM as compared to 100 μM. A concentration of 1 mM was required to decrease CFE to 10% of control (data not shown). Exposure of cells to formaldehyde for 5 hr remarkably decreased their survival to 32% CFE and 2% CFE at 100 or 300 μM formaldehyde, respectively (17). When bronchial cells were exposed to γ-rays, formaldehyde markedly in-

536

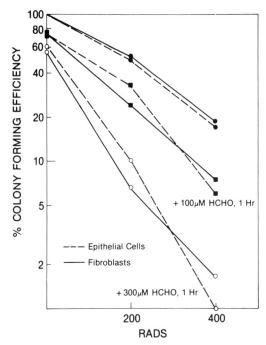

Fig. 5. Colony forming efficiency of human bronchial cells after exposure to γ-rays and formaldehyde. ●, cells exposed to γ-rays; ■, cells exposed to γ-rays followed by 100 μM formaldehyde for 1 hr; o, cells exposed to γ-rays followed by 300 μM formaldehyde for 1 hr.

creased the toxicity with a marked decrease in CFE in both cell types. Significant potentiation of toxicity was observed at 400 rads with concentrations of 100 μM formaldehyde at 200 rads and 400 rads with concentrations of 300 μM formaldehyde. In similarity the toxicity of 0.2 mM MNU, an essentially nontoxic dose, was synergistically increase by the simultaneous presence of 100 μM formaldehyde (17).

DISCUSSION

Studies have shown that several human tissues *in vitro* have the ability to metabolically convert potential carcinogenic compounds into their ultimate carcinogenic form (19). In addition, the metabolism in human tissues was generally identical to that ob-

served in animal tissues in which the compounds are carcinogenic;
a result suggesting that the compound may be a potential human
carcinogen.

Although N-nitrosamines have not been proven by epidemiological
studies to be causative agents in the induction of human cancer,
these compounds cause tumor formation in experimental animals.
In addition, N-nitrosamines often exhibit organotrophic effects
and animal species variation with regard to the carcinogenic potency (20). In cultured human tissues, this class of compounds
is also the only one so far to show marked organ differences in
the metabolism into ultimate reactive species that react with
cellular DNA (Table 1). The apparent lack of DNA binding in
certain tissues possibly may reflect qualitative or quantitative
differences that are below the detection limit of the assay.
Human fetal liver and esophagus did not activate DMNA to metabolites that bind to DNA, whereas fetal stomach activated several
N-nitrosamines to a higher extent than did cultured esophagus
(21). Slices of human lung and liver was reported to metabolize
DMNA (22,23) as measured by the formation of $(^{14}C)-CO_2$, and by
human liver *in vivo* by the presence of N7- and O^6-methylguanines
in DNA isolated from a liver of a person who died of DMNA posio-
ning (24).

Effects of N-nitroso compounds have been related to the degree
of alkylation in target tissue DNA and the ability of the tissue
to remove these lesions (25). Following metabolic activation of
DMNA or spontaneous hydrolysis of N-methyl-N'-nitrosourea, methylation of oxygens of DNA bases, e.g., O^6-guanine, occurs and these
modified bases are considered to be critical promutagenic lesions
in that they cause direct miscoding during DNA synthesis. Treatment of DNA *in vitro* with alkylating agents, i.e., N-methyl-N'-
nitrosourea, results in a ratio of O^6-methylguanine to N7-methyl-
guanine of ∿0.11 and similar levels have been found in hepatic
DNA of animals receiving high doses of N-nitrosamines (25). After
exposure of human bronchial cells to N-methyl-N'-nitrosourea the
ratio of O^6-methylguanine to N7-methylguanine was only 0.04 (17).
This fact indicates a fast removal of O^6-methylguanine, which is
in agreement with the observation that human tissues and cells
are approximately 10-fold more efficient than the corresponding

rat tissues and cells in removing this lesion by direct reversal repair. The presence of formaldehyde resulted in a dose dependent inhibition of removal of O^6-methylguanine (17).

Metabolism of DMNA leads to one to one stoichiometric generation of methylcarbonium ion and formaldehyde. Whereas the methylcarbonium ion formed in this reaction is thought to be responsible for carcinogenicity of N-nitrosamines; a possible contribution of formaldehyde has been largely neglected. Formaldehyde causes the formation of DNA-protein crosslinks and DNA SSB in human bronchial cells. The fact that the SSB could be accumulated in the presence of AraC and hydroxyurea suggests the involvement of excision repair of formaldehyde induced DNA lesions. Furthermore, formaldehyde inhibits repair of DNA damage caused by different chemical and physical carcinogens including ionizing radiation, UV-radiation, BPDE or N-methyl-N'-nitrosourea. The removal of O^6-methylguanine and the ligation of γ-ray-induced SSB seem to be preferentially sensitive, since significant inhibitory effects are obtained at 100 μM formaldehyde. A number of mechanisms may be involved in the inhibition of DNA repair by formaldehyde. The high reactivity of the chemical probably causes methylolation of chromatin or other proteins including enzymes critical to DNA repair processes. Following 1 hr incubation of bronchial cells with 1 mM (^{14}C)-formaldehyde, a 100-fold higher level of radioactivity is associated with protein as compared with DNA (17). Thus, the potentiating effect of formaldehyde on the cytotoxicity of γ-rays or N-methyl-N'-nitrosourea may depend on interaction with enzymes critical for the repair of the respective DNA lesions as demonstrated by the fact that O^6-methylguanine was removed at significant slower rates in formaldehyde exposed bronchial fibroblasts (17).

Since formaldehyde damages DNA, inhibits DNA repair, and potentiates the cytotoxicity of γ-rays or N-methyl-N'-nitrosourea in human bronchial cells, and since the formaldehyde may act in concert with physical and chemical agents (i.e. nitrosocompounds) we suggest that the mutagenic and carcinogenic effects of this chemical alone or in combination with other agents should be further investigated.

ACKNOWLEDGEMENTS

We thank H. Autrup, A.J. Fornace,Jr., J.F. Lechner and A.E. Pegg for valuable contributions to this work and Ms. R.-M. Jagerborn for secreterial assistance.

REFERENCES

1. Harris, C.C., Trump, B.F. and Stoner, G.D., Eds (1980) Culture of normal tissues and cells. Methods in Cell Biol. Academic press Inc., New York, Volumes 21A, 21B.

2. Lechner, J.F., Haugen, A., McClendon, I.A. and Pettis, E.W. (1982) Clonal growth of normal adult human bronchial epithelial cells in serum-free medium. In Vitro, 18, 633.

3. Maciag, T., Nemore, R.E., Weinstein, R. and Gilchrest, B.A. (1981) An endocrine approach to the control of epidermal growth: Serum-free cultivation of human keratinocytes. Science, 211, 1452.

4. Auerbach, C., Moutschen-Dahmen, M. and Moutschen, J. (1977) Genetic and cytogenetical effects of formaldehyde and related compounds. Mutat. Res. 39, 317.

5. Hemminki, K. (1981) Reactions of formaldehyde with guanosine. Toxicol. Lett., 9, 161.

6. Report of the formaldehyde panel (1982) Environ Health Perspect. 43, 139.

7. Waydhas, C., Weigl, K. and Sies, H. (1978) The disposition of formaldehyde and formate arising from drug N-demethylations dependent on cytochrome P-450 in hepatocytes and in perfused rat liver. Eur. J. Biochem. 89, 143.

8. Goldmacher, V.S. and Thilly, W.G. (1983) Formaldehyde is mutagenic for cultured human cells. Mutat. Res. 116, 417.

9. Swenberg, J.A., Kerns, W.D., Mitchell, R.I., Caralla, E.J. and Pavkov, K.L. (1980) Induction of squamous cell carcinomas of the rat nasal cavity by inhalation exposure to formaldehyde vapor. Cancer Res. 40, 3398.

10. Harris, C.C., Frank, A., Van Haaften, C., Kaufman, D., Connor, R., Jackson, F., Barret, L., McDowell, E. and Trump, B. (1976) Binding of (^{3}H)-benzo(a)pyrene to DNA in cultured human bronchus. Cancer Res. 36, 1011.

11. Bennet, R.A. and Pegg, A.E. (1981) Alkylation of DNA in rat tissues following administration of streptozotocin. Cancer Res. 41, 2786.

12. Kohn, K.W., Ewig, R.A.G., Erikson, L.C. and Zwelling, L.A. (1981) Measurement of strand breaks and crosslinks by alkaline elution. In DNA Repair, A Laboratory Manual of Research Procedures (Eds. E.C. Friedberg and P.C. Hanawalt), Marcel Dekker, New York, pp 379-401.

13. Fornace, A.J. Jr. (1982) Detection of DNA single strand breaks produced during the repair of damage by DNA-protein cross-linking agents. Cancer Res. 42, 145.

14. Grafström, R.C., Fornace, A.J. Jr., Autrup, H., Lechner, J.F. and Harris, C.C. (1983) Formaldehyde damage to DNA and inhibition of DNA repair in human bronchial cells. Science 220, 216.

15. Harris, C .C., Autrup, H., Stoner, G., McDowell, E., Trump, B. and Schafer, P. (1977) Metabolism of acyclic and cyclic N-nitrosamines in cultured human bronchi. J. Natl. Cancer Inst. 59, 1401.

16. Autrup, H. and Stoner, G.D. (1982) Metabolism of N-nitrosamines by cultured rat and human esophagus. Cancer Res. 42, 1307.

17. Grafström, R.C. and Harris, C.C., unpublished observations.

18. Ross, W.E. and Shipley, N. (1980) Relationship between DNA damage and survival in formaldehyde treated mouse cells. Mutat. Res. 79, 277.

19. Harris, C.C., Trump, B.F., Grafström, R.C. and Autrup, H. (1982) Differences in metabolism of chemical carcinogens in cultured human epithelial tissues and cells. J. Cellular Biochemistry, 18, 285.

20. Magee, P.N., Montesano, R. and Preussman, B. (1977) Chemical carcinogenesis. Am. Chem. Soc. Monogr. 173, 449.

21. Autrup, H., unpublished observations.

22. DenEngelse, L., Gibbink, M. and Emmelot, P. (1975) Studies on lung tumors. III. Oxidative metabolism of dimethylnitrosamines by rodent and human lung tissues. Chem. Biol. Interactions, 11, 535.

23. Montesano, R. and Magee, P.N. (1970) Metabolism of dimethylnitrosamine by human liver slices in vitro. Nature (London) 288, 173

24. Herron, D.C. and Shank, R.C. (1980) Methylated purines in human liver DNA after probable dimethylnitrosamine poisoning. Cancer Res. 40, 3116.

25. Pegg, A.E. (1983) Formation and removal of methylated nucleosides in nucleic acids of mammalian cells. In "Recent results in Cancer Research", (Ed. J. Nass), Vol. 84, pp 49-62, Springer-Verlag, Berlin.

© 1983 Elsevier Science Publishers B.V.
Extrahepatic Drug Metabolism and Chemical Carcinogenesis,
J. Rydström, J. Montelius and M. Bengtsson eds.

EARLY CHANGES IN GENE EXPRESSION DURING HEPATOCARCINOGENESIS

SNORRI S. THORGEIRSSON, PETER J. WIRTH AND RITVA P. EVARTS
Laboratory of Carcinogen Metabolism, National Cancer Institute, Bethesda, MD
20205 (U.S.A.)

INTRODUCTION

The carcinogenic process is traditionally divided into three phases: initiation, promotion and progression (1). Although this division of the carcinogenic process, particularly with respect to initiation and promotion, was first established in the mouse skin carcinogenesis system, the oncogenic process in several other tissues can clearly be divided into initiation and promotion (1). The rodent liver is one of the tissues in which initiation and promotion can be clearly separated and several experimental systems have been devised to study this process in vivo (1,2,3).

The initiation events in chemically induced tumorigenesis is generally believed to be the covalent interaction of the carcinogen with DNA in the target organ. This interaction appears to alter the information processing in the cell and cause changes in both gene expressions and phenotypic characteristics. These initiated cells will, under appropriate conditions (e.g. promotion), develop into malignant tumor cells (2). Therefore, the cellular changes (at least some of these changes) that are introduced during initiation are essential for the development of neoplasia since promotion with a "pure promoter" results in no tumor without the initiating events (1,2).

Relatively little is known about the gene products that control and maintain the initiated phenotype and how these products may change as a function of time during promotion and progression phases of the carcinogenic process. In order to determine the biochemical characteristics of the initiation stage it is necessary to isolate the initiated cells in sufficient quantity to allow for both biochemical and biological examination of these cells. It is in this respect that the liver offers many advantages over other systems used in the study of the mechanism of chemical carcinogenesis. The advantages of the liver model include: (1) Responsiveness to a broader spectrum of initiators and promoters than any other single tissue; (2) abundance, relative homogeneity and accessibility of liver tissues; (3) retention of cells representing the various stages of oncogenesis at the site of origin; and (4) availability of histochemical techniques for identifying the putative clones of early preneoplastic hepatocytes.

The present work is a part of our current studies on the mechanisms of chemical carcinogenesis using the rodent liver as our model system. In our initial studies we have focused on the separation and biological as well as biochemical characterization of the preneoplastic liver cells in the rat.

MATERIALS AND METHODS

Fischer rats, both newborn and weanling, were used for these studies. The experimental protocols used for hepatocarcinogenesis were those described by Solt and Farber (4), and Peraino et al. (5). Isolation of hepatocytes were performed according to the method of Seglen (6), and separation of different cells according to size was accomplished by elutriation technique (7). Separation of cells according to absence and/or presence of hepatocyte binding protein (asialoglycoprotein receptor) was accomplished by coating tissue culture plates with asialofetuin (8). The two-dimensional gel electrophoresis of total cellular proteins was performed according to the methods of Miller et al. (9).

RESULTS AND DISCUSSION

Foci of altered liver parenchymal cells are detectable relatively early in the various experimental protocols used in the rat (2). These foci are distinguished from surrounding normal liver tissue by a number of phenotypic markers, especially altered enzyme-histochemical reactions (2).

We have made the assumption that these enzyme "altered" foci and later hyperplastic nodules represent an early clonal outgrowth from initiated hepatocytes and would therefore be appropriate targets for the isolation and characterization of the initiation stage in hepatocarcinogenesis.

Five subpopulations of normal rat hepatocytes can be separated by elutriation or counterflow-centrifugation ranging from small (16-18 μm in diameter) diploid cells to large ($\geq$ 25 μm in diameter) polypoid cells (7). Earlier work by Wanson et al. (7) demonstrated that during treatment with hepatocarcinogen a selective increase in the large cell fraction in the liver was observed. Furthermore, early changes in the surface proteins in the hepatocytes have been observed upon treatment with liver carcinogen (Table 1; 10,11).

We have used these characteristics of the putative initiated cell as the basis for separation from the normal hepatocytes (Table 2). After collagenase perfusion and separation by elutriation into small and large cell fractions, further separation of the cells were done on the basis of presence or absence of surface receptor for asialofetuin by allowing the cells to attach to

TABLE 1

BINDING OF ASIALOOROSOMUCOID (ASOR) TO INTACT RAT HEPATOCYTES AND CELL HOMOGENATES

Tissue	ASOR-Bound (Percent of Control)
Normal liver[a]	100%
Neoplastic nodules	
3 days	38
14 days	36
90 days	37
PHC	5
Regenerating liver[b]	25

[a]ASOR bound to cell homogenate from untreated liver: 325 ± 21 pmoles per g liver (ref. 10).

ASOR bound to intact hepatocytes: $1000 \text{ ng}/10^7$ cells.

[b]Two days after partial hepatectomy (ref. 11).

TABLE 2

ISOLATION AND SEPARATION OF PRENEOPLASTIC RAT HEPATOCYTES

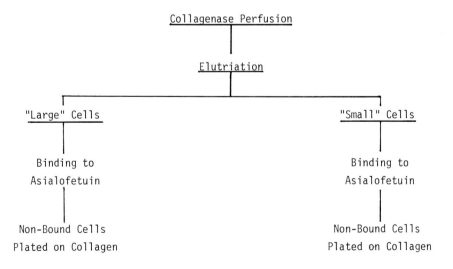

asialofetuin coated plates. Those cells that did not attach to the asialofetuin would by definition not have the surface receptor and fall under the
category of initiated cells. There is a strong correlation between the
absence of binding to asialofetuin receptor and the expression of γ-glutamyl-
transpeptidase (γ-GT).

One of the most striking in vivo characteristics of the initiated hepatocyte
is its capacity to replicate upon exposure to promoters such as phenobarbital
or 2,3,7,8-tetrachlorodibenzo-p-dioxin (TCDD) (1,2). To test the capacity of
the isolated and putative initiated cells to replicate in vivo we have transplanted these cells into the anterior chamber of the eye in weanling isogenic
rats (Figure 1). Preliminary data indicate that both normal and initiated
cells grow in the eye but the initiated cells have far greater capacity to
replicate than the normal cell. Furthermore, fully transformed cells (e.g.
hepatoma cells) proliferate rapidly when injected into the anterior chamber of
the eye and display all the characteristics of malignant cells (i.e. invasive-
ness, metastasis, etc.). It therefore appears that transplantation to the
anterior eye chamber may provide an important model for in vivo studies of the
development of malignancy in initiated cells.

Tumor markers such as γ-GT, glucose-6-phosphatase, and ATPase have been
extensively used in the study of hepatocarcinogenesis (2). However, these
markers are not stable and changes occur during the oncogenic process (2).
Since numerous changes in gene expression take place during the carcinogenic
process, it seems desirable to measure and/or examine as many changes as
possible in order to define those that most closely are associated with the
process, and more specifically to define changes in gene expression that are
characteristic of the different stages in tumor formation. We have attempted
to do this by using quantitative 2-D electrophoresis of total cellular proteins
to define the gene products that appear to be involved in the different stages
of the carcinogenic process.

After elutriation untreated normal hepatocytes and both small and large cells
from carcinogen treated rats are maintained in culture for 24 hours and then
pulse labeled for 4 hours with [^{14}C] amino acids. Total cellular proteins are
then separated on the basis of isoelectric point (pH 5-8) in the first dimension and molecular weight (15-200 K daltons) in the second dimension.
Relatively few qualitative protein differences (5-8) were observed among the
various cell types (normal hepatocytes vs small and large cells isolated from
carcinogen treated rats). In contrast, however, approximately 10-15% of the
proteins (polypeptides) were undergoing quantitative changes of at least 50%

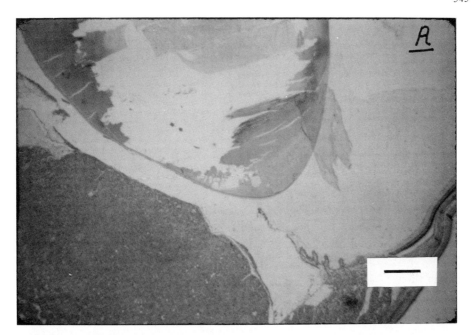

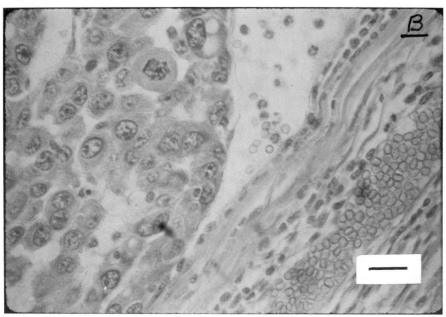

FIG. 1A. Rat hepatoma cells (7777) were injected into the anterior chamber of the right eye of a weanling rat. Animal was killed 5 days later. The tumor cells are seen in the left lower corner. Bar = 500 μm.

FIG. 1B. Higher magnification of the 7777 cells in the anterior chamber of the eye. Bar = 20 μm.

during the initiation stage. The changes (both qualitative and quantitative) which occur are distributed at all molecular weight sizes and at all pH values in the first dimension isoelectric focusing gel.

In summary, we have developed a system to separate the putative initiated (or preneoplastic) cells from livers of rats exposed to liver hepatocarcinogens. Both biological and biochemical characteristics of these cells are currently being studied.

REFERENCES

1. Pitot, H.C. and Sirica, A.E. (1980) Biochim. Biophys. Acta, 605, 191.
2. Emmelot, P. and Scherer, E. (1980) Biochim. Biophys. Acta, 605, 247.
3. Bannasch, P., Mayer, D. and Hacker, H.J. (1980) Biochim. Biophys. Acta, 605, 217.
4. Solt, D. and Farber, E. (1976) Nature, 263, 701.
5. Peraino, C., Staffeldt, E.F. and Ludeman, V.A. (1981) Carcinogenesis, 2, 463.
6. Seglen, P.A. (1972) Exp. Cell Res., 74, 450.
7. Wanson, J.C., Bernart, D., Penasse, W., Mosselmans, R. and Bannasch, P. (1980) Cancer Res., 40, 459.
8. Rubin, K., Oldberg, A., Hook, M. and Obrink, B. (1978) Exp. Cell Res., 117, 165.
9. Miller, M.J., Xuong, N.-H. and Geiduschek, P.E. (1982) J. Bacteriol., 151, 311.
10. Stockert, R.J. and Becker, F.F. (1980) Cancer Res., 40, 3632.
11. Howard, D.J., Stockert, R.J. and Morell, A.G. (1982) J. Biol. Chem., 257, 2856.

© 1983 Elsevier Science Publishers B.V.
Extrahepatic Drug Metabolism and Chemical Carcinogenesis,
J. Rydström, J. Montelius and M. Bengtsson eds.

MECHANISMS OF INITIATION AND PROMOTION OF CARCINOGENESIS IN MOUSE EPIDERMIS

Stuart H. Yuspa, M.D.

Laboratory of Cellular Carcinogenesis and Tumor Promotion, National Cancer
Institute, NIH, Bethesda, Maryland 20205, (U.S.A.)

INTRODUCTION

Studies performed in mouse skin have indicated that tumor induction by
chemicals can be subdivided into two distinct stages, initiation and promotion.
Initiation results from exposure to a classical mutagenic carcinogen and is
irreversible even after a single exposure. The permanently altered initiated
cell and its progeny may never form a tumor or in any way be recognizable in
the target tissue. Exposure to tumor promoters permits the expression of
the neoplastic change in initiated cells, and tumors develop. In contrast
to initiation, promoters must be given repeatedly to be effective; individual
exposures are reversible. Other model systems for chemical carcinogenesis have
shown a similar biology although the initiating and promoting agents involved
may be distinct for each tissue. Thus liver, esophagus, colon, bladder,
mammary gland and trachea of the rat, and lung and stomach of the mouse are
subject to multistage tumor induction. It is clear from this list that the
phenomenon occurs in the epithelium of complex tissues. In most, target
epithelial cells are organized in a stratifying or maturing arrangement usually
in a terminally differentiating lining epithelium. Such epithelia are often
composed of more than one cell type or of cells in differing biological states.
It is not clear if tissue complexity is a fundamental requirement for a
multistage mechanism or if other, less complex, organ sites have simply not
been adequately explored.

Tumors may also be induced in skin by repeated application of initiating
agents. Studies comparing tumor induction by initiator-promoter or by
repeated initiator application have suggested that the mechanism of cancer
induction by each protocol may be different. One stage protocols generally
yield de novo carcinomas or persistent papillomas while 2-stage protocols
yield mostly papillomas which regress (1,2). Carcinomas arise from papillomas
late in the 2-stage process often independently of continuous promoter treatment (3). This difference in the pattern of induction of preneoplastic and
malignant lesions is shown graphically in Fig. 1 where data from 3 separate
reports of skin tumorigenesis (1,3,4) are compared. When promoters are employed
to induce skin cancer there is a preponderance of benign lesions. Carcinogenesis involving promoters also differs from repeated initiator application

548

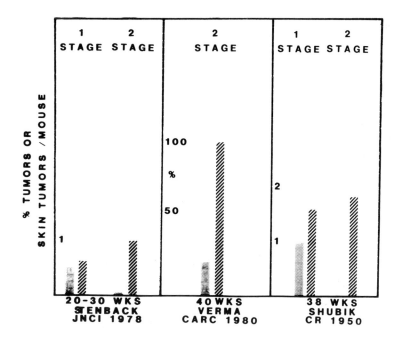

Figure 1.   Compilation of data on relative incidence of benign or malignant tumors produced by particular carcinogenesis protocols in mouse skin.   One stage protocols utilize repeated exposures to a polycyclic aromatic hydrocarbon.   Two stage protocols involve a single exposure to a polycyclic aromatic hydrocarbon followed by croton oil or TPA.   For details of these studies see references (1,3,4).

in strain susceptibility and in the types of chemicals which modify each process (5). Mechanistic studies in tumor promotion therefore must be directed at defining pathogenesis based upon the biology of cancer induction by the two-stage protocol, particularly with regard to the formation of benign lesions.

While conceptual advances in the biology of carcinogenesis have come
from whole animal studies, mechanistic studies are better performed under
less complex circumstances. Since mouse epidermis was so widely studied in
vivo, was readily available and had clearly separable stages in the transformation process, we have developed an in vitro model to study stages of
carcinogenesis in mouse epidermal cells. Over the last decade, results from
this and other laboratories have shown that mouse epidermal cell culture is
both a valid and useful model system to study normal epidermal function as
well as alterations associated with tumor initiation and promotion (6). To
facilitate experimental work a major advance in epidermal cell culture came
with the discovery that extracellular ionic calcium is a key regulator of
epidermal growth and differentiation (7). In medium with reduced calcium
concentrations (0.02 - 0.09 mM), epidermal basal cells are selectively culti-
vated. These cells have morphological, cell kinetic and marker protein
characteristics of basal cells and grow as a monolayer with a high proliferation rate. When the calcium concentration of culture medium is elevated to
levels found in most commercial preparations (1.2 - 1.4 mM), proliferation
ceases and terminal differentiation rapidly ensues with squamous differentiation and sloughing of cells occurring by 72-96 hours. This simple physiological manipulation has been useful in approaching questions regarding
initiation and promotion.

The Biological Nature of Initiation:

The monoclonal nature of benign skin tumors (8) suggests they are clonal
expansions of initiated cells. Growth kinetic studies performed on these
tumors indicate several differences from normal skin. The labeling index is
about 10 fold higher in both benign and malignant skin tumors (2). A striking
difference from normal is the presence of proliferating cells away from the
basement membrane zone in benign tumors whereas normal cells are obligated to
cease proliferation and initiate their program of terminal differentiation
upon leaving the basement membrane.

The ability to proliferate under conditions where normal cells are
obligated to differentiate would likely be an early event in transformation,
perhaps a key change in initiation. The responses of cultured basal cells to
increases in extracellular calcium resemble the changes observed in basal
cells in vivo as they migrate away from the basement membrane and commit to
differentiate. In cell culture therefore, it might be expected, in analogy to
in vivo data, that carcinogens could alter the basal cell response to calcium
induced terminal differentiation. Our laboratory has been studying this model

and some results are presented in Table 1 and have been published previously (9).

Basal cells exposed to carcinogens in vitro and subsequently induced to
differentiate by calcium formed foci which resisted terminal differentiation.
A number of initiating agents cause the induction of foci including N-methyl-
N'-nitro-N-nitrosoguanidine (MNNG), 7,12-dimethylbenzanthracene (DMBA),
benzo[a]pyrene (BP), 4-nitroquinoline-N-oxide (NQO), and N-acetoxyacetyl-
aminofluorene (AAF). In general the potency of each agent in vitro parallels
its potency as an initiator in mouse skin. Where studied, colony number observed for each agent was proportional to carcinogen dose (Table 1 and (9)).
Cells obtained from these colonies have typical keratinocyte morphology,
express differentiative functions, synthesize keratin proteins but fail to
cease proliferation when signaled to differentiate by Ca^{++}. Such cells are
generally not tumorigenic when tested early after selection in high Ca^{++}, but
but on prolonged subculture tumorigenic cell lines evolve. Similar foci can
be derived from cell cultures of mouse skin initiated in vivo by exposure to
7,12-dimethylbenz[a]anthracene and cultured in 0.02 mM calcium medium for
several weeks followed by selection in 1.2 mM calcium. In these experiments
control skin does not yield colonies (10). Malignant epidermal cells cultured
in the presence of a large excess of normal basal cells in 0.02 mM calcium
medium also continue to proliferate and form colonies when switched to 1.2
mM calcium while normal cells slough from culture as terminally differentiated squames (9). These results suggest that initiation of carcinogenesis
results in the ability of initiated cells to resist the signal to cease
proliferation in association with terminal differentiation. In normal skin
such a trait alone could not result in a tumor due to the strong regulatory
influences of surrounding normal cells (11).

The Biological Nature of Promotion:

The monoclonal origin of tumors, the suggestion of remodeling of the
epidermis with repetitive promoter exposure and the requirement for repeated
promoting stimuli prior to the development of tumors strongly suggest that
cell selection is involved in promotion (12). Analysis of the biochemical
changes in mouse skin produced by phorbol esters and in particular 12-0-
tetradecanoylphorbol-13-acetate (TPA) has been useful in formulating working
hypotheses on the mechanism of cell selection in tumor promotion. A large
number of changes occur in response to TPA (5). Several occur within a few
minutes (cyclic nucleotides, prostaglandins) others take hours (changes
in RNA and protein synthesis, polyamine synthesis, transglutaminase and

histidase activity, histone phosphorylation and phospholipid synthesis)
or up to 24 hours (DNA synthesis and synthesis of a histidine rich protein,
HRP). The hyperplasia induced by phorbol esters in mouse skin may persist for
weeks. Mediation of some responses via action at the cell membrane is likely,
and a receptor for TPA has been identified in mouse skin (13). The pleio-
trophic responses of skin to TPA exposure can be divided into major functional
groups relating to epidermal differentiation or proliferation. Many of these
changes occur with the same temporal sequence. Since differentiation and
proliferation are thought to be mutually exclusive in epidermis, and basal
cells appear to be the principle target for TPA action (14), considerable
heterogeneity must exist among basal cells in their program of induced
responses. It is these biochemical and biological observations that have
guided our studies to elucidate the mechanism of tumor promotion.

Our studies have been designed to elucidate the cellular basis for
selection with the hope that the results could explain selective clonal
expansion of differentiation-altered initiated cells. When the responsiveness
of basal cells to TPA was studied, it became clear that a portion of the population was induced to differentiate by the promoter (Fig 2). This could be
detected by morphological changes, measurement of the formation of cornified
squames and increase in the activity of the differentiation-specific enzyme
epidermal tranglutaminase (15,16). As terminally differentiated cells sloughed
from the culture dish, transglutaminase activity decreased. The basal cells
remaining after a brief TPA exposure were shown to be transiently resistant to
terminal differentiation when cultured in 1.2 mM calcium or when exposed
to TPA a second time (16). However, these cells were stimulated to proliferate
by the second TPA exposure. Thus two types of responses occur in epidermal
basal cells exposed to phorbol esters. In one population there is the induction
of terminal differentiation. In a second population, TPA stimulates proliferation and produces a transient block in response to a differentiation stimulus.
This latter cell type cannot be induced to differentiate by a second TPA
exposure if the interval between exposures is short. This is similar to the
response of mouse skin in vivo after several TPA exposures where proliferative
stimulation in the principle response. If the culture interval between
TPA exposures is prolonged (10 days), then heterogeneity in responsiveness
is restored (16). This is similar to findings in vivo where treatment
intervals are prolonged.

The pharmacological basis for epidermal heterogeneity could be explained
by studies of phorbol ester binding to membrane receptors. In mouse skin

552

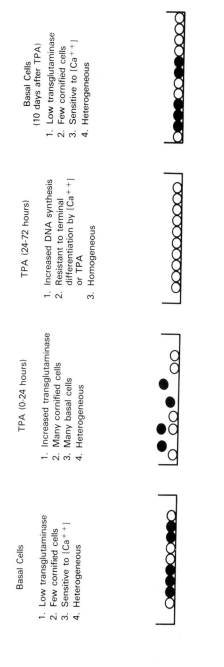

FIG 2

MECHANISM OF SELECTIVE REGENERATIVE HYPERPLASIA INDUCED BY TUMOR PROMOTERS IN MOUSE EPIDERMIS

Basal Cells

1. Low transglutaminase
2. Few cornified cells
3. Sensitive to [Ca^{++}]
4. Heterogeneous

TPA (0-24 hours)

1. Increased transglutaminase
2. Many cornified cells
3. Many basal cells
4. Heterogeneous

TPA (24-72 hours)

1. Increased DNA synthesis
2. Resistant to terminal differentiation by [Ca$^+$] or TPA
3. Homogeneous

Basal Cells
(10 days after TPA)

1. Low transglutaminase
2. Few cornified cells
3. Sensitive to [Ca^{++}]
4. Heterogeneous

Figure 2. Schematic presentation of the heterogeneous response pattern induced by phorbol ester tumor promoters in cultured mouse basal cells. Solid circles represent cells induced to differentiation while open circles are cells stimulated to proliferate. The proliferating cells are obviously precursors to the differentiating cells as seen in the right hand column. For experimental details see (16).

phorbol ester binding to membrane receptors is heterogeneous with at least 2 and possibly 3 classes of binding sites (17). In cultured keratinocytes, subclasses of binding sites can be elicited by inducing terminal differentiation with 1.2 mM Ca^{++} (18). When cells induced to differentiate by 1.2 mM Ca^{++} are simultaneously exposed to TPA, there is a marked acceleration of the differentiation response and a recruitment of cells into the differentiating pool (19). These findings suggest that the biological and receptor heterogeneity observed in skin is based on a difference in maturation state of epidermal cells. More mature cells respond by accelerated differentiation, while less mature cells are stimulated to proliferate. Studies with a limited number of differentiation-resistant initiated cell lines indicate that these cells are resistant to the differentiative influences of TPA but can be stimulated to proliferate by the promoter. These results are not influenced by the Ca^{++} concentration in the culture medium. The initiated cell lines also appear to have only a single phorbol ester binding component.

Conversion of Papillomas to Carcinomas:

The results obtained from studies in epidermal basal cell cultures suggest that phorbol esters produce a balanced and programmed heterogeneous response with regards to differentiation and proliferation. The net effect of this type of heterogeneity is to select for and to expand the proliferating population with each promoter exposure, thus remodeling the target tissue. Clonal selection of carcinogen-altered (differentiation-altered) cells would result if normal basal cells were induced to differentiate while altered (initiated) cells were among those which are stimulated to proliferate. Clonal expansion of initiated cells (with an altered program of differentiation) resulting from phorbol ester regulated cell selection would yield benign tumors which are the major product of two stage skin carcinogenesis. This model requires that a subsequent change in a papilloma cell is necessary for carcinoma development.

To examine the conversion of benign to malignant lesions, we produced papillomas on Sencar mouse skin by a standard initiation-promotion protocol. Groups of papilloma-bearing mice were subdivided after 10 weeks of TPA promotion into 5 groups of 30 animals each. One group received only topical acetone for the remainder of the experiment while the others received either topical TPA, topical MNNG, topical 4-NQO or systemic urethane once per week. The conversion rate from papilloma to carcinoma was then calculated during a 42 week experimental period (Fig. 3 and (20)). In controls without papillomas (uninitiated) the 3rd stage agents produced no or a very few tumors

554

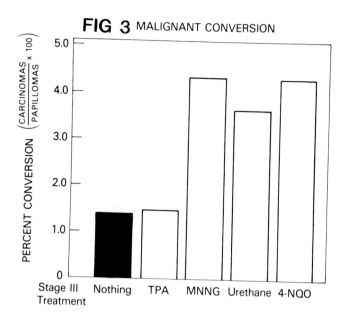

Figure 3. Conversion rate of papillomas to carcinomas in 3-stage carcinogenesis. Sencar mice were initiated with 20 µg DMBA (Stage 1) and promoted
for 10 weeks with 2.5 µg TPA once per week (Stage 2). Stage 3 treatments
were applied once per week as follows: acetone (nothing), 2.5 µg TPA,
120 µg MNNG topically, 250 µg 4-NQO topically, or 20 mg urethane intra-
peroneally. Papillomas and carcinomas were recorded weekly and confirmed
histologically at sacrifice. Data shown is the result at 52 weeks
calculated as cumulative carcinomas divided by maximum papilloma incidence
for each group.

(not shown). In papilloma bearing mice (Fig 3), the conversion rate was low
and the values identical with either continuous TPA or acetone exposure. Thus
TPA did not enhance conversion from benign to malignant lesions. All three
genotoxic carcinogens used in stage 3 markedly enhanced malignant conversion
(Fig 3) and also accelerated carcinoma development by up to 12 weeks (not
shown). These results indicate that malignant conversion may result from
further genetic change in papilloma cells. The ineffectiveness of TPA may be
due to its inactivity as a mutagen.

Table 1. Quantitation of Foci Resistant to Growth Inhibition and
Terminal Differentiation In High Calcium Medium

Treatment (Day 3)	Plates +/ Total Plates (%)	Control Colonies/ Plate	Survival Index	Corrected Colonies/ Plate
1. Control (0.1% ethanol	1/10 (10%)	0.1	1.00	0.1
MNNG (13.6 μM x 1 h)	2/8 (25%)	0.4	0.45	0.8
2. Control (0.1% ethanol)	0/12 (0)	0	1.00	0
MNNG (12 μM x 1 h)	3/12 (25%)	0.6	0.83	0.7
Benzo[a]pyrene (0.4 μM x 24 h)	5/12 (42%)	0.4	1.00	0.4
Benzo[a]pyrene (4.0 μM x 24 h)	2/12 (17%)	1.2	0.70	1.7

All groups were maintained for 14 days in low Ca^{++} and 4 weeks in high
Ca^{++} medium before fixation and rhodamine staining. For experimental
details see (9).

CONCLUSIONS:

   Multistage carcinogenesis in mouse skin appears to have at least 3 components
as demonstrated by our in vitro and in vivo studies. The initial alteration
produced by initiators has the characteristics of a genetic change resulting
in an uncoupling of the proliferative block associated with induced terminal
differentiation. The clonal expansion of this population is accomplished by
tumor promoters. In the case of phorbol esters, a receptor mediated selective
regenerative hyperplasia may be the underlying pharmacological response. The
result of these two stages is a premalignant lesion. The conversion of premalignant cells to carcinoma cells is not accomplished by the promoter but may
occur spontaneously at a low rate. This low conversion rate can be significantly enhanced by genotoxic carcinogens suggesting a further genetic change
is required. The high level of proliferation and the large proliferative
pool in papillomas may be associated with a finite spontaneous rate of genetic
change and malignant conversion in papillomas.

ACKNOWLEDGEMENTS

   I am indebted to my colleagues Drs. Henry Hennings, Ulrike Lichti and Molly
Kulesz-Martin for their contributions to these studies and for their dis-
cussions in formulating the conclusions. The technical assistance of Theresa
Ben and Anne Kilkenny and the secretarial assistance of Margaret Green are
also appreciated.

REFERENCES

1. Shubik, P. (1950) Cancer Res. 10: 713-717.

2. Burns, F.J., Vanderlaan, M., Sivak, A., and Albert, R.A. (1976). Cancer Res. 36: 1422-1427.

3. Verma, A.K. and Boutwell, R.K. (1980) Carcinogenesis 1: 271-276.

4. Stenback, F. (1978) Natl. Cancer Inst. Monograph 50: 57-70.

5. Yuspa, S.H. (1983) In: Goldsmith, L.A. (Ed.) Biochemistry and Physiology of the Skin, Vol II, Oxford University Press, New York, pp. 1115-1138.

6. Yuspa, S.H., Hawley-Nelson, P., Stanley, J.R., and Hennings, H. (1980) Transplant. Proc. 12: Suppl 1, 114-122.

7. Hennings, H., Michael, D., Cheng, C., Steinert, P., Holbrook, K., and Yuspa, S.H. (1980) Cell 19: 245-254.

8. Iannaccone, P.M., Gardner, R.L. and Harris, H. (1978) J. Cell Sci. 29: 249-269.

9. Kulesz-Martin, M., Koehler, B., Hennings, H., and Yuspa, S.H. (1980) Carcinogenesis 1: 995-1006.

10. Yuspa, S.H. and Morgan, D.L. (1981) Nature 293: 72-74.

11. Potten, C.S. and Allen, T.D. (1975) Differentiat. 3: 161-165.

12. Yuspa, S.H., Hennings, H., Lichti, U. (1981) J. Supramol. Struct. 17: 245-257.

13. Delclos, K.B., Nagle, D.S., and Blumberg, P.M. (1980) Cell 19: 1025-1033.

14. Lichti, U., Patterson, E., Hennings, H., and Yuspa, S.H. (1981) J. Cell Physiol 107: 261-270.

15. Yuspa, S.H., Ben, T.B., Hennings, H., and Lichti, U. (1980) Biochem. Biophys. Res. Commun. 97: 700-708.

16. Yuspa, S.H., Ben, T., Hennings, H. and Lichti, U. (1982) Cancer Res. 42: 2344-2349.

17. Dunn, J.A. and Blumberg, P.M. (1982) Proc. Am. Assoc. Cancer Res. 23: 100.

18. Dunn, J.A., Yuspa, S.H., and Blumberg, P.M. (1983) Proc. Am. Assoc. Cancer Res. 24: 111.

19. Yuspa, S.H., Ben, T., and Hennings, H. (1983) submitted for publication.

20. Hennings, H., Shores, R., Wenk, M.L. and Yuspa, S.H. (1983) Nature, in press.

© 1983 Elsevier Science Publishers B.V.
Extrahepatic Drug Metabolism and Chemical Carcinogenesis,
J. Rydström, J. Montelius and M. Bengtsson eds.

METABOLIC ACTIVATION OF AROMATIC AMINES AND THE INDUCTION OF LIVER, MAMMARY GLAND AND URINARY BLADDER TUMORS IN THE RAT

CHARLES M. KING, CHING Y. WANG, MEI-SIE LEE, JIMMIE B. VAUGHT, MASAO HIROSE
AND KENNETH C. MORTON
Department of Chemical Carcinogenesis, Michigan Cancer Foundation,
110 East Warren, Detroit, Michigan 48201 (U.S.A.)

INTRODUCTION

The susceptibilities of the liver, mammary gland and urinary bladder of the rat to aromatic amines have been used in attempts to identify and characterize those events crucial to their carcinogenic response to these agents. Tumor induction by aromatic amines appears to result from the combined effects of the distribution of the agent or its metabolites to the susceptible tissue, the production of reactive metabolites in the target cells, the replication of DNA altered by reaction with the carcinogen and the amplification of errors introduced by replication of the carcinogen-altered genome. Although the common structural feature of aromatic amines, an aromatic ring to which nitrogen is attached, may result in similar metabolic transformations among this class of compounds, differences in structure lead to disposition by different pathways and to products that differ in reactivity. Carcinogenic responses to these agents reflect these specificities. Our objective has been to employ metabolic differences due to structure, and biological systems that have different metabolic capacities, in order to clarify the mechanisms of action of the aromatic amines.

PATHWAYS OF METABOLIC ACTIVATION

Metabolic activation, as used here, refers to the metabolic production of derivatives that are capable of reaction with tissue macromolecules. Emphasis is given to those pathways that yield products that can alter nucleic acids, since active metabolites of aromatic amines that react with nucleic acids, both DNA and RNA, can also react with protein (FIGURE 1). However, metabolites that can react with protein (e.g. nitroso and quinone imine derivatives) can not necessarily react with nucleic acid (1,2,3).

N-Oxidized Metabolites. Attention has been focused on the reaction of N-oxidized arylamine derivatives with nucleic acids because these derivatives are often more carcinogenic than their arylamine precursors (4). At acid pH, many

558

FIGURE 1

METABOLIC FORMATION OF NUCLEIC ACID ADDUCTS

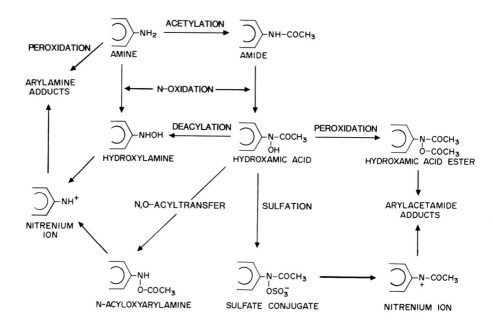

arylhydroylamines can react readily with nucleic acid on conversion to
nitrenium ions (5). The lability of these compounds and the question of the
extent of their reaction with nucleic acid under physiological conditions has
made it difficult to evaluate their role in the carcinogenic process.

The greater stability of the N-acetylated, N-oxidized derivatives, the arylhydroxamic acids, has facilitated both their detection in biological systems,
as well as their study in biochemical and biological experiments. Conjugation
of arylhydroxamic acids with sulfate can, in some cases (e.g. N-hydroxy-2-
acetylaminofluorene), yield products that react with nucleic acid at neutral
pH to give arylacetamide-substituted guanine adducts (2). An alternative
mechanism of activation of arylhydroxamic acids is by N,O-acyltransfer to give
N-acyloxyarylamines that can introduce arylamine substituents at C-8 of guanine derivatives (6,7,8). Whereas the sulfotransferase is a cytosolic enzyme
that is resistant to paraoxon, an organotriphosphate, both cytosolic and
microsomal arylhydroxamic acid N,O-acyltransferases have been identified (9).
The microsomal enzymes are inhibited by paraoxon, the cytosolic acyltransferases are not.

Oxidation of arylhydroxamic acids in vitro with both enzymatic and inorganic reagents has been shown to produce N-acetoxy-N-arylacetamide derivatives that can react with nucleic acids to give arylacetamide-substituted adducts (10). As yet, there is no evidence that these reactions occur in intact cells.

Peroxidative Activation of Arylamines. Zenser and his collaborators demonstrated that prostaglandin synthase preparations can metabolize benzidine to products that react with nucleic acids (11). Subsequent studies in our laboratory have shown that, while benzidine is highly active in this system, acetylation of one or both of its amino groups reduced adduct formation by more than 99% (12). Furthermore, 4,4'-methylene-bis(2-chloroaniline), an aryldiamine with a methylene bridge between the two aromatic rings of the compound, was not activated by prostaglandin synthase. The relatively small quantities of nucleotide adducts formed from 4-aminobiphenyl with this activation system resulted from reaction with cytidine. In contrast, adduct formation with nitrenium ions from the hydroxylamine or hydroxamic acids derived from 4-aminobiphenyl was with guanine and adenine.

MECHANISMS OF TUMOR INDUCTION

Liver. Rat liver is crucial to the response of all three organs considered here, in that it N-oxidizes amines and amides, a reaction believed to be required for tumor induction by these compounds (13). Thus, this organ is capable of the initial activation step and is not dependent on the metabolic capacity of other organs. Acetylation of aromatic amines also takes place in the liver; few differences are to be expected in the responses of rats treated with amines or acetamides (14). As indicated above, subsequent hepatic activation of the products of N-oxidation can occur as a consequence of sulfate conjugation, N,O-acyltransfer by cytosolic or microsomal enzymes, or deacylation of arylhydroxamic acids. The major DNA adducts are derived from pathways that yield arylamine-substituted products; arylacetamide-containing derivatives are present in minor quantities (15).

Paradoxically, both 4-aminobiphenyl, a nonhepatocarcinogen, and 2-aminofluorene, which does induce liver tumors in susceptible animals, primarily form rat liver DNA-arylamine adducts of the type that would be produced by reaction of the hydroxylamine or N-acyloxyarylamine derivatives. However, liver tumor induction is linked to the need for a complete carcinogen to elicit a hepatotoxic response, presumably to ensure that DNA alterations by the carcinogen will be fixed through replication. In attempting to account for the differences in the carcinogenic activities of the biphenyl and fluorene derivatives it was noted that the biphenyl derivatives are relatively nontoxic and do not exhibit a sulfate-dependence for macromolecular adduct formation (3). In contrast, administration of N-hydroxy-2-acetylaminofluorene produces liver necrosis that is associated with the production of macro-molecular adducts derived from activation of the carcinogen by sulfate conjugation (16). Moreover, sulfate conjugation levels are directly correlated with the LD_{50} of N-hydroxy-2-acetylaminofluorene in several strains of rats, and is also correlated with hepatocarcinogenicity in this and other species (17,18). Neoplastic nodules induced by this compound have lost their capacity to activate the hydroxamic acid by sulfate conjugation and, in so doing, have become resistant to its toxicity so that they can replace the liver cells that are killed by the carcinogen. Sulfate conjugation of N-hydroxy-2-acetylamino-fluorene may be regarded, therefore, as an important factor in amplifying genomic damage caused by other pathways (16).

Viewed alternatively, evidence that the arylamine-substituted DNA lesions may represent a genotoxic potential came from experiments that subjected female CD rats to sequential partial hepatectomy, a single treatment with N-hydroxy-4-acetylaminobiphenyl and prolonged administration of phenobarbital (19). The animals used in this study have little capacity for conjugation of the hydroxamic acid with sulfate. In addition, this carcinogen does not depend on sulfate conjugation for adduct formation, and it forms arylamine-substituted nucleic acid adducts in liver cells. Prior partial hepatectomy and subsequent phenobarbital treatment had been observed to enhance the tumor-igenic effects of other compounds. As shown in TABLE 1, these two supple-mentary treatments enhanced the formation of neoplastic nodules and gamma-glutamyltranspeptidase (GGT)-positive foci, although only a single rat devel-oped a hepatocellular carcinoma. These data support the idea that the intro-duction of arylamine substituents into rat liver DNA can elicit a neoplastic response under appropriate conditions, and, further, that an aromatic amine that induces liver cancer in rats does so because it introduces this type of lesion as well as eliciting DNA synthesis due to its hepatotoxic effects.

Mammary Gland. Immature female Sprague-Dawley rats readily develop tumors of the mammary gland when treated with a wide range of N-substituted aromatic compounds (20). Several characteristics of this organ make it a valuable adjunct to the liver in attempts to clarify the mechanisms by which aromatic amines induce tumors. There is a striking difference in the ability of this gland to metabolize these agents as compared to liver. Of the metabolic activation pathways that yield products that are capable of reaction with nucleic acid, only N,O-acyltransfer has been demonstrated (21,22); mammary gland does not have demonstrable sulfotransferase or deacylase activity (13).

TABLE 1

LIVER LESIONS INDUCED BY N-HYDROXY-4-ACETYLAMINOBIPHENYL IN CONJUNCTION WITH
PRIOR PARTIAL HEPATECTOMY AND SUBSEQUENT PHENOBARBITAL TREATMENT

A single i.p. injection of the carcinogen (C) in DMSO (S) was given 24 hours
after partial hepactectomy of female CD rats (19). Phenobarbital (PB) was
administered in the diet. The animals were sacrificed at 64 weeks.

Treatment	Effective Animals	Percentage of Rats with Neoplastic Nodules	Carcinoma	Number of GGT-Foci per sq. cm. liver section
PH C PB	23	74	4	1.97
PH S PB	18	17	0	0.68
PH C	19	11	0	0.13
PH S	18	0	0	0.10
C PB	19	21	0	0.74
S PB	19	5	0	0.43
C	20	5	0	0.06
S	19	0	0	0.21

Although a peroxidative capacity has been described (20), no definitive
nucleic acid adduct studies have been carried out with this system. Male
Sprague-Dawley derived rats, which sometimes develop mammary tumors in
response to aromatic amines, also have mammary gland acyltransferase (22).

As in the liver, the mammary gland has two cytosolic N,-O-acyltransferases
(21,22). The larger enmzyme is specific for formylated substrates and is
inhibited by paraoxon. Based on this inhibition, substrate specificities and
behavior on gel filtration, this enzyme is believed to be a microsomal component that is released during the homogenization process (9). The smaller cytosolic acyltransferase is resistant to paraoxon and esentially incapable of
activating N-hydroxy-N-formylaminoarenes (21). The relative activities of the
paraoxon-resistant liver and mammary acyltransferases are shown in TABLE 2.

Nucleic acid adducts isolated from the mammary tissue are compatible with
a reaction mechanism involving nitrenium ions generated from arylhydroxylamines or N-acyloxyarylamines. The N-acetyl moiety of N-hydroxy-2-acetyl-
aminofluorene is not incorporated into RNA of mammary gland (23); the DNA
contains a single adduct, i.e., guanine substituted at the C-8 position
through the amino group of 2-aminofluorene (24).

In addition to the more conventional methods of administering carcinogens in
tumor induction studies, such as i.p. injections or oral admimistration, it is
possible to induce tumors of the rat mammary gland with a single direct application of the compound by either a surgical technique or by injection. The

TABLE 2

RELATIONSHIP OF MAMMARY TUMOR INDUCTION TO METABOLIC ACTIVATION OF
ARYLHYDROXAMIC ACIDS BY CYTOSOLIC N,O-ACYLTRANSFERASE

The hydroxamic acids were given 8x i.p. (0.1 mmole/Kg) to immature female CD
rats. Tumor induction and liver gammaglutamyltranspeptidase ((GGT) foci were
determined at 42 weeks (21). Metabolic activation was determined using
partially purified, paraoxon-resistant cytosolic N,O-acyltransferase from
mammary gland or liver. The relative activities within each of these two
preparations are shown; these data do not permit comparison of the relative
levels of acyltransferase in these tissues.

Compound Administered[+]	Effective Animals	%Animals with Mammary Tumors	Relative Acyltransferase		GGT-Foci per sq. cm Liver
			Mammary	Liver	
N-hydroxy-AAF	29	59	48	1620	3.50
N-hydroxy-AABP	30	30	6.9	504	3.50
N-hydroxy-PABP	30	20	5.2	79	1.40
N-Hydroxy-FABP	20	7	(2.5	20	0.35
Solvent only	30	3	----	----	0.31

[+]N-Hydroxy-AAF, N-hydroxy-2-acetylaminofluorene; N-hydroxy-AABP, N-hydroxy-4-
acetylaminobiphenyl; N-hydroxy-PAP, N-hydroxy-4-propionylaminobiphenyl;
N-hydroxy-FABP, N-hydroxy-4-formylaminobiphenyl.

tumorigenic response is unlikely to be the result of physical effects, since
the response is compound-specific (25). Development of this technique by
Giganti and her collaborators has shown that direct application of N-hydroxy-
2-acetylaminofluorene, but not 2-acetylaminofluorene or N-2-fluorenylhydroxyl-
amine, produce mammary tumors at the site of treatment.

A subsequent study confirmed the inactivity of 2-acetylaminofluorene when
applied locally, and further demonstrated that the production of mammary gland
carcinomas by arylhydroxamic acid derivatives of N-2-fluorenylhydroxylamine
was dependent on the structure of the N-acyl moiety, i.e. the acetylated
derivative was more active than either the formyl or propionyl analogues (22).

Additional evidence in support of the participation of N,O-acyltransferase
in the production of mammary tumors came from experiments in which four
hydroxamic acids that differed in their activation potential by N,O-acyl-
transfer were administered i.p. (21). The tumorigenic response, the relative
activations by the paraoxon resistant liver and mammary gland acyltransferases, and the production of GGT-positive foci in the livers of these
animals is shown in TABLE 2. These findings support the conclusion that those
arylhydroxamic acids that are most readily activated by the paraoxon-resistant
acyltransferase of mammary gland are more potent tumorigens for this target

tissue. Furthermore, this specificity parallels the abilities of these compounds to elicit the formation of GGT-positive foci in the livers of the same animals, a process that is independent of sulfate conjugation as indicated above.

Collectively, these observations are consistent with the following mechanisms. The mammary gland of the immature female Sprague-Dawley rat is capable of activating arylhydroxamic acids by N,O-acyltransfer. When treated at the time the gland is undergoing DNA synthesis, errors are introduced into the genome as a consequence of replication of DNA modified by the introduction of arylamine-substituents via acyltransfer. Subsequently, these errors are amplified by hormonal influences on the mammary gland. Unlike the liver, which rarely undergoes cell division unless challanged by toxic agents, it is not necessary for a mammary carcinogen to be toxic to the target cells, since the normal physiological influences are sufficient to stimulate the cell division that is required for the carcinogenic process. In the male rat, the smaller number of target mammary cells and the lesser hormonal influence on this tissue less frequently results in tumor formation. Recognition of the involvement of this metabolic pathway in the induction of tumors in the mammary gland should aid in the more specific identification of the actual target cells involved in the process, as well as further delineation of the relationship of the paraoxon-sensitive and -resistant acyltransferases.

Urinary Bladder. In contrast to the hepatocarcinogenic process, and for unknown reasons, urinary bladder tumor formation in the rat decreased on exposure of replicating target cells to carcinogen (26). The role of urinary metabolites of bladder carcinogens for the induction of bladder tumors is strongly supported by the observation that the portion of rat or dog bladders protected from contact with urine that contains arylamine metabolites does not develop tumors. Since urinary, as compared to biliary, excretion is a function of the molecular weight of a compound and varies from species to species, the carcinogenic response of the bladder depends on both the structure of the aromatic amine and the excretion characteristics of the animal species. Rats appear to be less susceptible to bladder carcinogenesis by arylamines than dogs, monkeys, and humans. Among the known human bladder carcinogens, only high and prolonged doses of 2-aminonaphthalene is known to induce bladder tumors in rats (27). However, 2-acetylaminofluorene, phenacetin, o-anisidine, and p-chloro-o-phenylenediamine, that are not known to be associated with human bladder cancer, are able to induce bladder tumors in the rat (28-30). Both acetylated and nonacetylated N-hydroxy metabolites of bladder carcinogens are found in the urine of rats exposed to aromatic amines.

564

Administration of a variety of carcinogenic arylamines to dogs results in the formation of bladder tumors. Because dog liver cannot N-acetylate arylamines, many believe that N-acetylation is not required for bladder tumor induction. In contrast, administration of structurally analogous carcinogenic N-arylacetamides to dogs results in the formation of both liver and bladder tumors, with the susceptibility to bladder carcinogenesis being related to the relative ease of deacetylation by the dog enzyme (31). Evidence for the importance of nonacetylated amines in humans comes from a recent report that all but one of 23 bladder cancer patients with putative occupational exposure to chemicals were of slow acetylator phenotype (32).

Arylhydroxylamines and their conjugates have been proposed to be ultimate bladder carcinogens (33). Their effects on rat urothelial cells have been assessed in an in vitro system using unscheduled DNA synthesis (UDS) as an indicator of DNA damage that may be related to their abilities to induce tumors (34). The results (TABLE 3) have shown that the acetylated and nonacetylated N-hydroxy derivatives of 2-aminofluorene and 4-aminobiphenyl and the N-glucuronides of the corresponding arylhydroxylamines are able to induce UDS. The O-glucuronide of N-hydroxy-2-acetylaminofluorene, the only O-glucuronide examined, is not active in inducing UDS. It appears that rat urothelial cells may be able to activate arylhydroxamic acids either by deacetylation or by N,O-acyltransfer. The ability of rat urothelial cells to deacetylate 2-acetylaminofluorene has been shown (35). The poor response of rat urothelial cells to 2-aminonaphthalene derivatives comes either from low levels of adduct formation, or from the inability of these cells to repair N^2 and ring-opened deoxyguanosine adducts of the DNA that comprise approximately 80% of the adducts produced by N-hydroxy-2-aminonaphthalene (36). Thus, the

TABLE 3

ARYLAMINE-INDUCED UNSCHEDULED DNA SYNTHESIS IN PRIMARY RAT UROTHELIAL CELLS

Compound (10^{-5} M)	Grains/Nucleus $\pm$ Std. Dev.
N-Hydroxy-2-aminofluorene	51+9
N-Hydroxy-2-acetylaminofluorene	43+8
N-Glucuronide of N-hydroxy-2-aminofluorene	23+8
O-Glucuronide of N-hydroxy-2-acetylamimofluorene	1+3
N-Hydroxy-4-aminobiphenyl	18+8
N-Hydroxy-4-acetylaminobiphenyl	15+6
N-Glucuronide of N-hydroxy-4-aminobiphenyl	16+6
N-Hydroxy-2-aminonaphthalene	5+4
N-Hydroxy-2-acetylaminonaphthalene	4+4
N-Glucuronide of N-hydroxy-2-aminonaphthalene	4+3
Control	2+2

N-glucuronidation of arylhydroxylamines may simply facilitate the transport of active carcinogens to the bladder. The relative insensitivity to arylamines of the urothelial cells of rats, as compared to those of dogs and humans, may be due to the O-glucuronidation of arylhydroxamic acids which occur as a consequence of N-acetylation in the liver.

CONCLUSIONS

This paper offers examples of three divergent organ systems that afford opportunities to explore and exploit the multiple mechanisms by which N-substituted aromatic compounds induce tumors in the rat. Their use, in conjunction with compounds with closely related structures, reinforce the conclusion that members of this class of carcinogens are able to induce tumors as a consequence of a multiplicity of metabolic pathways and physiological influences. Recognition of this complexity will further both our attempts to evaluate the potential adverse effects of new compounds, as well as efforts to unravel those events that are crucial to the carcinogenic process.

ACKNOWLDEGEMENTS

The studies in this report from the A. Taubman Facility were supported by USPHS grants CA 23386 (CMK), CA 23800 (CYW) and CA 32303 (KCM) and an institutional grant from the United Foundation of Detroit. We wish to thank Christine Hendry for her assistance in the preparation of this manuscript.

REFERENCES

1. King, C.M. and Krick, E. (1965) Biochim. Biophys. Acta., 111, 147-153.
2. King, C.M. and Phillips, B. (1969) J. Biol. Chem., 244, 6209-6216.
3. King, C.M., Traub, N.R., Cardona, R.A. and Howard, R.B. (1976) Cancer Res., 36, 2374-2381.
4. Miller, E.C., Miller, J.A., and Hartman, H.A. (1961) Cancer Res., 31, 815-824.
5. Frederick, C.B., Mays, J.B., Ziegler, D.M., Guengerich, F.P. and Kadlubar, F. R. (1982) Cancer Res., 42, 2671-2677.
6. King, C.M., and Phillips, B. (1968) Science 159, 1351-1353.
7. Bartsch, H., Dworkin, M., Miller, J.A., and Miller, E.C. (1972) Biochim. Biophys. Acta., 286, 272-298.
8. King, C.M. (1974) Cancer Res., 34, 1503-1515.
9. Glowinski, I.B., Savage, Lee, M.-S. and King, C.M. (1983) Carcinogenesis, 4, 67-75.
10. Bartsch, H. and Hecker, E. (1971) Biochim. Biophys. Acta., 237, 567-578.
11. Mattammal, M.B., Zenser, T.V., and Davis, B.B. (1981) Cancer Res., 41, 4961-4966.

566

12. Morton, K.C., King, C.M., Vaught, J.B., Wang, C.Y., Lee, M.-S. and Marnett, L.J. (1983) Biochem. Biophys. Res. Commun. 111, 96-103.

13. Irving, C.C. (1979) in: A.C. Griffin and C.R. Shaw (Ed.), Carcinogens: Identification and Mechanisms of Action, Raven Press, New York p.p. 211-228.

14. King, C.M. and Glowinski, I.B. (1983) Environ. Health Perspec. 49, 43-50, 1983.

15. Kriek, E., and Westra, J.G. (1979) CRC Press, Inc., Boca Raton, Fa. p.p. 1-28.

16. Shirai, T. and King, C.M. (1982) Carcinogenesis 3, 1385-1391.

17. Irving, C.C. (1975) Cancer Res. 35, 2959-2961.

18. Gutmann, H.R. Malejka-Giganti, D., Barry, E.T. and Rydell, R.B. (1972) Cancer Res. 32, 1554-1561.

19. Shirai, T., Lee, M.-S., Wang, C.Y. and King, C.M. (1981) Cancer Res., 41, 2450-2456.

20. Malejka-Giganti, D, Ritter, C.L. and Ryzewski, C.N. (1983) Environ. Health Perspectives, 49, 175-183.

21. Shirai, T., Fysh, J.M., Lee, M-S., Vaught J.B. and King, C.M. (1981) Cancer Res., 41, 4346-4353.

22. Allaben, W.T., Weeks, C.E., Weis, C.C., Burger, G.T. and King, C.M. (1982) Carcinogenesis, 3, 233-240.

23. King, C.M., Traub, N.R., Lortz, Z.M., and Thissen, M.R. (1979) Cancer Res., 3369-3372.

24. Beland, F.A., Weiss, C.C., Fullerton, F.F. and Allaben, W.T. (1981) J. Supramol. Struct. Cell. Biochem. Suppl. 5, 169.

25. Malejka-Giganti, D. and Gutmann, H.R. (1975) (38980) Proc. Soc. Expl. Expl. Biol. Med., 150, 92-97.

26. Shirai, T. (1980) Cancer Res. 40, 3709-3712.

27. Hicks, R.M. and Chowaniec, J. (1977) Cancer Res., 37, 2943-2949, 1977.

28. Weisburger, E.K., Murthy, A.S.K., Fleischman, R.W., and Hagopian, M. (1980) Carcinogenesis 1, 495-499.

29. Isaka, H., Yoshii,H., Otsuji, A., Koike, M., Nagai, Y., Koura, M., Sugiyasu, K., and Kanabayashi, T. (1979) Gann, 70, 29-36.

30. Johansson, S.L. (1981) Int. J. Cancer 27, 521-529.

31. Lower, G.M., Jr., Nilsson, T., Nelson, C.E., Wolf, H., Gamsky, T.E., and Bryan, G.T. (1979) Environ. Health Perspectives 29, 71-79.

32. Cartwright, R.A., Glashan, R.W., Rogers, H.J., Ahmad,, R.A. (1982) Lancet, 842-845.

33. Kadlubar, F.T., Miller, D.A., and Miller, E.C. (1977) Cancer Res., 37, 805-814.

34. Wang, C.Y., Linsmaier-Bednar, E.M., Garner, C.D., and Lee, M.-S. (1982) Cancer Res. 42, 3974-3977.

35. Moore, B.P., Hicks, R.M., Knowles, M.A. and Redgrave, S. (1982) Cancer Res. 42, 642-648.

36. Kadlubar, F.F., Dooley, K.C., and Beland, F.A. (1980) Proc. Am. Assoc. Cancer Res., 21, 119.

© 1983 Elsevier Science Publishers B.V.
Extrahepatic Drug Metabolism and Chemical Carcinogenesis,
J. Rydström, J. Montelius and M. Bengtsson eds.

COMPARISONS OF BENZO(a)PYRENE METABOLISM AND DNA-BINDING BETWEEN SPECIES AND INDIVIDUALS: OBSERVATIONS IN RODENT TRACHEA AND HUMAN ENDOMETRIUM

DAVID G. KAUFMAN[1,2], MARC J. MASS[1], BONNIE B. FURLONG[2] AND B. HUGH DORMAN[1]
[1]Department of Pathology and [2]Cancer Research Center, University of North Carolina School of Medicine, Chapel Hill, North Carolina 27514 (U.S.A.)

INTRODUCTION

The respiratory epithelium of major airways, and the glandular epithelium of the endometrium are two common sites for the development of cancer in humans. Studies of carcinogenesis in the tracheobronchial epithelium have been extensively pursued in experimental models using rats and hamsters in vivo (1) and in culture including studies with human bronchial tissue (2). In contrast, relatively little attention has been given to experimental studies of carcinogenesis in endometrial tissue. This report describes studies investigating biological influences on the metabolism of benzo(a)pyrene (BP) and its binding to DNA in organ cultures of these two tissues. The goal of these studies is to determine whether observations of these features of carcinogenesis can eventually be utilized to identify tissues and individuals with particular susceptibility to the development of cancer.

Respiratory tract cancers can be induced with regularity in Syrian golden hamsters and Fischer 344 rats. Intratracheal instillation using BP-ferric oxide has been used to produce tracheobronchial epidermoid carcinomas in hamsters, but when applied to rats, no tracheobronchial epidermoid cancers have ever been reported (3-6). Instead, bronchiolo-alveolar cancers of the peripheral lung result from the administration of BP-ferric oxide to rats via the intratracheal route (3,4). Tumors resembling human lung cancers can be produced in rat or hamster tracheas when they are treated with carcinogens as heterotopic tracheal grafts, but in grafted hamster tracheas this requires a much lower dose (7,8).

Since clearance of BP from the respiratory tracts of rats and hamsters are similar, both species are exposed to equivalent doses of BP over time. Therefore, differences in exposure cannot explain the discrepancies in tumor incidence. For this reason we considered whether differences in the activation of BP in the tracheas of rats and hamsters could explain the marked differences in sensitivity of these two species to polynuclear hydrocarbon-induced neoplasia. Rats and hamsters were compared with respect to the BP metabolites produced in tracheal microsomes and organ cultures, and the specific activities of binding of BP to DNA in epithelial cells of tracheas maintained in organ culture.

The binding of carcinogens to DNA in target tissues of experimental animals appears to be associated with the transformation of these tissues by most, if not all, chemical carcinogens. Although the relationship between the binding of carcinogens to DNA in human tissues and the neoplastic transformation of these tissues is not known, the role of carcinogen binding to DNA is presumed to be similar to that in experimental animals. Recent studies have shown measurable levels of carcinogen binding to DNA of several human tissues in organ culture (9-11). BP is the carcinogen most commonly used in these studies, and the earlier results have shown that human tissues can metabolically activate BP to forms that bind to DNA. Studies of this type permit comparisons of metabolism and binding to be made between different individuals and between different human tissues. Experimental studies of this type are important for several reasons. Analysis of carcinogen binding in human tissues in vitro may suggest the potential importance of specific chemical carcinogens in human cancer. Comparisons of carcinogen metabolism and binding to DNA in tissues from humans and experimental animals may indicate the extent to which extrapolations between species may be valid. Also, fresh human tissue maintained in vitro for brief periods may preserve many of the characteristics of the tissue in vivo, thus providing the opportunity to examine how the normal properties of the tissue contribute to the process of carcinogenesis. Unlike other human tissues in which BP metabolism and binding to DNA has been studied, endometrium undergoes profound physiological changes in differentiation in response to changes in circulating hormone levels. This is reflected in variations in several physiological factors. Alterations of differentiation may influence levels of metabolism and of BP binding and thus alter the potential carcinogenic effects on the tissue. Therefore, the relationship between metabolism, DNA binding and various biological properties of the tissue appeared to be important subjects for identification of factors which might contribute to an increased risk for development of endometrial cancer.

MATERIALS AND METHODS

Tissue Obtainment.   Random-bred Syrian golden male hamsters or Fischer strain 344 male rats were anaesthetized using ether and tracheas were excised and opened longitudinally. Tracheas were placed in Ham's F-10 medium containing 10% calf serum, buffered to pH 7.4 with 0.25 M HEPES and sodium bicarbonate.

Human endometrial tissue was obtained from hysterectomy specimens of patients offering informed consent as described previously (12). The specimen was washed, minced into cubes, and incubated for 18 hr in a 5% CO_2 incubator at 37° in 5 ml of CMRL Medium 1066 supplemented with 10% heat-inactivated fetal bovine serum, 100 units penicillin per ml, 100 µg streptomycin per ml, 10 mM L-glutamine buffered with 28 mM HEPES, pH 7.4. For each specimen of endometrial tissue, the day of the menstrual cycle at the time of hysterectomy was determined morphologically by 2 pathologists using standard morphological criteria (12).

Exposure to BP for monooxygenase induction in tracheal organ cultures.
Media which was 5 µM in BP was routinely used for BP monooxygenase induction. Tissues placed in the culture medium but lacking BP served as uninduced controls. At the end of the 18 hr induction period, tracheas were removed from the medium containing BP, blotted to remove adherent fluid, transferred to new dishes containing medium without BP and incubated for an additional 4 hr.

Metabolites produced by organ cultures. Generally labeled (^{3}H)BP (25 Ci/mmole) was repurified and dissolved in acetone. Rat and hamster tracheas in organ culture were incubated with 1 µM (^{3}H)BP for 18 hr. A culture dish containing no tissue but containing 5 ml of medium with 1 µM (^{3}H)BP was used as a control. Fragments of human endometrial tissue were incubated for 18 hr and then extracted with organic solvents for analysis by high pressure liquid chromatography (HPLC). Ethyl acetate containing 0.08% butylated hydroxytoluene (BHT) was added to the mixture; BHT reduced the likelihood of further non-enzymatic oxidation of (^{3}H)BP and metabolites to BP-quinones during extraction. After the incubation the tissue was removed and the media was divided into 2 aliquots. The first was subjected to acetone/ethyl acetate extraction using acetone/ethyl acetate at ratios of solvent to medium of 1:2. The remaining aliquots were adjusted to pH 5 by the addition of an equal volume of 0.2 M sodium acetate buffer, pH 5. Aryl sulfatase (11 units) and ß-glucuronidase (1000 units) were added and incubated for 2 hr at 37°C to release BP metabolites conjugated with sulfate and glucuronic acid. Extraction with acetone/ethyl acetate followed.

HPLC Procedures. HPLC was performed on the residue obtained from acetone/ethyl acetate extracts dried under nitrogen. Samples were dissolved in absolute methanol containing authentic BP metabolites obtained from the Carcinogenesis Program of the National Cancer Institute. BP tetrols were synthesized. A 10 µl aliquot was injected into a high-pressure liquid chromatograph fitted with a a µBondapak C_{18} column. Metabolites were eluted at ambient temperature using a linear gradient of methanol/water beginning at 60% methanol and ending at 80% methanol. Metabolites were identified by chromatographic retention times. Therefore, it is possible that other unidentified metabolites were also present in the radioactively labeled peaks of identified metabolites.

DNA Isolation and Purification. Tracheal epithelial cells scraped from the cartilaginous supportive tissue or fragments of human endometrium were homogenized and extracted with phenol to remove protein and unreacted (³H)BP. After the phenol extraction, absolute ethanol was added to the aqueous phase, and the precipitate formed at -20°C was sedimented. The pellet was resuspended and traces of phenol were removed by ether extraction. RNA was removed with RNase and residual protein was hydrolyzed with proteinase K. Unbound (³H)BP was removed from the samples by extensive ether extractions and residual ether was evaporated with N_2. Samples were dialyzed, mixed with CsCl and DNA was banded in density gradients. Gradients were fractionated, and the DNA peak fractions were isolated and rebanded in a second CsCl gradient. Following rebanding, the DNA content and radioactivity in each fraction was determined and specific activities of (³H)BP binding were calculated.

RESULTS

Microsomes isolated from epithelial cells of tracheas incubated for 5 min with 0.25 µM to 20 µM (³H)BP converted less than 2% of the initial substrate added to oxygenated products. Microsomes from hamster tracheas cultured for 24 hr with unlabeled BP demonstrated a substrate-inducible BP monooxygenase activity. Apparent K_m values for control and BP-pretreated tracheas were between 1 µM and 2 µM. The apparent V_{max} values were 30.2 and 97 pmol/mg microsomal protein/min for the constitutive and induced BP monooxygenases, respectively ($p < 0.001$). It was not possible to measure the activity of BP monooxygenase in microsomes from epithelial cells of rat tracheas (i.e., the activity was below the limit of detection). Activity was undetectable in 10,000 g supernatants from homogenates of control rat tracheas, but was detectable if the rat tracheas were exposed to 5 µM BP for 24 hr in organ culture. The K_m values calculated from Lineweaver-Burk plots of BP monooxygenase from 10,000 g supernatants from epithelial cells of hamster and rat tracheas incubated for 24 hr in the presence of 5 μM BP were equivalent. In contrast, the V_{max} values are 6.3 and 13.5 pmol/mg protein/min for BP monooxygenase in rat and hamster tracheas, respectively; these values are significantly different (p<0.05).

Acetone/ethyl acetate extractable metabolites produced during incubation of hamster tracheal microsomes co-chromatographed with the 9,10-diol, 4,5-diol, 7,8-diol, BP quinones, 3 and 9-hydroxy BP. A metabolite chromatographing between the 9,10-diol and the 4,5-diol was noted but was not identified. Greater than half of the radioactivity co-chromatographed with BP quinones and BP-phenols. Since BHT was present, it is not likely that the BP-quinones arose from spontaneous oxidation of BP-phenols during the extraction steps. Rat tracheal microsomes produced entirely different quantities and proportions of acetone/ethyl acetate-soluble BP metabolites. Most of the radioactivity co-chromatographed with 3-hydroxy BP. Small peaks corresponded to BP-quinones and the 9,10-diol, but some metabolites could not be identified.

Secondary metabolic processes were observed by incubating (^{3}H)BP with whole tracheas in organ culture. Acetone/ethyl acetate soluble products of BP metabolism represent about 35% of the products released into the medium by hamster tracheal organ cultures. Exposing organ culture medium to β-glucuronidase and aryl sulfatase released another 30%. The 9,10-diol was the major metabolite not conjugated with glucuronic acid or sulfate. BP-phenols were the next most abundant class of metabolites and they were good substrates for conjugation. BP-quinones and 7,8-diol were present largely as glucuronide or sulfate esters. BP-tetrols were produced in small quantity; after exposure to β-glucuronidase and aryl sulfatase their quantity did not increase. Metabolites more polar than BP-tetrols represented about 20% of the metabolites present after exposure to the deconjugating enzymes. During the 24 hr incubation the total quantity of water-soluble plus acetone/ethyl acetate-soluble metabolites produced were 3.7 pmol/mg tissue for rat tracheas, and 7.8 pmol/mg tissue for hamster tracheas. The 9,10-diol was the major acetone/ethyl acetate extractable metabolite but β-glucuronidase and aryl sulfatase treatment of the rat tracheal organ culture medium released a large quantity of BP-phenols into the acetone/ethyl acetate phase of the medium; the BP-phenols represented 40% of the total metabolites identified. Before treatment of the medium with β-glucuronidase and aryl sulfatase, BP-phenols made up about 25% of the acetone/ethyl acetate-soluble metabolites.

BP-quinones, 7,8-diol, and 4,5-diol comprised the remaining metabolites in the organ culture medium in which rat tracheas were incubated. BP-tetrols represented only about 1 % of the total products identified. The ratio of acetone/ethyl acetate-soluble metabolites produced by tracheas in organ culture recovered after incubation of the culture medium with β-glucuronidase and aryl sulfatase varied from 1.1 to 22 for hamster tracheas as compared to rat tracheas. The largest ratio representing the biggest difference between hamster and rat metabolites is that for BP-tetrol; hamster tracheas produce 22-fold more BP-tetrols than do rat tracheas.

Binding of (H^3)BP to DNA in epithelial cells of rat and hamster tracheas. The quantity of metabolites which bound to DNA of tracheas in culture was determined in DNA purified on isopyknic CsCl gradients. The mean binding level for rats was 1.55×10^{-4} pmol (^3H)BP bound/μg DNA/24 hr. A level of 1.23×10^{-4} pmol/μg DNA/24 hr was observed in BP-pretreated tracheas and a level of 0.91×10^{-4} pmol/μg DNA/24 hr was found in DNA from control rat tracheas. BP-pretreatment of hamster tracheas increased binding more than 2-fold from 16.9×10^{-4} to 42.6×10^{-4} pmol/μg DNA/24 hr. The mean level of binding of (^3H)BP was 26.7×10^{-4} pmol/μg DNA/24 hr. Therefore, the mean value for (^3H)BP binding to DNA in hamster tracheas was 17-fold greater than it was for rat tracheas.

BP Metabolism and Binding to DNA in Human Endometrial Tissue. Twenty-six specimens of human endometrium were used for studies of (^3H)BP metabolism in organ cultures. All were obtained from hysterectomy specimens where histologic studies confirmed that the endometrial tissue was normal. Three of the patients were postmenopausal. For the 23 premenopausal patients the menstrual cycle stage at the time of surgery was determined both from the medical history and histologic observations. Cultures produced derivatives of (^3H)BP which cochromatographed with authentic BP metabolite standards. The (^3H)BP metabolites identified in the acetone/ethyl acetate extract included: BP-sulfate conjugate, 7,10/8,9-tetrol, 9,10-diol, 4,5-diol, 7,8-diol, 1,6-Q, 3,6-Q, 6,12-Q, 9-OH-BP and 3-OH-BP. A large variation was observed between metabolite profiles produced by the individual endometrial specimens.

The mean values of individual metabolites in BP-metabolite profiles for 8 smokers did not differ from the mean values of the 15 non-smokers (P>0.1). Metabolite profiles were analyzed with respect to the menstrual cycle and a number of metabolites were found to vary according to the time in the menstrual cycle. These variations did not coincide with the proliferative and secretory phases of the cycle. For example, the BP-sulfate conjugate and 9,10-diol were elevated and the BP-phenols and quinones were decreased in the middle portion of the cycle. The metabolite profiles from the 3 postmenopausal patients' endometrial specimens were compared to the profiles from the 23 premenopausal patients. The proportion of BP-sulfate conjugates in the metabolite profiles from the 3 postmenopausal patients were found to be near the lower range of values for this metabolite. The average value for the BP-sulfate conjugates for these 3 specimens was found to be significantly different than the mean for the 23 premenopausal specimens.

Purified human endometrial DNA formed a well-defined band when centrifuged to equilibrium in a second CsCl gradient and UV absorbance was coincident with radioactivity. Background levels of radioactivity and UV absorbance were very low in other fractions. The specific activities of (^{3}H)BP binding to DNA derived from individual specimens showed minimal differences between duplicate samples. The range of specific activities of (^{3}H)BP binding to human endometrial DNA obtained from 41 individual human specimens varied from 1 to 70 DPM/μg DNA or nearly two orders of magnitude. Between these extremes, specimens display a smooth monophasic progressive increase in specific activities without clustering at any binding level and 88% have specific activities of 30 DPM/μg DNA or less.

The variation of (^{3}H)BP binding to the DNA of human endometrial specimens was evaluated as a function of the menstrual cycle. Specimens were grouped among 3 categories according to their position in the menstrual cycle at the time of tissue obtainment: 1) early and mid-proliferative, 2) late proliferative and early secretory, or 3) mid- and late secretory. The highest levels of (^{3}H)BP binding were found in specimens obtained between days 10 and 21 of the menstrual cycle, corresponding to the late proliferative and early secretory stages; 16 specimens had an average specific activity of 25 DPM/μg DNA. The lowest levels of binding were observed in the mid- and late secretory segments of the menstrual cycle between days 21 and 28, where 10 specimens had an average specific activity of 7 DPM/μg DNA. In the early and mid-proliferative phases, days 1 to 10 of the menstrual cycle, the average specific activity calculated from 11 specimens was 15 DPM/μg DNA. Statistical analysis showed that the mean binding level in the late proliferative and early secretory phases of the cycle is significantly higher than the mean binding level in the mid-and late secretory phases.

Endometrial specimens from 4 post menopausal women were analyzed for (^{3}H)BP binding to DNA. Because one of these patients had been maintained on estrogen replacement therapy prior to hysterectomy and was biologically different from the other patients who had entered a natural menopause, her specimen was excluded from this group. Specific activities in the remaining 3 postmenopausal patients ranged from 3 to 8 DPM/μg DNA with an average value of 5 DPM/μg DNA. This average level is less than one-third the average specific activity of 17 DPM/μg DNA found for (^{3}H)BP binding in the 37 premenopausal patients. Statistical analysis showed that the mean binding level in premenopausal tissue is significantly higher than the mean binding level for postmenopausal tissue. The binding level observed in the one excluded postmenopausal specimen was 27 DPM/μg DNA, a value consistent with levels of binding observed in the late proliferative and early secretory phases of the normal menstrual cycle.

DISCUSSION

   Microsomes isolated from normal or BP-treated hamster tracheas metabolized BP, but only microsomes from BP treated rat tracheas, not controls, had measurable metabolizing activity and this was lower than for hamsters (13). Metabolites produced by microsomes from these two species differed from metabolites generated by intact organ cultures. HPLC profiles of metabolites generated by hamster and rat tracheal organ cultures also differed significantly. Of particular note was a 22-fold greater quantity of metabolites co-chromatographing with 7,8,9,10-BP-tetrol in the organic extractable component of ß-glucuronidase and sulfatase-treated medium from hamster tracheal organ cultures. Comparable to the metabolism studies, binding of ^{3}H-BP to DNA was also determined in the epithelial cells of the tracheal organ cultures. Binding of ^{3}H-BP to hamster tracheal DNA was 17-fold greater than for rat tracheal DNA, in close agreement with the difference between species for the principal breakdown product of BP-diolepoxide. These results demonstrate that the species difference in susceptibility to carcinogenesis in the tracheobronchial epithelium between rats and hamsters could be explained primarily or completely by the differences in the metabolism of this carcinogen in this tissue. If these observations can be extrapolated to human beings it may be possible to define individual risk to a given exposure to a carcinogen, and contribute to prevention of lung cancer.

   Studies of BP metabolism and DNA binding with organ cultures of human endometrium were designed to investigate individual variations in the processes. There was a 75-fold range in levels of binding of BP to DNA in endometrial specimens (14). This is comparable to the range of BP binding levels seen earlier in specimens of human bronchus, esophagus, and colon (9-11). A large variation between individuals was also observed in the activity of BP metabolism and in the proportions of metabolites formed. Both BP metabolism and DNA binding were found to be influenced by the hormonal status of the patient at the time the endometrial tissue was obtained. Endometrial tissue obtained during the portion of the menstrual cycle when estrogen levels are highest, generated larger proportions of metabolites co-chromatographing with 9,10-diol BP and monohydroxy BP-sulfate conjugates whereas the proportions of BP-phenols and quinones were lower. Specimens from postmenopausal women, with low estrogen levels, had greatly reduced monohydroxy-BP-sulfate conjugates (15). Levels of binding of BP to DNA were higher during the proliferative phase in premenopausal women when estrogen levels are elevated, as compared to levels observed in mid and late secretory phase. BP binding levels in endometrial tissue from women in normal menopause were low. These results indicate that hormonal status, and, in particular, the state of estrogenization, is an important factor influencing BP metabolism and DNA binding in endometrial tissue in organ culture. These observations may suggest testable hypotheses regarding determination of individual susceptibility for endometrial cancer.

ACKNOWLEDGEMENTS

Supported by grant CA32239 from the National Cancer Institute. Fellowships supported M.J.M (ES07017), B.B.F. (CA09156) and B.H.D. (Chemical Industry Institute of Toxicology). An RCDA (CA00431) from NCI supported D.G.K.

REFERENCES

1. Nettesheim, P. and Greisemer, R.A. (1978) Experimental models for studies of respiratory tract carcinogenesis. Pathogenesis and Therapy of Lung Cancer, C. C. Harris (Ed.) Marcel Dekker, New York, pp. 75-188.

2. Harris, C.C. and Autrup, H., Stoner, G.D., Yang, S.K., Leutz, J.C., Gelboin, H.V., Selkirk, J.C., Conner, R. J., Barrett, L.A. and Jones, R.T. (1977) Metabolism of benzo(a)pyrene and 7,12-dimethylbenz(a)anthracene in cultured human bronchus and pancreatic duct. Cancer Res., 37, 3349-3355.

3. Blair, W.H. (1974) Chemical Induction of lung carcinomas in rats. In: Karbe, E. and Parks, J.F. (Eds.) Experimental Lung Cancer: Carcinogenesis and Bioassays, Springer-Verlag, Berlin, pp. 199-206.

576

4. Schreiber, H., Martin, D.H. and Pazmino, N. (1975) Species differences in the effect of benzo(a)pyrene-ferric oxide on the respiratory tract of rats and hamsters. Cancer Res., 35, 1654-1661.

5. Blair, W.H., Otero, N. and Rao, H. (1973) Development of lung neoplasms in rats treated with 7,12-dimethylbenzanthracene. Proc. Am. Assoc. Cancer Res., 14, 497.

6. Shreiber, H., Nettesheim, P. and Martin, D.H. (1972) Rapid development of bronchiolo-alveolar squamous cell tumors in rats after intratracheal injection of 3-methylcholanthrene. J. Natl. Cancer Inst. 49, 541-546.

7. Nettesheim, P., Greisemer, R.A., Martin, D.H. and Caton, J.E. (1977) Induction of preneoplastic and neoplastic lesions in grafted hamster tracheas continuously exposed to benzo(a)pyrene. Cancer Res. 37, 1272-1278.

8. Mossman, B. T. and Craighead, J. E. (1978) Induction of neoplasms in hamster tracheal grafts and 3-methylcholanthrene-coated Lycra fibers. Cancer Res., 38, 3717-3722.

9. Autrup, H., Harris, C.C., Trump, B.F. and Jeffrey, A.M. (1978) Metabolism of benzo(a)pyrene and identification of the major benzo(a)pyrene-DNA adducts in cultured human colon. Cancer Res., 38, 3689-3696.

10. Harris, C.C., Autrup, H., Conner, R., Barrett, L.A., McDowell, E.M. and Trump, B.F. (1976) Interindividual variation in binding of benzo(a)pyrene to DNA in cultured human bronchus. Science, 194, 1067-1069.

11. Harris, C.C., Autrup, H., Stoner, G.D., Trump, B.F., Hillman, E., Schafer, P.W., Jeffrey, A.M. (1979) Metabolism of benzo(a)pyrene, N-nitrosodimethylamine, and N-nitrosopyrrolidine, and identification of the major carcinogen-DNA adducts formed in cultured human esophagus. Cancer Res., 39, 4401-4406.

12. Kaufman, D.G., Adamec, T.A., Walton, L.A., Carney, C.N., Melin, S.A., Genta, V.M., Mass, M.J., Dorman, B.H., Rodgers, N.T., Photopulos, G.J., Powell, J. and Grisham, J.W. (1980) Studies of human endometrium in organ culture. Methods Cell Biol., 21B, 1-27.

13. Mass, M.J., and Kaufman, D.G. (1983) A comparison between the activation of benzo(a)pyrene in organ cultures and microsomes from the tracheal epithelium of rats and hamsters. Carcinogenesis, 4, 297-303.

14. Dorman, B.H., Genta, V.M., Mass, M.J., and Kaufman, D.G. (1981) Benzo(a)pyrene Binding to DNA in Organ Cultures of Human Endometrium. Cancer Res., 41, 2718-2722.

15. Mass, M.J., Rodgers, N.T., Kaufman, D.G. (1981) Benzo(a)pyrene Metabolism in Organ Cultures of Human Endometrium. Chem.-Biol. Interactions, 33, 195-205.

© 1983 Elsevier Science Publishers B.V.
Extrahepatic Drug Metabolism and Chemical Carcinogenesis,
J. Rydström, J. Montelius and M. Bengtsson eds.

MECHANISMS INVOLVED IN MULTISTAGE CHEMICAL CARCINOGENESIS IN MOUSE SKIN

T. J. SLAGA

The University of Texas System Cancer Center, Science Park - Research Division,
P.O. Box 389, Smithville, TX 78957 (U.S.A.)

INTRODUCTION

Investigations using the mouse skin tumorigenesis model has contributed
greatly to our understanding that chemical carcinogenesis is a multistage
process. It is now well known that skin tumors in mice can be induced by the
sequential application of a subthreshold dose of a carcinogen (initiation stage)
followed by repetitive treatment with a weak or noncarcinogenic promoter
(promotion stage). After a discussion of the important aspects of skin tumor
initiation and promotion, results will be presented to show that the tumor
promotion stage can be operationally and mechanistically further divided into at
least two stages. In addition, during the progression from benign to malignant
tumors there are further alterations in the differentiation capacity of epidermal cells.

INITIATION

The initiation stage in mouse skin can be accomplished by a wide variety of
direct acting carcinogens or procarcinogens and is essentially an irreversible
stage which as data suggests probably involves a somatic mutation in some aspect
of epidermal differentiation (1). We have recently found that skin tumor initiation probably occurs in dark basal keratinocytes since a good correlation exists
between the degree of tumor initiation and the number of dark cells present in
the skin (Slaga, T.J. and Klein-Szanto, A.J.P. Unpublished results). The dark
basal keratinocytes are present in the skin in large numbers during embryo-
genesis, in moderate numbers in newborns, in low numbers in young adults, and
in very low numbers in old adults which suggest that these cells may be epidermal stem cells (2). The initiating potential of mouse skin decreases with
the age of the mouse to the point that it is very difficult to initiate mice
greater than one year of age when the number of dark basal keratinocytes are
extremely rare. The critical molecular target of skin tumor initiators is
probably DNA in the epidermal stem cells since there is a good correlation
between the skin tumor initiating activities of several polycyclic aromatic
hydrocarbons (PAH) and their ability to bind covalently to epidermal DNA (1).
In addition, potent inhibitors of PAH tumor initiation such as certain antioxidants (butylated hydroxytoluene and butylated hydroxyanisole), flavones

(7,8-benzoflavone and 5,6-benzoflavone), vitamins (A, C, and E), noncarcinogenic PAHs (dibenz(a,c)anthracene, benzo(e)pyrene, and pyrene), and 2,3,7,8-tetra-chlorodibenzo-p-dioxin decrease the level of the PAH bound to epidermal DNA (1).

PROMOTION

The tumor promotion stage in mouse skin can be accomplished by a wide variety of weak or noncarcinogenic agents and is initially reversible but later becomes irreversible. Phorbol esters such as 12-O-tetradecanoyl-phorbol-13-acetate (TPA), teleocidin A,anthralin, 1-fluoro-2, 4-dinitrobenzene, benzo(e)pyrene, benzoyl peroxide and tobacco smoke condensate are examples of tumor promoters with moderate to strong activity. Skin tumor promoters bring about a number of important epigenetic changes in the skin such as membrane alterations, inflamma-tion, epidermal hyperplasia, and an increase in ornithine decarboxylase (ODC) activity, polyamines, prostaglandins, protease activity, cAMP independent protein kinase activity and dark basal keratinocytes as well as other embryonic charac-teristics in adult skin (1). In addition, the skin tumor promoters cause a decrease in epidermal superoxide and catalase activities as well as a decrease in the number of glucocorticoid receptors and a decreased response of G_1 chalone in adult skin (1,3,4). The phorbol ester tumor promoters and teleocidin A-induced changes appear to be mediated by their interaction with specific membrane receptors whereas many of the other promoters do not act through this receptor but may involve a free radical mechanism (1,5).

In order to have a better understanding of the differences in initiating and promoting agents, Table I compares the biological properties of these agents.

TABLE I

COMPARISON OF BIOLOGIC PROPERTIES OF INITIATING AND PROMOTING AGENTS

Initiating Agents	Promoting Agents
1. Usually carcinogenic by them-selves; however, some chemicals such as benzo(a)pyrene diol-epoxide and urethane act as pure initiating agents	1. Either are weak or noncarcinogenic by themselves
2. Must be given before promoting agent	2. Must be given after initiating agent
3. Single exposure is sufficient	3. Requires prolonged treatment
4. Action is irreversible and additive	4. Action is reversible (at early stage) and not additive
5. No apparent threshold	5. Appears to be threshold

TABLE I (Cont.)

6. Are electrophiles or yield electrophiles that bind covalently to cell macromolecules	6. No evidence of covalent binding but bind physically to receptors and/or work through a free radical mechanism
7. Mutagenic	7. Not mutagenic

A number of inhibitors and modifiers of skin tumor promotion have been very useful in our understanding of what cellular events are important in skin tumor promotion (1). In general, the majority of known inhibitors of skin tumor promotion are agents that inhibit the promoter-induced hyperplasia, ODC activity and polyamine levels, prostaglandins, and dark basal keratinocytes (1). In addition, skin tumor promotion can be counteracted by a number of antioxidants, vitamins, and cAMP or agents that elevate endogenous levels of cAMP (1). Although putrescine and prostaglandin E_2 and F_{2d} do not promote skin tumors, they effectively enhance TPA promotion (1). Table 2 summarizes the effects of fluocinolone acetomide (FA), retinoic acid (RA), tosyl phenylalamine chloromethyl ketone (TPCK), difluoromethylornithine (DFMO), butylated hydroxyanisole (BHA), vitamins C and E, selenium, and cyproterone acetate (CPA) on TPA promotion and TPA-induced epidermal hyperplasia, dark basal keratinocytes, and polyamine levels (1, Slaga and Davidson Unpublished results).

TABLE 2

EFFECTS OF FA, RA, DFMO, TPCK, BHA, CPA, VITAMIN E AND C, AND SELENIUM ON TUMOR PROMOTION AND TPA-INDUCED EPIDERMAL HYPERPLASIA, DARK KERATINOCYTES, AND POLYAMINE LEVELS

Inhibitor	TPA Promotion	Relative Ability (%) to Counteract		
		TPA-Induced Hyperplasia	TPA-Induced Dark Cells	TPA-Induced ODC and Polyamine Levels
FA	100	100	100	20
RA	80	0	0	85
TPCK	70	0	70	10
DFMO	55	0	0	95
BHA	95	0	0	85
Vitamin E	80	?	?	?
Vitamin C	60	0	0	?
CPA	95	60	?	0
Selenium	80	?	?	?

MULTISTAGE PROMOTION

We have recently found that skin tumor promotion can be operationally and
mechanistically further divided into at least two stages (6,7). This was
possible because we found that mezerein induced many of the cellular events
similar to TPA but mezerein was a weak or nonpromoting agent (6). We rational-
ized that TPA must be inducing some additional cellular event(s) that mezerein
could not effectively induce. In order to test this, we initiated mice and
gave limited treatment of TPA which would not promote and then treated the mice
repetitively with mezerein. As shown in Table 3, this regimen was an effective
way of inducing tumors.

TABLE 3

TWO-STAGE PROMOTION[a]

	Initiation		Promotion			Relative Tumor Response
1. DMBA	—1wk→	TPA		32X	→	100
2. DMBA	—1wk→	Mezerein(4μg)		32X	→	2
			Stage I	Stage II		
3. DMBA	—1wk→	TPA —4X→	Acetone	28X →		0
4. DMBA	—1wk→	TPA —4X→	Mezerein(4μg)	28X →		85

[a]The mice were initiated with 10 mmoles of 7,12-dimethylbenz(a)anthracene (DMBA)
and promoted with 2μg of TPA.

Both stages of promotion show a good dose-response relationship. It should
be emphasized that only one application of a first stage promoter is required
and this stage is irreversible for 4 - 6 weeks (1). Besides TPA and 12-deoxy-
phorbol-13-decanoate, which are known promoters, nonpromoters such as 4-0-methyl
TPA, calcium ionophore A23187, hydrogen peroxide as well as wounding are effective stage I promoters (1). These agents plus wounding increase the number of
dark basal keratinocytes (stem cells?) which suggest that these cells are
important in the first stage of promotion. Prostaglandin E_2 specifically
enhances stage I of promotion whereas putrescine specifically enhances stage
II of promotion (1). Stage I of promotion can be inhibited by FA, TPCK, and
vitamin E which also counteracted the TPA-induced dark basal keratinocytes.
These dark cells are normally present in high numbers in embryonic skin (20 -
50 % of basal cells) but are present in low numbers in adult skin (<3 % of basal
cells). Papillomas and carcinomas also have a large number of these dark

cells (6). As discussed earlier, the dark cells appear to be the critical
target cells of the tumor initiator and the first stage promoters stimulate
these cells to rapidly divide by both a direct and indirect mechanism (Slaga
and Klein-Szanto Unpublished results).

The second stage of promotion is initially reversible but later becomes
irreversible. A number of weak or nonpromoting agents such as mezerein and
12-deoxyphorbol-13-2,4,6-decatrienoate are effective second stage promoters (1).
Although mezerein by itself is not able to increase the number of dark cells
or decrease the level of glucocorticoid receptors, it can effectively maintain
these conditions after TPA treatment in a two-stage promotion protocol (9).
Stage II of promotion can be inhibited by FA, RA, DFMO, BHA, CPA, and vitamins
E and C which counteract either the mezerein-induced ODC, cell proliferation
and/or as yet unidentified events (7,9 and Slaga Unpublished results). Based
on these results with inhibitors, polyamines and epidermal cell proliferation
as well as some unidentified event(s) appear to be important events in stage II
of promotion.

PROGRESSION

The initiation-promotion protocol either by single stage promotion or by two-
stage promotion induces a large number of benign papillomas followed by a low
number of malignant squamous cell carcinomas in comparison to the total number of
papillomas. A complete carcinogenesis protocol (repetitive applications of a
carcinogen) induces a low level of papillomas followed by a large number of carcinomas. Although the initiation-promotion protocol is less effective than the
complete carcinogenesis protocol in causing carcinomas, the initiation-promotion
protocol allows one to critically examine the differences in papillomas and carcinomas as well as to study the factors involved in the progression of papillomas
to carcinomas. We have found that all squamous cell carcinomas lack several
differentiation product proteins such as high molecular weight keratins(60,000-
62,000) and filaggrin but are positive for gamma glutamyltransferase (GGT) whereas only about 20% of the papillomas generated by a initiation-promotion protocol
have a similar condition (10,11, and Mamrack and Slaga Unpublished results).
Before visible tumors appear using the initiation-promotion protocol these
conditions appear to be normal which suggest that these changes are very late
responses. We have recently found (also, Yuspa and Coworkers, personal communication) that if papillomas are treated once with an initiating dose of N-methyl-
N-nitrosoquanidine (MNNG) we can significantly increase the conversion of
papillomas to carcinomas possibly by a genetic mechanism (Slaga Unpublished
results). This type of treatment (initiation-promotion-initiation) gives a

carcinoma response similar to complete carcinogenesis, i.e. giving a carcinogen such as DMBA or MNNG repetitively which probably supplies initiating and promoting influences continuously. Table 4 describes some important characteristics of either tumor initiation, promotion, initiation-promotion, initiation-promotion-initiation, or complete carcinogenesis.

TABLE 4

A COMPARISON OF TUMOR INITIATION, PROMOTION, INITIATION-PROMOTION, INITIATION-PROMOTION-INITIATION, AND COMPLETE CARCINOGENESIS IN MOUSE SKIN

A. Tumor Initiation

  1. Causes initial alteration in differentiation capacity of epidermal stem cell population (First Mutation?).

  2. Since there is no stimulation of stem cell population by promoter, natural turn-over of altered stem cell population is normally too slow for tumor formation.

  3. In rare cases, a few papillomas appear after very long latency period.

  4. No second alteration in differentiation capacity of stem cells so no carcinoma formation.

B. Promotion

  1. Rapid stimulation of stem cell population by tumor promoter.

  2. Continuous promotion can sometimes lead to low level of benign papillomas after long latency period if spontaneous first alteration in differentiation capacity of stem cells occurs. However, this is a low frequency occurrence.

  3. Even lower frequency of carcinoma formation because the probability of further alterations in differentiation capacity of stem cells is extremely rare.

C. Initiation-Promotion

  1. Initiation causes first alteration in differentiation capacity of stem cell population.

  2. Rapid stimulation of altered stem cell population by promoter.

  3. A large number of papillomas appear after very short latency period.

  4. Low level of carcinomas occur in comparison to papillomas because additional alterations in differentiation capacity of stem cells has to occur by spontaneous means (genetic changes?).

D. Initiation-Promotion-Initiation

  1. Same as C except that treatment of papillomas with initiator leads

to greater frequency of appearance of additional alterations of stem
cell population (loss of high molecular weight keratins and filaggrin
and appearance of GGT).

2. High level of papillomas and carcinomas.

E. Complete Carcinogenesis

1. This type of treatment leads to continuous exposure of initiating and
promoting agents from carcinogen.

2. Because of additive nature of initiation, high frequency of initial
alteration in differentiation capacity of stem cell population.

3. Rapid stimulation of altered stem cell population by promotion component
of carcinogen.

4. Low level of papillomas because high frequency of additional alterations
in differentiation capacity of stem cells leads directly to large number
of carcinomas.

Chart 1 summarizes the sequence of events as well as important aspects of
multistage chemical carcinogenesis in mouse skin.

CHART 1 (Summary)

MULTISTAGE CHEMICAL CARCINOGENESIS IN MOUSE SKIN

INITIATION

1. Probably occurs in stem cells (dark cells).

2. Covalent binding of initiator to DNA in stem cells leading to
permanent alteration in differentiation capacity.

3. Round or two of cell division needed to fix altered state.

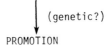

(genetic?)

PROMOTION

Stage I

1. Only one application of TPA is necessary and is irreversible for
4 - 6 weeks.

2. Nonpromoting agents such as calcium ionaphore (A23187), 4-O-methyl
TPA, H_2O_2 and wounding can act as Stage I promoters.

3. The above agents stimulate the initiated stem cell (dark cell)
population by a direct and indirect mechanism.

4. Number of glucocorticoid receptors are decreased.

5. Prostaglandins stimulate Stage I and FA, TPCK, and vitamin E inhibit
Stage I.

584

CHART 1 (Cont.)

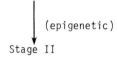

(epigenetic)

Stage II

1. Multiple applications of mezerein or similar agents are required.

2. Reversible at first but becomes irreversible.

3. Mezerein can maintain stem cell proliferation and decrease in gluco-corticoid receptors but cannot induce these events by itself.

4. Most of the biochemical events shown to be important in tumor pro-motion occur in Stage II.

5. Stimulated by putrescine and inhibited by FA, RA, DFMO, BHA, CPA, and vitamins C and E.

6. Polyamines and cell proliferation important events in Stage II.

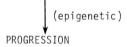

(epigenetic)

PROGRESSION

Benign Papillomas

1. Large number of dark cells.

2. Loss of glucocorticoid receptors.

3. High level of polyamines and prostaglandins.

4. Approximately 80% of papillomas have high molecular weight keratins and filaggrin and are negative for GGT. 20% have reverse condition.

5. Some papillomas are reversible while others are irreversible.

6. Treatment of papillomas with MNNG increases the conversion of papillomas to carcinomas.

(genetic?)

Carcinomas

1. Large number of dark cells.

2. All lack glucocorticoid receptors.

3. All lack high molecular weight keratins and filaggrin (differentiation proteins).

4. All positive for GGT.

5. High level of polyamines and prostaglandins.

CHART 1 (Cont.)

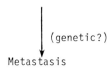

(genetic?)

Metastasis

1. Normally low but certain agents such as MNNG can increase metastatic potential.

ACKNOWLEDGEMENTS

Supported by Public Health Service grant CA 34890 from the National Cancer Institute.

REFERENCES

1. Slaga, T.J., Fischer, S.M., Weeks, C.E., Klein-Szanto, A.J.P. and Reiners, J. (1982) J. Cellular Biochem., 18, 207.

2. Klein-Szanto, A.J.P. and Slaga, T.J. (1981) Cancer Res., 41, 4437.

3. Solanki, V., Rana, R.S. and Slaga, T.J. (1981) Carcinogenesis 2, 1141.

4. Davidson, K.A. and Slaga, T.J. (1982) J. Invest. Dermatol., 79, 378.

5. Solanki, V. and Slaga, T.J. (1981) Proc. Natl. Acad. Sci. U.S.A., 78, 2544.

6. Slaga, T.J., Fischer, S.M., Nelson, K. and Gleason, G.L. (1980) Proc. Natl. Acad. Sci. U.S.A., 77, 3659.

7. Slaga, T.J., Klein-Szanto, A.J.P., Fischer, S.M., Weeks, C.E., Nelson, K. and Major, S. (1980) Proc. Natl. Acad. Sci. U.S.A., 77, 2251.

8. Klein-Szanto, A.J.P., Major, S.M. and Slaga, T.J. (1980) Carcinogenesis, 1, 399.

9. Davidson, K.A. and Slaga, T.J. (1983) Cancer Res., (In press).

10. Nelson, K.G. and Slaga, T.J. (1982) Cancer Res., 42, 4176.

11. Klein-Szanto, A.J.P., Nelson, K.G., Shah, Y. and Slaga, T.J. (1983) J. Natl. Cancer Inst., 70, 161.

© 1983 Elsevier Science Publishers B.V.
Extrahepatic Drug Metabolism and Chemical Carcinogenesis,
J. Rydström, J. Montelius and M. Bengtsson eds.

NMRI NU/NU MOUSE SKIN FIBROBLASTS: REGAIN OF ARYLHYDROCARBON HYDROXYLASE INDUCIBILITY OF TRANSFORMED CELL LINES AFTER A TUMOR PHASE

MARIITTA LAAKSONEN[1], RAUNO MÄNTYJÄRVI[1], OSMO HÄNNINEN[2] AND ASTA RAUTIAINEN[1]
Departments of [1]Clinical Microbiology and [2]Physiology, University of Kuopio,
Kuopio, Finland

INTRODUCTION

Cell culture- adult animal system provides a model in which the different steps of carcinogenesis can be studied from transformation to tumor formation. Our previous studies have shown that secondary cultures of newborn NMRI *nu/nu* (nude) mouse skin fibroblasts can be adapted for focus formation assay by using 3-methylcholanthrene (3-MC) as a reference carcinogen, and that these cells contain carcinogen-metabolizing monooxygenase system (1). These cells are also responsive to focus formation induced with a DNA tumor virus, SV_{40}, which is affected by low levels of carcinogenic chemicals (2).

In this work we have studied the activity of aryl hydrocarbon hydroxylase (E.C. 1.14.14.2) in some established cell lines originated from transformation experiments with SV_{40}, 3-MC or their combination.

MATERIALS AND METHODS

Cell cultures. Primary fibroblast cultures were prepared by trypsinization from minced skin preparations of newborn *nu/nu* mouse as described by Laaksonen *et al.* (1). SV_{40}, 3-MC and combination transformation experiments were performed as described earlier (1,2). Cell lines were established by growing out cells from representative foci.

Enzyme assay. Aryl hydrocarbon hydroxylase (AHH) activity was measured as described by Nebert and Gelboin (3). Induction agent was benz(a)anthracene (BA). The cells were treated in the logarithmic growth phase at 13 μM BA for 24 hours. Cell protein was determined by the method of Lowry *et al.* (4) using bovine serum albumin as a standard.

RESULTS AND DISCUSSION

The carcinogen-metabolizing enzyme complex was present in the secondary nude mouse fibroblast cultures (NuF), and it was also inducible by benz(a)anthracene (Table 1). The cell lines showed no AHH activity at basal state either before or after the tumor phase. A cell line transformed by 3-MC alone ($NuMC_2$) showed very high inducible AHH activity. This cell line was not, however,

TABLE 1.

ARYLHYDROCARBON HYDROXYLASE ACTIVITY IN SECONDARY FIBROBLAST CULTURES AND
IN ESTABLISHED CELL LINES ORIGINATED FROM NMRI NU/NU (NUDE) MOUSE

Cultured cells	AHH, pmol/mg protein/min		
	Basal activity[a]	BA-induced[a]	BA-induced[b]
NuF	3.5	6.3	
$NuMC_2$	BDL	25.4	Not tumorigenic
$NuSV_{40}$	BDL	BDL	4.1
$NuMCSV_{40}$ I	BDL	BDL	1.5
$NuMCSV_{40}$ III	BDL	1.3	0.5

[a]Cell cultures from transformed foci
[b]After a reculture from tumor
 BDL = below detection level

tumorigenic when tested in adult mouse. The two cell lines transformed by
combination of SV_{40} and 3-MC ($NuMCSV_{40}$I and $NuMCSV_{40}$III) had inducible AHH
activity after reculturing from a tumor. One of them also had inducible
activity before tumor formation but the other one did not. A similar finding
was obtained from the cell line transformed by SV_{40} alone ($NuSV_{40}$).

The results indicate that at least some established cell lines regain AHH
inducibility after an *in vivo* tumor phase. The growth in an animal may thus
renormalize the intracellular AHH control system so that it becomes responsive
to polycyclic aromatic hydrocarbons.

REFERENCES

1. Laaksonen, A.M., Mäntyjärvi, R.A. and Hänninen, O.O.O. (1983),
   Medical biol., 61, 59

2. Laaksonen, M., Mäntyjärvi, R. and Hänninen, O. (1982) in: Hietanen, E.,
   Laitinen, M. and Hänninen, O. (Ed.), Cytochrome P-450, Biochemistry,
   Biophysics and Environmental Implications, Elsevier Biomedical Press
   B.V., pp. 801-804.

3. Nebert, D.W. and Gelboin, H.V. (1968), J. Biol. Chem., 243, 6242.

4. Lowry, O.H., Rosebrough, A.L., Fare, A.D. and Randall, R.J. (1951),
   J. Biol. Chem., 193, 265.

© 1983 Elsevier Science Publishers B.V.
Extrahepatic Drug Metabolism and Chemical Carcinogenesis,
J. Rydström, J. Montelius and M. Bengtsson eds.

MODULATING EFFECTS OF 2,3,7,8-TETRACHLORODIBENZO-p-DIOXIN ON SKIN CARCINOGENESIS
INITIATED BY 7,12-DIMETHYLBENZ(a)ANTHRACENE IN CF-1 SWISS MICE.

PIERRE LESCA

Laboratoire de Pharmacologie et de Toxicologie Fondamentales, 205 route de
Narbonne, 31400, Toulouse, France.

INTRODUCTION

Polycyclic aromatic hydrocarbons (PAH) such as benzo(a)pyrene (BP), 7,12-di-
methylbenz(a)anthracene (DMBA)... are transformed by several enzymes (cytochrome P-450-dependent monooxygenases and epoxide hydrolase) to chemically inert as
well as reactive metabolites. The latter are able, after binding to cellular
macromolecules (proteins, RNA, DNA), to initiate toxic, mutagenic and carcinogenic processes. A lot of investigations have demonstrated that the nature as
well as the amount of reactive metabolites bound to critical macromolecules
play a key-role in the carcinogenic development. But, another important question concerns the influence of the activation rate of PAHs, *in vivo*, on the extent of DNA damages and the appearance of tumors. From previous investigations
it could be inferred that a slow activation of DMBA might be more noxious, for
the skin cells, than the quick formation of a considerable amount of reactive
metabolites (1). This problem is now considered by studies using an induction-
initiation-promotion carcinogenesis model with CF-1 Swiss mice.

MATERIALS AND METHODS

2,3,7,8-Tetrachlorodibenzo-p-dioxin (TCDD), a very potent inducer of aryl hydrocarbon hydroxylase (AHH) has been used for the modulation, on a large scale,
of the activity of this enzyme. 1 ng to 1 µg of TCDD was applied on the back of
20 mice.

Skin microsomal AHH activity and [3H]BP covalent binding to DNA, *in vitro*.
After 24 hrs of induction by TCDD the skin microsomes were prepared and used
for the AHH determination and binding of [3H]BP metabolites to DNA, *in vitro*(2).

Carcinogenesis experiments. DMBA (10 or 25 µg) was applied 24 hrs after induction by TCDD. Promotion was carried out by a two-fold weekly treatment of 12-0-
tetradecanoylphorbol-13-acetate (TPA)(10 µg) during 20 weeks.

RESULTS AND DISCUSSION

Table 1 shows that a dose-dependent relationship exists between the increasing dose of TCDD applied to skin mice and the induction of AHH activity of
skin microsomes as well as the *in vitro* binding of the ultimate carcinogenic

590

TABLE 1

MODULATION BY TCDD OF SKIN MICROSOMAL AHH ACTIVITY AND DNA-BINDING OF
BP-7,8-DIOL-9,10-EPOXIDE, *IN VITRO*.

Treatment µg/mouse	AHH activity pmol 3-OHBP/min/mg prot.	Ratio to untreated	BPDE-binding pmol/mg DNA
no TCDD	0.88	1	0.9
TCDD 0.001	9.30	10.6	5.5
TCDD 0.01	20.00	22.8	6.8
TCDD 0.1	53.00	60.0	17.0
TCDD 1	54.00	61.0	20.0

metabolite BP-7,8-diol-9,10-epoxide (BPDE) to DNA.

In vivo, with respect to the appearance of tumors, a dual effect of TCDD is observed, Figure 1, when 25 µg/mouse of DMBA were applied to the skin. It appears that an optimal rate of DMBA activation exists which corresponds to the highest number of tumors. The only observed anticarcinogenic effect for the highest doses of TCDD is the rule when only 10 µg DMBA were applied to the skin.

Many other experiments are needed to explain these apparently conflicting results and we are now studying the eventual connection between the DNA damages and the different phases of the cell cycle.

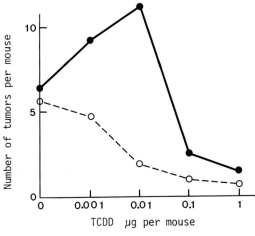

Fig. 1. Modulating effects of TCDD on skin carcinogenesis by DMBA, ●———● 25 µg/mouse, o————o 10 µg/mouse.

REFERENCES

1. Lesca, P. (1981) Carcinogenesis, 2, 199.
2. Legraverend, C., Mansour, B., Nebert, D.W. and Holland, J.M. (1980)
   Pharmacology, 20, 242

© 1983 Elsevier Science Publishers B.V.
Extrahepatic Drug Metabolism and Chemical Carcinogenesis,
J. Rydström, J. Montelius and M. Bengtsson eds.

ROLE OF DIETHYLSTILBESTROL (DES) QUINONE FORMATION IN HAMSTER KIDNEY TUMOR INDUCTION

Joachim G. Liehr, Beverly B. DaGue and Annie M. Ballatore

Analytical Chemistry Center and Department of Biochemistry and Molecular Biology, University of Texas Medical School at Houston, Houston, Texas 77025

The present study of formation and reactivity of DES quinone was undertaken to elucidate the mechanism of initiation and promotion of tumors by DES. DES is a complete carcinogen, i.e., no co-carcinogen treatment is required for the induction of renal clear cell carcinoma in male Syrian hamster (1). DES quinone has been postulated previously to be a short-lived reactive metabolite involved in tumor induction by DES (2,3). It has been postulated (4) to be formed by peroxidase which has been found (5) by Metzler and McLachlan to be present in male Syrian hamster kidney. It has been postulated to be formed in situ, in the kidney (2,3).

DES   ## DES quinone

DES quinone was synthesized by oxidation with silver oxide in aprotic solvents. It was found to rearrange spontaneously in aqueous systems to β-dienestrol (β-DIES). At 23°C, the half-life of DES quinone in methanol was 77 min. and in water 44 min. β-DIES is one of the major metabolites of DES found (6) in vivo and in vitro. L-Ascorbic acid readily reduced DES quinone to an equimolar mixture of cis- and trans-DES (7). The large amounts of β-DIES and cis-DES found (6) in DES metabolism studies, suggest that DES quinone may be a major metabolite of DES, although its reactivity may have prevented its detection in vivo. In vitro, DES was found to be readily oxidized to DES quinone by horseradish peroxidase or a crude preparation of uterine peroxidase from estrogen-treated ovariectomized rat. Peroxidases are known (8) to be induced by estrogens and are located preferentially in tissues dependent on estrogen for growth.

DES quinone must be considered to be (one of) the carcinogenic metabolite(s) of DES. Without enzyme mediation, DES quinone binds to calf thymus DNA at levels significantly above binding levels of DES to DNA (3). The binding of DES quinone to DNA may be assisted by initial non-covalent interaction of DES

592

quinone with DNA. The highly planar structure of DES quinone, identified in nuclear magnetic resonance studies, is thought to facilitate such interactions.

These experiments confirm earlier postulates (2,9) by Metzler and McLachlan of DES quinone as a reactive intermediate based on their findings (9) that DES binding to protein and DNA is mediated by mouse uterine peroxidase catalyzed oxidation.

ACKNOWLEDGEMENT

Financial Support was provided by an NIH, National Cancer Institute Grant (CA27539).

REFERENCES

1. Kirkman, H. (1959) Natl. Cancer Inst. Monograph, No. 1, 1.

2. Metzler, M. and McLachlan, J.A. (1978) in: Neubert, D., Merker, H.J., Nau, H. and Langman, J. (Eds.), Role of Pharmacokinetics in Prenatal and Perinated Toxicology, Georg Thieme Verlag, Stuttgart, Germany, p. 157.

3. Liehr, J.G., DaGue, B.B., Ballatore, A.M. and Sirbasku, D.A. (1982) in: Sato, G.H., Pardee, A.B. and Sirbasku, D.A. (Eds.), Cold Spring Harbor Conferences on Cell Proliferation, Vol. 9: Growth of Cells in Hormonally Defined Media, Cold Spring Harbor Laboratory, Cold Spring Harbor, NY, p. 445.

4. Liao, S. and Williams-Ashman, H.G. (1962) Biochim. Biophys. Acta., 59, 705.

5. McLachlan, J.A., Metzler, M. and Lamb, J.C. (1978) Life Sci., 23, 2521.

6. Metzler, M. (1981) CRC Critical Reviews Biochem., 10, 171.

7. Liehr, J.G., Wheeler, W.J. and Ballatore, A.M. (1983) in: Meyskens, F.L. and Prasad, K.N. (Eds.), Proceedings of the First International Symposium on the Modulation and Mediation of Cancer by Vitamins. S. Karger Publishers, Basel, Switzerland, in press.

8. Lyttle, C.R. and DeSombre, E.R. (1977) Proc. Natl. Acad. Sci. USA, 74, 3162.

9. Metzler, M. and McLachlan, J.A. (1978) Biochem. Biophys. Res. Commun., 85, 874.

© 1983 Elsevier Science Publishers B.V.
Extrahepatic Drug Metabolism and Chemical Carcinogenesis,
J. Rydström, J. Montelius and M. Bengtsson eds.

IN VITRO CULTIVATION OF EMBRYONIC RAT TONGUE CELLS AND INDUCTION OF GGT POSITIVE CLONES BY BENZO(a)PYRENE : A GOOD MODEL SYSTEM FOR ORAL CARCINOGENESIS STUDIES

K.V.KESAVA RAO, A.V.D'SOUZA AND S.V.BHIDE

Carcinogenesis Division, Cancer Research Institute

Tata Memorial Centre, Parel, Bombay - 400 012, (INDIA)

INTRODUCTION

Malignant transformation in culture of fibroblastic cells or epithelial cells derived from different sources have been described extensively (1,2,3,4). However, for want of a suitable model, in-depth studies to elucidate the mechanism of oral carcinogenesis, are hampered. In the present paper we wish to report the feasibility of developing a simple in vitro model system for oral carcinogenesis studies. GGT was utilized as a histochemical marker for carcinogen-induced changes to indenify the early events in primary mixed cell cultures of embryonic rat tongue by benzo (a) pyrene. Evidence is presented for the existence of a carcinogen dose-related cell specificity in the induction of GGT - stained areas, which will help to assess and understand the carcinogen altered cell populations and their role as potential precursors in the development of oral cancer.

MATERIALS AND METHODS

Media. Dulbecco's modification of Eagle's medium supplemented with 10% FBS (Flow Laboratories, U.K.) and gentamycin at 50 ug/ml was used in all experiments. The cells were maintained in 50 mm corning glass petridishes and were incubated at 37°C with an atmosphere of 5% CO_2 in air.

Primary cultures and carcinogen treatment.

Setting up of primary cultures of embryonic rat tongue and carcinogen treatment was carried out as described earlier (5).

GGT-assay. Assay for the GGT-activity was carried out by the histochemical method of Rutenburg et al (6). After GGT-activity staining, the petridishes were held under refrigeration over night, then nuclei were counter stained with hematoxylin and pictures were taken.

RESULTS

Fine fragments of embryonic rat tongue when suspended in complete medium and transferred to glass petridish attach to the surface of the vessel. Cells slowly

Abbreviations used : FBS = Fetal Bovine Serum, BP = Benzo(a)pyrene,
GGT = Gamma-Glutamyl Transpeptidase.

594

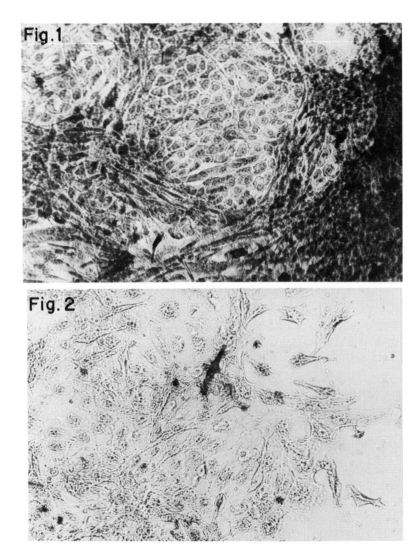

Fig. 1.   Photomicrograph of mass fibroblast and epithelial cell outgrowth from explants.

Fig. 2.   GGT activity in control cell cultures.

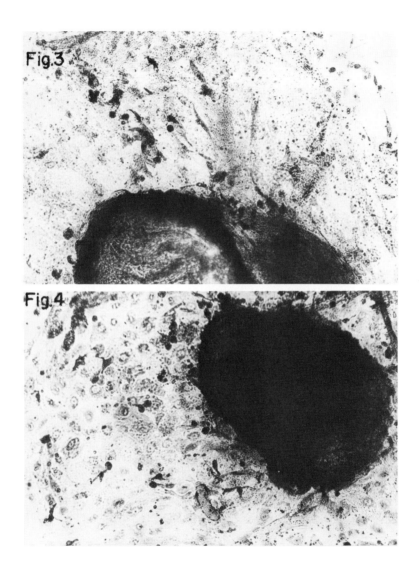

Fig.3.   GGT-activity in cell cultures treated with BP at 2.5 ug/ml.

Fig.4.   GGT- activity in cell cultures treated with BP at 10.0 ug/ml.

596

start migrating and by 72 hr outgrowth of cells with fibroblastic and epithelial cell morphology was obtained from several explants. After 6th day of planting the explants, petridishes were full with mass cultures (Fig.1.) Since GGT is considered as one of the important early markers for pre-neoplasic cells (7,8), it was felt interesting to treat cells at different concentrations of BP and see which are the cells that stain histochemically for GGT activity.The untreated mixed cell cultures, when stained for GGT activity, showed very few small areas with little back ground activity (Fig.2). In cultures treated with BP at 2.5 ug/ml clear cut regions of cells with fibroblastic morphology were intensely stained for GGT activity. No staining was observed in cells with epithelial cell morphology (Fig. 3). At 10 ug/ml of BP almost all cells with fibroblast morphology were eliminated from cultures and cells with epithelial cell morphology showed positive staining for GGT activity (Fig. 4).

Understanding early events during carcinogenesis and their role in the carcinogenic process remains a major challenge and important goal even today. Recently, Solt and Shklar (8) reported that GGT-stained plaques in DMBA treated hamster buccal pouch can be the potential precursors for the development of squamous epithelial neoplasms. If this observation is extrapolated to the present study, it is likely that at lower carcinogen concentration cells with fibroblast morphology and at relatively higher concentration cells with epithelial morphology may become the potential precursors, for the development of neoplasia, thus suggesting for the first time the possibility of existance of a carcinogen dose-related cell specificity in chemical carcinogenesis in heterogenous cell populations.

REFERENCES
1. Berwald, Y. and Sachs, L. (1965) J.Natl.Cancer Inst,.35, 641.
2. Heidelberger, C. (1973) Advan.Cancer Res., 18, 317.
3. Kakunaga, T. (1978) Proc.Natl.Acad.Sci. (USA) , 75, 1334.
4. Milo, G.E. et al., (1981) Cancer Res., 41, 5096.
5. Kesava Rao, K.V. et al., (1983) Neoplasma, 30, 35.
6. Rutenburg, A.M. et al., (1969) J.Histochem. Cytochem., 17,517.
7. Farber, E. and Cameron, R. (1980) Advan.Cancer Res.,31,125.
8. Solt, D.B. and Shklar, G. (1982) Cancer Res., 42, 285.

© 1983 Elsevier Science Publishers B.V.
Extrahepatic Drug Metabolism and Chemical Carcinogenesis,
J. Rydström, J. Montelius and M. Bengtsson eds.

RABBIT ALVEOLAR MACROPHAGE - MEDIATED MUTAGENESIS OF POLYCYCLIC AROMATIC HYDROCARBONS IN V79 CHINESE HAMSTER CELLS

LENNART ROMERT[1] AND DAG JENSSEN[2]

[1]Division of Cellular Toxicology, [2]Division of Toxicological Genetics, Wallenberg Laboratory, University of Stockholm, S-106 91 Stockholm, Sweden

When particles are inhaled and deposited in the alveoli of the mammalian lung, they are phagocytosed by pulmonary alveolar macrophages (PAM). Contaminated air such as industrial air pollution and tobacco smoke is frequently associated with airborne particles. Such particles often function as carriers of combustion products which are found to be both mutagenic (1) and carcinogenic (2). The extraction and biotransformation of these products within PAM and the possible transfer of their activated forms into surrounding tissues may play an important role in chemically induced lungcancer. The present study was initiated to investigate the role which particle phagocytosis by PAM plays in the metabolic pathway of particle-bound chemicals to mutagenic and carcinogenic products. To study this, rabbit PAM-preparations (3) were used as a metabolizing device in combination with V79 Chinese hamster cells, as a mutational indicator system according to earlier describtion (4). The number of induced gene mutations in the locus for HGPRT was studied using reseeding technique (5).

The capacity for bioactivation of benzo[a]pyrene (B[a]P), its 7,8-diol (7,8-diol) and 2-amino-anthracene (2-AA) by PAM was investigated. Because of the high variation between different PAM-preparations, a statistically significant effect of the three compounds could only be demonstrated in a series of four or five experiments. The mutagenic effect is illustrated in figure 1. Experiments were performed to find out the way in which the phagocytic process could effect the bioactivation of polycyclic aromatic hydrocarbons (PAH). The results from different experiments (of which one is illustrated in figure 2) showed that PAM-mediated mutagenesis of the 7,8-diol was enhanced five to tenfold if PAM were fed with opsonized particles. Since it has been established (6) that the promoting agent 12-O-tetradecanoylphorbol 13-acetate (TPA) can stimulate a series of reactions that closely resemble changes occurring after ingestion of particles, it was also of interest to examine the influence of TPA on PAM-mediated mutagenesis. Preliminary results indicated (figure 2) that TPA could enhance the PAM-mediated mutagenesis of the 7,8-diol about ten times. TPA in combination with particle-ingestion, investigated in the same experiment (figure 2), suggested a synergistic way of action.

The mechansim by which the phagocytosis by PAM or TPA enhanced the mutagenicity of the 7,8-diol, as detected in cocultivated V79 cells, is not known. Beside the suggestion that the bioactivation of 7,8-diol is stimulated in PAM by the phagocytic process or by

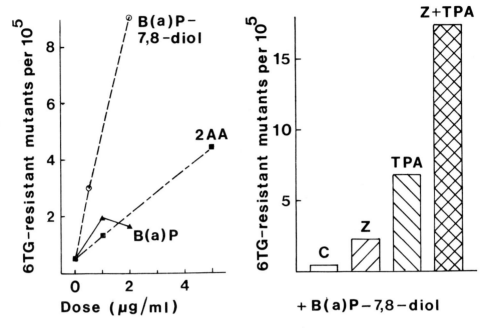

Fig.1. Mutagenicity in V79 Chinese hamster cells cocultivated with PAM and treated for 70 hours with 2AA (■, B[a]P (▲) or B[a]P-7,8-diol (O).

Fig.2. Mutagenicity in the V79/PAM system (see fig.1) after treatment with 0.75 µg/ml B[a]P-7,8-diol (24h) only (C) or in combination with Zymsan-particles (Z) and/or TPA.

TPA, speculation leads to other possible explanation. Increased uptake, due to extensively binding of the 7,8-diol to the particles or as a direct result of the phagocytic process, provide explanations, which have to be investigated. Whether the potentiating effect of TPA indicated here, can be connected with its promoting activity in vivo, have to be investigated further.

REFERENCES

1. Alink, G.M., H.A.Smit, J.J.van Houdt, J.R.Kolkman and J.S.M.Boleij (1983) Mutagenic activity of airborne particulates at non-industrial locations, Mutation Res., 116, 21-34.
2. Epstein, S.S., K.Fiyi and S.Asahina (1979) Carcinogenicity of a composite organic extract of urban particulate atmospheric pollutants following subcutaneous injection in infant mice., Environ. Res., 19, 163-176.
3. Romert, L., V.Bernson and B.Petterson (1983) The oxidative metabolism and phagocytotic capacity of pulmonary alveolar macrophages. Effects of air pollutants., accepted for publication in J. Toxicol. Environ. Health.
4. Romert, L. and D.Jenssen (1983) Rabbit alveolar macrophage-mediated polycyclic aromatic hydrocarbons in V79 Chinese hamster cells., Mutation Res., in print.
5. Jenssen, D., B.Beije and C.Ramel (1979) Mutagenicity testing on Chinese hamster V79 cells treated in the in vitro liver perfusion system. Comparative investigation of different in vitro metabolizing systems with dimethylnitrosamine and benzo(a)pyrene., Chem.-Biol. Interact., 27, 27-39.
6. Hoidal, J.R., J.E.Repine, G.D.Beall, F.L.Rasp and J.G.White (1978) The effect of phorbol myrestate acetate on the metabolism and ultrastructure of human alveolar macrophages., Am. J. Pathol., 91, 469-482.

© 1983 Elsevier Science Publishers B.V.
Extrahepatic Drug Metabolism and Chemical Carcinogenesis,
J. Rydström, J. Montelius and M. Bengtsson eds.

INHIBITORY EFFECTS OF SOME THIOL COMPOUNDS ON THE METABOLIC ACTIVATION OF DI-
METHYLNITROSAMINE(DMN) AND DIMETHYLHYDRAZINE(DMH) IN GUINEA-PIG HEPATOCYTES
AND ENTEROCYTES

STANISLAV YANEV[1], GABRIELE HAUBER[2], MICHAEL SCHWENK[2] AND HERBERT REMMER[2]

[1]Dept. of Drug Toxicology, Inst. of Physiology, Bulg.Acad.Sci., 1113 Sofia
(Bulgaria) and [2]Inst. of Toxicology, Univ. of Tübingen, 7400 Tübingen(FRG)

It is well known that there are multiple pathways for DMN metabolism, only
some of them being cyt-p-450-dependent. On the other hand, the difference in
the organ sensitivity to some cancer-inducing agents/like DMH-produced colon
cancer/ is explained with the different rates of metabolic activation of these
compounds. Therefore, the usage of different metabolic inhibitors is of great
importance for the better understanding of the mechanisms of carcinogenesis.

It has been shown that Disulfiram, Diethyldithiocarbamate(DDC) and CS_2 inhibit the metabolic activation of some carcinogens,e.g. DMH to azomethane and
azoxymethane, thus preventing colon neoplasia(1) and DMN to reactive metabolites, protecting the liver from necrosis and cancer (2).

The aim of this study was to compare the inhibitory effects of potassium
ethylxanthogenate(PEX), an oxygen analog of DDC, with that of DDC upon DMN
and DMH metabolism in guinea-pig hepatocytes and enterocytes.

MATERIALS AND METHODS

Female guinea-pigs, weighing 250-300 g, were used. Isolated hepatocytes and
enterocytes were obtained by the modified methods of Baur et al.(3) and
Weiser(4), respectively.

RESULTS AND DISCUSSION

PEX selectively blocked the DMN hepatocytes metabolism. The I_{50} value for
inhibition of DMN-demethylation by PEX was much lower than that for inhibition
of aminopyrine-demethylation/Table 1/. The same was found for the DDC.

TABLE 1

DMN, AP AND HCHO METABOLISM IN HEPATOCYTES ($^{14}CO_2$-PRODUCTION)
Inhibitory effects of PEX and DDC / I_{50} values in mM /

	DMN(16.5 mmM)	AP(2.7 mmM)	HCHO(2.5 mM)
PEX	0.045	3.6	no effect
DDC	0.037	1.0	no effect

The inhibition of the rat liver microsomal DMN-demethylation by PEX was non-competitive. Blocking the DMN-metabolism PEX prevented the covalent binding of DMN-metabolites to hepatocytes proteins and DNA /Table 2/.

TABLE 2

HEPATOCYTES - DMN COVALENT BINDING (^{14}C-)

	DNA (cpm/e_{260})	PROTEIN (cpm/mg)
CONTROLS	42.1±3.2	2663.0±45.0
PEX (1 mM)	14.2±1.4	395.0±28.0
DDC (1 mM)	10.3±1.1	415.0±31.0

The DMH metabolism tested by $^{14}CO_2$-production in isolated guinea-pig intestinal and colon cells showed ten times higher rate in the colon cells. PEX and DDC blocked the DMH metabolism only in the colon cells/Table 3/. The present data provided supporting evidence for the observed in vivo protective effect

TABLE 3

ENTEROCYTES DMH-DEMETHYLATION($^{14}CO_2$)/ pmoles/mg/45 min /

	Intestinal cells	Colon cells
Controls	25.9+2.2	261.3±11.2
PEX (1 mM)	26.0±3.4	61.8±8.4
DDC (1 mM)	24.9±2.8	93.6±7.3

of PEX and DDC on the development of colon cancer after DMH treatment (5).

The inhibitory effects of PEX on the metabolism of DMN and DMH in hepatocytes and enterocytes might be due to their own metabolism leeding to reactive metabolites which disturb the function of the cyt-p-450 system (6).

REFERENCES
1. Fiala, E.S., Bobotas, G., Kulakis, C. and Weisburger, J.H. (1977) Xenobiotica, 7, 5.
2. Schmähl, D., Krüger, F.W., Habs, M. and Diehl, B. (1976) Z. Krebsforsch., 85, 271.
3. Baur, H., Kasperek, S. and Pfaff, E. (1975) Hoppe-Seyler's Z. Physiol. Chem., 356, 827.
4. Weiser, M.M. (1973) J.Biol.Chem., 248, 2536.
5. Wattenberg, L.W. (1977) J.Natl.Cancer Inst., 58, 395.
6. Yanev, S., Frank, H. and Remmer, H. (1983) Biochem.Pharmacol./in press/.

© 1983 Elsevier Science Publishers B.V.
Extrahepatic Drug Metabolism and Chemical Carcinogenesis,
J. Rydström, J. Montelius and M. Bengtsson eds.

ACCUMULATION OF CARCINOGENS AND DRUGS IN CELLS
AS DETERMINED BY FLUORESCENCE MICROSCOPY

ERICH ZEECK AND HERBERT KOWITZ
Universität Oldenburg, P.O.Box 2503,D 2900 Oldenburg, Germany

INTRODUCTION

From several laboratories it is reported that fetal calf serum
and biologically active phorbol esters stimulate the uptake of
different substances in cells (1 - 4). On the acceleration of the
transport of benzo(a)pyrene (BP) into cells as determined by fluorescence microscopy will be reported here. Moreover the uptake of
mopidamol, a drug against cancer, in cultured cells is considered.

MATERIALS AND METHODS

The cells used were human fibroblasts GM 3349 (Institute of Medical Research, Camden,N.J.) and human embryo fibroblasts FH 112
(skin) and FH 122(lung) (Seromed, Munich). The cells were grown
in HAM F12 medium (Seromed) containing 10% fetal calf serum (Boeh-
ringer,Mannheim). BP (Roth, Karlsruhe) was dissolved in glycerol
(p.a., Merck, Darmstadt) (saturated solution at 25°C). 4ß-phorbol-
12,13-dibutyrate (PDBu) (Sigma, Munich) was dissolved in HAM F12
medium without serum, $2 \cdot 10^{-8}$M. For the addition of BP the saturated glycerol solution (freshly prepared) was added (1o%) to the
growth medium. Mopidamol ($2,2^{'}2^{''},2^{'''}$-((4-piperidinoimido-(5,4-d)
-pyrimidine-2,6-diyl)dinitrilo-tetraethanol) is the active component of the drug Rapenton (Thomae,Biberach).

The cells were grown on the cover glass of special culture chambers (tissue culture chambers, C.A. Greiner,Nürtingen).

The measurements were performed with a Zeiss microscope photo-
meter with RCA 8850 photomultiplier and Ortec-Brookdeal photon
counter. The intensity of fluorescence emission at 405 nm with a
fluorescence excitation at 365 nm was taken as a measure for the
BP concentration.

RESULTS

When BP is added to cultured cells, the BP uptake reaches a maximum at about 12 hours. This holds when serum is present in the

culture medium. Levels of 10 to 20% serum have been reported to inhibit the transformation of C3H/10T1/2 cells by carcinogenic hydrocarbons (5). When cells are incubated with HAM F12 medium without serum for 5 min. at 37°C then the addition of BP leads to a rapid accumulation of BP by the cells, the maximum is reached within about 6 min. The effect of incubation with this medium without serum is not compensated by the presence of serum during the addition of BP: When immediately after incubation the medium is changed, the new medium contains 10% serum and 10% glycerol saturated with BP. The foregoing period of exposition to a medium without serum is sufficient to cause the acceleration of BP uptake.

Incubation with HAM F12 medium containing PDBu without serum caused the same effects as incubation with HAM F12 alone, presence of serum (10%) together with PDBu prevented the acceleration of BP uptake.

In addition to polycyclic aromatic hydrocarbons many substances that are used in drugs show bright fluorescence, and their transport into cells can be observed by fluorescence microscopy. This holds e.g. for mopidamol, a drug used against cancer. When applicated to the cultured fibroblasts GM 3349 this substance is accumulated mainly in cells which are just in the phase of cell division, an effect which may be of influence on the action of this drug.

REFERENCES

1. Lee, L.S. and Weinstein, I.B. (1979), Membrane effects of tumor promoters: Stimulation of sugar uptake in mammalian cell cultures, J. Cell Physiol. 99, pp. 451 - 460.

2. Wrighton, S.A. and Mueller, G.C. (1982), Rapid acceleration of deoxyglucose transport by phorbol esters in bovine lymphocytes, Carcinogenesis 3, pp, 1415 - 1418.

3. Hennings, H., Yuspa, S.H., Michael, D. and Lichti, U. (1978), Modification of epidermal cell response to 12-O-tetradecanoyl-phorbol-13-acetate by serum level, culture temperature and pH, in: Slaga,T.J., Sivak, A. and Boutwell, R.K. (Ed.),Carcinogenesis, Vol. 2, Mechanisms of Tumor Promotion and Cocarcinogenesis, Raven Press, New York.

4. Rozengurt, E. and Heppel, L.A. (1975), Serum rapirly stimulates ouabain-sensitive Rb^+ influx in quiescent 3T3 cells, Proc.Natl. Acad. Sci. USA 72, pp. 4492 - 4495.

5. Bertram, S.J. (1977), Effects of serum concentration on the expression of carcinogen-induced transformation in the C3H/10T1/2 cell line, Cancer Res. 37, pp. 514 - 523.

© 1983 Elsevier Science Publishers B.V.
Extrahepatic Drug Metabolism and Chemical Carcinogenesis,
J. Rydström, J. Montelius and M. Bengtsson eds.

PREDICTION OF CARCINOGENIC AND MUTAGENIC POTENCIES USING THE PLS METHOD

Ulf Edlund, Sven Hellberg[*], Dan Johnels[*], Bo Nordén and Svante Wold
Research Group for Chemometrics and Department of Organic Chemistry, Umeå
University, S-901 87 Umeå, Sweden.

The use of the Partial Least Squares method (PLS)(1) for quantitative prediction of biological activities from the chemical structure is illustrated by
two examples.

A Y-block consisting of biological activities (toxicity, carcinogenicity, mutagenicity etc.) and an X-block consisting of descriptors of chemical structure
(lipophilicity, electron distribution and different measures of molecular size)
are represented by separate Principal Components-like models (PC). The dimen-
sionality of the models is estimated by crossvalidation (2). These PC-like
models are related to each other by linear models.

The method is illustrated by two examples:

1. Prediction of the carcinogenic potency of eleven polycyclic aromatic hydrocarbons (PAH) having a bay region (3).

In the PAH example the chemical descriptors consist of a. theoretical data:
Pullman indices, resonance energies etc. and experimental data: absorption
spectral parameters, HPLC retention indices etc. and b. simplified C-13 NMR
parameters. A plot of carcinogenicity against predicted carcinogenicity using
the descriptors a. is showed in Fig. 1.

2. Analysis of four mutagenicity tests and one toxicity test for a set of seven
   one and two carbon halogenated hydrocarbons (4).

In the second example the halogenated hydrocarbons were characterized by log P
(octanol/water), molar refractivity, molar volume and atomic charges. All
together eleven descriptors were used. A plot of one of the mutagenicity tests
against the predictions is showed in Fig. 2.

604

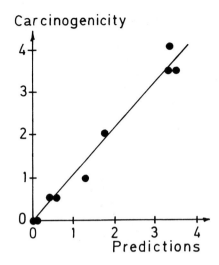

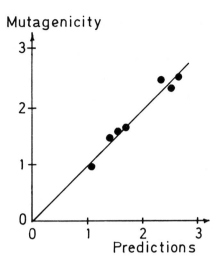

Fig. 1. Plot of observed carcinogenicity against predicted
carcinogenicity for PAH.

Fig. 2. Plot of observed mutagenicity against predicted mutagenicity
for the halogenated hydrocarbons.

REFERENCES

1. Wold S., Albano C., Dunn III W.J., Esbensen K., Hellberg S., Johansson E.
   and Sjöström M., Proc. IUFOST Conf. " Food research and data analysis ",
   Oslo 1982 (H. Martens Ed.), Elsevier, Amsterdam, 1983.

2. Wold S., Technometrics, 20 (1978), 397.

3. Nordén B. Edlund U., Johnels D. and Wold S., Quant. Struct. -Act. Relat.,
   in press.

4. Dunn III W.J., Wold S., Edlund U., Hellberg S. and Gasteiger J., in manuscript.

© 1983 Elsevier Science Publishers B.V.
Extrahepatic Drug Metabolism and Chemical Carcinogenesis,
J. Rydström, J. Montelius and M. Bengtsson eds.

BENZO(A)PYRENE METABOLISM IN HUMAN HAIR FOLLICLE CELLS: POSSIBLE INDICATORS

FOR INDIVIDUAL DIFFERENCES IN SUSCEPTIBILITY TO CHEMICAL CARCINOGENS

MATH W.A.C. HUKKELHOVEN, LISETTE W.M. VROMANS AND ALPHONS J.M. VERMORKEN
Research Unit for Cellular Differentiation and Transformation, University of
Nijmegen, Geert Grooteplein Noord 21, 6525 EZ Nijmegen, The Netherlands

Differences in the biological response to carcinogens, especially polycyclic
aromatic hydrocarbons (PAH), have been described among species, individuals,
tissues and cell-types (1,2). The existence of interspecies variation precludes
direct extrapolation of data obtained in experimental animals to the human situation. Therefore the use of human biopsy tissue is important in studies involved
in chemical carcinogenesis. However, for population studies the choice of human
biopsy tissue is very limited. Since interindividual variation in carcinogen
metabolism seems to be primarily under genetic control (3), these population
studies should allow to detect high risk populations.

Although interindividual variation can result from every step in chemical carcinogenesis, e.g. metabolic activation, binding to DNA, repair of damaged DNA
and promotion of initiated cells, most efforts have been spent to correlate differences in carcinogen metabolism to susceptibility to carcinogens. Lymphocytes
have been used frequently for this purpose, but unfortunately the results have
been ambiguous (4,5). We have proposed that human hair follicles are a convenient biopsy-tissue for identifying individuals with increased risk for developing
chemically induced cancer (6). They are of epithelial origin which is important
since most human malignancies are carcinomas. Moreover, they are available from
a large number of individuals and can be plucked without medical qualifications
and risks of adherent side-effects.

Up till now the following results with this novel biopsy tissue in human carcinogenesis have been obtained:

1 Human hair follicles have been shown able to metabolise benzo(a)pyrene (BP),
  the most studied prototype compound for PAH, to a range of organic solvent-
  soluble metabolites including tetrols, dihydrodiols, quinones and phenols as
  analysed by high performance liquid chromatography (7). See Fig. 1.

2 Human hair follicle cells can be cultured (8) which enables the study of other
  parameters in the process of chemical carcinogenesis, such as induction of
  carcinogen-metabolising enzymes, DNA-binding, mutation studies etc. For this
  purpose a specially constructed culture dish has been developed (9). See Fig.
  2. The device (Epicult[®], now commercially available from Sanbio B.V., The

606

Netherlands) allows to fix a bovine eye lens capsule, a basement membrane-
like extracellular matrix which forms the growth substrate for the hair follicle keratinocytes.

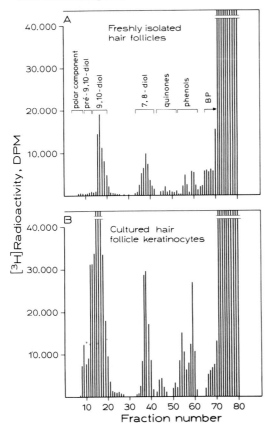

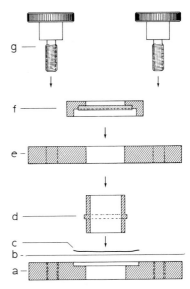

Fig. 1. HPLC-analysis of organic solvent-
soluble metabolites of ^{3}H-BP formed by freshly isolated hair follicles (A) and cultured
hair follicle keratinocytes (B).

Fig. 2. Schematic drawing of the
culture dish (Epicult) used for
culturing hair follicle keratinocytes. Essentially, the bottom of
the dish (a) is covered by a small
piece of foil (b). Then the central cylinder (d) on which the
lens capsule (c) is stuck, is placed on the bottom. The dish is
completed by placing the upper
part of the dish (e) and by fixing the various parts by means of
2 screws (g). The glass centre of
the lid (f) allows microscopic
examination of the cultures.

3 Metabolism of BP to dihydrodiol-derivatives, the direct precursors of the
  suspected ultimate carcinogens of PAH, the diol-epoxides, has been shown to
  be genetically determined for a large part in hair follicles (10). This was
  concluded from an analysis of BP-metabolism in monozygotic twins, dizygotic
  twins and pairs of unrelated individuals (see Fig. 3).

4 The response of BP-metabolism in cultured hair follicle keratinocytes towards

pre-exposure to PAH is comparable with that in cultured epithelial cells of the human bronchus, the target-tissue for PAH-induced neoplasia (11,12). Moreover, BP-metabolism to organic solvent-soluble and water soluble metabolites is qualitatively and quantitatively comparable between both tissues. It was found that in both cell-types pre-exposure to benz(a)anthracene (BA) resulted in an induction of phenolic BP-metabolites while the formation of dihydrodiols was not enhanced. This is in contrast with murine (strain C3Hz) epithelial cells where both phenolic as well as dihydrodiol DP-metabolites were induced after pre-treatment with BA.

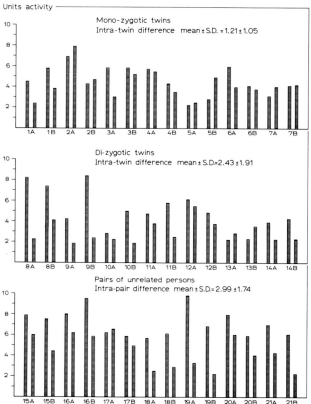

Fig. 3. Formation of ^{3}H-BP-dihydrodiols in freshly isolated hair follicles from 7 monozygotic twins, 7 dizygotic twins and 7 pairs of unrelated individuals. Each pair was assayed two times. Note the increasing intra-pair difference in the sequence: monozygotic twins, dizygotic twins, pairs of unrelated individuals.

5 Recently, sensitive microassays have been developed for quantitation of aryl hydrocarbon hydroxylase and epoxide hydratase, two key-enzymes in metabolic activation and detoxification of PAH (13,14).

608

Using freshly isolated hair follicles and cultured hair follicle keratinocytes of groups of patients with lung or laryngeal cancer, we are presently investigating which enzymatic parameters are relevant and whether or not other biochemical end-points can serve as a standard for determination of individual susceptibility to carcinogens (Supported by the Netherlands Cancer Society).

REFERENCES

1 Autrup, H. (1982) Drug Metab. Rev., 13, 603.

2 Harris, C.C., Trump, B.F., Grafstrom, R.C. and Autrup, H. (1982) J. Cell. Biochem., 18, 285.

3 Nebert, D.W., Eisen, H.J., Negishi, M., Lang, M.A. and Helmeland, L.M. (1981) Ann. Rev. Pharmacol. Toxicol., 21, 431.

4 Kellermann, G., Shaw, C.R., Luyten-Kellermann, M. (1973) N. Engl. J. Med., 289, 936.

5 Atlas, S.A., Vesell, E.S. and Nebert, D.W. (1976) Cancer Res., 36, 4916.

6 Vermorken, A.J.M. and Bloemendal, H. (1979) in: Boelsma, E. and Rümke, Ph. (Eds.), Tumour Markers: Impact and Prospects, Elsevier/North-Holland Biomedical Press, Amsterdam, pp. 305-326.

7 Hukkelhoven, M.W.A.C., Dijkstra, A.C. and Vermorken, A.J.M. (1983) J. Chromatogr. Biomed. Applic., 276, in the press.

8 Weterings, P.J.J.M., Vermorken, A.J.M. and Bloemendal, H. (1981) Br. J. Derm., 104, 1.

9 Hukkelhoven, M.W.A.C., Vermorken, A.J.M. and Bloemendal, H. (1980) Prep. Biochem., 10, 473.

10 Hukkelhoven, M.W.A.C., Vermorken, A.J.M., Vromans, E. and Bloemendal, H. (1982) Clin. Genet., 21, 53.

11 Hukkelhoven, M.W.A.C., Vromans, E., Vermorken, A.J.M. and Bloemendal, H. (1982) Toxicol. Lett., 12, 41.

12 Hukkelhoven, M.W.A.C., Vromans, E., Vermorken, A.J.M. and Bloemendal, H. (1982) Anticancer Res., 2, 89.

13 Hukkelhoven, M.W.A.C., Vromans, E.W.M., Vermorken, A.J.M., van Diepen, C. and Bloemendal, H. (1982) Anal. Biochem., 125, 370.

14 Hukkelhoven, M.W.A.C., Vromans, E.W.M., Vermorken, A.J.M. and Bloemendal, H. (1982) FEBS Lett., 144, 104.

Correspondence: Dr. A.J.M. Vermorken

© 1983 Elsevier Science Publishers B.V.
Extrahepatic Drug Metabolism and Chemical Carcinogenesis,
J. Rydström, J. Montelius and M. Bengtsson eds.

ELUCIDATION OF THE ANTINEOPLASTIC POTENCY OF VITAMIN C ON BENZO(a)PYRENE INDUCED TUMORS IN RATS

GEORGE KALLISTRATOS[1], ERHARD FASSKE[2], ANDREAS DONOS[1],
VASSILIKI KALFAKAKOU-VADALOUKA[1] AND ANGELOS EVANGELOU[1]

[1]Department of Experimental Physiology,Faculty of Medicine,University of Ioannina (Greece) and [2]Department of Pathology,Research Institute for Experimental Biology and Medicine D-2061-Borstel FRG.

INTRODUCTION

The results concerning the effect of Vitamin C for the prevention and treatment of malignant diseases are very conflicting. Several studies indicate a positive effect of Vitamin C for the prevention and treatment of different types of animal and human cancer(1-6).

Contrarywise, investigations reporting that Vitamin C could not suppress tumor induction caused by a number of carcinogens , as well as, high doses of Vitamin C therapy to benefit patients with advanced cancer have been also published (7-8).

Since the above mentioned contradictory results are all based on experimental and clinical investigations , it might be assumed that Vitamin C has a diverse action against malignancy, varying from total regression of tumors up to no effect or even stimulation of tumor growth (9).

In order to contribute to the elucidation of the biological effect of ascorbic acid in malignancy, the Antineoplastic potency (Ap) of Vitamin C against Benzo(a)pyrene induced tumors in Wistar rats has been determined.

MATERIALS AND METHODS

For the determination of the Carcinogenic potency (Cp) of Benzo-(a)pyrene (BaP), twenty seven 8 week-old female Wistar rats were treated with a single s.c. injection of 10mg BaP dissolved in 1ml tricaprylin. According to the following relation Cp is define as:

$$Cp = \frac{\text{PERCENTAGE OF TUMOR INDUCTION}}{\text{MEAN SURVIVAL TIME IN DAYS}} \times 100$$

For the elucidation of the Antineoplastic potency of Vitamin C on BaP induced tumors, thirty female Wistar rats were also treated with 10mg BaP in 1ml tricaprylin (2nd GROUP).

Vitamin C was orally administered as a 2.5g % solution added to the drinking water of the rats which was sweetened with 2g % sugar.

RESULTS

Few weeks after the s.c. administration of the BaP carcinogen ,a tumor was formed locally in the area where the BaP solution was injected. The BaP-induced tumors were gradually increased in size and weight; They were larger and heavier compared with the 2nd GROUP treated with Vitamin C. The rats died because of the malignancy between 153-252 days after the s.c. injection of BaP.(TABLE 1)

According to the experimental results , the Carcinogenic potency of Benzo(a)pyrene was determined through the following calculations

$$Cp_{BaP-rats} = \frac{100}{191.52} \times 100 = 52.21$$

where $\bar{X}control$ 191.52 days, standard deviation 27.825 and n=27 rats.

In the second GROUP where Vitamin C was orally administered to the rats , a prolongation of their mean survival time occured which was 224.33 days, that means 32.81 days longer than the control group without Vitamin C. This difference of survival time , is statistically significant according to the t-student test p 0.01.

The average Vitamin C intake was 500mg/rat/day (375-625mg Vit.C). The total amount of Vitamin C administered orally to the rats during the whole period of the experiment , with a mean survival time of 224 days was :

500mg X 224 days = 112g Vitamin C/rat/mean survival time

This amount of Vitamin C corresponds approximately 50 % of their body weight.

The Carcinogenic potency (Cp) of BaP in the presence of Vitamin C was calculated:

$$Cp_{BaP+Vit.C-rats} = \frac{100}{224.33} \times 100 = 44.58$$

where $\bar{X}_{Vit.C}$ was 224.33 days, with a standard deviation of 63.62 and n 30 rats.

Consequently , under the mentioned experimental conditions , the oral administration of Vitamin C to the Wistar rats treated with BaP, caused a reduction of the Carcinogenic potency of the carci-

TABLE 1

HISTOLOGY AND WEIGHTS OF THE BaP INDUCED TUMORS IN PRESENCE AND ABSENCE OF VITAMIN C

GROUPS and compounds administered	number of rats	tumor induction n %	tumor weight mean (max-min)	H I S T O L O G Y	n	%
1.GROUP Control 10mg BaP in 1ml tricaprylin	27	27 100	110 (25-270)	Fibrosarcoma Rhabdomyosar. Undiff.sarc. mixed tumors	9 7 10 1	33 26 37 4
2.GROUP 10mg BaP in 1ml tricaprylin + Vit.C orally	30	30 100	89 (18-158)	Fibrosarcoma Rhabdomyosar. Undiff.sarc. mixed tumors no histology[a,b]	15 6 4 3 2	50 20 13 10 7

[a]Cannibalism,[b]still alive

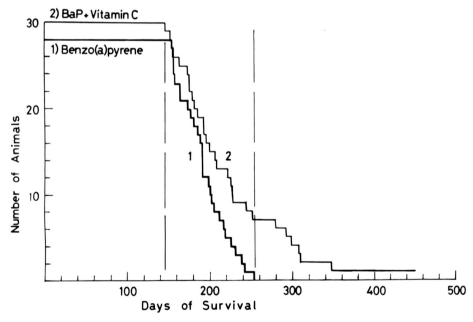

FIGURE 1
LIFE PROLONGATION OF WISTAR RATS TREATED WITH A SINGLE s.c.INJECTI-
ON OF 10mg BaP AND SIMULTANEOUS ORAL ADMINISTRATION OF VITAMIN C
(GROUP 2). CONTROL GROUP 1 WITHOUT VITAMIN C.

nogen from 52.21 to 44.58.

Therefore, the Antineoplastic potency (Ap) of Vitamin C on BaP-induced tumors in Wistar rats was

$$52.21 - 44.58 = 7.63 \text{ units, or expressed as}$$

a ratio $\quad 52.21 \; / \; 44.58 = 1.17$

It must be pointed out that the analysis of the mortality curve of the Vitamin C treated group (FIGURE 1) also revealed that in the case of four rats, ascorbic acid was practically ineffective. If the beneficial effect of Vitamin C is taken into consideration only for the remaining population of the 26 rats, then the mean survival time will increased to 235.5 days, the Cp for BaP will decrease to 42.46 and the statistical significance will be p 0.001.

The Antineoplastic potency of Vitamin C could probably be improved by combining this anticarcinogen with other potent antineoplastic agents.

ACKNOWLEDGEMENTS

We thank Mrs U.Kallistratos and Miss E.Goula for the technical assistance and Hoffmann-La Roche Basel for the supply of Vitamin C.

REFERENCES

1. Cameron,E. and Pauling,L.(1974) Chem.Biol.Interact.9,273-283.

2. Morishige,F.and Murata,A.(1979) J.Intl.Acad.Prev.Med. 5,47-52.

3. Murata,A.(1980) 3rd Intl.Vit.C.Symp.Sao Paolo Brazil 7-10 Sept.

4. Pipkin,G.,Schlegel,J.V.,Nishimura,R. and Schultz,G. (1969) Proc.Soc.Exp.Biol.Med. 131,522-524

5. Raineri,R.and Weisburger,J.H.(1975)Ann.N.Y.Acad.Sci.258,181-189

6. Kallistratos,G. and Fasske,E.(1980) Folia Biochim.Biol.Graeca 17,4-144.

7. Soloway,M.S.,Cohen,S.M.,Dekernion,J.B. and Persky,L.(1975) J.Urol. 113,483-486

8. Creagan,E.T.,Moertel,C.G.,O´Fallon,J.R.,Schutt,A.J.,O´Connell,M. Rubin,J. and Frytak,S.(1969) New England J.Med. 301,687.

9. Kallistratos,G.,Fasske,E.,Donos,A.and Vadalouka-Kalfakakou,V. (1982) Proc.2nd Ann.Cancer Symp.NFRC-Cancer Res.Ass.Brunel Sept.1-2,U.K.

© 1983 Elsevier Science Publishers B.V.
Extrahepatic Drug Metabolism and Chemical Carcinogenesis,
J. Rydström, J. Montelius and M. Bengtsson eds.

BRONCHIOLAR EPITHELIAL CELL NECROSIS AND SELECTIVE IMPAIRMENT OF PULMONARY MICROSOMAL MONOOXYGENASES IN MICE BY NAPHTHALENE AND 1,1-DICHLOROETHYLENE

THEODORE E. GRAM, KLAAS R. KRIJGSHELD, SAMUEL S. TONG, EDWARD G. MIMNAUGH, MICHAEL A. TRUSH, AND MICHAEL C. LOWE
Biochemical Toxicology Section, Laboratory of Medicinal Chemistry and Pharmacology, National Cancer Institute, NIH, Bethesda, MD 20205 (U.S.A.)

INTRODUCTION

The existence and biochemical mechanisms of organ-specific toxicity are the subject of heightened interest among toxicologists. In the present report, we describe conditions under which naphthalene and 1,1-dichloroethylene (DCE) produce selective damage to mouse lung without morphologic or enzymatic evidence of nephro- or hepatotoxicity.

MATERIALS AND METHODS

Male C57BL/6J mice weighing about 25 g were injected with a single intraperitoneal dose of naphthalene (225 mg/kg) or DCE (125 mg/kg) dissolved in olive oil; controls received olive oil. Groups of animals were sacrificed at various times thereafter ranging from 1 day to 42 days and lung, kidney, and liver were removed for light microscopic or enzymatic study as described previously (1). Lungs were fixed by tracheal infusion followed by immersion in fixative.

RESULTS AND DISCUSSION

Effects of naphthalene. Injection of a single dose of naphthalene into mice produced a significant (30-70%) and prolonged (8-15 days) impairment in pulmonary microsomal monooxygenase activities without altering these activities in liver microsomes. The time course of naphthalene-induced morphologic damage to bronchiolar epithelium paralleled compromises in pulmonary monooxygenase activity. No concomitant alterations in hepatic morphology were observed. Maximum inhibition of enzyme activity occurred about 3 days after naphthalene administration; 7-ethoxyresorufin O-deethylase activity was reduced to about 30% of control values whereas NADPH cytochrome c reductase and cytochrome P-450 were reduced about 50%. Benzphetamine N-demethylase and aryl hydrocarbon hydroxylase (AHH) in lung were less affected. Inhibited activities remained at relatively constant levels between days 3 and 8 and by day 15, there was a clear trend returning toward controls.

Histologically, the pulmonary non-ciliated bronchiolar epithelial (Clara) cell was the primary target of naphthalene toxicity. At early time points and at low magnifications, it appeared as if the entire bronchiolar epithelium was undergoing necrosis and sloughing into the lumen. However, higher magnifications revealed residual ciliated epithelium. It is important to note that 15 days after a single dose of naphthalene, 4 of the 6 enzymes examined remained below control values; histologically, at 15 days, Clara cells appeared to be regenerating but were abnormal both in number and appearance.

Effects of DCE. A single dose of DCE injected into mice caused a reduction of cytochrome P-450 levels and related monooxygenases in lung microsomes with no corresponding changes in liver and kidney. Examination of the lung tissue by light microscopy revealed necrosis restricted to the Clara cells. In contrast, liver and kidney were relatively unaffected by DCE treatment, as indicated both by lack of changes in microsomal monooxygenase activities and morphology. Maximal inhibition of pulmonary monooxygenases occurred 2-4 days after dosing and did not return to control levels until about day 21. Cytochrome P-450, NAPDH cytochrome c reductase, benzphetamine N-demethylase, and ethoxyresorufin-0-deethylase activities activities were reduced to about 50% of control levels while AHH activity was less severely affected. By contrast, coumarin 7-hydroxylase in lung microsomes was reduced to 10% of control 4 days after DCE. The delayed return of lung microsomal P-450-linked enzyme activities (21 days) was paralleled by a correspondingly slow reappearance of bronchiolar Clara cells.

It is of interest that DCE, a selective Clara cell toxin, reduced the activity of coumarin 7-hydroxylase in mouse lung to ~10% of control levels within 4 days. This confirms the finding of Devereux and Fouts (2) in purified cell populations from rabbit lung that the specific activity of coumarin 7-hydroxylase in Clara cells was 42 times that of type II cells. Other pulmonary monooxygenases were less restricted to Clara cells; Clara cell/type II cell ratios were about 4 for AHH and about 1.5 for NADPH cytochrome c reductase (2). Urade et al (3) in 1982 also found coumarin 7-hydroxylase activity to be highly concentrated in Clara cells purified from mouse lung.

REFERENCES

1. Tong, S.S. et al (1982) Expt. Molec. Pathol., 37, 358.
2. Devereux, T. and Fouts, J.R. (1981) in: Jakoby, W.B. (Ed.), Methods in Enzymology, Academic Press, New York, pp. 147-153.
3. Urade, Y., et al (1982) Biochem. Biophys. Res. Commun., 105, 567.

© 1983 Elsevier Science Publishers B.V.
Extrahepatic Drug Metabolism and Chemical Carcinogenesis,
J. Rydström, J. Montelius and M. Bengtsson eds.

EFFECT OF INDUCERS OF AHH ON PROLIFERATION OF MITOGEN-STIMULATED
HUMAN LYMPHOCYTES. BENZANTHRACENE-INDUCED INCREASE IN PROLIFERA-
TION OF CELLS SHOWING LOW RESPONSE TO MITOGEN AND ITS TOXICITY
IN CELLS SHOWING HIGH RESPONSE TO MITOGEN.

ANDRZEJ L. PAWLAK, KRZYSZTOF WIKTOROWICZ AND RENATA MIKSTACKA
Institute of Human Genetics, Polish Academy of Sciences, Strze-
szyńska 30/36, 60-479 Poznań /Poland/

INTRODUCTION

Changes in proliferation and viability of cells may affect the
assessment in vitro of inducibility of aryl hydrocarbon hydroxylase /AHH/ by methylcholanthrene/MC/-type inducers and by aminophylline. Several of the MC-type inducers of AHH are known as
complete carcinogens, which exhibit also promoting activity /1/.
In reference to aminophylline no data indicating its promoting
activity are available.

MATERIALS AND METHODS

The effect of benz/a/anthracene /BA/ on blast transformation was
studied in mitogen-stimulated peripheral blood mononuclear cells
/PBMC/ from 53 healthy donors. Isolation of PBMC and cell cultures
were performed as described earlier /2/. Spectrofluorimetric measurement of activity of AHH was based on estimation of fluorescent
products of metabolism of benzo/a/pyrene in suspension of cells/3/.
Blastogenesis was estimated on the basis of morphological criteria
/4/. Incorporation of thymidine into DNA was studied in triplicate
cultures of 0.2 ml aliquots of cell suspension on microplates at
$37^{\circ}C$ in 5% CO_2-air chamber. ^{3}H-thymidine /0.5 uCi; UVVVR Prague,
specific activity 20 Ci/mmole/ was added to the culture 3 h before
the harvest /5/. BA and MC in acetone and aminophylline diluted
with culture medium were added to cell cultures.

RESULTS AND DISCUSSION

In 53 pairs of control and BA-treated cultures no significant
effect of BA /2 uM/ on per cent values of blast cells was noted
with the paired test of Wilcoxon /p=0.05/. In 13 pairs of control
and BA-treated cultures with low mean percentage of blast cells

/below 60/, the per cent values of lymphoblasts in BA-induced cultures were higher than in control cultures. This effect may be due to promoting activity of BA, and is thought to correspond to the recent finding that the cells resistant to mitogenic effects of phorbol esters remain sensitive to the promoting effects of these compounds /6/. On the other hand, the decrease in the number of blast cells in BA-induced cultures /toxic effect/ was noted only in cultures characterized by the higher mean values of blast cells in pairs of control and BA-treated cultures. The increase in toxicity of BA with the higher mean values of blast cells may correspond to the correlation between stimulation of lymphocytes by mitogen and DNA repair induced in these cells by treatment with N-acetoxy-2-acetylaminofluorene /7/.

The slight decrease in the per cent values of blast cells and in the number of viable cells was noted in cultures treated for 24 h with aminophylline /0.7mM/. The presence of BA /2 μM/ seems to counteract this effect of aminophylline.

Aminophylline /0.7mM/ decreased incorporation of thymidine both in control and in BA/2 μM/-treated cells. At concentrations 5 μM and higher BA and MC caused decrease in thymidine incorporation.

ACKNOWLEDGEMENTS

The authors thank Mrs. Aleksandra Walczak for her skillful technical assistance. The work was supported by Polish Academy of Sciences within the projects 09.7.3.1.2.2 and 10.5.02.1.

REFERENCES

1. Mondal, S., Brankow, D.W. and Heidelberger, C.H./1976/ Cancer Res., 36, 2254.

2. Mikstacka, R.M. and Pawlak, A.L. /1981/ Bull.Acad.Polon.Sci., Ser.Sci.biolog., 29, 201.

3. Pawlak, A.L., Wiktorowicz, K. and Duczmal-Szewczuk, B. /1982/ Cancer Lettr., 17, 95.

4. Steffen, J., Dopierała, G. and Stolzmann, W. /1966/ Post.Hig. Med.Dośw., 20, 485.

5. Chen, H.W., Heiniger, H.J. and Kandutsch, A.A. /1975/ Proc.Natl. Acad.Sci.US 72, 1950.

6. Colburn, N.N., Wendel, E.J. and Abruzzo, G. /1981/ Proc.Natl. Acad.Sci.US 78, 6912.

7. Pero, R.W. and Östlund, C. /1980/ Mutation Res., 73, 349.

© 1983 Elsevier Science Publishers B.V.
Extrahepatic Drug Metabolism and Chemical Carcinogenesis,
J. Rydström, J. Montelius and M. Bengtsson eds.

BENZO(A)PYRENE METABOLIZING ENZYMES AND LYMPHOCYTE STIMULATION IN PATIENTS WITH BRONCHIAL CARCINOMA

CHRISTEL BLUHM AND EDGAR E. OHNHAUS
Dept. of Internal Medicine, University of Essen,
Hufelandstr. 55, D-4300 Essen 1 (FRG)

INTRODUCTION

Polycyclic aromatic hydrocarbons (PAHs), e.g. benzo(a)pyrene, are environmental chemical carcinogens and constituents of cigarette smoke. They exert their mutagenic and carcinogenic activity only after biotransformation, generally by microsomal monooxygenases (MO). The resulting carcinogenic intermediate metabolites are detoxified by glutathione S-transferases (GST). Epoxide hydrolase (EH) is involved in both toxifying and detoxifying processes.

MATERIAL AND METHODS

Patients. 94 patients with bronchial carcinoma (66 smokers, 15 non smokers) and tuberculosis (13 smokers) undergoing surgical resection were included in this study.

Assays. MO activity (Ethoxycoumarin O-deethylase) was determined according to Ullrich and Weber (1). EH activity was measured with $[^3H]$-benzo(a)pyrene 4,5-oxide as substrate (2), and for GST the assay by Habig et al. was used with 2,4-dinitrochlorbenzene as substrate (3). Lymphocyte stimulation (4) was carried out with benzo(a) pyrene (BP), 3-methylcholanthrene (3-MC), and with three different mitogens, concanavalin A (Con A), phytohemagglutinin (PHA), and pokeweed mitogen (PWM).

RESULTS

Table 1 shows the stimulation index (SI) in lymphocytes from patients with different lung diseases compared with healthy volunteers. Smoking patients with bronchial carcinoma had a significantly lower SI following Con A and PHA than smokers with tuberculosis. Treatment with BP and 3-MC showed no differences.

TABLE 1

Lymphocyte Stimulation Index (SI)

SI: $[^3H]$-thymidine incorporation after mitogen treatment /$[^3H]$-thymidine incorporation without mitogen

Patients	Con A	PHA	PWM	BP	3-MC
Healthy vol. (S)	31.7± 1.8	49.6±4.7	10.4±1.4	2.1±0.3	2.4±0.3
Healthy vol.(NS)	40.8± 7.2	79.6±14.0	16.8±3.1	4.4±1.0	2.0±0.2
Tuberculosis (S)	45.3±12.4 }a	112.7±12.5 }b	23.0±4.1	7.3±3.1	2.1±0.4
Tumor (S)	29.3± 2.2	63.5± 4.8	20.8±2.0	4.4±0.6	1.9±1.5
Tumor (NS)	40.3± 5.9	80.2± 1.4	13.4±1.8	4.2±1.3	1.9±0.4

Comparison of bracketed values by unpaired Student t-test:
a) $p < 0.05$ b) $p < 0.001$

As shown in table 2 there was no significant difference in the activities of EH and GST in lung tissue. MO activity was significantly higher in patients with tuberculosis, which may have been due to the treatment of these patients by a drug combination including rifampicin for about six months before surgery.

TABLE 2

BENZO(A)PYRENE METABOLIZING ENZYMES IN HUMAN LUNG TISSUE

Patients	Enzyme activities (pmol product $\times$ mg^{-1} $\times$ min^{-1})		
	EH	GST	MO
Tumor (NS)	937±147	87003±12262	1.23±0.53
Tumor (S)	1050± 94	94978± 7801	0.94±0.24 }a
Tuberculosis (S)	1315±225	85486±16682	2.46±0.87

Comparison of bracketed values by unpaired Student t-test:
a) $p < 0.05$

REFERENCES

1. Ullrich, V. and Weber, P. (1976) Hoppe-Seyler's Z. Physiol. Chem. 353, 1171-1177
2. Schmassmann, H.U., Glatt, H.R., Oesch, F. (1976) Anal. Biochem. 74, 94-104
3. Habig, W.H., Pabst, M.J., Jakoby, W.B. (1974) J. Biol. Chem. 249, 7130-7139
4. Grosse-Wilde, H., Baumann, P., Netzel, B., Kolb, H.J., Mempel, W., Wank, R., Albert, E.D. (1973) Transpl. Proc. V,4, 1567-1571

© 1983 Elsevier Science Publishers B.V.
Extrahepatic Drug Metabolism and Chemical Carcinogenesis,
J. Rydström, J. Montelius and M. Bengtsson eds.

STUDIES ON A NASAL CAVITY CARCINOGEN: METABOLISM AND BINDING OF PHENACETIN IN THE MUCOSA OF THE UPPER RESPIRATORY TRACT

EVA BRITTEBO[1] AND MARIA ÅHLMAN[2]

[1]Department of Pharmacology, Biomedicum, SLU, Box 573, S-751 23 Uppsala, and [2]Section of Organic Chemistry, Environmental Toxicology Unit, Wallenberg Laboratory, University of Stockholm, S-106 91 Stockholm (Sweden).

INTRODUCTION

Recent studies have demonstrated that peroral administration of the analgesic drug phenacetin induces tumours in the nasal cavity in experimental animals (1, 2). Since a growing number of chemicals are known to be metabolized by the nasal mucosa (3-5) it was considered of interest to examine the distribution and metabolism of phenacetin in the respiratory system of rats.

MATERIALS AND METHODS

Chemicals. $(1-^{14}C\text{-ethyl})$-phenacetin was prepared from p-acetylaminophenol in a one step reaction with $(1-^{14}C)$-ethyliodide (12.1 MBq, 2.12 GBq/mmol) (6). The reaction was carried out in ethanol containing sodium-ethoxide. Phenacetin (5.6 MBq, 2.12 GBq/mmol) was isolated after preparative TLC.

Experiments. The distribution of (^{14}C)-phenacetin in Sprague-Dawley rats was studied by whole-body autoradiography and microautoradiography. In addition, slices of selected tissues were incubated in culture medium containing (^{14}C)-phenacetin and the rate of $^{14}CO_2$ formation was determined.

RESULTS

Five minutes after an i.v. injection of (^{14}C)-phenacetin a high and selective uptake of radioactivity had taken place in the nasal- and tracheo-bronchial mucosa, whereas a low uniformly distributed radioactivity was present in the other tissues. In the nose, the labelling was most pronounced in the mucosa of the ethmoturbinates, whereas the radioactivity was low in the mucosa covering the naso- and maxillo-turbinates. By extraction of tissue-sections with organic solvents it was possible to remove the homogeneously distributed radioactivity in the tissues, whereas the labelling of the mucosa of the respiratory tract was non-extractable and thus probably represented firmly bound metabolites. Micro-autoradiography of the nasal region showed that the highest amount of tissue-bound radioactivity was present in the subepithelial glands (Bowman's glands) located beneath the olfactory epithelium of the ethmoturbinates and septum. The olfactory epithelium was also labelled, whereas the respiratory and squamous epithelia showed only low amounts of radioactivity. The lateral nasal gland close to the maxillary sinus contained a high amount of tissue-bound radioactivity.

The rapid localization of metabolites in the mucosa of the respiratory tract suggests that a local metabolism of phenacetin takes place. Incubations with slices from the nasal mucosa confirmed that phenacetin was metabolized by this tissue. In comparison with other tissues such as the liver, lung and kidney, the highest metabolic rate was found in the nasal mucosa. Addition of metyrapone or SKF 525A decreased the rate of $^{14}CO_2$ production by the nasal mucosa, indicating the participation of a cytochrome P-450-dependent monooxygenase. Autoradiography of tissue-pieces incubated with ^{14}C-phenacetin showed that radioactivity was selectively localized in the nasal- and tracheo-bronchial mucosa.

In conclusion, the results of the present investigation demonstrate that the nasal cavity carcinogen phenacetin is metabolized by the nasal mucosa to products which subsequently bind to various glands and epithelia of the tissue. The nasal cavity tumours induced by phenacetin have been suggested to have a glandular and epithelial origin (1). The observed in situ-metabolism of phenacetin may therefore play an important role in the pathogenesis of phenacetin-induced tumours of the upper respiratory tract.

ACKNOWLEDGEMENTS

Supported by the Swedish Council for Planning and Coordination of Research.

REFERENCES

1. Isaka, H., Yoshi, H., Otsuji, A., Koike, M., Nagai, Y., Koura, M., Sugiyasu, K. and Kanabayashi, T. (1979) Gann, 70, 29.

2. Johansson, S.L. (1981) Int. J. Cancer, 27, 521.

3. Brittebo, E.B., Löfberg, B. and Tjälve, H. (1981) Chem.-Biol. Interactions, 34, 209.

4. Brittebo, E.B. and Tjälve, H. (1981) Carcinogenesis, 2, 959.

5. Brittebo, E.B. (1982) Acta Pharm. Tox., 51, 227.

6. Vogel, A.I. (1964) A textbook of practical organic chemistry, 3rd edn, Longmans, Greene & Co., Ltd., London, p. 997.

© 1983 Elsevier Science Publishers B.V.
Extrahepatic Drug Metabolism and Chemical Carcinogenesis,
J. Rydström, J. Montelius and M. Bengtsson eds.

METABOLISM AND BINDING OF CHLOROBENZENE IN THE MUCOSA OF THE UPPER RESPIRATORY TRACT

INGVAR BRANDT AND EVA BRITTEBO

Department of Pharmacology, SLU, Uppsala Biomedical Centre, Box 573,
S-751 23 Uppsala, Sweden.

INTRODUCTION

Chlorobenzene is known to induce bronchiolar and hepatic necrosis in mice (1). Whereas the liver damage caused by halogenated aromatic hydrocarbons is believed to be due to formation in situ of chemically reactive metabolites (2, 3), it is not known whether the pulmonary toxicity is mediated by metabolites formed within the lung or by metabolites which have reached the lung via the blood from the liver. In the present investigation, the in vivo and in vitro metabolism and binding of chlorobenzene in the respiratory system were studied in mice.

MATERIALS AND METHODS

Chemicals. Uniformly labelled ^{14}C-chlorobenzene (31 mCi/mmol) was obtained from Amersham International plc, England.

Experiments. The distribution of ^{14}C-chlorobenzene (CB) in C57 Bl-mice was studied by autoradiography. CB is a volatile compound which can be evaporated from thin tissue-sections by heating. This procedure was used to register the localization and binding of non-volatile radioactivity (metabolites) in the respiratory tract. In addition, tissue sections were extensively washed with organic solvents to remove un-bound radioactivity, leaving only tissue-bound radioactivity (metabolites).

In addition, in vitro-experiments with slices of selected tissues were performed in culture medium containing CB. The ability of the tissues to form CB-metabolites which could not be extracted from the tissues by extensive organic solvent extraction was determined.

RESULTS

Autoradiograms obtained from mice i.v. injected with ^{14}C-chlorobenzene
showed that a selective uptake of non-volatile metabolites had taken place in
the nasal and tracheo-bronchial mucosa already 1 min after injection. Autoradiograms prepared with tissue sections which had been extensively washed with
organic solvents showed that parts of the radioactivity in the nasal and tracheo-
bronchial mucosa could not be extracted from the tissues. Autoradiography of
lung tissue incubated with ^{14}C-chlorobenzene in vitro gave similar results.
Quantitative measurements with tissue-slices incubated in vitro showed that the
formation of non-extractable metabolites was most pronounced in the nasal mucosa. The formation of non-extractable metabolites by the nasal mucosa and
lung in vitro was inhibited by metyrapone, piperonylbutoxide and SKF 525A,
indicating the participation of the cytochrome P-450 system.

In conclusion, the results indicate that the toxic action of chlorobenzene in
the bronchial mucosa may involve an in situ formation of reactive products,
which become firmly bound to the tissue constituents. The high binding of
metabolites in the nasal mucosa suggests that also this tissue may be a site of
toxic action of chlorobenzene.

ACKNOWLEDGEMENTS

Financial support was provided by the Swedish Council for Planning and Coordination of Research.

REFERENCES

1. Reid, W.D., Ilett, K.F., Glick, J.M. and Krishna, G. (1973) Am. Rev.
   Resp. Dis., 107, 539.
2. Reid, W.D., Cristie, B., Krishna, G., Mitchell, J.R., Moskowitz, J. and
   Brodie, B.B. (1971) Pharmacology, 6, 41.
3. Monks, T.J., Lau, S.S. and Gillette, J.R. (1982) 8th European workshop
   on drug metabolism, Sart Tilman, Belgium, Sept. 5-9, p. 113.

© 1983 Elsevier Science Publishers B.V.
Extrahepatic Drug Metabolism and Chemical Carcinogenesis,
J. Rydström, J. Montelius and M. Bengtsson eds.

THE RENAL METABOLISM OF A GLUTATHIONE CONJUGATE OF THE CARCINOGEN HEXACHLORO-1:3-BUTADIENE: EVIDENCE FOR THE FORMATION OF A MUTAGENIC METABOLITE IN THE RAT KIDNEY

TREVOR GREEN, JOHN A NASH, JENNY ODUM AND EDWIN F HOWARD
Imperial Chemical Industries PLC, Central Toxicology Laboratory, Alderley Park, Macclesfield, Cheshire, SK10 4TJ, UK

INTRODUCTION

Hexachloro-1:3-butadiene (HCBD) is a potent nephrotoxin and renal carcinogen. Short term tests including the Ames assay have failed to predict the carcinogenicity of HCBD. This study was undertaken to investigate the metabolic activation of HCBD in the rat in relation to the observed organ specificity, and to explain the failure of the Ames assay to predict the genotoxicity of this compound.

METHODS

In vivo metabolism. Male 200g Alderley Park rats were each given a single oral dose of C-14 HCBD (200 mg/kg:250 μCi) and urine collected for 24 hr. Bile was collected for 24 hr from rats given a similar dose of HCBD. Metabolites were separated by HPLC and identified by GC-MS.

In vitro renal metabolism. Thin slices of rat renal cortex were incubated under O_2 with 0.5 mM of the glutathione or N-acetyl cysteine conjugate of HCBD. Ammonia and pyruvate were determined in the medium at intervals for up to 5 hr.

Mutagenicity assay. The HCBD conjugates were tested using the standard Ames assay except that rat kidney S9 or β-lyase plus acylase replaced rat liver S9.

RESULTS

In vivo metabolism. The major biliary metabolite (40%) of HCBD is a glutathione conjugate. A sulphenic acid metabolite of HCBD has been identified in urine (Fig 1).

In vitro renal metabolism. The GSH and N-acetyl cysteine conjugates of HCBD were metabolised by rat kidney slices to give pyruvate (and lactate), ammonia (Table 1) and a reactive fragment.

Ames assay. Both conjugates of HCBD were potent mutagens in the assay when activated by rat kidney S9, or in the case of the N-acetyl cysteine conjugate when activated by β-lyase plus acylase (Table 2).

Fig 1   The metabolic activation of hexachlorobutadiene in the kidney

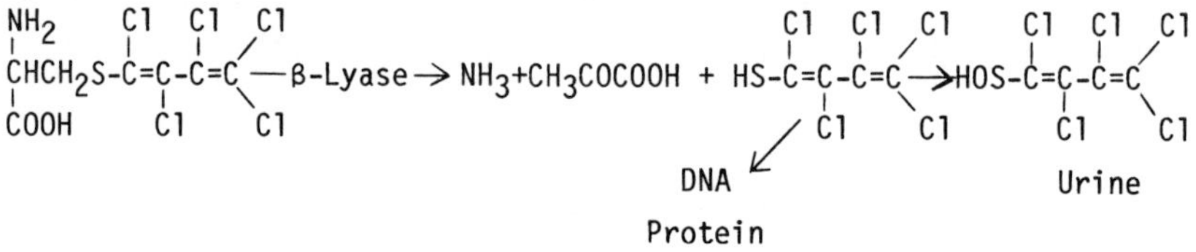

$$NH_2 \quad Cl \quad Cl \quad Cl$$
$$CHCH_2S-C=C-C=C \quad -\beta\text{-Lyase} \rightarrow NH_3+CH_3COCOOH + HS-C=C-C=C \rightarrow HOS-C=C-C=C$$
$$COOH \quad Cl \quad Cl$$

(Cl Cl Cl, Cl Cl ; Cl Cl, Cl Cl)

DNA / Protein   Urine

TABLE 1

MUTAGENICITY OF THE N-ACETYL CYSTEINE-HCBD CONJUGATE

	Salmonella typhimurium TA100 revertants/plate			
Activation	None	Rat kidney S9	β-Lyase	β-Lyase + acylase
Conc μg/plate				
0	56±8	74±11		
0.2	45±5	106±6		
2.0	57±11	216±22	102±9	228±21
2.0	52±6	428±16		
50	65±5	153±20		

TABLE 2

METABOLISM OF HCBD CONJUGATES TO NH_3 AND PYRUVATE BY RAT KIDNEY SLICES

	nmol Metabolites/mg slice					
Conjugate (10mM)	1 hr		3 hr		5 hr	
	NH_3	Pyruvate	NH_3	Pyruvate	NH_3	Pyruvate
Control	4.4	0.38	11.2	0.49	13.5	0.55
GSH-HCBD	7.6	0.93	18.2	1.53	27.0	2.5
N-Ac-Cyst HCBD	9.4	0.47	12.9	1.01	19.0	3.55

DISCUSSION

The results show that HCBD is metabolised in the liver to give a GSH conjugate which is excreted in bile. This conjugate when dosed orally is highly nephrotoxic (data not shown) suggesting readsorption from the gut and transport to the kidney. Renal metabolism of this conjugate has been shown to occur via the enzyme β-lyase giving a reactive fragment (Fig 1) which is both nephrotoxic and highly mutagenic. Evidence for the structure of this fragment has been obtained by the identification of a urinary sulphenic acid metabolite of HCBD. The Ames assay fails to detect HCBD because it fails to reproduce this complex metabolic process.

© 1983 Elsevier Science Publishers B.V.
Extrahepatic Drug Metabolism and Chemical Carcinogenesis,
J. Rydström, J. Montelius and M. Bengtsson eds.

DOSE- AND SEX-RELATED VARIATION IN THE DISPOSITION AND HEPATIC EFFECTS OF CINNAMYL ANTHRANILATE IN THE MOUSE.

JOHN CALDWELL, ANDREW ANTHONY, IAN A. COTGREAVE, SUSAN A. SANGSTER AND
J. DAVID SUTTON
Department of Pharmacology, St. Mary's Hospital Medical School, London W2 1PG,
England.

Cinnamyl anthranilate (CA) is a synthetic food flavour and fragrance agent. There is currently some concern over the potential risk to man from its use as it produced liver tumours in mice following administration of very large doses. However, it is not a carcinogen in rats, nor is it a mutagen in a variety of tests. It would be expected that CA would be metabolized by hydrolysis to cinnamyl alcohol and anthranilic acid. The former is a GRAS compound, while the latter was not carcinogenic in an NCI bioassay in rats and mice.

The use of very high doses of a compound in a toxicity test can cause a "kinetic overload", in which the metabolism and pharmacokinetics are distorted relative to the situation obtaining at normal doses. The tissues may thus be exposed to different compounds at very high doses than at low doses, with the consequence that effects seen at very high doses may not occur at low doses.

We now report on studies designed to examine the disposition and hepatic effects of CA in the C3B6F1 mouse, in relation to dose, to provide a pharmacokinetic critique of the toxicity tests of CA in this species.

Following oral administration of CA (500mg/kg) to C3B6F1 mice, peak plasma levels of unchanged CA were reached in 30 min and were higher in males (5.7μg/ml) than in females (1.5μg/ml). Unchanged CA in urine accounted for 0.3-0.4% of dose. Anthranilic acid (ca. 17%) and hippuric acid (ca. 35%; the major metabolite of cinnamyl alcohol) were present in urine, with higher recoveries in females.

Groups of male and female C3B6F1 mice were given 0, 10, 100, 1000, 5000, 15000 and 30000 ppm CA in the diet. After 4 days, the CA-containing diet was removed and urine collected for 24h. This contained, in increasing concentration with dose, CA (more in males) and hippuric and anthranilic acids (more in females).

Further groups of male and female mice were given these diets for 19 days and then killed. Relative liver weight and microsomal cytochrome P-450 increased with increasing dose above 1000ppm, more markedly in females than males although the maximal response (2-fold) was the same in both sexes. Microsomal protein content was unchanged. The results are presented in the Table.

	Cinnamyl anthranilate content of the diet (ppm)						
	0	10	100	1000	5000	15000	30000
FEMALES							
Relative liver weight (%)	5.2	4.9	5.1	5.3	5.6	7.3	8.4
Microsomal protein (mg/g liver)	25.9	31.2	32.1	26.7	29.2	27.0	23.8
Cytochrome P-450 (nmol/mg protein)	0.34	0.37	0.44	0.41	0.51	0.45	0.72
MALES							
Relative liver weight (%)	4.5	4.4	4.4	6.0	6.8	8.1	8.6
Microsomal protein (mg/g liver)	22.8	26.9	30.2	20.6	25.9	26.1	25.4
Cytochrome P-450 (nmol/mg protein)	0.41	0.40	0.43	0.49	0.57	0.62	0.80

SDS-PAGE of the microsomes revealed the dose-dependent induction of a protein of 72kd (possibly NADPH-cytochrome P-450 reductase) and a cytochrome P-450 isozyme of 53kd. Aniline hydroxylase activity in the 9000xg supernatant was unaltered by CA dosing, as was p-nitroanisole O-methylation activity in female mice. In males, this latter is significantly reduced at doses of 5000 ppm and above.

In these studies, CA has been shown to cause liver hypertrophy and microsomal enzyme induction. These effects are seen at the higher doses, above 1000ppm, and are not detected at lower doses, suggesting that they may be mediated by unchanged CA, whose hydrolysis has been shown to be saturated at high doses. The association of these hepatic effects and enhancement of liver tumours in mice suggests that CA resembles the so-called promoting agents e.g. phenobarbitone, rather than alkylating agents such as the nitrosamines.

ACKNOWLEDGEMENTS
Supported by grants from F.E.M.A. and R.I.F.M., U.S.A. We are grateful to Dr. A.R. Boobis for the SDS-PAGE analysis, and to Drs. B.K. Barnard, R.A. Ford and P. Shubik for helpful discussion. We thank Prof. R.L. Smith for his encouragement.

AUTHOR INDEX

Åhlman, M.   619
Ahotupa, M.   223,245,305
Aitio, A.   223
Alexandrov, V.A.   515
Ålin, P.   153,171
Amrhein, C.A.   489
Anderson, M.W.   459
Andersson, B.   113
Anisimov, V.N.   515
Anthony, A.   213,625
Åstrand, I.-M.   171
Åström, A.   375
Aune, T.   25

Baars, A.J.   243
Bakke, J.   257
Balk, L.   95,225
Ball, L.M.   267,295
Ballatore, A.M.   591
Baron, J.   73
Belvedere, G.   193
Bend, J.R.   25,253,351,459
Bengtsson, M.   363
Bespalov, V.G.   515
Betner, I.   251
Bhide, S.V.   593
Bianco, M.T.   303
Bigger, C.A.H.   439
Birberg, W.   95,221
Blanck, A.   249,373,375
Blomstedt, M.   267
Bluhm, C.   617
Bondon, A.   201
Boobis, A.R.   207
Borm, P.   315,319
Bowes, S.   311
Bowman, C.M.   227
Boyd, J.A.   105
Brandt, I.   267,621
Breimer, D.D.   243
Bresnick, E.   419
Brittebo, E.   619,621
Brown, M.I.   489
Bryngelsson, C.   521
Bryngelsson, T.   521
Busk, L.   205

Caderni, G.   309
Caldwell, J.   213,625
Cautreels, W.   201
Cerutti, P.   499
Chipman, J.K.   275
Christou, M.   449
Cooper, C.S.   429
Cotgreave, I.A.   625
Cristodoulides, L.G.   189
Croft, J.E.   25

D'Souza, A.V.   593
DaGue, B.B.   591
Dao, T.L.   315
Davi, H.   201
Davies, D.S.   207
de Long, M.J.   181
Decken, A. von der   523
DePierre, J.W.   95,185,209
211,225,375
Di Simplicio, P.   303
Digernes, V.   215
Dipple, A.   439
Dolara, P.   309
Domin, B.A.   43,253
Donos, A.   609
Dorman, B.H.   567

Edlund, U.   603
Ehrenberg, A.   469
Eisen, H.J.   379
Eling, T.E.   105
Elovaara, E.   29,239,241
Engström, K.   239
Eriksson, L.   297,373
Eriomin, A.N.   39
Evangelou, A.   609
Evarts, R.P.   541

Fang, W.-F.   57
Farber, E.   11,297
Fasske, E.   609
Flesher, J.W.   237
Frankhuijzen-Sierevogel, A.   319
Friedberg, T.   163
Friedman, J.   499
Furlong, B.B.   567

Georgellis, A. 247
Glaumann, H. 67
Glowinski, I.B. 507
Goldman, P. 283
Goldstein, M. 89
Golly, I. 235
Gottlieb, K. 227
Gower, J.D. 299
Grafström, R.C. 527
Gram, T.E. 613
Gräslund, A. 469
Green, T. 623
Grover, P.L. 429
Guengerich, F.P. 73
Gustafsson, B.E. 257,267,295
Gustafsson, J-Å. 67,89,205,
257,267,295,373,375,401
Guthenberg, C. 153,171,191

Haaparanta, T. 67,89
Haglund, L. 67,89
Hallberg, E. 371
Hällström, I. 249
Halpert, J. 67,211,251
Hänninen, O. 587
Hansson, T. 373,375
Harris, C.C. 527
Harrison, D.E. 423
Hauber, G. 599
Hawke, R. 23
Heinonen, T. 29,307
Hellberg, S. 603
Hemminki, K. 511
Hewick, D. 293
Hietanen, E. 177,245,305,307
Hincal, F. 233
Hines, R.N. 419
Hirom, P.C. 275
Hirose, M. 557
Hlavica, P. 235
Hofman, G. 315
Hoppenkamps, R. 183
Howard, E.F. 623
Huckle, K.R. 513
Huggins, C. 3
Hukkelhoven, M.W.A.C. 605
Hulshoff, A. 315,319
Hunt, J.M. 479
Hutt, A.J. 213

Ichihara, K. 229,231
Ishihara, K. 231
Iversen, O.H. 215

Jakoby, W.B. 73
Jansen, M. 243
Järvisalo, J. 29
Jefcoate, C.R. 449
Jenssen, D. 597
Jensson, H. 153,187
Jergil, B. 211
Jerina, D.M. 337
Jernström, B. 469
Johnels, D. 603

Kahn, C. 207
Kaipainen, P. 27
Kaku, M. 231
Kalfakakou-Vadalouka, V. 609
Kallama, S. 511
Kallistratos, G. 609
Kardy, A.M. 237
Kärenlampi, S.O. 425
Kaufman, D.G. 567
Kawabata, T.T. 73
Keller, G.M. 449
Kesava Rao, K.V. 593
Ketterer, B. 189
King, C.M. 557
Klaude, M. 523
Klippert, P. 315,319
Knapp, S.A. 73
Knutson, J.C. 409
Köhler, C. 89
Korsakov, M.V. 515
Kowitz, H. 601
Kozak, C.A. 425
Krauss, R.S. 105
Krijgsheld, K.R. 613
Kusunose, E. 229,231
Kusunose, M. 229

Laaksonen, M. 587
Laishes, B.A. 479
Lalley, P.A. 425
Lang, M. 27
Larsen, G. 267
Larsson, R. 113
Lau, P.P. 57
Laurén, S. 29
Lee, I.P. 351
Lee, M.-S. 557
Legraverend, C. 423,425
Lesca, P. 589
Levy, J. 419
Lewtas, J. 295

Liehr, J.G. 591
Likhachev, A.J. 515
Lindeke, B. 113
Linnainmaa, K. 177
Lipkin, M. 131
Ljungquist, E. 219
Lodovici, M. 309
Löf, A. 219
Lowe, M.C. 613
Lund, J. 401
Lycksell, P.-O. 469

Mackenzie, P.I. 379
Mäki, M. 307
Manchester, D.K. 227
Månér, S. 225
Mannervik, B. 153,171,187,191
Mäntyjärvi, R. 587
Mäntylä, E. 177,223,245
Marnett, L.J. 489
Marti, E. 201
Mason, M.E. 389
Mass, M.J. 567
Mattison, D.R. 337,363
Meerman, J.H.N. 143
Meijer, J. 95,221
Metelitza, D.I. 39
Meyer, D.J. 189
Mikstacka, R. 615
Milbert, U. 163
Millburn, P. 275
Mimnaugh, E.G. 613
Mingels, M.-J. 315,319
Moldéus, P. 113
Möller, L. 267
Møller, M. 507
Montelius, J. 123
Morgenstern, R. 185
Morreal, C.E. 325
Morton, K.C. 557
Moschel, R.C. 439
Mukhtar, H. 351
Mulder, G.J. 143
Myers, S.R. 237

Nagayama, J. 351
Naldini, A. 303
Napalkov, N.P. 515
Nash, J.A. 623
Näslund, B. 251
Nebert, D.W. 27,379,423,425
Negishi, M. 379
Neims, A. 23
Neville, A.M. 429

Newaz, S.N. 57
Nightingale, M.S. 337
Nilsson, L. 267
Noordhoek, J. 315,319
Nordén, Å. 521
Nordén, B. 469,603
Nordenskjöld, M. 113
Nordqvist, M. 219
Nyan, O. 189

O'Hare, M. 429
Odum, J. 623
Oesch, F. 163
Ogita, K. 229,231
Ohmachi, T. 51
Ohnhaus, E.E. 617
Okey, A.B. 389
Olsson, M. 191
Omiecinski, C. 419
Orsén, I. 517
Oshinsky, R.J. 57
Ovsyannikov, A.I. 515

Pacifici, G.M. 33
Papadopoulos, D. 247
Parker, N.B. 227
Pasanen, M. 217
Pawlak, A.L. 615
Payvar, F. 401
Pelkonen, O. 217
Pero, R.W. 509,521
Phillips, D.H. 429
Philpot, R.M. 25,43,253
Pilotti, Å. 95,221
Plummer, S. 207
Poellinger, L. 401
Poirier, M.C. 479
Poland, A. 409
Popovic, I.G. 515
Prochaska, H.J. 181
Prough, R.A. 489
Pue, M.A. 275

Rafter, J.J. 267,295
Rahimtula, A. 113
Rane, A. 33
Rautiainen, A. 587
Raynor, L. 23
Redick, J.A. 73
Reed, G.A. 105
Remmel, R.P. 283
Remmer, H. 599
Renwick, A.G. 311

Robertson, I.G.C.   25
Romert, L.   597
Rømyhr, O.   215
Roomi, W.   297
Ross, D.   113
Ruscetti, F.W.   423
Rydström, J.   123,247,363,371

Sagami, I.   51
Salley, F.F.   57
Sangster, S.A.   213,625
Savela, K.   511
Sawicki, J.T.   439
Schelin, C.   211
Schuster Bruce, R.   189
Schwenk, M.   599
Seidegård, J.   95,209,247,509
Serabjit-Singh, C.J.   25,43,253
Siegers, C.-P.   183
Silbergeld, E.K.   337
Sims, P.   429
Singh, G.   23
Sinha, D.K.   325
Sivarajah, K.   105
Slaga, T.J.   577
Smith, R.L.   213
Söderkvist, P.   205
Spiewak, J.   297
Ståhlberg, M.-L.   307
Stansbury, K.H.   237
Stralka, D.J.   57
Strobel, H.W.   57
Struble, C.   257
Sutton, J.D.   625
Suzuki, K.   351
Swallow, W.H.   429

Takizawa, K.   337
Talalay, P.   181
Tan, Q.H.   131
Thies, E.   183
Thorgeirsson, S.S.   507,541
Tishchenko, I.V.   39
Toftgård, R.   205,519
Tomatis, L.   515
Tong, S.S.   613

Törnquist, S.   519
True, B'A.   479
Trush, M.A.   613
Tukey, R.H.   379
Turner, C.R.   449
Tursi, F.   193

Usanov, S.A.   39

Vainio, H.   29,177,193,239,245
Vainiotalo, S.   241
Vaught, J.B.   557
Vella, L.M.   389
Vermorken, A.J.M.   605
Vigny, P.   429
Vromans, L.W.M.   605

Wallace, R.B.   73
Walles, S.A.S.   517
Wang, C.Y.   557
Warholm, M.   153
Warren, B.L.   43
Watanabe, M.   51
Weston, A.   429
Wick, D.G.   73
Wiklund, L.   519
Wiktorowicz, K.   615
Wills, E.D.   299
Wilson, N.M.   449
Wilson, S.   293
Wirth, P.J.   541
Wold, S.   603
Wolf, C.R.   163
Wrange, Ö.   401

Yagi, H.   337
Yalçin, S.   171,187
Yamamoto, K.   401
Yamamoto, S.   229
Yanev, S.   599
Younes, M.   183
Yuspa, S.H.   547

Zedeck, M.S.   131
Zeeck, E.   601
Zimmerman, R.   499
Zitting, A.   241